D1614015

Paediatric Pulmonary Function Testing

Progress in Respiratory Research

Vol. 33

Series Editor   *Chris T. Bolliger*, Cape Town

Paediatric Pulmonary Function Testing

Volume Editors   *Jürg Hammer*, Basel
                     Ernst Eber, Graz

80 figures, 27 in color, and 41 tables, 2005

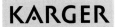

Basel · Freiburg · Paris · London · New York ·
Bangalore · Bangkok · Singapore · Tokyo · Sydney

Prof. Dr. med. Jürg Hammer
Head
Division of Intensive Care
and Pulmonology
University Children's Hospital Basel
Römergasse 8
4005 Basel, Switzerland

Prof. Dr. med. Ernst Eber
Respiratory and Allergic
Disease Division
Paediatric Department
Medical University of Graz
Auenbruggerplatz 30
8036 Graz, Austria

Library of Congress Cataloging-in-Publication Data

Paediatric pulmonary function testing / volume editors, Jürg Hammer, Ernst
Eber.
        p. ; cm. – (Progress in respiratory research, ISSN 1422-2140 ; v.
33)
   Includes bibliographical references and indexes.
   ISBN 3-8055-7753-2 (hard cover : alk. paper)
   1. Pediatric respiratory diseases.   2. Pulmonary function tests.   3.
Pulmonary function tests for newborn infants.
   [DNLM: 1. Respiratory Function Tests–methods–Child.   2. Respiratory
Function Tests–methods–Infant.   3. Respiratory Physiology–Child.   4.
Respiratory Physiology–Infant.   5. Respiratory Tract
Diseases–diagnosis–Child.   6. Respiratory Tract
Diseases–diagnosis–Infant.   WF 141 P126 2005] I. Hammer, Jürg. II. Eber,
Ernst. III. Title. IV. Series.

RJ433.5.P8P34 2005
618.92′2–dc22

2004020307

Bibliographic Indices. This publication is listed in bibliographic services, including Current Contents® and Index Medicus.

Drug Dosage. The authors and the publisher have exerted every effort to ensure that drug selection and dosage set forth in this text are in accord with current recommendations and practice at the time of publication. However, in view of ongoing research, changes in government regulations, and the constant flow of information relating to drug therapy and drug reactions, the reader is urged to check the package insert for each drug for any change in indications and dosage and for added warnings and precautions. This is particularly important when the recommended agent is a new and/or infrequently employed drug.

© Copyright 2005 by S. Karger AG,
P.O. Box, CH–4009 Basel (Switzerland)
www.karger.com
Printed in Switzerland on acid-free paper by
Reinhardt Druck, Basel
ISBN 3–8055–7753–2, ISSN 1422–2140

Contents

Foreword

To date thirty-two volumes have been published in the *Progress in Respiratory Research* Series. All but two have dealt with adult pulmonology. The two volumes dedicated to paediatric pulmonology were volume 17 on *Paediatric Respiratory Disease* published as far back as 1981, and volume 22 on *Lung Function in Children and Adolescents* published in 1987. Both these volumes have been very successful. In particular, the volume on lung function has been sold for many years. Since I took over as Editor-in-Chief of the series, I have had numerous and constant enquiries about a new book on paediatric lung function. These requests have finally led to the recruitment of two well-known paediatric pulmonologists who enthusiastically endorsed the idea of editing a new volume. And here it is: volume 33 of the series on *Paediatric Pulmonary Function Testing* edited by Prof. Jürg Hammer, Basel, Switzerland, and Prof. Ernst Eber, Graz, Austria.

True to the vision of the series, the book concentrates on recent advances in the field and authors have been encouraged to include the latest references of 2004 as well. Coupled with the known speed of production of the Publisher, S. Karger AG, the provided information is cutting edge and will guarantee an enduring success of the book. With the advent of many new testing techniques this volume is not just an updated version of previously described methods, but pretty revolutionary in its content. The editors were further able to unite a 'who's who' in the field with global representation of chapter authors. My congratulations to the editors as well as to all chapter authors for a great book!

C.T. Bolliger, Series Editor

Preface

Although attempts to measure pulmonary function have been made even in infants for over 100 years, objective methods to assess pulmonary function in the paediatric age group have been very limited until recently. Infants and preschool children are generally too young to understand and perform the manoeuvres necessary for conventional pulmonary function testing. The lack of cooperation and the size of the subjects in this age group demand miniaturization and special adjustments of both methods and apparatus. While some 40 years ago many of the methods developed for the assessment of pulmonary function in adults, such as plethysmography, were adapted for use in infants and children, new tests, such as passive respiratory mechanics and the rapid thoraco-abdominal compression technique, have been developed specifically for use in infants. Recent advances in technology and diagnostic tools have dramatically increased the armamentarium of paediatric pulmonologists to assess the respiratory system of their patients. Improved knowledge of molecular processes and innovations in the analysis of exhaled air have further amplified the possibilities to diagnose lung diseases and evaluate treatment effects by measuring novel biological markers in exhaled air or breath condensate.

It was the purpose of this book to bring together experts and researchers in paediatric pulmonary function testing to contribute their knowledge and expertise for a comprehensive overview of the most recent developments in this field.

The book is divided into four sections. The first section reviews the current lung function tests used in infants and toddlers, who are by nature unable to cooperate with any testing procedure. It describes the methodologies, provides normal values when available and advice for data interpretation by discussing the expected changes in the most

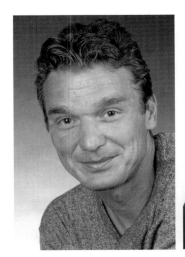
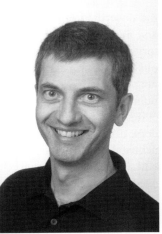

Jürg Hammer, Basel   Ernst Eber, Graz

common paediatric respiratory diseases. Some of these new techniques are now close to clinical application. Nevertheless, infant pulmonary function testing is not widely available yet and limited to a few but steadily growing number of experienced centres. Infant pulmonary function testing will provide objective measures in epidemiological and clinical studies, but it still has not found its place in the clinical management of the individual infant. Despite all advances, there are still considerable problems that prevent pulmonary function testing from playing the same diagnostic role in the management of infants with respiratory disorders as it does in older children or adults. These problems include the need for sedation, at least for some of the tests, and consequently the reservations against frequent or repetitive testing. Other issues are the acceptability of such investigations for the parents, and the lack of appropriate reference data for growth and development.

The second section deals with the classic adult-type pulmonary function tests and their application in the semi-cooperative or even cooperative older child. It discusses age-related technical issues and the limitations of the methodological standards and guidelines of these tests which are usually established for adults. In addition, it describes their clinical usefulness in children and looks at the problem of reference data in this population.

The third section covers tests which assess the respiratory system beyond the usual measurements of pulmonary mechanics, lung volumes, and bronchial responsiveness. These include investigations such as the measurements of respiratory muscle function, work of breathing, diffusing capacity, and inflammatory markers in exhaled air and breath condensate.

The fourth part is devoted to the clinical usefulness of the described pulmonary function tests for the diagnosis and management of the most common paediatric respiratory disorders. This part is unique since the very few previous books on paediatric respiratory function testing have not included any discussions on the clinical value of pulmonary function testing in diagnosing and/or managing children with asthma, cystic fibrosis, neuromuscular disorders, after lung or bone marrow transplantation, or after neonatal lung disease. The book ends with the most important aspects of pulmonary function testing in neonatal and paediatric intensive care units, a very promising field where infant pulmonary function testing may eventually have a major impact on the clinical management of the individual and usually very ill patient.

Our vision for this issue was to provide those involved in treating infants and children with respiratory disorders with a practical, up-to-date textbook which reviews in detail the substantial technical and methodological progress that was accomplished in paediatric pulmonary function testing in the past. Further, it was our goal to discuss the recent advances in respiratory physiology and pathophysiology, and to review the diagnostic value of paediatric pulmonary function tests at the present time.

We hope that this book will further promote the development and application of paediatric pulmonary function tests to provide us with the necessary tools to treat children with respiratory disorders to the best of our knowledge.

We are grateful to S. Karger AG, Switzerland and to Chris Bolliger, Editor of the *Progress in Respiratory Research* series, for stimulating us to edit a comprehensive book on paediatric pulmonary function testing, which will doubtless emphasize the special and unique aspects of assessing infants and children with respiratory problems and draw attention to the fact that children are not simply 'small adults'.

We are thankful to all authors for accepting such a short production time (all chapters have been written in the first six months of 2004) and for their efforts to make this an updated state-of-the-art textbook on paediatric pulmonary function testing.

Finally, we would like to thank both our wives and children for their patience and tolerance with two very crazy and dedicated paediatric pulmonologists (and intensivists).

Jürg Hammer, Ernst Eber,
Volume Editors

Introduction

Hammer J, Eber E (eds): Paediatric Pulmonary Function Testing.
Prog Respir Res. Basel, Karger, 2005, vol 33, pp 2–7

....

The Peculiarities of Infant Respiratory Physiology

Jürg Hammer[a]   Ernst Eber[b]

[a]Division of Paediatric Intensive Care and Pulmonology, University Children's Hospital Basel,
Basel, Switzerland; [b]Respiratory and Allergic Disease Division, Paediatric Department,
Medical University of Graz, Graz, Austria

Abstract

This chapter summarizes the most important developmental changes in respiratory physiology that occur from infancy to adolescence. The first year of life is characterized by major changes in the shape and stiffness of the rib cage. Infants have to adopt a breathing strategy to dynamically elevate their end-expiratory lung volume above that passively determined by the outward recoil of the rib cage and the inward recoil of the lung. This strategy is necessary to maintain an adequate lung volume and to prevent airway closure in the presence of reduced outward recoil of the highly compliant chest wall, which is achieved by three mechanisms: (a) a higher respiratory rate with insufficient time to exhale to the elastic equilibrium volume level, (b) laryngeal adduction during exhalation to increase the resistance to airflow, and (c) maintenance of diaphragmatic muscle tone during expiration. Other important differences relate to the increased compliance of the upper and lower airways which render children susceptible to dynamic airway collapse, especially during vigorous respiration. The elastic recoil of the lung provides little support for the airways to remain open during tidal breathing in infancy, and increases until adolescence due to alveolarization and maturation of elastic fibres. Any decrease in airway diameter results in a dramatic increase in resistance to breathing due to the smaller airway size of infants, since the resistance to airflow is inversely related to the fourth power of the airway radius. The diaphragm acts less efficiently because of the highly compliant chest wall and a more horizontal insertion at the rib cage. It is also poorly equipped to sustain high workloads due to the lower numbers of fatigue-resistant type I muscle fibres in the first year of life. The differences in respiratory physiology between infants and older children and adolescents explain the higher susceptibility of infants to more severe manifestations of respiratory diseases. Knowledge of the developmental changes occurring in the different components of the respiratory system is essential for the correct assessment of respiratory compromise in children.

Introduction

There are a number of physiological and anatomical reasons why infants are less able to cope with a given stress to the respiratory system than are older children and adults [1, 2], and disorders of any of the components of the ventilatory pathway may contribute to this (table 1). Probably the most notable difference clinically is that the basal metabolic rate is higher in infants than in adults. On a body weight basis, the oxygen consumption is 2–3 times higher than in the adult, decreasing gradually from around 7 ml/kg/min at birth to the adult value of 3–4 ml/kg/min. The normal resting state in infants is already one of high respiratory and cardiovascular activity compared with that of the adult [3]. In addition, infants have a larger surface area to body weight ratio and higher energy requirements for growth [4]. Coupled with a lower functional residual capacity, infants and children consequently have less respiratory reserve. It is

Table 1. Physiological reasons for the increased susceptibility of infants for respiratory compromise in comparison to adults

Cause	Physiological or anatomical basis
Metabolism ↑	O_2 consumption ↑
Risk of apnoea ↑	Immaturity of control of breathing
Airway resistance ↑	
Upper airway resistance ↑	Nose breathing
	Large tongue
	Airway size ↓
	Collapsibility ↑
	Pharyngeal muscle tone ↓
	Compliance of upper airway structures ↑
Lower airway resistance ↑	Airway size ↓
	Collapsibility ↑
	Airway wall compliance ↑
	Elastic recoil ↓
Lung volume ↓	Numbers of alveoli ↓
	Lack of collateral ventilation
Efficiency of respiratory muscles ↓	Efficiency of diaphragm ↓
	Rib cage compliance ↑
	Horizontal insertion at the rib cage
	Efficiency of intercostal muscles ↓
	Horizontal ribs
Endurance of respiratory muscles ↓	Respiratory rate ↑
	Fatigue-resistant type I muscle fibres ↓

the purpose of this chapter to provide the basic knowledge of why the infant's respiratory tract is not just a miniature version of the adult respiratory tract.

Development of the Respiratory System

Embryologically, the lungs begin as a ventral outpouching of the foregut, namely the laryngotracheal groove, during the 4th week of gestation. Each of the structural components – airways, alveoli, and blood vessels – grows differently with respect to increase in number as well as in size [5, 6]. This non-isotropic or dysanaptic growth pattern has been confirmed by lung function tests in cross-sectional surveys of infants and children, since considerable remodelling of the respiratory tract occurs even after birth [7, 8]. The bronchial system, as far as its branching pattern is concerned, is nearly fully developed long before alveolar development begins. By the 7th week of gestation all segmental bronchi are present, and the characteristic branching pattern of conducting airways is complete by the 16th week of gestation. The terminal bronchioli grow further to form alveolar ducts and eventually primitive alveoli at about the 6th month of gestation. Alveoli appear as early as at 32 weeks of gestation; however, most alveoli

are added through multiplication after birth until about the age of 3 years. Later in life, the increase in lung volume is mainly due to expansion of alveoli. It is conceivable that the lung and airways grow isotropically as soon as alveolar multiplication is complete, probably from the age of 2–3 years on [9].

Central Control of Breathing

Control of breathing during the transition from the fetal state to the breathing child is very different from that in adults [10]. A considerable amount of maturation of control of breathing occurs in the last few weeks of gestation, which explains the high prevalence of apnoea in infants born prematurely. The breathing pattern of newborn infants is irregular with considerable breath-to-breath variability and periodic breathing at times, especially in those born prematurely. The neural basis for chemoreceptor-mediated ventilatory responses is present in the fetus. However, the qualitative and quantitative responses to hypercapnia or hypoxia are different from the adult response. Infants with apnoea were observed to exhibit a decreased and variable sensitivity to hypercapnia [11, 12]. In response to hypoxia, the fetus was used to decrease his activity including breathing movements during intrauterine life while adults respond to hypoxia with increased respiratory efforts. In addition, the fetus was used to arterial oxygen tensions in the umbilical vein of about 25–35 mm Hg. Complete postnatal adaptation of the peripheral chemoreceptors to arterial oxygen tensions in the range of 80–90 mm Hg does not happen instantaneously after birth and requires time. Especially premature infants are not able to sustain the physiological hyperventilatory response to hypoxemia for a prolonged period [13, 14]. Changes in sleep state have also a much more profound influence on the breathing pattern than later in life [15]. Hence, the newborn infant is much more vulnerable to any noxious stimuli and disturbances of the respiratory control mechanisms than older children [16].

Upper and Lower Airways

In the newborn, nasal breathing is obligatory or at least strongly preferential due to the configuration of the upper airways. The epiglottis is relatively large, floppy, and positioned high in the pharynx so that it is in contact with the soft palate, thereby favouring nasal over mouth breathing [17]. In addition, the relatively large tongue occupies most of the oropharynx which makes oral respiration even more difficult. Nevertheless, mouth breathing can occur if the nasal passages are obstructed [18, 19]. However, it is less efficient than in the older child or adult. The configuration of the upper airways changes with growth. Over the first 2 years of life, the larynx and hydatid bone move down the posterior portion of the tongue, which facilitates buccal respiration and the development of speech.

The resistance of the nasal passages in the newborn and the adult is approximately 50% of total airway resistance. The larynx, trachea and bronchi are considerably more compliant than in the older child or adult, thus making the infant's airway highly susceptible to distending and compressive forces [20]. In addition, the activity of the genioglossus and other muscles responsible for maintaining upper airway patency is decreased in infants [21]. Thus, with any obstruction of the upper airway, significant dynamic inspiratory collapse of upper airway structures can occur during forceful inspirations which further adds to the obstruction already present. With lower airway obstruction, forced expiratory efforts result in increased intrathoracic pressure, and dynamic expiratory lower airway collapse occurs, further limiting expiratory flow (e.g., worsening of upper or lower airway obstruction in the crying child). Understanding this phenomenon of

dynamic airway collapse is particularly important in treating agitated children with upper or lower airway obstruction. It explains why sedatives or other efforts to relieve anxiety and reduce crying in infants and children are effective in minimizing dynamic airway collapse, which exaggerates the airway obstruction caused by the underlying pathology.

The airways of a child are relatively large in comparison with those of an adult [22]. However, in absolute terms they are small, and minor changes in the airway radius create a much larger increase in resistance to airflow in the infant than in the adult [23, 24], since the resistance increases by the fourth power of any reduction in radius. In the adult lung, about 80% of the resistance to airflow may be attributed to airways greater than 2 mm in diameter, because the peripheral airways provide a large cross-sectional area and thus contribute little (less than 20%) to total airway resistance. Conversely, small peripheral airways contribute about 50% to the total airway resistance in the infant lung. As airway diameter and length increase with age and growth, airway resistance falls tremendously from birth to adulthood [11, 25]. Therefore, diseases that affect the small airways and cause large changes in peripheral resistance may be clinically silent in an adult, but can cause significant problems in infants (e.g., bronchiolitis).

Chest Wall

Because of its shape, high compliance, and deformability, the contribution of the rib cage to tidal breathing is limited in newborns and infants. The sternum is soft and thus only provides an unstable base for the ribs. The highly compliant ribs are horizontally placed, and the intercostal muscles are poorly developed, so that the bucket-handle motion upon which thoracic respiration depends is impossible. Thus, the potential to increase the thoracic cross-sectional area is limited. The angle of insertion of the dome-shaped diaphragm at the lower ribs is more horizontal than it is in older children. Hence, contraction of the diaphragm during inspiration will tend to move the lower rib cage inward. The intercostal muscles and the diaphragm are antagonists at the costal margin, and the balance of control over the costal margin depends on the arch of the diaphragm. If the diaphragm is flat (e.g., pulmonary hyperinflation), it wastes energy by constricting the costal margin – an essentially forced expiratory act – instead of exerting its force by drawing air into the thorax with inspiration. This paradoxical inward motion of the costal margin

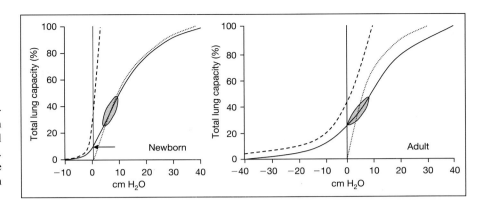

Fig. 1. Comparison of the static pressure-volume curves of the respiratory system (—), of the lung (•••), and the chest wall (---) between the newborn and the adult. Tidal breathing (filled loop) is kept above the elastic equilibrium of the respiratory system in the neonate (arrow) [adapted from 45].

with inspiration is called Hoover sign and is a common symptom in children with marked peripheral airway obstruction and hyperinflation [26, 27].

The highly compliant chest wall is easily distorted, so that under conditions of respiratory impairment much energy is wasted by sucking in ribs rather than air. The loss in tidal volume is made up by greater expenditure in the work of breathing, even under normal conditions. This paradoxic inward movement of the chest wall during inspiration is a common sign of almost every disorder causing respiratory distress in infants, but is most pronounced in upper airway obstruction. By 1 year of age, the rib cage contribution to tidal breathing is similar to that of the adolescent, suggesting that major developmental changes in rib cage shape, compliance, and deformability take place during infancy [28]. The compliance of the chest wall equals that of the lung only by the 2nd year of life [29].

The newborn and infant have high chest wall compliance, at least 5 times higher than that of the lung, contrary to the adult [30]. Since the balance between chest and lung recoil pressure determines the static resting volume of the lung, the infant reaches equilibrium at a relatively much lower lung volume than the adult (fig. 1). Breathing at tidal volumes overlapping closing volumes will result in airway closure and areas of ventilation-perfusion mismatch [31]. Hence, the oxygen reserve in the lung is reduced. Normally, however, infants are constantly reestablishing lung volumes with crying and movement. In addition, the infant actively elevates the end-expiratory lung volume above the elastic equilibrium volume by expiratory braking [32]. This is achieved by several mechanisms: (1) high respiratory rate with insufficient time to exhale to the elastic equilibrium volume, (2) laryngeal adduction during exhalation to increase the resistance to airflow, and (3) postinspiratory diaphragmatic muscle activity.

By the end of the 1st year of life active elevation of the end-expiratory volume decreases [33], and the rib cage contribution to tidal breathing has approached adult characteristics [28].

Respiratory Muscles

The diaphragm is the most important breathing muscle, and any disease or physiological process which impairs diaphragmatic function will predispose the individual to respiratory failure (e.g., surgery, abdominal distension, hyperinflation of the lungs). The proportion of respiration performed by the diaphragm increases dramatically in REM sleep, because then the phasic and tonic inhibition of intercostal muscles causes the rib cage to move in an uncoordinated way and out of phase with the diaphragm. In addition, loss of respiratory muscle tonic activity (including electrical activity of the diaphragm at end expiration) leads to a decrease in functional residual capacity during REM sleep [34]. The work of breathing in REM sleep is therefore high [35]. Since the infant spends a great deal of time asleep, and the predominant sleep state is REM [36], there are considerable periods when ventilation is less than optimal in even the normal situation.

At birth, the respiratory muscles appear histochemically to be poorly equipped to sustain high workloads, and the majority of the muscle mass are type II 'fast-twitch' fibres. Maturational changes in the respiratory musculature occur, with increased mass and a progressive increase in the fatigue-resistant type I muscle fibres, to approach adult values within the first year of life [37]. In addition, premature infants have to undergo a considerable amount of maturational changes in respiratory muscle coordination of the upper airway muscles and the diaphragm which make them susceptible to obstructive sleep apnoea [38, 39].

Lung Parenchyma

The elastic tissue in the septa of the alveoli surrounding the conducting airways provides the elastic recoil which enables the airways to remain open. Early in life there are few relatively large alveoli that provide little support for the airways, which are thus able to collapse easily. Alveolar addition continues throughout early childhood by septal division, providing more elastic recoil and a decreased tendency for airway collapse with increasing age [40]. Elastic recoil increases until adolescence and declines again with aging. Collateral pathways of ventilation (intra-alveolar pores of Kohn and bronchoalveolar canals of Lambert) do not appear until 3–4 years of age [41, 42], which excludes alveoli beyond obstructed airways to be ventilated by these alternate routes and predisposes the infant to the development of atelectasis. Hypoxemia and hypercapnia occur early and can become profound quickly in infants.

The lung is not fully developed at birth. By the 16th week of gestation, all the non-respiratory airways are present. Most respiratory airways appear between the 16th week of gestation and birth. Alveolar development starts relatively late in the 7th month of intrauterine life. Postnatally, the gas exchange areas grow at a faster rate than the conducting system. The alveoli, as they exist in the adult, do not begin to appear until about 8 weeks of age. In the newborn, the terminal bronchioles give rise to respiratory bronchioles, transitional ducts and terminal saccules. By 2 months of age, alveolar multiplication begins and continues to about 2–3 years of age [9, 43–44]. With the increase in alveolar number, the elastic fibres are still not mature. The distribution and concentration of elastic fibres do not reach adult values until adolescence.

Conclusion

The considerable differences in respiratory physiology between infants and adults explain why infants and young children have a higher susceptibility to more severe manifestations of respiratory diseases, and why respiratory failure is a common problem in neonatal and paediatric intensive care units. The appreciation of the peculiarities of paediatric respiratory physiology is not only essential for correct assessment of any ill child, but also for correct interpretation of any pulmonary function test performed in this population.

References

1 Newth CJL: Respiratory disease and respiratory failure: Implications for the young and the old. Br J Dis Chest 1986;80:209–217.
2 Newth CJL: Recognition and management of respiratory failure. Pediatr Clin North Am 1979;26:617–643.
3 Cook CD, Cherry RB, O'Brian D, Kalberg P, Smith CA: Studies of respiratory physiology in the newborn infant. I. Observations on normal premature and full-term infants. J Clin Invest 1955;34:975–982.
4 Kennaird DL: Oxygen consumption and evaporative water loss in infants with congenital heart disease. Arch Dis Child 1976;51: 34–41.
5 Reid LM: Lung growth in health and disease. Br J Dis Chest 1984;78:113–134.
6 Burri PH: Fetal and postnatal development of the lung. Annu Rev Physiol 1984;46:617–628.
7 Zapletal A, Motoyama EK, Van de Woestijne KP, Hunt VR, Bouhuys A: Maximum expiratory flow-volume curves and airway conductance in children and adolescents. J Appl Physiol 1969;26:308–316.
8 Lanteri CJ, Sly PD: Changes in respiratory mechanics with age. J Appl Physiol 1993;74: 369–378.
9 Merkus PJFM, ten Have-Opbroek AAW, Quanjer PH: Human lung growth: A review. Pediatr Pulmonol 1996;21:383–397.

10 Givan DC: Physiology of breathing and related pathological processes in infants. Semin Pediatr Neurol 2003;10:271–280.
11 Gerhardt T, Bancalari E: Apnea of prematurity. I. Lung function and regulation of breathing. Pediatrics 1984;74:58–62.
12 Frantz ID, Adler SM, Thach BT, Taeusch HW: Maturational effects on respiratory responses to carbon dioxide in premature infants. J Appl Physiol 1976;41:41–45.
13 Rigatto H, Brady JP, de la Torre-Verduzco R: Chemoreceptor reflexes in premature infants. I. The effect of gestational and postnatal age on the ventilatory response to inhalation of 100% and 5% oxygen. Pediatrics 1975;55: 604–613.
14 Sankaran K, Wiebe H, Seshia MMK, Boychuck RB, Cates D, Rigatto H: Immediate and late ventilatory response to high and low O_2 in preterm infants and adult subjects. Pediatr Res 1979;13:875–878.
15 Finer NN, Abroms IF, Taeusch HW: Ventilation and sleep states in newborn infants. J Pediatr 1976;89:100–108.
16 Schläfke ME: Atmungsregulation und Entwicklung, pathophysiologische Aspekte. Pneumologie 1997;51:398–402.
17 Moss ML: The veloepiglottic sphincter and obligate nose breathing in the neonate. J Pediatr 1965;67:330–331.

18 Swift PG, Emery JL: Clinical observations on the responses to nasal occlusion in infancy. Arch Dis Child 1973;48:947–951.
19 Rodenstein DO, Perlemuter N, Stanescu DC: Infants are not obligatory nasal breathers. Am Rev Respir Dis 1985;131:343–347.
20 Deoras KS, Wolfson MR, Searls RL, Hilfer SR, Shaffer TH: Developmental changes in tracheal structure. Pediatr Res 1991;30:170–175.
21 Gauda EB, Miller MJ, Carlo WA, DiFiore JM, Johnsen DC, Martin RJ: Genioglossus response to airway occlusion in apneic versus non-apneic infants. Pediatr Res 1987;22: 683–687.
22 Engel S: The Child's Lung: Developmental Anatomy, Physiology, and Pathology. London, Arnold, 1947.
23 Eckenhoff JE: Some anatomic considerations of the infant larynx influencing endotracheal anesthesia. Anesthesiology 1951;12:401–410.
24 Hogg JG, Williams J, Richardson JB, Macklem PT, Thurlbeck WM: Age as a factor in the distribution of lower airway conductance and in the pathologic anatomy of obstructive lung disease. N Engl J Med 1970;282:1283–1287.
25 Stocks J, Godfrey S: Specific airway conductance in relation to postconceptional age during infancy. J Appl Physiol 1977;43:144–154.

26 Klein M: Hoover sign and peripheral airways obstruction. J Pediatr 1992;120:495–496.

27 Hoover CF: The functions of the intercostal muscles. JAMA 1919;73:17–20.

28 Hershenson MB, Colin AA, Wohl MEB, Stark AR: Changes in the contribution of the rib cage to tidal breathing during infancy. Am Rev Respir Dis 1990;141:922–925.

29 Papastamelos C, Panitch HB, England SE, Allen JL: Developmental changes in chest wall compliance in infancy and early childhood. J Appl Physiol 1995;78:179–184.

30 Gerhardt T, Bancalari E: Chest wall compliance in full-term and premature infants. Acta Paediatr Scand 1980;69:359–364.

31 Mansell A, Bryan AC, Levison H: Airway closure in children. J Appl Physiol 1972;33:711–714.

32 Kosch PC, Stark AR: Dynamic maintenance of end-expiratory lung volume in full-term infants. J Appl Physiol 1987;45:18–23.

33 Colin AA, Wohl MEB, Mead J, Ratjen FA, Glass G, Stark AR: Transition from dynamically maintained to relaxed end-expiratory volume in human infants. J Appl Physiol 1989;67:2107–2111.

34 Martin RJ, Okken A, Rubin D: Arterial oxygen tension during active and quiet sleep in the normal neonate. J Pediatr 1979;94:271–274.

35 Muller N, Gulston G, Cade D, Whitton J, Froese AB, Bryan MH, Bryan ACL: Diaphragmatic muscle fatigue in the newborn. J Appl Physiol 1979;46:688–695.

36 Gabriel M, Albani M, Schulte FJ: Apneic spells and sleep states in preterm infants. Pediatrics 1975;57:142–147.

37 Keens TG, Bryan AC, Levison H, Ianuzzo CD: Developmental pattern of muscle fiber types in human ventilatory muscles. J Appl Physiol 1978;44:909–913.

38 Waggener TB, Frantz ID 3rd, Cohlan B, Stark AR: Mixed and obstructive apneas are related to ventilatory oscillations in premature infants. J Appl Physiol 1989;66:2818–2826.

39 Miller MJ, Carlo WA, DiFiore JM, Martin RJ: Airway obstruction during periodic breathing in premature infants. J Appl Physiol 1988;64:2496–2500.

40 Bryan AC, Mansell AL, Levison H: Development of the mechanical properties of the respiratory system; in Hudson WA (ed): Development of the Lung. New York, Dekker, 1977.

41 Boyden EA: Notes on the development of the lung in infancy and childhood. Am J Anat 1967;121:749–762.

42 Boyden EA: Development of the human lung; in Brennemann's Practice of Pediatrics. Hagerstown, Harper & Row, 1975, vol 4, chap 64.

43 Zeltner TB, Caduff JH, Gehr P, Pfenninger J, Burri PH: The postnatal development and growth of the human lung. I. Morphometry. Respir Physiol 1987;67:247–267.

44 Zeltner TB, Burri PH: The postnatal development and growth of the human lung. II. Morphology. Respir Physiol 1987;67:269–282.

45 Agostoni E: Volume-pressure relationships of the thorax and lung in the newborn. J Appl Physiol 1959;14:909–913.

Prof. Dr. med. Jürg Hammer, Head
Division of Intensive Care and Pulmonology
University Children's Hospital Basel
Römergasse 8
CH–4005 Basel (Switzerland)
Tel. +41 61 685 65 65
Fax +41 61 685 50 59
E-Mail juerg.hammer@unibas.ch

Measurements of Pulmonary Function in Infants and Small Children

Hammer J, Eber E (eds): Paediatric Pulmonary Function Testing.
Prog Respir Res. Basel, Karger, 2005, vol 33, pp 10–19

Tidal Breathing Measurements

Karin C. Lødrup Carlsen[a]   Kai-Håkon Carlsen[b]

[a]Section of Allergology and Pulmonology, Department of Paediatrics,
Women-Child-Division, Ullevål University Hospital, Oslo, [b]Voksentoppen BKL,
National Hospital, Oslo, Norway

Abstract

Tidal breathing measurements have been used for some time to evaluate lung development during infancy, to diagnose respiratory diseases, to assess the effect of treatment, and also to predict respiratory diseases in subjects who for some reason cannot perform voluntary forced respiratory manoeuvres. However, standardization of measurements is required, and a discussion on interpretation of findings, scientific and clinical value of such measurements, as well as establishment of reference values across ages is needed. The present chapter will briefly discuss these issues in very young children.

Non-interventional tidal breathing measurements may be obtained in any subject, regardless of respiratory state or arousal state, provided the subject is quietly breathing. This may be ascertained in both in- and out-patient settings with dedicated staff carefully trained to obtain a safe and comfortable surrounding for child and guardian.

In principle there are two ways to measure tidal breathing parameters; by tidal flow and/or volume measures (often as loops) obtained through a pneumotachograph or an ultrasonic flow-sensor via a face mask, or by respiratory inductive plethysmography by use of bands around the chest and abdomen. Most studies have applied face masks and pneumotachographs, but recently also ultrasonic flow-meters have become available for such measurements.

The clinical value of tidal breathing measurements depends upon the question asked. Several studies have demonstrated tidal flow-volume (TFV) loops to be valuable as a screening and diagnostic tool for separating upper from lower airway diseases, and many studies have demonstrated typical patterns of the flow-volume (or flow-time) traces in patients with bronchial obstruction. The most commonly reported parameter in relationship to bronchial obstruction is the ratio of time to reach peak expiratory flow to total expiratory time, although several other parameters have been proposed. TFV loops have been used for diagnosis of obstructive airway disease, but have been shown to be less valuable for the early diagnosis of diseases such as cystic fibrosis. Reduced lung function early in life (in the neonatal period or in early infancy) has been associated with later development of recurrent wheeze or asthma, but it is unlikely that TFV loops will be useful to predict obstructive airway disease at an individual level. Tidal breathing parameters have been important in clinical epidemiological research, as well as for objective measurements of response to medication in young children, too young to cooperate with forced manoeuvres.

Due to the complex physiological functions regulating breathing, TFV measures probably represent both respiratory mechanics as well as control of breathing. When employing such measurements, it is important to be familiar with the factors that might influence results, to ensure qualified interpretation of results. However, the measurements are relatively easily obtained provided the child is in a comfortable setting and relaxes. One of the main advantages of tidal breathing measurements is the possibility to obtain objective measures of lung function in infants and young children with respiratory disease without the need for sedation. Lung function by tidal breathing measurements may contribute as one of several objective measures for

Table 1. Tidal breathing parameters in healthy children

	n	Age mean ± SD (range)	t_{PTEF}/t_E mean ± SD (95% CI)	Vt (ml) mean ± SD (95% CI)	RR mean ± SD (95% CI)	Comments
Lødrup Carlsen et al. [67]	802	2.7 ± 0.9 days	0.32 ± 0.11	24.8 ± 4.6	58.9 ± 14	awake newborns
Stocks et al. [19]	23	6.4 ± 0.8 weeks	0.33 ± 0.10	36.1 ± 4.8	42.9 ± 7.3	full term, natural sleep
Stocks et al. [19]	49	6.8 ± 1.0 weeks	0.32 ± 0.08	40.1 ± 5.6	45.8 ± 9.4	full term, sedated
Yuksel et al. [59]	60	2 (1–12) days	0.38 ± 0.06			full term, natural sleep
Stick et al. [33]	19	58 (33–114) h	0.44 ± 0.11		46.6 ± 6.3	full term, natural sleep
Stick et al. [33]	19		0.47 ± 0.14[1]		50.3 ± 14.4	full term, natural sleep
Carlsen et al. [11]	26	34 ± 19 months	0.36 (0.33–0.39)	10.9 (9.8–11.9)	34.2 (28.2–40.3)	
Van der Ent et al. [25]	120	4.8 ± 1.2 years	0.45 ± 0.08[2]			awake
Van der Ent et al. [25]	106	8.0 ± 1.1 years	0.41 ± 0.07[2]			awake

Vt = tidal volume; t_{PTEF}/t_E = time to reach peak tidal expiratory flow/total expiratory time; RR = respiratory rate; CI = confidence interval.
[1] Respitrace (no face mask).
[2] Data given in original paper as Tme/Te.

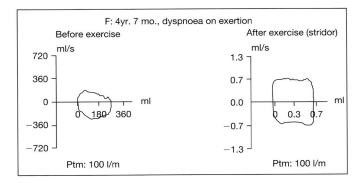

Fig. 4. TFV loops before and after exercise in a girl with exercise-induced stridor due to (later verified by endoscopy) laryngotracheomalacia.

Diagnosis

It was early suggested that TFV loops could be used as a method to screen for laryngotracheal disease [7], and the method has proven valuable also recently for monitoring treatment of tracheobronchomalacia [53] and as a screening and diagnostic procedure in noisily breathing infants [54]. Similarly, we have used TFV loops as a diagnostic tool for separating upper from lower airway disease, as shown in figure 4 in a girl with exercise-induced stridor before and immediately after intense running for 5 min. Although TFV measurements have been studied in various lower respiratory tract diseases such as cystic fibrosis [25, 42, 55], chronic lung disease of the newborn [56] and gastro-oesophageal reflux [57], most interest has nevertheless been associated with obstructive airway disease (OAD) in infancy and early childhood.

No clear cut-off value has been found that can discriminate between children with and without OAD, and there is a relatively large variation in tidal breathing parameters among both healthy children and children with respiratory disease. Table 1 reports some tidal breathing parameters from healthy children related to age. Although relatively similar values of reduced mean t_{PTEF}/t_E (0.16–0.22) have been reported in young asymptomatic children with OAD [11, 58] in some studies, van der Ent et al. [25] reported a higher mean t_{PTEF}/t_E of 0.30 before application of a β_2-agonist in children older than 3 years. This was however significantly lower than among control children (mean t_{PTEF}/t_E = 0.41). Furthermore, Yuksel et al. [59] found significantly reduced neonatal t_{PTEF}/t_E in children who subsequently developed recurrent wheeze compared to those who were still healthy at 1 year (median, range: 0.35, 0.30–0.44 vs. 0.41, 0.30–0.52, respectively). In children with (acute) bronchial obstruction, lower values still have been found (0.08–0.19) in acute bronchiolitis [24] and after histamine provocation [60], respectively. However, overlapping t_{PTEF}/t_E ranges in subjects with and without OAD in most studies limit the value of using TFV measures as a diagnostic test. Other studies have not been able to detect differences between healthy children and children with cystic fibrosis [55] or in those patients with lower respiratory tract infections or asthma [61].

Repeated Measurements after Intervention

Although there is a lack of standardization of bronchial provocation or reversibility testing employing TFV measures,

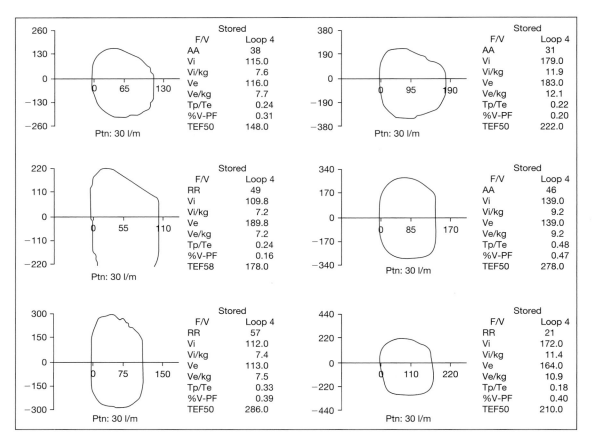

Fig. 5. TFV loops in a 22-month-old girl with suspected exercise-induced asthma. The left hand curves are measured prior to any treatment, the right hand curves after 5 weeks intense medical treatment. Top curves are baseline, middle curves immediately after attempted 5 min running (which she was not able to complete the first time), and the bottom curves 15 min after bronchodilator therapy. The investigations demonstrate broncho-protection after medical treatment compared to the initial investigation. Initially, the girl gave up running after approximately 3 min, with rapidly worsening clinically detectable bronchial obstruction. She had no symptoms during the second investigation.

several reports indicate that additional valuable information may be gained by such measurements. First of all, possible effects of medication may be objectively assessed in acute disease [24], as well as in stable conditions [11], such as after treatment with inhaled corticosteroids [62]. A few studies have found different responses to β_2-agonists by tidal breathing parameters in asymptomatic children with OAD compared with children without OAD [11, 26, 58], and children with gastro-oesophageal reflux were found to be less likely to respond to bronchodilators than other children with OAD [57]. On the other hand, a few studies have assessed bronchial provocation in children by tidal breathing, demonstrating mean decreases in tidal ratios after histamine [25, 60] and methacholine [63], respectively. Although the response to a bronchodilator (without clinically detectable bronchial obstruction) has not yet been investigated for its diagnostic value, one study demonstrated a close correlation between eosinophil activation (measured by serum eosinophil cationic protein) and the degree of bronchodilator response in infants and children shortly after the onset of OAD [58]. It remains to be seen whether or not children with a high degree of bronchodilator response very early in life (with or without eosinophil activation) are more likely to have asthma later in childhood. Since no agreement has been reached upon how to assess reversibility of airway obstruction in very young children, we have suggested crude definitions of responders, non-responders, and paradoxal responders [26, 45], based upon an improvement of greater than two standard deviations (SD), a less than 2 SD change, or a greater than 2 SD reduction of $t_{\mathrm{PTEF}}/t_{\mathrm{E}}$ of the curves selected, respectively from before to after medication.

In a clinical setting, we also use TFV loops to assess exercise-induced asthma in children too young to perform regular spirometry, as demonstrated in figure 5. However, well-conducted studies are warranted before any firm conclusions as to validity and diagnostic yield can be determined in such a setting. It remains to be seen whether TFV measurements together with other laboratory tests may improve our diagnostic and predictive capability in young children with OAD.

Although reduced lung function in early life has been associated with later OAD in several studies [52, 59, 64, 65], the predictive value for individual children has so far not been elucidated. With the large intra-individual variations within groups of healthy children as well as children with respiratory diseases, it is unlikely that such measurements will be sensitive enough to be of practical use for most healthy neonates. However, for research such measurements have been found to be of great value, such as documenting reduced lung function as a result of maternal smoking during pregnancy [34, 35, 66].

Tidal Breathing Measurements during Physical Exercise Testing

As already mentioned, a place for tidal breathing measurements during exercise in children and adults with chronic lung diseases has recently been found. Although these measurements require cooperation during exercise such as treadmill run, and thus cannot be used in children below 6–7 years of age, it should be mentioned that such measurements are increasingly used in research settings as well as in clinical practice. The use of TFV loops measured during increasing exercise until maximum exercise load compared to the pre-exercise maximum expiratory and inspiratory flow-volume loops, gives valuable information about pulmonary limitations to physical exercise and oxygen uptake, as well as to the possibility to improve physical performance through physical training [10].

However, it should be underlined that such measurements cannot be performed in infants and preschool children.

Conclusion

The interest in tidal breathing lung function measurements has increased over the last two decades, and such measurements have been found useful for research as well as for clinical purposes. Although much work still remains to be done in order to define their value in individual patients, we believe that such measurements are valuable supplements to the medical history, clinical examination and other laboratory tests within the field of paediatric respiratory medicine.

References

1 Deming J, Hanner JP: Respiration in infancy. II. A study of the rate, volume and character of healthy infants during the neonatal period. Am J Dis Child 1936;51: 823–831.

2 Bouhuys A: The clinical use of pneumotachograph. Acta Med Scand 1957;159:91–103.

3 Hyatt RE BL: The flow volume curve. A current perspective. Am Rev Respir Dis 1973; 107:191–199.

4 Takishima T, Grimby G, Graham W, Knudson R, Macklem PT, Mead J: Flow -volume curves during quiet breathing, maximum voluntary ventilation and forced vital capacities in patients with obstructive lung disease. Scand J Respir Dis 1967;48:384–393.

5 Adler SM, Wohl ME: Flow-volume relationship at low lung volumes in healthy term newborn infants. Pediatrics 1978;61: 636–640.

6 Morris MJ, Lane DJ: Tidal expiratory flow patterns in airflow obstruction. Thorax 1981; 36:135–142.

7 Abramson AL, Goldstein MN, Stenzler A, Steele A: The use of the tidal breathing flow volume loop in laryngotracheal disease of neonates and infants. Laryngoscope 1982;92: 922–926.

8 Refsum HE, Foenstelien E: Exercise-associated ventilatory insufficiency in adolescent athletes; in Oseid S, Edwards AM (eds): The Asthmatic Child in Play and Sport. London, Pitman, 1983, pp 128–139.

9 Babb TG, Rodarte JR: Estimation of ventilatory capacity during submaximal exercise. J Appl Physiol 1993;74:2016–2022.

10 Johnson BD, Weisman IM, Zeballos RJ, Beck KC: Emerging concepts in the evaluation of ventilatory limitation during exercise: The exercise tidal flow-volume loop. Chest 1999;116: 488–503.

11 Carlsen KH, Lødrup Carlsen KC: Tidal breathing analysis and response to salbutamol in awake young children with and without asthma. Eur Respir J 1994;7: 2154–2159.

12 Lødrup-Carlsen KC, Carlsen KH: Lung function in awake healthy infants: The first five days of life. Eur Respir J 1993;6: 1496–1500.

13 Wauer J, Leier TU, Henschen M, Wauer RR, Schmalisch G: In vitro validation of an ultrasonic flowmeter in order to measure the functional residual capacity in newborns. Physiol Meas 2003;24:355–365.

14 Cernelc M, Suki B, Reinmann B, Hall GL, Frey U: Correlation properties of tidal volume and end-tidal O_2 and CO_2 concentrations in healthy infants. J Appl Physiol 2002;92:1817–1827.

15 Hammer J, Reber A, Trachsel D, Frei FJ: Effect of jaw-thrust and continuous positive airway pressure on tidal breathing in deeply sedated infants. J Pediatr 2001;138:826–830.

16 Bates JH, Schmalisch G, Filbrun D, Stocks J: Tidal breath analysis for infant pulmonary function testing. ERS/ATS Task Force on Standards for Infant Respiratory Function Testing. European Respiratory Society/ American Thoracic Society. Eur Respir J 2000;16:1180–1192.

17 Richardson P: Lung mechanics: A discussion of methods for measurements in newborn infants. Arkos 1989;December:15–21.

18 Frey U, Stocks J, Sly P, Bates J: Specification for signal processing and data handling used for infant pulmonary function testing. ERS/ATS Task Force on Standards for Infant Respiratory Function Testing. European Respiratory Society/American Thoracic Society. Eur Respir J 2000;16:1016–1022.

19 Stocks J, Dezateux CA, Jackson EA, Hoo AF, Costeloe KL, Wade AM: Analysis of tidal breathing parameters in infancy: How variable is TPTEF:TE? Am J Respir Crit Care Med 1994;150:1347–1354.

20 van der Ent CK, Brackel HJL, Mulder P, Bogaard JM, Brackel HJ: Improvement of tidal breathing analysis in children with asthma by on-line automatic data processing. Eur Respir J 1996;9:1306–1313.

21 Morris MJ, Madgwick RG, Collyer I, Denby F, Lane DJ: Analysis of expiratory tidal flow patterns as a diagnostic tool in airflow obstruction. Eur Respir J 1998;12:1113–1117.

22 Lodrup KC, Mowinckel P, Carlsen KH: Lung function measurements in awake compared to sleeping newborn infants. Pediatr Pulmonol 1992;12:99–104.

23 Djupesland PG, Lodrup Carlsen KC: Nasal airway dimensions and lung function in awake, healthy neonates. Pediatr Pulmonol 1998;25:99–106.

24 Lodrup Carlsen KC, Carlsen KH: Inhaled nebulized adrenaline improves lung function in infants with acute bronchiolitis. Respir Med 2000;94:709–714.

25 van der Ent CK, Brackel HJL, van der Laag J, Bogaard JM: Tidal breathing analysis as a measure of airway obstruction in children three years of age and older. Am J Respir Crit Care Med 1996;153:1253–1258.

26 Lodrup Carlsen KC, Pettersen M, Carlsen KH: Is bronchodilator response in two year old children associated with asthma risk factors? Pediatr Allergy Immunol, in press.

27 Cohn MA, Rao AS, Broudy M, Birch S, Watson H, Atkins N, et al: The respiratory inductive plethysmograph: A new non-invasive monitor of respiration. Bull Eur Physiopathol Respir 1982;18:643–658.

28 Adams JA: Respiratory inductive plethysmography; in Stocks J, Sly PD, Tepper RS, Morgan WJ (eds): Infant Respiratory Function Testing. London, Wiley, 1996.

29 Manczur T, Greenough A, Hooper R, Allen K, Latham S, Price JF, et al: Tidal breathing parameters in young children: Comparison of measurement by respiratory inductance plethysmography to a facemask pneumotachograph system. Pediatr Pulmonol 1999;28:436–441.

30 Newth CJL, Hammer J: Measurements of thoraco-abdominal asynchrony and work of breathing in children; in Hammer J, Eber E (eds): Paediatric Pulmonary Function Testing. Prog Respir Res. Basel, Karger, 2005, vol 33, pp 148–156.

31 Allen JL, Wolfson MR, McDowell K, Shaffer TH: Thoracoabdominal asynchrony in infants with airflow obstruction. Am Rev Respir Dis 1990;141:337–342.

32 Allen JL, Greenspan JS, Deoras KS, Keklikian E, Wolfson MR, Shaffer TH: Interaction between chest wall motion and lung mechanics in normal infants and infants with bronchopulmonary dysplasia. Pediatr Pulmonol 1991;11:37–43.

33 Stick SM, Ellis E, Le Souëf PN, Sly P: Validation of respiratory inductance plethysmography (Respitrace) for the measurement of tidal breathing parameters in newborns. Pediatr Pulmonol 1992;14:187–191.

34 Stick SM, Burton PR, Gurrin L, Sly PD, LeSouef PN: Effects of maternal smoking during pregnancy and a family history of asthma on respiratory function in newborn infants. Lancet 1996;348:1060–1064.

35 Lødrup Carlsen KC, Jaakkola JJ, Nafstad P, Carlsen KH: In-utero exposure to cigarette smoking influences lung function at birth. Eur Respir J 1997;10:1774–1779.

36 Springer C, Godfrey S, Vilozni D, Bar-Yishay E, Noviski N, Avital A: Comparison of respiratory inductance plethysmography with thoracoabdominal compression in bronchial challenges in infants and young children. Am J Respir Crit Care Med 1996; 154:665–669.

37 Sivan Y, Deakers TW, Newth CJ: Thoracoabdominal asynchrony in acute upper airway obstruction in small children. Am Rev Respir Dis 1990;142:540–544.

38 Hunter JM, Sperry EE, Ravilly S, Colin AA: Thoracoabdominal asynchrony and ratio of time to peak tidal expiratory flow over total expiratory time in adolescents with cystic fibrosis. Pediatr Pulmonol 1999;28:199–204.

39 Anonymous: Respiratory function measurements in infants: Measurement conditions. American Thoracic Society/European Respiratory Society. Am J Respir Crit Care Med 1995;151:2058–2064.

40 Lodrup Carlsen KC, Stenzler A, Carlsen KH: Determinants of tidal flow volume loop indices in neonates and children with and without asthma. Pediatr Pulmonol 1997;24: 391–396.

41 Frey U, Silverman M, Suki B: Analysis of the harmonic content of the tidal flow waveforms in infants. J Appl Physiol 2001;91:1687–1693.

42 Colasanti RL, Morris MJ, Madgwick RG, Sutton L, Williams EM: Analysis of tidal breathing profiles in cystic fibrosis and COPD. Chest 2004;125:901–908.

43 Banovcin P, Seidenberg J, Von der HH: Assessment of tidal breathing patterns for monitoring of bronchial obstruction in infants. Pediatr Res 1995;38:218–220.

44 Kayaleh RA, Dutt A, Khan A, Wilson AF: Tidal breath flow-volume curves in obstructive sleep apnea. Am Rev Respir Dis 1992;145: 1372–1377.

45 Lodrup Carlsen KC: Tidal breathing at all ages. Monaldi Arch Chest Dis 2000;55: 427–434.

46 Tangsrud SE, Carlsen KC, Lund-Petersen I, Carlsen KH: Lung function measurements in young children with spinal muscle atrophy; a cross sectional survey on the effect of position and bracing. Arch Dis Child 2001;84: 521–524.

47 McKiernan BC, Dye JA, Rozanski EA: Tidal breathing flow-volume loops in healthy and bronchitic cats. J Vet Internal Med 1993;7: 388–393.

48 Herholz C, Tschudi P, Gerber H, Moens Y, Straub R: Ultrasound spirometry in the horse: A preliminary report on the method and the effects of xylazine and lobeline hydrochloride medication. Schweiz Arch Tierheilkd 1997; 139:558–563.

49 Lodrup Carlsen KC, Stenzler A, Carlsen KH: Determinants of tidal flow volume loop indices in neonates and children with and without asthma. Pediatr Pulmonol 1997;24: 391–396.

50 Seddon PC, Davis GM, Coates AL: Do tidal expiratory flow patterns reflect lung mechanics in infants? Am J Respir Crit Care Med 1996;153:1248–1252.

51 van der Ent CK, van der Grinten CP, Meessen NE, Luijendijk SC, Mulder PG, Bogaard JM: Time to peak tidal expiratory flow and the neuromuscular control of expiration. Eur Respir J 1998;12:646–652.

52 Young S, Arnott J, Le Souëf PN, Landau LI, Le Souef PN: Flow limitation during tidal expiration in symptom-free infants and the subsequent development of asthma. J Pediatr 1994;124:681–688.

53 Reiterer F, Eber E, Zach MS, Muller W: Management of severe congenital tracheobronchomalacia by continuous positive airway pressure and tidal breathing flow-volume loop analysis. Pediatr Pulmonol 1994;17: 401–403.

54 Filippone M, Narne S, Pettenazzo A, Zacchello F, Baraldi E: Functional approach to infants and young children with noisy breathing: validation of pneumotachography by blinded comparison with bronchoscopy. Am J Respir Crit Care Med 2000;162:1795–1800.

55 Ranganathan SC, Goetz I, Hoo AF, Lum S, Castle R, Stocks J: Assessment of tidal breathing parameters in infants with cystic fibrosis. Eur Respir J 2003;22:761–766.

56 Greenough A, Zhang YX, Yuksel B, Dimitriou G: Assessment of prematurely born children at follow-up using a tidal breathing parameter. Physiol Meas 1998;19:111–116.

57 Sheikh S, Goldsmith LJ, Howell L, Hamlyn J, Eid N: Lung function in infants with wheezing and gastroesophageal reflux [see comments]. Pediatr Pulmonol 1999;27:236–241.

58 Lodrup Carlsen KC, Halvorsen R, Ahlstedt S, Carlsen KH: Eosinophil cationic protein and tidal flow volume loops in children 0–2 years of age. Eur Respir J 1995;8:1148–1154.

59 Yuksel B, Greenough A, Giffin F, Nicolaides KH: Tidal breathing parameters in the first week of life and subsequent cough and wheeze. Thorax 1996;51:815–818.

60 Cutrera R, Filtchev SI, Merolla R, Willim G, Haluszka J, Ronchetti R: Analysis of expiratory pattern for monitoring bronchial obstruction in school-age children. Pediatr Pulmonol 1991; 10:6–10.

61 Clarke JR, Aston H, Silverman M: Evaluation of a tidal expiratory flow index in healthy and diseased infants. Pediatr Pulmonol 1994;17: 285–290.

62 Devulapalli CS, Haaland G, Pettersen M, Carlsen KH, Lodrup Carlsen KC: Inhaled steroids in young children: A cohort study. Effect on lung function. Eur Respir J 2004;23: 869–875.
63 Benoist MR, Brouard JJ, Rufin P, Delacourt C, Waernessyckle S, Scheinmann P: Ability of new lung function tests to assess methacholine-induced airway obstruction in infants. Pediatr Pulmonol 1994;18:308–316.
64 Halonen M, Stern D, Taussig LM, Wright A, Ray CG, Martinez FD: The predictive relationship between serum IgE levels at birth and subsequent incidences of lower respiratory illnesses and eczema in infants. Am Rev Respir Dis 1992;146:866–870.

65 Martinez FD, Morgan WJ, Wright AL, Holberg CJ, Taussig LM: Diminished lung function as a predisposing factor for wheezing respiratory illness in infants. N Engl J Med 1988;319:1112–1117.
66 Hoo AF, Henschen M, Dezateux C, Costeloe K, Stocks J: Respiratory function among preterm infants whose mothers smoked during pregnancy. Am J Respir Crit Care Med 1998;158: 700–705.
67 Lødrup Carlsen KC, Magnus P, Carlsen KH: Lung function by tidal breathing in awake healthy newborn infants. Eur Respir J 1994;7: 1660–1668.

Karin C. Lødrup Carlsen
Head, Section of Allergology and
Pulmonology, Department of Paediatrics
Women-Child-Division
Ullevål University Hospital, NO–0407
Oslo (Norway)
Tel. +47 22 11 87 65
Fax +47 22 11 86 63
E-Mail kclo@uus.no

Hammer J, Eber E (eds): Paediatric Pulmonary Function Testing.
Prog Respir Res. Basel, Karger, 2005, vol 33, pp 20–33

··

Respiratory Mechanics

Stephanie D. Davis[a]   Monika Gappa[b]   Margaret Rosenfeld[c]

[a]Division of Pediatric Pulmonology, University of North Carolina, Chapel Hill, N.C.;
[b]Department of Paediatric Pulmonology and Neonatology, Medizinische Hochschule Hannover,
Hannover, Germany; [c]Division of Pulmonary Medicine, Children's Hospital and Regional Medical
Center, Seattle, Wash., USA

Abstract

In infants, indices of respiratory mechanics may be evaluated through passive measurements when the respiratory muscles are relaxed or during dynamic measurements when they are actively contracting. The passive respiratory mechanics techniques evaluate the compliance and resistance of the entire respiratory system, and the respiratory system components cannot be partitioned. Passive measurements may be obtained through single or multiple occlusion techniques. Dynamic respiratory mechanics techniques allow the assessment of the compliance and resistance of the lung through transpulmonary pressure measurements obtained by esophageal manometry. Published reference data are limited to single-center studies, are laboratory specific and should be interpreted with caution. Despite the number of published research studies evaluating these techniques in various disease states, the applicability of these measurements to the individual is limited at this time. Future studies using standardized equipment and protocols will help define the clinical utility of these techniques in the individual infant.

In adults and older children, compliance and resistance are usually inferred indirectly from the results of standard lung function tests. Because lung function tests requiring cooperation cannot be performed in infants, techniques have been devised to measure compliance and resistance directly. In fact, compliance and resistance were the first pulmonary function parameters to be measured in infants,

with published studies dating back to the 1950s [1, 2]. This chapter will review (1) respiratory mechanics physiology in infancy, (2) passive and dynamic measurement techniques, (3) available reference data, (4) published literature assessing these measures in infants with disease, and (5) clinical applications.

Physiology

Commonly Measured Indices of Respiratory Mechanics

Respiratory mechanics measurements include compliance, resistance, and the time constant of the respiratory system. Compliance is defined as change in volume divided by change in pressure ($\Delta V/\Delta P$) (fig. 1). The compliance or the elastic recoil of the total respiratory system (C_{rs}) includes the compliance of the chest wall (C_{cw}) and the compliance of the lungs (C_L). Depending on where this change in pressure is measured, the different components of the C_{rs} can be assessed separately. In young infants, C_{cw} is high because of the instability of the rib cage, so C_{rs} is mainly dependent on C_L. As the infant ages, the rib cage becomes more stable and C_{cw} contributes more to C_{rs} [2–4].

Resistance is equal to change in pressure divided by change in flow ($\Delta P/\Delta V'$). Resistance of the respiratory system (R_{rs}) reflects the sum of the resistances of the airways, lung tissue, and chest wall. The components of R_{rs} may also be evaluated individually based on where the pressure change is measured. In the infant, the upper airway

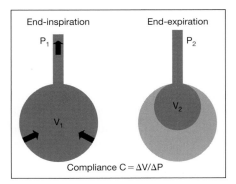

Fig. 1. V_1 and V_2 represent the lung volumes at end-inspiration and end-expiration, respectively. P_1 and P_2 represent the airway opening pressures at end-inspiration and end-expiration, respectively. In this schematic, compliance is defined as change in volume divided by change in pressure ($\Delta V/\Delta P$) between end-inspiration and end-expiration.

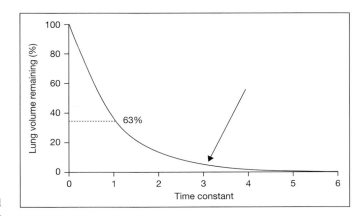

Fig. 2. The time constant is the product of respiratory system resistance and compliance ($T_{rs} = R_{rs} \times C_{rs}$). In this schematic, the expiratory time constant is the time taken for the lung to deflate to 63% of its original volume. After 3 time constants, lung emptying is 95% complete (arrow). (Modified from Taussig LM, Helms PJ: Introduction; in Stocks J, Sly PD, Tepper RS, Morgan WJ (eds): Infant Respiratory Function Testing, 1996. Reprinted by permission of Wiley-Liss, Inc. a subsidiary of John Wiley & Sons, Inc.)

contributes significantly to R_{rs}. Any condition leading to nasal congestion, such as upper respiratory tract infections, will substantially increase nasal resistance and thus, respiratory resistance. Loss of upper airway muscle tone following sedation with chloral hydrate may also increase upper airway resistance. Thus, measurements should be performed during a time when the infant is free of upper respiratory tract infections, and factors affecting the upper airway must be evaluated when interpreting results [2–4].

The time constant (T_{rs}) is the product of respiratory system compliance and resistance ($C_{rs} \times R_{rs}$). One expiratory time constant represents the amount of time required for a 63% decrease in volume (fig. 2). If an infant has stiff lungs or is poorly compliant, T_{rs} will be low, so exhalation occurs quickly and the infant is tachypneic. If an infant has increased airway resistance, T_{rs} is prolonged, so exhalation occurs slowly and the infant has a prolonged expiratory phase [3, 5].

Equation of Lung Motion

In 1916, Roher described an 'equation of motion' for the lungs and three different forces that lead to lung movement or the driving pressure of the respiratory system. These three different forces relate to the pressure needed (1) to prevail over the elastic properties of the lung (Pel), (2) to prevail over the resistive properties of the airways (Pres), and (3) to lead to acceleration of movement within the lung (Pin) [2, 3, 5].

$$Ptot = Pel + Pres + Pin.$$

The pressure needed to prevail over the elastic properties of the respiratory system is related to volume change. The pressure needed to prevail over airway resistance is

related to flow, and the pressure needed to lead to acceleration is related to inertance. The equation of motion can now be rewritten as the following:

$$Pdr = (1/C \times V) + (R \times V') + (I \times Acc),$$

where Pdr is the driving pressure, C is compliance with its reciprocal 1/C (elastance), V is volume, R is resistance, V' is flow, I is inertance, and Acc is acceleration or rate of flow. When studying respiratory mechanics, there are several assumptions. The first assumption is that inertance contributes very little to the equation or is negligible; therefore, this factor is eliminated. This assumption may not apply to infants with higher respiratory rates than adults. Assuming that inertance is negligible, the driving pressure of the respiratory system is dependent mainly on the compliance and resistive properties of the lungs. A second assumption is that the lung can be described as a single, linear system. This assumption may not be true when evaluating infants with lung disease and multiple compartments of air trapping [2, 3, 5].

Respiratory mechanics can be assessed through passive or dynamic measurements. Passive measurements are obtained during a brief pause in spontaneous respiration during which the respiratory muscles are relaxed and pressures can equilibrate [3]. During dynamic measurements, the infants are breathing spontaneously and the respiratory muscles are contracting [6]. The physiologic background of these two different types of measurements is described below (fig. 3).

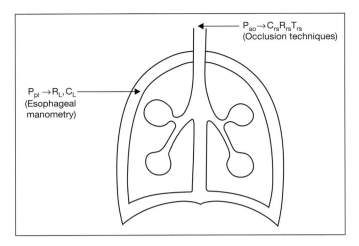

$$P_{ao} \rightarrow C_{rs}R_{rs}T_{rs}$$
(Occlusion techniques)

$$P_{pl} \rightarrow R_L, C_L$$
(Esophageal manometry)

Fig. 3. During passive respiratory mechanics measures, total respiratory system compliance (C_{rs}), resistance (R_{rs}), and time constant measures (T_{rs}) are calculated by measuring airway opening pressures (P_{ao}). The compliance and/or resistance of the chest wall, lung, or airway cannot be evaluated separately with passive respiratory mechanics maneuvers. During dynamic measurements, assessment of the resistance (R_L) and compliance (C_L) of the lung is possible due to transpulmonary pressure measurements. Transpulmonary pressure is equivalent to the difference between the pressure measured at the airway opening (P_{ao}) and the pleural pressure (P_{pl}).

Passive Respiratory Mechanics

When applying passive respiratory mechanics techniques, airflow, volume, and pressure are analyzed when there is no activity of the respiratory muscles. C_{rs}, R_{rs} and T_{rs} are calculated. The compliance and/or resistance of the chest wall, lung, or airway cannot be evaluated separately with these maneuvers. However, in the case of the young infant, the compliance of the chest wall is so high that this component adds little to C_{rs}.

Passive respiratory mechanics techniques or the occlusion techniques are applied by performing an occlusion maneuver at a lung volume above functional residual capacity (FRC). These occlusion maneuvers result in a brief respiratory pause if the Hering-Breuer inflation reflex can be induced. When an infant's airway is occluded above FRC, stretch receptors in the chest wall are activated, leading to a short apnea and relaxation of the respiratory muscles. During relaxation, inspiration is inhibited and exhalation is prolonged. During the occlusion, there is no airflow and pressures can equilibrate such that the airway opening pressure reflects the pressure within the alveoli. Since the pressure of the respiratory system equilibrates during the maneuver, the airway

opening pressure represents the elastic recoil of the total respiratory system.

The assumptions of this technique are that (1) the respiratory system is a single, linear compartment; (2) inertance is negligible; (3) the respiratory muscles are completely relaxed during occlusion and exhalation; (4) the pressure equilibrates throughout the respiratory system during the occlusion, and (5) compliance and resistance measures do not change during the exhalation part of the tidal breath. The validity of these assumptions may be questionable in infants with lung disease and even in healthy infants [2, 3].

Dynamic Respiratory Mechanics

Dynamic respiratory mechanics are evaluated during spontaneous breathing with ongoing respiratory muscle activity. Unlike passive respiratory mechanics measures where the components of the respiratory system cannot be partitioned, dynamic respiratory mechanics measurements allow assessment of the resistance and compliance of the lung if transpulmonary pressure is measured. Transpulmonary pressure is equivalent to the difference between the pressure measured at the airway opening and the pleural pressure (fig. 3). An esophageal catheter is inserted nasally and an approximate measure of pleural pressure changes [7] can be recorded. By measuring airflow, lung volume, and transpulmonary pressure changes, dynamic respiratory mechanics may be assessed.

Alveolar and intrapleural pressures change throughout the tidal breathing cycle. At end-inspiration and end-expiration, alveolar pressure is zero since there is no airflow and no pressure changes. At end-inspiration, the intrapleural pressure is negative or subatmospheric due to the opposing forces of the lungs and chest wall. During mid-inspiration, the alveolar pressure becomes negative to initiate airflow into the lungs. The pressure change within the alveoli during the mid-inspiratory part of the tidal breath depends on airway resistance (P = resistance × flow). Therefore, in an infant with airway obstruction due to bronchiolitis, asthma, or cystic fibrosis, this pressure change within the alveoli will be greater compared to healthy subjects in order to overcome the increased airway resistance.

During tidal breathing, the elastic recoil of the lung is the driving force for exhalation, causing an increase in alveolar pressure, which leads to the expiratory flow of the tidal breath. The intrapleural pressure is less negative during mid-expiration compared to mid-inspiration secondary to the need to overcome both the resistance of the lung tissue and the airways to create exhalation. This difference in pleural pressure during the different phases of tidal breathing contributes to hysteresis of the pressure-volume curve. Hysteresis is defined as the property of the respiratory system where more pressure is needed to inflate the lung compared to the pressure needed to deflate the lung. Dynamic lung compliance reflects these changes in volume and pressure that occur during spontaneous breathing [2, 5, 6].

The assumptions of the dynamic respiratory mechanics measurements are the following: (1) inertance is considered negligible. During dynamic measurements, this assumption may not be true in infants who breathe at higher respiratory rates compared to adults; therefore, the force required to move the lungs may be greater. (2) The lung is analyzed as a single compartment. This assumption may not be true due to the theory of frequency dependence. This theory states that flow may be present within the airways of the lung despite the presence of no airflow at the airway opening. (3) Esophageal pressure simulates pleural pressure changes. First, improper placement of the esophageal catheter may lead to erroneous results. In addition, due to paradoxical rib cage movement noted in some infants, the intrapleural pressure changes may differ depending on location within the thoracic cavity [4]. Premature infants, healthy infants during REM sleep, and infants with airway obstruction display evidence of paradoxical rib cage movement. (4) The compliance and resistance measures are constant throughout the inspiratory and expiratory components of the tidal breath. The elastic forces are assumed to be equivalent, but opposite when assessing mid-inspiratory and mid-expiratory tidal volumes. This assumption may not be true in infants with obstructive airway disease [2, 4, 6].

Techniques

Passive Respiratory Mechanics (fig. 4)

The two most common methods for measuring passive respiratory mechanics are the single and multiple occlusion techniques. In 1976, Olinsky et al. [8] were the first to assess respiratory mechanics using brief occlusion maneuvers. A less common method, the weighted spirometry technique, has also been described when assessing passive respiratory mechanics [9–11]. For the occlusion techniques, the Hering-Breuer reflex must be invoked to elicit relaxation of the respiratory system, thus allowing accurate assessment of respiratory mechanics measurements. To perform these techniques, airflow, pressure and volume changes at the mouth must be recorded and analyzed. This

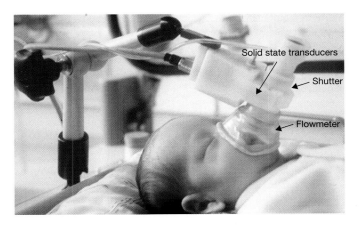

Fig. 4. This photograph demonstrates a sedated infant undergoing an occlusion technique. The equipment used for the occlusion techniques includes a shutter, flowmeter, and transducers.

section will review the methodology of both the single and multiple occlusion techniques.

Preparing the Infant for the Study

Prior to performing the occlusion techniques, the infant should be weighed and measured. Except for very young infants, sedation is usually required, most commonly with chloral hydrate. Sleep deprivation and performing the technique at naptime in the older infant may facilitate effective sedation. Infants must be screened for the presence of risk factors for sedation, such as upper airway obstruction or significant concomitant diseases.

The infant should be in the supine position with his or her head and neck slightly extended for the measurements. To promote extension a roll or head ring should be placed under the infant's neck. A facemask is placed around the infant's nose and mouth. The dead space of the facemask should be recorded. Putty is often placed around the facemask to prevent air leaks (fig. 4) [3].

Equipment

The equipment needed to perform these techniques must measure flow, volume, and airway opening pressure accurately as described in detail in previous manuscripts created by the European Respiratory Society/American Thoracic Society Task Force on Standards for Infant Respiratory Function Tests [12–14]. Commercial devices are available that perform the single occlusion technique, but not the multiple occlusion technique. There is one commercially available device that performs a double occlusion technique [15]. When performing measurements with these devices, the user should adhere to standard guidelines.

Table 1. Equipment for occlusion techniques (details of the equipment have been described previously [3, 12])

Equipment	Details
Computer	Should sample at a rate of 100–200 Hz
Pressure transducers	Appropriate range for airway opening pressures encountered
Amplifiers	
Pneumotachograph or flowmeter	Ability to measure flows over a linear and appropriate range based on the infant's weight
Shutter/valve	Low dead space
Face mask and putty	Noncompliant or 'stiff'
Monitoring device	Ability to monitor heart rate and oxygen saturation
Suction/resuscitation equipment/oxygen	Should be easily accessible if needed
Neck roll or head ring	
Manometer for calibration	Calibration over a pressure range up to 35 cm H_2O or 3.5 kPa
Calibrated syringe	

A list of equipment for these procedures is given in table 1 [3, 12].

The equipment should be calibrated daily and ideally before each study. To perform calibration, a pressure manometer should be used to ensure accurate airway opening pressure measurements. The range calibrated should include values as high as 3.5 kPa. In addition, the pneumotachograph or flowmeter should be calibrated over appropriate flow ranges. Flow ranges based on weight have been published [12]. Not only should the flowmeter be able to measure these ranges, but calibration should also reflect these values.

The dead space of the face mask should be low, allowing the infant to comfortably breathe into the circuit. The brand and size of the face mask should be documented. An overly soft facemask may dampen pressure changes; a stiffer mask will promote more accurate measurements. The occlusion valve or shutter should also have a low dead space to prevent increased work of breathing during the maneuver. This low dead space is especially important in the small infant. During the occlusion, the valve should close quickly, be airtight and quiet to prevent the infant from awakening. An airtight occlusion is essential to allow for pressurization and accurate measurements [3, 12].

The flowmeter should be linear, have minimal dead space and should be heated to prevent condensation. The transducers should also reflect the airway opening pressure measured. The computer should display flow, volume and airway opening pressure during the measurements. A time-based tracing of these parameters is ideal to monitor for air leaks and stability of tidal breathing [3, 12].

The infant's vital signs should be monitored continuously from the time of administration of the sedative to recovery from sedation. Resuscitation equipment should be immediately available along with oxygen and suction. The technicians performing the measurement should be certified in resuscitation.

Single Occlusion Technique

During the single breath occlusion technique, the infant's airway is briefly occluded at the end-inspiratory part of the tidal breath. Induction of the Hering-Breuer reflex leads to respiratory system relaxation during the occlusion and immediately after the occlusion is released. This simple technique allows measurement of the C_{rs}, R_{rs}, and T_{rs}.

Detailed Methods

Prior to performing the single breath occlusion technique, the user should check for leaks in the system. To check for a leak, tidal breathing is recorded for approximately 20–30 s to assure stability. Once stability is obtained, the infant's airway is briefly occluded at the end-inspiratory part of the tidal breath. After occlusion, at least 5 tidal breaths are collected. A leak is present if there is no plateau during the occlusion, or the airway opening pressure is not maintained. A leak is also present if the tidal breathing 'steps up', or there is a volume shift after the occlusion. Once the user is assured that no leak is present, the single breath technique can be performed.

To perform the single breath technique: (1) At least 5 tidal breaths are collected prior to the occlusion to assure stability of the end-expiratory level. (2) The occlusion should be initiated by rapidly closing the valve or shutter at the infant's airway at the end-inspiratory part of the tidal breath or within 3 ml of the beginning of exhalation. (3) The length of the occlusion should be at least 400 ms. Very brief occlusions may not induce the Hering-Breuer reflex and an adequate plateau may not be obtained. Occlusions that are too long may lead to the infant inspiring early after release of the occlusion. (4) The occlusion should be stopped once an adequate plateau has been reached. The occlusion should also be stopped if the infant inspires against the closed valve, and the length of the occlusion should not exceed 1,500 ms. (5) Three to five acceptable maneuvers should be obtained for analysis [3, 12].

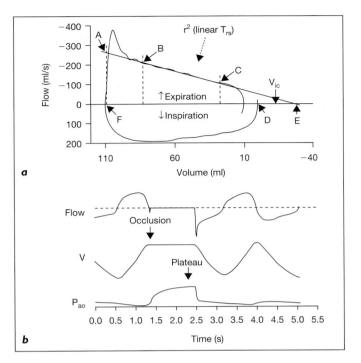

Fig. 5. Passive flow-volume curve obtained during the single-breath occlusion technique. A: Extrapolation of the time constant slope to the 'pseudoflow.' The time constant (T_{rs}) is analyzed from the slope between points B and C. Point D is the end-expiratory level prior to occlusion (occ). E is the extrapolation of the time constant slope to the point where flow is equivalent to zero on the volume axis. F is the release of the occlusion. The volume of intercept (V_{ic}) is measured between points D and E. The second schematic represents flow, volume (V), and airway opening pressure (P_{ao}) measures versus time. (Fletcher M, Baraldi E, Steinbrugger B: Passive Respiratory Mechanics; in Stocks J, Sly PD, Tepper RS, Morgan WJ (eds): Infant Respiratory Function Testing, 1996. Reprinted by permission of Wiley-Liss, Inc. a subsidiary of John Wiley & Sons, Inc.)

Data Analysis

To assess C_{rs} ($\Delta V / \Delta P$), the change in pressure is calculated as the difference between atmospheric pressure and the plateau achieved during the occlusion. The change in volume is the difference between the point where the extrapolated slope crosses the x-axis (no flow) and the point when the shutter or valve is released leading to the relaxed exhalation (fig. 5).

T_{rs} is calculated from the slope of the linear decay and is equivalent to the change in volume divided by the change in flow. Since the time constant is equal to the product of resistance and compliance, resistance can then be calculated from this equation. R_{rs} can also be analyzed by back extrapolating the slope of the linear decay to the point where the occlusion is released. This point represents the change in flow or pseudoflow occurring at the time the shutter is released. R_{rs} is then equal to the change in pressure measured at the airway opening divided by this change in flow or pseudoflow. Once the resistance is calculated using either methodology, the resistance of the device should be subtracted from this value to obtain accurate results [3, 12].

Data acceptability has been reported in detail elsewhere [3, 12], but will be reviewed below.

In a technically acceptable maneuver

1. The decay of the exhalation should be linear and smooth without glottic closure, early inspiration or braking. There will be flow transients at the beginning of the linear decay and the slope used for the time constant analysis should not include these transients or the early inspiration noted at the end of the exhalation. The transients represent the unpressurized pneumotachograph. Linearity may not occur in infants with lung disease due to different compartments of the respiratory system emptying at different times (fig. 6).
2. The relaxed exhalation should be linear for at least 40% of the curve with an $r^2 > 0.99$, based on least-squares linear regression analysis.
3. The occlusion plateau should occur for at least 100 ms with a standard deviation or variability of <0.1 cm H_2O or <10 Pa.
4. The tidal breathing should be stable prior to the occlusion to exclude the presence of leaks or drift.
5. During the occlusion, there should be no flow through the pneumotachograph or flowmeter.
6. The volume of intercept should be <3 ml/kg. The volume of intercept is the difference between the end-expiratory level of the prior tidal breath and the point where the extrapolated slope crosses the x-axis.

The mean value plus the standard deviation should be reported based on at least three acceptable maneuvers.

Multiple Occlusion Technique

During the multiple occlusion technique, the airway opening is briefly occluded at different volumes above the end-expiratory level. During these occlusions, the airway opening pressure and the volume are measured. The pressure and volume measurements are recorded on an x-y plot and the slope is analyzed. The slope represents the C_{rs} [3, 12].

Detailed Methods

Leaks around the mask should be checked as described above for the single occlusion technique. Once it has been

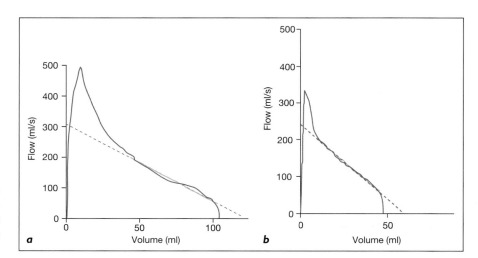

Fig. 6. Schematic *a* represents an unacceptable single breath occlusion passive flow-volume curve due to the alinearity of the exhalation. Schematic *b* is an acceptable maneuver with a linear exhalation.

established that there are no leaks present, the performance of the multiple occlusion technique may commence. If the infant awakens prior to completing full data collection, the analysis will not be accurate. To perform this technique: (1) Tidal breathing is collected prior to the occlusion to assure stability of the end-expiratory level. (2) Once tidal breathing is stable, the infant's airway opening should be occluded at end-inspiration or early expiration. (3) Occlusions should be between 400 and 1,500 ms. The length of the occlusion depends on the individual infant and may even need to be adjusted in the same individual during a study. (4) The plateau should be at least 100–200 ms. Two hundred milliseconds is preferable, but a 100-ms plateau may be necessary in an infant with tachypnea. (5) Once occlusion is complete, the infant should be allowed to achieve a stable end-expiratory level by collecting at least 5–10 tidal breaths. The number of tidal breaths collected will depend on the individual infant. (6) At least 5 occlusions should be performed at end-inspiration or the beginning of end-expiration. (7) Once these higher volume occlusions are performed, occlusions should be performed at progressively lower volumes. Establishing predefined points where the occlusions should occur during exhalation is preferred. (8) Ten occlusions at different lung volumes should be collected and analyzed [3, 12].

Data Analysis

During the multiple occlusion technique, C_{rs} represents the relationship of the lung volume change and the airway opening pressure change measured at the time of the occlusion. The volume change is calculated as the difference between the baseline volume or the end-expiratory level and the volume at the time of the occlusion. The pressure change at the airway opening is calculated as the difference between atmospheric pressure and the pressure at the time of the occlusion plateau. The compliance measurements are calculated several times at the different predefined occlusion points. These measurements are then plotted on an x-y diagram comparing the relationship of the volume and pressure changes, and regression analysis is performed. This type of analysis (versus simply taking a mean of each compliance value performed at different predefined occlusion points) is critical to account for the infant dynamically elevating his or her FRC. The intercept of the regression line accounts for the infant breathing at this elevated FRC, thus providing a more accurate measurement of compliance. Without accounting for this physiologic phenomenon, the compliance measure would be underestimated.

Details about multiple occlusion data analysis and technical acceptability have been published elsewhere [3, 12].

A brief review, as published previously, is detailed below.

1. The user should establish that the end-expiratory level is stable, and that the change in the end-expiratory level pre and post occlusion is less than 10%.
2. The plateau should be at least 100 ms with a change in pressure between the start and end of the plateau of less than 2%.
3. Regression line should have an $r^2 > 0.95$.
4. At least six acceptable occlusions should be analyzed over an appropriate pressure range, as previously recommended [12].

Modifications of the Occlusion Techniques

In the section below, alternative methods of measuring passive respiratory mechanics in the infant are discussed.

The weighted spirometry technique, expiratory volume clamping, and the assessment of compliance from near total lung capacity will be reviewed.

Weighted Spirometry

This technique evaluates compliance from a lung volume above resting FRC by applying a weight to the spirometer. The infant breathes against this positive pressure imposed by the weight, thus elevating FRC, and compliance is assessed from this lung volume. Compliance is calculated by dividing the increase in lung volume by the increase in pressure imposed by the weight. The compliance of the circuit must be subtracted from the total compliance measured to obtain the C_{rs}. The compliance of the circuit should be small to prevent an alteration of the respiratory mechanics since the infant breathes against this weight.

Very little has been published about this technique since the early 1990s [3, 9–11].

Expiratory Volume Clamping

This technique allows recruitment of the Hering-Breuer reflex and an elevation of the lung volume by having the infant breathe against an occluded expiratory valve for three to five tidal breaths. Analysis may then be performed through the single or multiple occlusion technique once the occlusion is released. In addition, analysis may be performed during the expiratory volume clamping by evaluating the slope of the volume and pressure changes that occur during the procedure. Due to the introduction of the raised volume technique, expiratory volume clamping has not been a popular method recently [3, 16].

Assessing Compliance from Near Total Lung Capacity

As described in the raised volume thoracoabdominal compression technique [see chapter by Modl and Eber, 17, this volume], the infant's lungs are inflated to a preset pressure (i.e. 30 cm H_2O or 3 kPa), the infant is allowed to passively exhale, and after several inflation-passive deflation maneuvers, the infant exhibits a respiratory pause. By performing this technique, pressure-volume curves may be obtained from an elevated lung volume that is near total lung capacity. Once the pause is induced, the infant's lungs are inflated again to a preset pressure, and the infant is allowed to passively exhale while multiple occlusions are performed. This novel technique was recently described in 49 healthy infants, and the compliance was calculated from the slope of the pressure-volume curve [18].

Dynamic Respiratory Mechanics

The assessment of dynamic respiratory mechanics occurs in the spontaneously breathing infant. In the past, this type of maneuver has typically involved the placement of an esophageal catheter in order to measure transpulmonary pressure. Transpulmonary pressure is defined as the difference between airway opening pressure and pressure measured within the pleural space. Since pressure measurements within the pleural space are not possible, an esophageal catheter is used to simulate these pressure changes. Other techniques that measure dynamic respiratory mechanics involve the use of body plethysmography, forced oscillation, and interrupter resistance techniques. These latter three techniques will be discussed in other chapters in this book. This section will review the equipment and methodology needed to perform dynamic respiratory mechanics measurements using an esophageal catheter. With these techniques, flow, volume, and transpulmonary pressure changes are measured during spontaneous breathing to assess respiratory mechanics [2, 6, 7].

Preparing the Infant for the Study

Preparing the infant for the study requires a protocol similar to that described in the section 'Passive Respiratory Mechanics'.

However, for dynamic respiratory mechanics measurements involving the assessment of transpulmonary pressure changes, the esophageal catheter may be placed when the infant is awake or sedated. Timing of placement is the individual laboratory's preference; however, sedated infants may tolerate this procedure better than awake infants. Correct placement of the esophageal catheter must be verified as described below.

Equipment

Equipment is needed that measures flow, volume, and transpulmonary pressure changes. Table 2 summarizes this equipment. Calibration of the equipment should be performed on a daily basis and ideally, before studying each subject. When calibrating the pressure transducers, the manometer should be set to reflect the appropriate range of pressures encountered for both the esophageal catheter and the airway opening. As in the occlusion methods, the pneumotachometer or flowmeter should be calibrated to reflect appropriate flow ranges as documented in previous reports [6, 7].

The dead space of the face mask, flowmeter and circuit should be minimal to promote comfortable tidal breathing. The shutter, as in the occlusion methods, should not be

Table 2. Equipment for dynamic respiratory mechanics techniques (details of the equipment have been described previously [6, 7])

Equipment	Details
Computer	Should sample at a rate of 100–200 Hz
Pressure transducers	Appropriate range for pressures encountered at the esophageal catheter and the airway opening
Esophageal catheters	Balloon or microtip transducer
Pneumotachograph or flowmeter	Ability to measure flows over a linear and appropriate range based on the infant's weight
Shutter/valve	Low dead space
Facemask and putty	Firm facemask
Monitoring device	Ability to monitor heart rate and oxygen saturation
Suction/resuscitation equipment/oxygen	Should be easily accessible if needed
Neck roll or head ring	
Manometer for calibration	
Calibrated syringe	

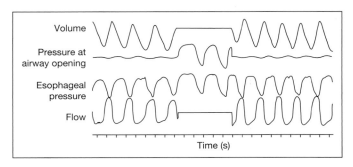

Fig. 7. This schematic demonstrates an occlusion test during dynamic respiratory mechanics measurements. Volume, airway opening pressure, esophageal pressure, and flow are measured. An occlusion test should be performed prior to any testing to assure that the pressure at the airway opening accurately reflects the esophageal pressure changes. (Davis GM, Stocks J, Gerhardt T, Abbasi S, Gappa M: Measurement of dynamic lung mechanics in infants; in Stocks J, Sly PD, Tepper RS, Morgan WJ (eds): Infant Respiratory Function Testing, 1996. Reprinted by permission of Wiley-Liss, Inc. a subsidiary of John Wiley & Sons, Inc.)

noisy and close rapidly. There should be no leaks around the shutter. Close monitoring of vital signs is mandatory as described in the occlusion section.

Esophageal Balloon or Catheter Placement

Correct placement of the esophageal balloon or catheter is critical for accurate transpulmonary pressure measurements. The esophageal pressure measurements reflect pressure changes in the pleural space due to close apposition of the esophagus to the pleura. This assumption has been questioned because pleural pressure changes may vary based on location within the thoracic cavity due to paradoxical chest wall movement (common in young infants) or airway obstruction [4]. The changes in the esophageal pressure will vary depending on the size of the tidal breath and the compliance or resistance of the respiratory system. In an infant with pulmonary disease, the esophageal pressure changes will be increased due to the amount of pressure needed to overcome either a less compliant lung or an increase in airway resistance [7].

There are several options when selecting the device used to measure esophageal pressure changes. These options include an esophageal balloon, a liquid-filled catheter, or a catheter tip pressure transducer. The advantages and disadvantages of these options are reviewed in detail in a previous publication [7]. The microtransducer catheter has

been reported to be reliable in evaluating transpulmonary pressure, and due to its simplicity may guarantee more accurate results compared to esophageal balloons or liquid-filled catheters [19]. When choosing the esophageal manometry device, adhering to previously published guidelines is essential, and if using an esophageal balloon, documentation of the characteristics of the balloon should be included in published data. Correct placement of the manometry device within the esophagus is essential for accurate measurements. The device should first be placed in the stomach then withdrawn to the esophagus. Details regarding verification of esophageal placement have been previously described [7]. Once esophageal placement is achieved, an occlusion test must be performed to ensure correct placement [7].

To perform an occlusion test (fig. 7), a shutter or valve located near the infant's airway is closed for two to three tidal breaths. The infant breathes against this occlusion, and the pressures at the airway opening and within the esophagus are recorded. To assure that the pressure changes at the airway opening accurately reflect the esophageal pressure changes, the ratio of esophageal pressure/airway opening pressure should be 1.00 ± 0.05. If this ratio is significantly greater than 1, there may be a leak, or equilibration may not have occurred between the two measures due to obstructed airways. If the ratio is significantly less than 1, the esophageal pressure changes may not reflect pleural pressure changes due to improper placement or equipment, or because of the inability of the manometer device to accurately reflect changes within the pleura (due to characteristics of the infant's chest wall). In certain infants, the ratio of 1.00 + 0.05 may not be possible. Due to the effect that minor physiologic changes can have on the esophageal manometry device, an occlusion test should be performed regularly during the testing period [7].

Measuring Dynamic Lung Mechanics Using an Esophageal Balloon

Once the esophageal manometry device has been correctly positioned and the occlusion test has been passed, data recording for dynamic lung mechanics measurements may commence. During these measurements, tidal volume, flow and pressure changes at the airway opening and esophagus are recorded. Stable tidal breathing should be verified during spontaneous breathing. Stability is not present if the tidal volume drifts or if the tidal breaths appear irregular. When recording data, the user should verify all physiologic parameters as described in detail in a previous publication [6]. To verify reproducibility, repeat measures should be performed at a set interval. If a therapeutic intervention is administered to the infant and measures are repeated, an occlusion test should be performed to verify accuracy of the measurements after the intervention [6].

Data Analysis

During dynamic respiratory mechanics measurements using an esophageal catheter, compliance and resistance of the lung are assessed using measures of volume, flow, and transpulmonary pressures. These measures are assessed over a number of tidal breaths. There are several different methods of analysis: (1) the Mead-Whittenberger technique [20, 21]; (2) the least-squares regression technique [22]; (3) the multiple linear regression technique [23]; and (4) the Mortola-Saetta technique [24]. These techniques have been described in detail in a previous publication; however, they will be reviewed briefly below [6].

The Mead-Whittenberger technique [20, 21] was used most often prior to the advent of computerized techniques. Using this analysis method, one assumes that flow is equal to zero at end-inspiration and end-expiration. Dynamic compliance is then calculated by measuring the change in volume between end-inspiration and end-expiration and measuring the change in transpulmonary pressure between these two points. In addition, the elastic recoil is assumed to be equal, but opposite at the mid-volumes (mid-inspiration and mid-expiration). Under this assumption, dynamic resistance can then be calculated by measuring the change in transpulmonary pressure between mid-inspiration and

mid-expiration and measuring the change in flow between these two points [6].

With the least-squares regression technique, dynamic compliance is calculated in a fashion similar to the Mead-Whittenberger technique. However, for the calculation of resistance, the elastic forces of the driving pressure are subtracted from the transpulmonary pressure to obtain the pressure that overcomes resistance. This resistance pressure is plotted against the corresponding flow, and the slope of this line represents lung resistance. The Mortola-Saetta method is simply a modification of the least-squares method [6].

The multiple linear regression technique is a computerized technique that analyzes flow, transpulmonary pressure, and volume over the respiratory cycle. These parameters are analyzed as a linear model, and the resistance and elastance (compliance is the reciprocal of this component) of the lung are calculated. The advantage of the computerized techniques is that several data points are used when calculating results as opposed to the Mead-Whittenberger technique. When using the computerized methods, the user should review each tidal breath to assure technically acceptable results are included in the analysis [6].

When reporting results, the mean and standard deviation of each parameter should be given. The parameters analyzed include respiratory rate, tidal volume, lung resistance and lung compliance. When reviewing data, at least 10 and up to 50 tidal breaths should be analyzed. Depending on the analysis technique used, the r^2 of the slope of the line should be reported. Data showing evidence of cardiac artifact, excessive drift, leak, sigh, breath-holding, or esophageal spasm should be discarded [6].

Reference Data

Only limited normative data from small, single-center studies are available for respiratory mechanics measurements. Because equipment is not standardized, measurements are laboratory specific and should be interpreted with caution. Most reference data are available from only a limited age range, i.e., from neonates and healthy preterm infants. In addition, few reports are available of measurements using different techniques in the same subjects [2, 25–27], so that reference values derived using one technique cannot be assumed to apply to measurements using a different technique. Until a multicenter study utilizing standardized equipment to evaluate respiratory mechanics measurements in a large, population-based cohort is completed, existing normal values cannot be considered definitive. Once appropriate reference data are available, results should be reported as z-scores. Z-scores accurately reflect a test result abnormality, independent of the variability of the parameter.

Measured values can be reported as absolute values or normalized for body size. There is no consensus regarding adjustment of measurement values for size. Correction is often based on length or body weight. The relationship between C_{rs} or R_{rs} and length is nonlinear and the regression line does not pass through the origin, so that dividing by length is an inappropriate method with which to correct for body size [3]. Correction for weight may be misleading in preterm infants because their highly compliant chest wall results in a higher ratio of C_{rs} to weight than in term infants [3]. Similarly, children with poor nutritional status due to chronic respiratory disease may have an altered relationship between age, weight, height, and lung volume so that correction for weight is questionable. The most rational basis for comparison may be the lung volume at which the measurements were obtained [2].

Reported values for C_{rs} per kilogram body weight in neonates and infants range from 9.1 to 15.7 ml/kPa/kg [2, 3, 8–11, 16, 28–37]. Hanrahan et al. [38] reported that normal C_{rs} values for healthy infants ranged between 5.4 and 16.05 ml/cm H_2O. Regression equations for the relationship of length to C_{rs} have also been published [2, 3, 29, 38–40].

Dynamic lung compliance values for newborns (pre- and full-term) and infants range from 11.2 to 20.4 ml/kPa/kg, and specific dynamic compliance ranges from 0.4 to 0.8 ml/kPa/ml volume of thoracic gas, measured either by helium dilution or plethysmography [2, 6, 8, 37, 41–52].

R_{rs} is a highly variable measurement. In addition, it is highest in preterm infants and newborns, decreasing during later infancy. Reported normal values from small studies range from 7.4 kPa/l/s in <2 week old preterm infants [30] to 2.7 to 3.9 kPa/l/s in studies of term infants up to 24 months of age [3, 16, 28, 29, 38, 40]. Specific airway conductance is recommended as a more constant parameter over age [(airway resistance $\times$ thoracic gas volume)$^{-1}$] [2]. Specific airway conductance ranges from 0.03/kPa $\cdot$ s at birth in term infants to 0.02/kPa $\cdot$ s in older children [2].

Respiratory Mechanics Measurements in Disease States

Respiratory mechanics measurements have contributed to the understanding of lung development in both health and disease. Within the context of research protocols, these techniques have provided important data on a wide variety of infant pulmonary diseases as well as diseases with secondary pulmonary involvement, such as congenital

heart disease or achondroplasia. Many of these studies are summarized by Fletcher et al. [3]. Respiratory mechanics measurements have been used to investigate the efficacy of antenatal steroids [53] and surfactant therapy [54–57] in preterm neonates with infant respiratory distress syndrome, and of systemic [58] and inhaled [59] corticosteroids in bronchopulmonary dysplasia. Garg et al. [60] demonstrated persistent abnormalities in dynamic pulmonary compliance and airway resistance in survivors of extracorporeal membrane oxygenation (ECMO) at 6 months of age.

A number of investigators have assessed responses to bronchodilators [61–63] and methacholine [64] utilizing passive respiratory mechanics measurements. Dynamic mechanics measurements have been used to assess the effectiveness of salbutamol delivery from a metered dose inhaler versus jet nebulizer [65]. C_{rs} and R_{rs} were assessed in a large cohort of HIV-infected infants [66]. In infants with cystic fibrosis, specific compliance and specific conductance have been shown to be abnormal even prior to the onset of symptoms [11, 67, 68]. In a longitudinal study of infants with achondroplasia, Tasker et al. [69] showed that with growth, these infants demonstrated increased airway resistance and marked reductions in C_{rs}. In children with congenital heart disease, a significant inverse relationship was found between pulmonary vascular engorgement and C_{rs} [70], and reduced C_{rs} associated with left-to-right shunts and pulmonary hypertension was rapidly improved after cardiac surgery [71]. Finally, passive respiratory mechanics measurements have been used to demonstrate an association between maternal smoking and infant lung function [37, 38, 72].

Clinical Applications

Measurements of passive and dynamic respiratory mechanics are difficult to interpret due to the lack of reliable reference values, and information on inter- and intrasubject variability. In addition, dynamic respiratory mechanics measurements have not been standardized. Thus, while they have contributed valuable data within the context of research studies, their applicability to the evaluation of individual patients is limited at this time. Table 3 summarizes advantages and disadvantages of the passive and dynamic techniques.

Compliance is interpreted differently in acute versus chronic lung disease [2]. Short-term changes in compliance during the course of acute lung disease, when the intrinsic elastic recoils of the respiratory system are assumed to be constant, reflect changes in the gas exchange

Table 3. Advantages and disadvantages of respiratory mechanics measurements

	Passive techniques	Dynamic techniques
Advantages	Commercially available equipment (Single and double occlusion technique) Noninvasive Simple, quick measurement Well tolerated Compliance fairly reproducible	Allow evaluation of lung compliance and resistance
Disadvantages	Assumption of pressure equilibration between airway opening and alveoli not valid in severely obstructed patients	No commercially available equipment Requires esophageal balloon placement Esophageal pressure not accurately measured with chest wall deformities or severe airway obstruction Techniques not standardized
	Resistance highly variable and dominated by upper airway resistance Requires sedation Rigorous criteria required for reporting only technically acceptable data Lack of reliable reference values Lack of data on inter- and intrasubject variability Limited utility for routine clinical use	

surface or lung volume. In chronic lung disease, changes in compliance may be a reflection of changes in elastic recoil.

R_{rs} is dominated by upper airway resistance, particularly in infants. Therefore, modest changes in lower airway resistance in response to treatment may be missed, and a bronchodilator response will be detected only with large changes in peripheral airway resistance.

References

1 Polgar G, Promadhat V: Pulmonary function testing in children: Techniques and standards. Philadelphia, Saunders, 1971, pp 170–180, 254?.
2 ATS and ERS: Respiratory mechanics in infants: Physiologic evaluation in health and disease. Am Rev Respir Dis 1993;147:474–496.
3 Fletcher M, Baraldi E, Steinbrugger B: Passive respiratory mechanics; in Stocks J, Sly PD, Tepper RS, Morgan WJ (eds): Infant Respiratory Function Testing. New York, Wiley, 1996, pp 283–327.
4 England SJ: Current techniques for assessing pulmonary function in the newborn and infant: Advantages and limitations. Pediatr Pulmonol 1988;4:48–53.
5 Taussig LM, Helms PJ: Introduction; in Stocks J, Sly PD, Tepper RS, Morgan WJ (eds): Infant Respiratory Function Testing. New York, Wiley, 1996, pp 1–18.

6 Davis GM, Stocks J, Gerhardt T, Abbasi S, Gappa M: Measurement of dynamic lung mechanics in infants; in Stocks J, Sly PD, Tepper RS, Morgan WJ (eds): Infant Respiratory Function Testing. New York, Wiley, 1996, pp 259–281.
7 Coates A, Stocks J, Gerhardt T: Esophageal manometry; in Stocks J, Sly PD, Tepper RS, Morgan WJ (eds): Infant Respiratory Function Testing. New York, Wiley, 1996, pp 241–258.
8 Olinsky A, Bryan AC, Bryan MH: A simple method of measuring total respiratory system compliance in newborn infants. S Afr Med J 1976;50:128–130.
9 Merth IT, Quanjer PH: Respiratory system compliance assessed by the multiple occlusion and weighted spirometer method in non-intubated healthy newborns. Pediatr Pulmonol 1990;8:273–279.

10 Tepper RS, Pagtakhan R, Taussig LM: Noninvasive determination of total respiratory system compliance in infants by the weighted-spirometer method. Am Rev Respir Dis 1984;130:461–466.
11 Tepper RS, Hiatt PW, Eigen H, Smith J: Total respiratory system compliance in asymptomatic infants with cystic fibrosis. Am Rev Respir Dis 1987;135:1075–1079.
12 Gappa M, Colin AA, Goetz I, Stocks J: ERS/ATS Task Force on standards for infant respiratory function testing. European Respiratory Society/American Thoracic Society. Passive respiratory mechanics: the occlusion techniques. Eur Respir J 2001;17:141–148.
13 Frey U, Stocks J, Coates A, Sly P, Bates J: Specifications for equipment used for infant pulmonary function testing. ERS/ATS Task Force on standards for infant respiratory function testing. European Respiratory Society/American Thoracic Society. Eur Respir J 2000;16:731–740.

14 Frey U, Stocks J, Coates A, Sly P, Bates J: Specifications for signal processing and data handling used for infant pulmonary function testing. ERS/ATS Task Force on standards for infant respiratory function testing. European Respiratory Society/American Thoracic Society. Eur Respir J 2000;16:1016–1022.

15 Goetz I, Hoo AF, Lum S, Stocks J: Assessment of passive respiratory mechanics in infants: Double versus single occlusion? Eur Respir J 2001;17:449–455.

16 Grunstein MM, Springer C, Godfrey S, Bar-Yishay E, Vilozni D, Inscore SC, Schramm CM: Expiratory volume clamping: A new method to assess respiratory mechanics in sedated infants. J Appl Physiol 1987;62:2107–2114.

17 Modl M, Eber E: Forced expiratory flow-volume measurements; in Hammer J, Eber E (eds): Paediatric Pulmonary Function Testing. Progress in Respiratory Research. Basel, Karger, 2005, vol 33, pp. 34–43.

18 Tepper RS, Williams T, Kisling J, Castile R: Static compliance of the respiratory system in healthy infants. Am J Respir Crit Care Med 2001;163:91–94.

19 Gappa M, Pilgrim L, Jackson E, Costeloe K, Stocks J. A new microtransducer catheter for measuring esophageal pressure in infants. Pediatr Pulmonol 1996;22:117–124.

20 Mead J, Whittenberger JL: Physical properties of human lungs measured during spontaneous respiration. J Appl Physiol 1953;5:779–796.

21 Davis GM, Coates AL: Pulmonary mechanics; in Hillman BC (ed): Pediatric Respiratory Disease: Diagnosis and Treatment. Philadelphia, Saunders, 1993, pp 1–12.

22 Stocks J, Thomson A, Wong C, Silverman M: Pressure-flow curves in infancy. Pediatr Pulmonol 1985;1:32–39.

23 Bhutani VK, Sivieri EM, Abbasi S, Shaffer TH: Evaluation of neonatal pulmonary mechanics and energetics: A two-factor least mean square analysis. Pediatr Pulmonol 1988;4:150–158.

24 Mortola JP, Saetta M: Measurements of respiratory mechanics in the newborn: A simple approach. Pediatr Pulmonol 1987;3:123–130.

25 Ratjen F, Zinman R, Stark AR, Leszczynski LE, Wohl MEB: Effect of changes in lung volume on respiratory system compliance in newborn infants. J Appl Physiol 1989;67:1192–1197.

26 Guslits BG, Wilkie RA, England SJ, Bryan AC: Comparison of methods of measurement of compliance of the respiratory system in children. Am Rev Respir Dis 1987;136:727–729.

27 Gerhardt T, Reifenberg L, Duara S, Bancalari E: Comparison of dynamic and static measurements of respiratory mechanics in infants. J Pediatr 1989;114:120–125.

28 Rabbette PS, Fletcher ME, Dezateux CA, Soriano-Brucher H, Stocks J. Hering-Breuer reflex and respiratory system compliance in the first year of life: A longitudinal study. J Appl Physiol 1994;76:650–656.

29 Masters IB, Seidenberg J, Hudson I, Phelan PD, Olinsky A: Longitudinal study of lung mechanics in normal infants. Pediatr Pulmonol 1987;3:3–7.

30 Gappa M, Rabbette PS, Costeloe KL, Stocks J: Assessment of passive respiratory compliance in healthy preterm infants: A critical evaluation. Pediatr Pulmonol 1993;15:304–311.

31 Mortola JP, Hemmings G, Matsuoka T, Saiki C, Fox G: Referencing lung volume for measurements of respiratory system compliance in infants. Pediatr Pulmonol 1993;16:248–253.

32 Fletcher ME, Hoo AF, Stocks J, Dezateux CA, Costeloe KL, Rabbette PS: Changes in weight corrected respiratory compliance with age in preterm infants. Am J Respir Crit Care Med 1994;149:A693.

33 Stocks J, Gappa M, Rabbette PS, Hoo AF, Mukhtar Z, Costeloe KL: A comparison of respiratory function in Afro-Caribbean and Caucasian infants. Eur Respir J 1994;7: 11–16.

34 Le Souef PN, England SJ, Bryan AC: Passive respiratory mechanics in newborns and children. Am Rev Respir Dis 1984;129: 727–729.

35 Migdal M, Dreizzen E, Praud JP, Vial M, Dehan M, Chambille B, Gaultier C: Compliance of the total respiratory system in healthy preterm and full-term newborns. Pediatr Pulmonol 1987;3:214–218.

36 Young S, Arnott J, O'Keeffe PT, Le Souef PN, Landau LI: The association between early life lung function and wheezing during the first 2 years of life. Eur Respir J 2000;15: 151–157.

37 Milner A, Marsh M, Ingram D, Fox G, Susiva C: Effects of smoking in pregnancy on neonatal lung function. Arch Dis Child Fetal Neonatal Ed 1999;80:8–14.

38 Hanrahan J, Brown R, Carey V, Castile R, Speizer F, Tager I: Passive respiratory mechanics in healthy infants. Am J Respir Crit Care Med 1996;154:670–680.

39 Thomson AH, Beardsmore CS, Silverman M: The total compliance of the respiratory system during the first year of life. Bull Eur Physiopathol Respir 1985;21:411–416.

40 Gutkowski P, Migdal M: Predicted values of pulmonary mechanics parameters in children under 2 years. Pneumonol Pol 1987;LV:65–70.

41 Stocks J: The functional growth and development of the lung during the first year of life. Early Hum Dev 1977;1:285–309.

42 Gerhardt TO, Hehre D, Feller R, Reifenberg L, Bancalari E: Pulmonary mechanics in normal infants and young children during first 5 years of life. Pediatr Pulmonol 1987;3:309–316.

43 Polgar G, Weng TR: The functional development of the respiratory system from the period of gestation to adulthood. Am Rev Respir Dis 1979;120:625–695.

44 Schmalisch G, Wauer RR: Percentiles for quantification of interindividual parameter distributions in lung function tests; in Grauel EL, Syllm-Rapoport I, Wauer RR (eds): Research in Perinatal Medicine. Leipzig, Thieme, 1986, pp 116–129.

45 Quanjer PH, Stocks J, Polgar G, Wise M, Karlberg J, Borsboom G: Compilation of reference values for lung function measurements in children. Eur Respir J 1989;2(suppl 4): 184s–261s.

46 Cook CD, Helliesen PJ, Agathon S: Relation between mechanics of respiration, lung size, and body size from birth to young adulthood. J Appl Physiol 1958;13:349–352.

47 Cook CD, Sutherland JM, Segal S, Cherry RB, Mead J, Mcllroy MB, Smith CA: Studies of respiratory physiology in the newborn infant. II. Measurements of mechanics in respiration. J Clin Invest 1957;37:440–448.

48 Swyer PR, Reiman RC, Wright JJ: Ventilation and ventilatory mechanics in the newborn. J Pediatr 1960;56:612–617.

49 Chu JS, Dawson P, Klaus M, Sweet AY: Lung compliance and lung volume measured concurrently in normal full-term and premature infants. Pediatrics 1964;34:525–532.

50 Phelan PD, Williams HE: Ventilatory studies in healthy infants. Pediatr Res 1969;3: 425–432.

51 Kreiger I: Studies on mechanics of respiration in infancy. Am J Dis Child 1963;105:51–60.

52 Howlett G: Lung mechanics in normal infants with congenital heart disease. Arch Dis Child 1972;47:707–715.

53 McEvoy C, Bowling S, Williamson K, Stewart M, Durand M: Functional residual capacity and passive compliance measurements after antenatal steroid therapy in preterm infants. Pediatr Pulmonol 2001;31: 425–430.

54 Pfenninger J, Aebi C, Bachmann D, Wagner BP: Lung mechanics and gas exchange in ventilated preterm infants during treatment of hyaline membrane disease with multiple doses of artificial surfactant (exosurf). Pediatr Pulmonol 1992;14:10–15.

55 Baraldi E, Pettenazzo A, Filippone M, Magagnin GP, Saia OS, Zacchello F: Rapid improvement of static compliance after surfactant treatment in preterm infants with respiratory distress syndrome. Pediatr Pulmonol 1993;15:157–162.

56 Kelly E, Bryan H, Possmayer F, Frndova H, Bryan C: Compliance of the respiratory system in newborn infants pre- and postsurfactant replacement therapy. Pediatr Pulmonol 1993;15:225–230.

57 Couser RJ, Ferrara TB, Wheeler W, McNamara J, Falde B, Johnson K, Hoekstra RE: Pulmonary follow-up 2.5 years after a randomized, controlled, multiple dose bovine surfactant study of preterm newborn infants. Pediatr Pulmonol 1993;15:163–167.

58 Brundage KL, Mohsini KG, Froese AB, Walker CR, Fisher JT: Dexamethasone therapy for bronchopulmonary dysplasia: Improved respiratory mechanics without adrenal suppression. Pediatr Pulmonol 1992;12: 162–169.

59 Cloutier MM: Nebulized steroid therapy in bronchopulmonary dysplasia. Pediatr Pulmonol 1993;15:111–116.

60 Garg M, Kurzner SI, Bautista DB, Lew CD, Ramos AD, Platzker ACG, Keens TG: Pulmonary sequelae at six months following extracorporeal membrane oxygenation. Chest 1992;101:1086–1090.

61 Rotschild A, Solimano A, Puterman M, Smyth J, Sharma A, Albersheim S: Increased compliance in response to salbutamol in premature infants with developing bronchopulmonary dysplasia. J Pediatr 1989;115:984–991.

62 Brundage KL, Mohsini KG, Froese AB, Fisher JT: Bronchodilator response to ipratropium bromide in infants with bronchopulmonary dysplasia. Am Rev Respir Dis 1990;142:1137–1142.

63 Denjean A, Guimaraes H, Migdal M, Miramand JL, Dehan M, Gaultier C: Dose-related bronchodilator response to aerosolized salbutamol (albuterol) in ventilator-dependent premature infants. J Pediatr 1992;120:974–979.

64 Benoist MR, Brouard JJ, Rufin P, Delacourt C, Waernessyckle S, Scheinmann P: Ability of new lung function tests to assess methacholine-induced airway obstruction in infants. Pediatr Pulmonol 1994;18:308–316.

65 Gappa, M, Gärtner M, Poets C, von der Hardt H: Effects of salbutamol delivery from a metered dose inhaler versus jet nebulizer on dynamic lung mechanics in very preterm infants with lung disease. Pediatr Pulmonol 1997;23:442–448.

66 Platzker AC, Colin AA, Chen XC, Hiatt P, Hunter J, Koumbourlis AC, Schluchter MD, Ting A, Wohl ME: Thoracoabdominal compression and respiratory system compliance in HIV-infected infants. Am J Repir Crit Care Med 2000;161:1567–1571.

67 Mohon RT, Wagener JS, Abman SH, Seltzer WK, Accurso FJ: Relationship of genotype to early pulmonary function in infants with cystic fibrosis identified through neonatal screening. J Pediatr 1993;122:550–555.

68 Clayton RG Sr, Diaz CE, Bashir NS, Panitch HB, Schidlow DV, Allen JL: Pulmonary function in hospitalized infants and toddlers with cystic fibrosis. J Pediatr 1998;132: 405–408.

69 Tasker RC, Dundas I, Laverty A, Fletcher M, Lane R, Stocks J: Distinct patterns of respiratory difficulty in young children with achondroplasia: A clinical, sleep, and lung function study. Arch Dis Child 1998;79:99–108.

70 Davies CJ, Cooper SG, Fletcher ME, Hatch DJ, Helms PJ, Gordon I, Stocks J: Total respiratory compliance in infants and young children with congenital heart disease. Pediatr Pulmonol 1990;8:155–161.

71 Baraldi E, Filippone M, Milanesi O, Magagnin G, Vencato F, Barbieri P, Pellegrino PA, Zacchello F: Respiratory mechanics in infants and young children before and after repair of left-to-right shunts. Pediatr Res 1993;34:329–333.

72 Dezateux C, Stocks J, Wade AM, Dundas I, Fletcher ME: Airway function at one year: Association with premorbid airway function, wheezing, and maternal smoking. Thorax 2001;56:680–686.

Stephanie D. Davis, MD
Division of Pediatric Pulmonology
130 Mason Farm Road
5130 Bioinformatics Bldg., CB # 7220
Chapel Hill, NC 27599
Tel. +1 919 966 1055
Fax +1 919 966 6179
E-Mail sddavis@med.unc.edu

Hammer J, Eber E (eds): Paediatric Pulmonary Function Testing.
Prog Respir Res. Basel, Karger, 2005, vol 33, pp 34–43

....

Forced Expiratory Flow-Volume Measurements

Manfred Modl   Ernst Eber

Respiratory and Allergic Disease Division, Paediatric Department, Medical University of Graz, Austria

Abstract

In cooperative subjects, voluntary forced expiratory maneuvers are a generally accepted tool for the diagnosis and management of lung diseases. The development of special techniques rendered forced expiratory maneuvers possible in infants as well. With the tidal volume rapid thoracoabdominal compression technique, valuable physiological, pathophysiological, and epidemiological data have been obtained. However, the fact that this technique operates in the tidal volume range, and therefore assesses lung function only for a small part of the vital capacity, limits its clinical value. Recent data suggest that the raised volume rapid thoracoabdominal compression technique may provide the investigator with a more sensitive diagnostic tool for the assessment of pulmonary function. This technique allows for highly reproducible measurements over an extended volume range, resembling voluntary forced vital capacity maneuvers of cooperative subjects. Despite the growing experience with this relatively new technique several methodological issues have to be resolved before recommending it for widespread use. Future directions must focus on the standardization of equipment and protocols, and on the establishment of reference values.

Introduction

Forced expirations from total lung capacity to residual volume are one of the most frequently used clinical tests for the assessment of pulmonary function in cooperative children and adults [1, 2]. As infants and young toddlers do not cooperate with pulmonary function testing special techniques have been developed which allow forced expirations to be measured in this age group as well. Two methods are currently established, namely the forced deflation and the rapid thoracoabdominal compression (RTC) techniques. The forced deflation technique applies a negative pressure to the airways resulting in a rapid deflation of the lung. This maneuver, however, requires an artificial airway, and hence remains restricted to intubated infants [see 3]. RTC maneuvers can be performed in spontaneously breathing infants. The technique applies a positive external pressure to the chest wall and abdomen of the infant, thereby rapidly squeezing air out of the lungs. This can either be done in the tidal volume range (tidal volume RTC technique) or over an extended volume range by raising lung volume above tidal inspiration through an inflation procedure prior to the RTC maneuver (raised volume RTC technique).

Physiological Background

The basis for the comprehension of forced expiratory maneuvers relies on the physiological concept of flow limitation, which dates from Fry et al. [4] who demonstrated that forced expiratory flows increase with increasing expiratory effort to a point beyond which a further increase in intrapleural pressure does not cause an additional increase in airflow; at this point forced expiration becomes effort-independent. This phenomenon has been explained by different theories; the two most widely accepted ones are briefly summarized below.

(1) The equal pressure point hypothesis [5]: During forced expirations expiratory muscles generate a positive intrapleural pressure. Together with the elastic recoil pressure of the lung, the resulting intra-alveolar pressure represents the driving force of expiration. At any instant there is a point along the airways where the pressure inside equals the pressure outside the airway (equal pressure point). Downstream (towards the mouth) of this segment transmural pressure becomes negative and causes a compression of the airway. At higher lung volumes, where elastic recoil pressures are high, this dynamic airway compression occurs in more central compartments which are less compliant due to their cartilaginous matrix. At lower lung volumes, however, this equal pressure point moves upstream (towards the alveoli) and dynamic compression reaches more compliant and collapsible airways. Thus, dynamic compression of these airways determines maximal expiratory airflow and makes forced expiration effort-independent.

(2) The wave speed theory [6]: The wave speed is the speed at which a pressure pulse wave propagates in a compliant tube. In the respiratory system flow limitation occurs at a point in the airway where expiratory flow equals the wave speed within this tube. The flow at wave speed (Vc) is directly proportional to the area (A) and inversely proprotional to the compliance (dP/dA) of the tube's cross section, and inversely proportional to the density (ρ) of the fluid within the system [$Vc = (A^3 \, dP/\rho \, dA)^{0.5}$]. At high lung volumes the flow-limiting site in the airways corresponds to the second and third generation of bronchi. As lung volume decreases during forced expiration, the airway caliber decreases, the flow-limiting site moves towards the alveoli, and hence maximal airflow decreases. At low lung volumes the density dependence of airflow is smaller and viscosity dependence becomes the predominant mechanism, thereby limiting forced expiratory flow [7].

Lung function techniques which try to imitate voluntary forced expirations in uncooperative infants should be able to reach flow limitation; this is particularly important in healthy subjects.

Measurement Conditions

Measurements of lung function with the RTC techniques require special equipment that meets current recommendations for infant respiratory function testing [8]. Well-trained personnel with particular patience in the handling of very young subjects and with special skills in respiratory physiology is a prerequisite to obtain accurate measurements and to ensure the infant's safety. Any apparatus must be clean and any component of the equipment that comes into contact with the infant must be sterilized. Forced expiratory maneuvers with the RTC techniques are performed while the infant sleeps. For this purpose tests are performed at a time of day when the infant usually sleeps. Prior to lung function testing, the child should be kept awake for at least 2–3 h. Measurements of body weight and length are done routinely before the tests. The infant is fed and subsequently sedated with orally administered chloral hydrate (usually 50–100 mg/kg body weight); alternatively, midazolam can be used (0.1–0.5 mg/kg body weight, either orally or rectally). During lung function measurements the infant is lying in the supine position, with the head supported in the midline and the neck slightly extended to stabilize upper airways and to prevent glottic closure [9]. Heart rate and oxygen saturation are continuously monitored throughout the whole procedure. With a sedated infant the laboratory should be prepared for the potential need of cardiopulmonary resuscitation.

Tidal Volume RTC Technique

Background

In 1978, Adler and Wohl [10] introduced a new technique for generating forced expirations in spontaneously breathing infants by applying positive thoracoabdominal pressures through a box surrounding the infant's body. This technique has been advanced by Taussig et al. [11] by the implementation of an inflatable jacket that is tightly wrapped around the infant's chest and abdomen. Rapidly filling the jacket with compressed air produces an external pressure source that generates a forced expiration from end-tidal inspiration.

Equipment

The infant breathes through a sealed face mask held over mouth and nose (fig. 1). The dead space of the mask should be kept minimal. A pneumotachograph, ideally linear from 0 to 150 liters/min, is connected to the mask and measures airflow. The squeeze jacket consists of a rapidly inflatable and expandable inner layer within a rigid outer layer; it is wrapped tightly around the infant's chest and abdomen, extending from the axillae to the upper thighs, with the arms remaining outside to achieve sufficient pressure transmission [12]. Care must be taken that the jacket is not wrapped so tightly as to restrict tidal breathing or so loosely as to cause insufficient pressure transmission across the chest wall. Through a wide-bore tubing of at least 25-mm internal diameter the inner layer is connected to a 50- to

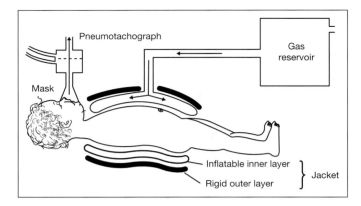

Fig. 1. Schematic illustration of equipment used for the tidal volume RTC technique.

100-liter gas reservoir filled with compressed air [8]. The jacket pressure (Pj) plateau is reached within 100 ms after opening the valve to the gas reservoir, and jacket inflation must be maintained until forced expiration is complete. Data collection and analysis are usually performed on a computer with a minimum sampling rate of 200 Hz [8].

Procedure

Initially, the transmission of the Pj to the intrapleural space is estimated. This can be done noninvasively by occluding the airway opening at the end of an inspiratory maneuver. After the airway opening pressure (Pao), measured at the infant's mouth, reaches a plateau, the jacket is rapidly inflated while the airway remains closed; once a second plateau in Pao occurs, the airway is opened and the jacket is deflated. The changes in Pao, which indirectly reflect changes in intrapleural pressure, are related to Pj and expressed as percent driving pressure for the RTC maneuver. Ideally, at least 50% of the Pj should be transmitted to the intrapleural space.

Forced expirations are generated by rapidly inflating the jacket at end-tidal inspiration, after a stable end-expiratory functional residual capacity (FRC) level of the preceding tidal breaths has been observed on a screen. The minimal Pj needed for generating forced expirations is determined from a run of maneuvers beginning with a Pj of 2–3 kPa; subsequently, pressure increments of 1–2 kPa are applied stepwise until the flow at FRC ($V'_{max, FRC}$) no longer increases. The Pj that produces the highest $V'_{max, FRC}$ without evidence of negative effort dependence is then used to generate forced expirations [8, 13]. When jacket transmission characteristics are good, pressures of around 4–5 kPa are usually sufficient. The obtained partial expiratory flow-volume

(PEFV) curves are generally quantified in terms of the maximal expiratory flow at FRC of the preceding tidal breath ($V'_{max, FRC}$) (fig. 2).

PEFV curves are accepted for analysis provided: (1) a stable FRC level of at least five tidal breaths prior to the RTC maneuver has been recorded; (2) peak expiratory flow is rapidly reached within the initial portion of the PEFV curve (within the first 30% of the volume of the previous tidal breath); (3) irregularities of the PEFV curve shape due to glottic closure are lacking; (4) forced expirations continue to a point below FRC, and (5) no shifts of the PEFV curve occur (i.e., no leaks at the face mask) [8]. Mean values and standard deviations (SD) or coefficients of variation for $V'_{max, FRC}$ are calculated from a series of three to five technically acceptable PEFV curves [8].

Normal Values and Data Interpretation

Although recent publications suggested other parameters to be superior in the detection of lung function changes [14, 15], $V'_{max, FRC}$ still is the most widely accepted parameter for the quantification of PEFV curves [8, 16, 17]. $V'_{max, FRC}$ mainly represents the function of smaller, more peripheral airways [11, 16]. Several research groups published normative data and found significant correlations between $V'_{max, FRC}$ and body length [18–20]. The main problem of presenting valid normative data, however, is the lack of standardized equipment. In addition, the investigated subjects from various centers differ with regard to ethnic, social and age-related factors, so that reported reference values are only applicable to that specific laboratory. In a first attempt to present multicenter data, measurements from two groups have been pooled and demonstrated nonlinear relationships between $V'_{max, FRC}$ and both body weight and length [8, 20–22]. Furthermore, significant gender differences were found, and the best correlations were detected for $V'_{max, FRC}$ and age after taking gender into account [8]. More recently, data from 459 healthy infants from three centers have been published which indicate that gender, age and body length are important predictors of $V'_{max, FRC}$ [23]. Despite these attempts, however, no widely acceptable reference data are currently available. With regard to data presentation, it is not recommended to use percent predicted values, but rather SD scores (z scores), which indicate a normal range for $V'_{max, FRC}$ [8, 23]. In addition, each lung function laboratory should ascertain whether published reference equations and the derived scores are applicable to their own laboratory.

The shape of the PEFV curve provides information on actual airway function as well as on data acceptability. Unacceptable data may stem from delayed chest

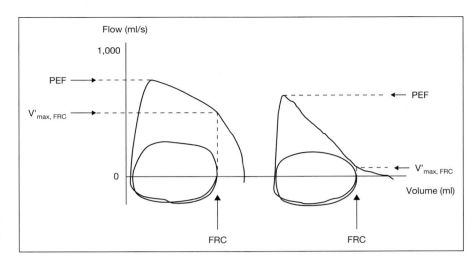

Fig. 2. PEFV curves from an infant with normal lung function (convex curve shape; left) and from an infant with bronchiolitis (concave curve shape; right). PEF = Peak expiratory flow.

compression, early inspiratory efforts or glottic closure [16]. A convex curve shape reflects normal airway caliber whereas concavity indicates bronchial obstruction [24] (fig. 2); plateaus in PEFV curves result from central airway obstructions such as tracheal stenosis or tracheomalacia [25–27].

Applications

Since its introduction, the tidal volume RTC technique has been widely adopted and used in numerous physiological, epidemiological and clinical studies [10–15, 17–56]. The results from these investigations have extended the understanding of lung growth and airway physiology in infancy [10, 11, 17, 18, 20, 33–37], have helped to detect and quantitate abnormal airway function during respiratory diseases [25–32, 38, 41, 42], have contributed to the development of treatment concepts for airway diseases [15, 43–51], and have been used to study the mechanisms underlying recurrent wheeze and the development of obstructive lung disease in early childhood [14, 22, 37, 39, 40, 52–56].

Limitations

The major disadvantage of the tidal volume RTC technique is the lack of a reliable volume landmark for the measurement of $V'_{max, FRC}$. FRC varies dynamically depending on sleep state, degree of sedation, respiratory rate, and changes in airway caliber [57–59]. This is the most likely reason for the high variability reported for $V'_{max, FRC}$ [11, 16, 18–20, 24, 59–64]. During serial assessments, $V'_{max, FRC}$ will often be measured at different absolute lung volumes. This is particularly important if

responses to bronchodilator therapy or other interventions are assessed. FRC levels increase as a consequence of airway narrowing. Bronchodilation may result in reduction of hyperinflation; airflow will then be measured at a lower lung volume than before the intervention. As a consequence, the effect of bronchodilator medication might be disguised and the clinical value of an intervention underestimated. Correspondingly, a bronchoconstrictor response might be underestimated by the reverse mechanism, too.

Another important concern is whether or not physiologically determined flow limitation is reached, a problem that may be more relevant in healthy infants than in patients with airway obstruction [13, 16, 17, 24, 29, 61]. Furthermore, it has been shown that pressure transmission from the jacket to the pleural space and to the airways declines with decreasing lung volume [11, 13]. The transmission of pressure to the airway may also depend on respiratory muscle activity. Kerem et al. [65] demonstrated that forced expiratory flows after end-inspiratory airway occlusion prior to the RTC maneuver exceed those obtained with the traditional procedure. They speculated that relaxation of respiratory muscles due to the activation of the Hering-Breuer reflex might be the major cause of this phenomenon. The influence of respiratory muscle activity at lower lung volumes, however, has not been investigated systematically so far.

In contrast to voluntary full vital capacity maneuvers, with the tidal volume RTC technique pulmonary function is assessed only for a small part of the vital capacity. As $V'_{max, FRC}$ mainly represents the function of peripheral airways, important information on more central airways may be missed [66].

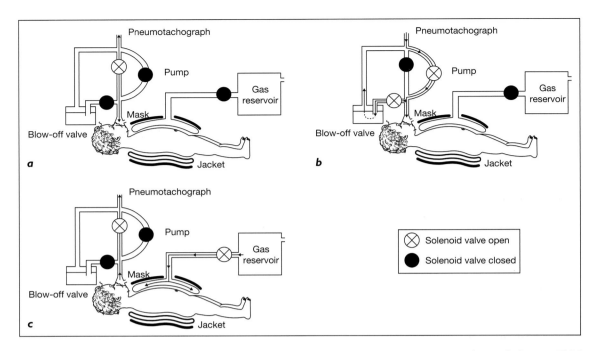

Fig. 3. Schematic illustration of equipment used for raised volume RTC maneuvers: pumping technique. *a* Tidal breathing through the main solenoid valve to the pneumotachograph. *b* 'Inflation' procedure through activation of the pumping system until a predetermined airway pressure, measured via a port in the face mask, is reached. *c* 'Squeeze' maneuver by opening the solenoid valve to the gas tank (for detailed comments see text).

Raised Volume RTC Technique

Background

In adults, forced expirations over the full vital capacity range have been found to provide more information on airway function than partial expiratory maneuvers [67]. In spontaneously breathing infants, first attempts to raise lung volume above the tidal volume range were made using a volume clamping technique. With this technique, tidal expirations are prevented by occluding the airway through a one-way valve so that progressive inspirations produce cumulative increases of the end-expiratory volume level [68]. The variability of lung volume at end-inspiration according to the number and the force of inspiratory efforts, however, limits the usefulness of this method. More recently, new techniques have been developed which raise lung volume by inflating the lungs to a given airway pressure. This can be performed using either a pump [62–64] or an external air supply [69–74].

Pumping Technique
Equipment
The pumping system requires a complex apparatus consisting of a modified diaphragm pump, a variable blow-off valve and several electronically controlled solenoid valves (fig. 3). The use of positive pressures for lung inflation demands special care with the application of the mask to obtain a leak-free system. The mask needs to be held firmly over the mouth and nose with particular attention to avoid obstruction of the upper airways. The face mask carries a port to measure Pao. The pump is situated within a circuit, produces an output flow of at least 11 liters/min and up to 20 liters/min, and must be able to stop pumping within 200 ms after switch-off. The variable blow-off valve is activated at the end of an inflation maneuver when lung volume, set by a predetermined airway pressure, is reached to limit the inspiratory pressure for patient safety. Alternatively, this can be done without a blow-off valve using an electronic signal from the Pao transducer that stops the pumping procedure. The solenoid valves are activated serially through a complex computer-operated system to obtain the desired sequence of tidal breathing, lung inflation and forced expiration. Rebreathing during unrecorded tidal breathing is minimized by an intermittent fresh gas flow within the circuit. The basic equipment for the compression maneuver remains the same as described for the tidal volume RTC technique.

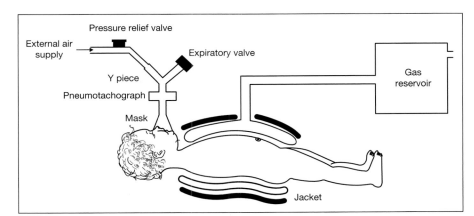

Fig. 4. Schematic illustration of equipment used for raised volume RTC maneuvers: multiple inflation technique (for detailed comments see text).

Procedure

The raised volume RTC maneuver with the pumping technique is illustrated in figure 3a–c. Initially, the infant breathes room air through a face mask and pneumotachograph. To raise lung volume, the pumping system is activated after a tidal expiration while the main solenoid valve closes simultaneously. Room air is drawn in through the pneumotachograph and inflates the infant's lungs until a predetermined airway pressure, measured at the infant's mouth, is reached. Once this pressure is achieved, the blow-off valve is activated, no more air enters through the pneumotachograph, and the pump is switched off. Then rapid jacket inflation is triggered; forced expiration starts after a short time delay (50 ms). This time delay between opening the solenoid valve to the jacket and the main solenoid valve to the pneumotachograph allows the jacket to be fully inflated prior to the onset of forced expiration. To facilitate relaxation of respiratory muscles due to the Hering-Breuer inflation reflex, usually three inflation maneuvers, the first two followed by passive expirations, precede each thoracoabdominal compression [62–64, 75].

Multiple Inflation Technique
Equipment

The face mask and the pneumotachograph are connected to a Y piece (fig. 4). The Y piece has an inspiratory limb which receives a constant bias flow from an external air supply, and an expiratory limb which can be closed repeatedly using a valve. The gas supply is adjustable and should be able to produce an airflow of up to 20 liters/min. A safety pressure relief valve controls the inflation pressure within the system and is activated if a predetermined airway pressure, measured at the infant's mouth, is reached.

Procedure

After tidal breathing through the pneumotachograph repeated occlusions of the expiratory limb at a frequency approximating the infant's respiratory rate are performed. This results in a progressive rise of the pressure within the system, and inflates the lungs above the tidal volume range until a predetermined airway pressure is reached. A subsequent release of the valve allows passive expiration to proceed. In order to ensure a constant inflation volume, inflations are held until a plateau on airway pressure and volume tracings is observed. At least 4–5 such augmented breaths are recommended to induce relaxation of the respiratory muscles prior to jacket inflation [76, 77]. Subsequently, forced expiration is initiated as described for the tidal volume RTC and the pumping techniques.

Methodological Aspects

Pressure transmission characteristics are most commonly assessed at end-tidal inspiration as described for the tidal volume RTC technique [63, 64, 75, 76]. Transmission pressures of 2–2.5 kPA have been suggested to be sufficient to achieve flow limitation in all infants [75]. The optimal Pj assessed during tidal volume RTC is valid for the subsequent application on raised volume RTC, provided the jacket has not been adjusted between the tests [77]. If only raised volume RTC is used, forced expirations are repeated with increasing Pj until the highest volumes or flows are obtained from a run of maneuvers beginning with a Pj of 2–3 kPa [72]. The optimal inflation pressure is subject of an ongoing discussion. Most centers use inflation pressures of 3 kPa [62–64, 71, 72, 74, 75], occasionally 2 kPa were used in order to minimize risks like potential volutrauma in very small infants [70]. Currently, pressures of 3 kPa are recommended to enable comparisons of results between

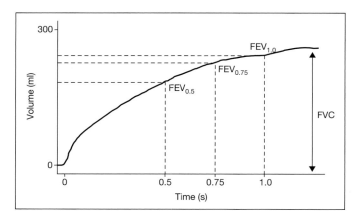

Fig. 5. Volume-time curve generated from raised lung volume as defined by 3 kPa inflation pressure.

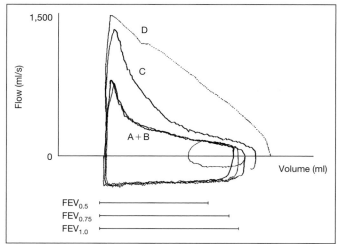

Fig. 6. Flow-volume curves with a concave shape, generated from raised lung volume as defined by 3 kPa inflation pressure (pumping technique) in an infant with bronchiolitis. Curves A + B, following a tidal loop, demonstrate the inflation-effected increase of lung volume followed by passive expirations. Curve C demonstrates the squeeze-effected forced expiratory flow-volume curve from the same elevated lung volume. Curve D illustrates a superimposed flow-volume curve from a normal infant matched for height and weight. Horizontal bars under the volume axis stand for the dimensions of timed volumes.

centers, unless there are specific contraindications [78]. The optimal airflow for the lung inflation maneuver so far remains an unresolved issue; reported values range from 11 to 20 liters/min [62, 63, 72–74]. For the multiple inflation method inspiratory flows of 1.5 times the peak tidal inspiratory flow have been recommended [69].

Data Analysis and Interpretation

As forced expirations start from predetermined lung volumes via a given inflation pressure, the raised volume RTC technique allows for measurements of volume-time parameters (fig. 5). The commonly reported parameters are forced vital capacity (FVC) and forced expiratory volumes at 0.4, 0.5, 0.75, and 1 s ($FEV_{0.4}$, $FEV_{0.5}$, $FEV_{0.75}$, and $FEV_{1.0}$), respectively [62–64, 70, 73–78]. In very young infants and in those with tachypnea, however, calculation of values like FVC and $FEV_{1.0}$ is often not feasible because of inspiratory efforts occurring before the end of the 1st second of expiration [63, 64, 69, 74, 79]; in such cases the use of $FEV_{0.4}$ [70, 74] or $FEV_{0.75}$ [63, 64] has been recommended for data analysis. More recently, forced expiratory flow parameters have been employed. Amongst these, forced expiratory flows at 50, 75 and 85% of FVC (FEF50, FEF75, and FEF85), and forced expiratory flow between 25 and 75% of FVC (FEF25–75) are the most frequently used [71–73, 76, 77, 79]. Recently, forced expiratory flows, in particular FEF50, have been reported to better discriminate between normal and abnormal airway function than timed volumes [79]. Timed volume measurements, however, are more reproducible than forced expiratory flows; the within-subject variability of FEV parameters has been found to be ≤5% [62–64], which is comparable to quality standards of voluntary lung function tests in school-age children and adults [1, 2].

As noted for the tidal volume RTC technique, the shape of the forced expiratory flow-volume curve provides information on actual airway function (fig. 6) as well as on data acceptability. Technically acceptable maneuvers are those without the occurrence of a leak during lung inflation, and with a smooth forced expiratory loop without evidence of early inspiratory effort or glottic closure. The peak expiratory flow should be rapidly reached within the initial 10% of expired volume. The best three curves defined as those with the highest FEV values with a variability of less than 10% are used for reporting results. As flow parameters are related to lung volume, they should only be determined if an infant breathes out fully towards residual volume.

Normal Values

Recently, reference equations based on 155 healthy infants from two centers have been published [72]. This study demonstrated a strong, nonlinear relationship of forced expiratory flows and volumes with body length. For FEF75, there was also a significant effect of gender with males having lower flows than females. However, the main problem with normal values for the raised volume RTC technique is the lack of standardized equipment. Thus, for the time being data should be presented in absolute numbers.

Applications

The raised volume RTC technique has only been applied in a limited number of studies so that available data are relatively sparse. Most of these investigations were mainly concerned with the evaluation of technical issues [62, 63, 69, 73–75, 77, 80, 81]; some examined the ability of this technique to detect normal and abnormal airway function, respectively [71, 72, 76, 79, 82–84]; others were focused on physiological and pathophysiological questions [75, 85–90]. The first clinical trials were performed to investigate bronchodilator responsiveness in infants with acute bronchiolitis, and in infants with recurrent wheeze, respectively [64, 91].

Limitations

Forced expiratory maneuvers with the raised volume RTC technique require a relatively complex equipment for lung inflation. Laboratories currently applying this technique use different pressure sources to raise lung volume above the tidal volume range. This makes the comparison of data between centers rather difficult, and also prevented the establishment of appropriate reference values so far. Another disadvantage of this technique is that the applied pressures during lung inflation require firm holding of the mask on the infant's face to avoid leaks, which necessitates adequate sedation in any case, and may cause problems with airway patency. Furthermore, gastric distention may occur due to positive pressure application through the face mask, which potentially decreases lung volumes. This phenomenon clearly depends on the magnitude of applied pressures and the number of inflation maneuvers performed [62]. Other potential problems like pneumothorax, respiratory insufficiency or apnea have not been reported so far. The raised volume RTC technique offers potential advantages over the tidal RTC technique; however, both techniques do not allow a separate assessment of the contributions of airway diameter and airway wall mechanics, and thus cannot definitely identify the site of changes in lung function.

References

1 Quanjer PH, Tammeling GJ, Cotes JE, Pedersen OF, Peslin R, Yernault JC: Lung volumes and forced ventilatory flows. Report Working Party Standardization of Lung Function Tests, European Community for Steel and Coal. Official Statement of the European Respiratory Society. Eur Respir J 1993;6(suppl 16):5–40.

2 American Thoracic Society: Standardization of Spirometry 1994 Update. Am J Respir Crit Care Med 1995;152:1107–1136.

3 Hammer J, Newth CJL: Pulmonary function testing in the neonatal and paediatric intensive care unit; in Hammer J, Eber E (eds): Paediatric Pulmonary Function Testing. Prog Respir Res. Basel, Karger, 2005, vol 33, pp 266–281.

4 Fry DL, Ebert EV, Stead WW, Brown CC: The mechanics of pulmonary ventilation in normal subjects and patients with emphysema. Am J Med 1954;16:80–97.

5 Mead J, Turner JM, Macklem PT, Little JB: Significance of the relationship between lung recoil and maximum expiratory flow. J Appl Physiol 1967;22:95–108.

6 Dawson SV, Elliot EA: Wave speed limitation on expiratory flow – A unifying concept. J Appl Physiol 1977;43:498–515.

7 Shapiro AH: Steady flow in collapsible tubes. J Biomech Eng 1977;99:126–147.

8 Sly PD, Tepper R, Henschen M, Gappa M, Stocks J: Tidal forced expirations. ERS/ATS Task Force on Standards for Infant Respiratory Function Testing. Eur Respir J 2000;16:741–748.

9 Reed WR, Roberts JL, Thach BT: Factors influencing regional patency and configuration of the human infant upper airway. J Appl Physiol 1985;58:635–644.

10 Adler S, Wohl ME: Flow-volume relationship at low lung volumes in healthy term newborn infants. Pediatrics 1978;61:636–640.

11 Taussig LM, Landau LI, Godfrey S, Arad I: Determinants of forced expiratory flows in newborn infants. J Appl Physiol 1982;53:1220–1227.

12 Steinbrugger B, Lanigan A, Raven JM, Olinsky A: Influence of the 'squeeze jacket' on lung function in young infants. Am Rev Respir Dis 1988;138:1258–1260.

13 LeSouef PN, Hughes DM, Landau LI: Effect of compression pressure on forced expiratory flow in infants. J Appl Physiol 1986;61:1639–1646.

14 Sheikh S, Goldsmith LJ, Howell L, Parry L, Eid N: Comparison of lung function in infants exposed to maternal smoking and in infants with a family history of asthma. Chest 1999;116:52–58.

15 Sheikh S, Castile R, Hayes J, McCoy K, Eid N: Assessing bronchodilator responsiveness in infants using partial expiratory flow-volume curves. Pediatr Pulmonol 2003;36:196–201.

16 LeSouef PN, Castile R, Turner DJ, Motoyama E, Morgan WJ: Forced expiratory maneuvers; in Stocks J, Sly PD, Tepper RS, Morgan WJ (eds): Infant Respiratory Function Testing. New York, Wiley-Liss,1996, pp 379–409.

17 Morgan WJ, Geller DE, Tepper RS, Taussig LM: Partial expiratory flow-volume curves in infants and young children. Pediatr Pulmonol 1988;5:232–243.

18 Tepper RS, Morgan WJ, Cota K, Wright A, Taussig LM: Physiologic growth and development of the lung during the first year of life. Am Rev Respir Dis 1986;134:513–519.

19 Hanrahan JP, Tager IB, Castile RG, Segal MR, Weiss ST, Speizer FE: Pulmonary function measures in healthy infants: Variability and size correction. Am Rev Respir Dis 1990;141:1127–1135.

20 Tepper RS, Reister T: Forced expiratory flows and lung volumes in normal infants. Pediatr Pulmonol 1993;15:357–361.

21 Stocks J, Henschen M, Hoo A-F, Costeloe K, Dezateux CA: The influence of ethnicity and gender on airway function in preterm infants. Am J Respir Crit Care Med 1997;156:1855–1862.

22 Hoo A-F, Henschen M, Dezateux C, Costeloe K, Stocks J: Respiratory function among preterm infants whose mothers smoked during pregnancy. Am J Respir Crit Care Med 1998;158:700–705.

23 Hoo AF, Dezateux C, Hanrahan JP, Cole TJ, Tepper RS, Stocks J: Sex-specific prediction equations for V'maxFRC in infancy. Am J Respir Crit Care Med 2002;165:1084–1092.

24 LeSouef PN, Hughes DM, Landau LI: Shape of forced expiratory flow-volume curves in infancy. Am Rev Respir Dis 1988;138:590–597.

25 Tepper RS, Eigen H, Brown J, Hurwitz R: Use of maximal expiratory flows to evaluate central airways obstruction in infants. Pediatr Pulmonol 1989;6:272–274.

26 Panitch HB, Keklikian EN, Motley RA, Wolfson MR, Schidlow DV: Effect of altering smooth muscle tone on maximal expiratory flows in patients with tracheomalacia. Pediatr Pulmonol 1990;9:170–176.

27 Thomson AH, Beardsmore CS, Firmin R, Leanage R, Simpson H: Airway function in infants with vascular rings: Preoperative and postoperative assessment. Arch Dis Child 1990; 65:171–174.

28 Godfrey S, Bar-Yishay E, Arad I, Landau LI, Taussig LM: Flow-volume curves in infants with lung disease. Pediatrics 1983;72:517–522.

29 Tepper RS, Morgan WJ, Cota K, Taussig LM: Expiratory flow limitation in infants with bronchopulmonary dysplasia. J Pediatr 1986; 109:1040–1046.

30 Prendiville A, Green S, Silverman M: Airway responsiveness in wheezy infants: Evidence for functional beta adrenergic receptors. Thorax 1987;42:100–104.

31 Beardsmore CS, Bar-Yishay E, Maayan C, Yahav Y, Katznelson D, Godfrey S: Lung function in infants with cystic fibrosis. Thorax 1988;43:545–551.

32 Tepper RS, Hiatt P, Eigen H, Scott P, Grosfeld J, Cohen M: Infants with cystic fibrosis: Pulmonary function at diagnosis. Pediatr Pulmonol 1988;5:15–18.

33 LeSouef PN, Geelhoed GC, Turner DJ, Morgan SEG, Landau LI: Response of normal infants to inhaled histamine. Am Rev Respir Dis 1989; 139:62–66.

34 Stick SM, Turnbull S, Chua HL, Landau LI, LeSouef PN: Comparison of airway responsiveness to histamine between infants and older children. Am Rev Respir Dis 1990;142: 1143–1146.

35 Stick SM, Turner DJ, LeSouef PN: Lung function and bronchial challenges in infants: Repeatability of histamine and comparison with methacholine challenges. Pediatr Pulmonol 1993;16:177–183.

36 Henderson AJW, Young S, Stick SM, Landau LI, LeSouef PN: The effect of salbutamol on histamine-induced bronchoconstriction in healthy infants. Thorax 1993;48:317–323.

37 Young S, O'Keeffe PT, Arnott J, Landau LI: Lung function, airway responsiveness, and respiratory symptoms before and after bronchiolitis. Arch Dis Child 1995;72:16–24.

38 Beardsmore C: Respiratory physiological measurements in infants with cystic fibrosis. Pediatr Pulmonol 1991;7:38–41.

39 Young S, LeSouef PN, Geelhoed GC, Stick SM, Turner KJ, Landau LI: The influence of a family history of asthma and parental smoking on airway responsiveness in early infancy. N Engl J Med 1991;324:1168–1173.

40 Young S, Sherrill DL, Arnott J, Diepeveen D, Le Souef PN, Landau LI: Parental factors affecting respiratory function during the first year of life. Pediatr Pulmonol 2000;29:331–340.

41 Clayton RG, Diaz CE, Bashir NS, Panitch HB, Shidlow DV, Allen JL: Pulmonary function in hospitalized infants and toddlers with cystic fibrosis. J Pediatr 1998;132:405–408.

42 Hartmann H, Seidenberg J, Noyes JP, O'Brien L, Poets CF, Samuels MP, Southall DP: Small airways patency in infants with apparent life-threatening events. Eur J Pediatr 1998; 157:71–74.

43 Hiatt P, Eigen H, Yu P, Tepper RS: Bronchodilator responsiveness in infants and young children with cystic fibrosis. Am Rev Respir Dis 1988;137:119–122.

44 Hughes DM, LeSouef PN, Landau LI: Effect of salbutamol on respiratory mechanics in bronchiolitis. Pediatr Res 1987;22:83–86.

45 Prendiville A, Green S, Silverman M: Paradoxical response to nebulized salbutamol in wheezy infants, assessed by partial expiratory flow-volume curves. Thorax 1987;42: 86–91.

46 Springer C, Bar-Yishay E, Uwayyed K, Avital A, Vilozni D, Godfrey S: Corticosteroids do not affect the clinical or physiological status of infants with bronchiolitis. Pediatr Pulmonol 1990;9:181–185.

47 Sly PD, Lanteri CJ, Raven JM: Do wheezy infants recovering from bronchiolitis respond to inhaled salbutamol? Pediatr Pulmonol 1991;10:36–39.

48 Tepper RS, Rosenberg D, Eigen H, Reister T: Bronchodilator responsiveness in infants with bronchiolitis. Pediatr Pulmonol 1994; 17:81–85.

49 Panitch HB, Allen JL, Alpert BE, Schidlow DV: Effects of CPAP on lung mechanics in infants with acquired tracheobronchomalacia. Am J Respir Crit Care Med 1994;150: 1341–1346.

50 Henderson AJ, Arnott J, Young S, Warshawski T, Landau LI, LeSouef PN: The effect of inhaled adrenaline on lung function of recurrently wheezy infants less than 18 months old. Pediatr Pulmonol 1995;20:9–15.

51 Hofhuis W, van der Wiel EC, Tiddens HAWM, Brinkhorst G, Holland WPJ, de Jongste JC, Merkus PJFM: Bronchodilation in infants with malacia or recurrent wheeze. Arch Dis Child 2003;88:246–249.

52 Martinez FD, Morgan WJ, Wright AL, Holberg CJ, Taussig LM: Diminished lung function as a predisposing factor for wheezing respiratory illness in infants. N Engl J Med 1988;319:1112–1117.

53 Martinez FD, Morgan WJ, Wright AL, Holberg C, Taussig LM: Initial airway function is a risk factor for recurrent wheezing respiratory illnesses during the first three years of life. Am Rev Respir Dis 1991;143:312–316.

54 Stick SM, Arnott J, Turner DJ, Young S, Landau LI, LeSouef PN: Bronchial responsiveness and lung function in recurrently wheezy infants. Am Rev Respir Dis 1991;144:1012–1015.

55 Martinez FD, Wright AL, Taussig LM, Holberg CJ, Halonen M, Morgan WJ: Asthma and wheezing in the first six years of life. N Engl J Med 1995;332:133–138.

56 Adler A, Ngo L, Tosta P, Tager IB: Association of tobacco smoke exposure and respiratory syncytial virus infection with airways reactivity in early childhood. Pediatr Pulmonol 2001; 32:418–427.

57 Bryan AC, England SJ: Maintenance of elevated FRC in the newborn: Paradox of REM sleep. Am Rev Respir Dis 1984;129:209–210.

58 Stark AR, Cohlan BA, Waggener TB, Frantz ID, Kosch PC: Regulation of end-expiratory lung volume during sleep in premature infants. J Appl Physiol 1987;62:1117–1123.

59 Maxwell DL, Prendiville A, Rose A, Silverman M: Lung volume changes during histamine-induced bronchoconstriction in recurrently wheezy infants. Pediatr Pulmonol 1988;5: 145–151.

60 Wall MA, Misley MC, Dickerson D: Partial expiratory flow-volume curves in young children. Am Rev Respir Dis 1984;129:557–562.

61 England SJ: Current techniques for assessing pulmonary function in the newborn and infant: Advantages and limitations. Pediatr Pulmonol 1988;4:48–53.

62 Turner DJ, Stick SM, LeSouef KL, Sly PD, LeSouef PN: A new technique to generate and assess forced expiration from raised lung volume in infants. Am J Respir Crit Care Med 1995;151:1441–1450.

63 Modl M, Eber E, Weinhandl E, Gruber W, Zach MS: Reproducibility of forced expiratory flow and volume measurements in infants with bronchiolitis. Pediatr Pulmonol 1999; 28:429–435.

64 Modl M, Eber E, Weinhandl E, Gruber W, Zach MS: Assessment of bronchodilator responsiveness in infants with bronchiolitis – A comparison of the tidal and the raised volume rapid thoracoabdominal compression technique. Am J Respir Crit Care Med 2000;161:763–768.

65 Kerem E, Reisman J, Gaston S, Levison H, Bryan AC: Maximal expiratory flows generated by rapid chest compression following end-inspiratory occlusion or expiratory clamping in young children. Eur Respir J 1995;8:93–98.

66 Gappa M: Cautious enthusiasm. Pediatr Pulmonol 1999;28:391–393.

67 Michoud MC, Ghezzo H, Amyot R: A comparison of pulmonary function tests used for bronchial challenges. Bull Eur Physiopathol Respir 1982;18:609–621.

68 Grunstein MM, Springer C, Godfrey S, Bar-Yishay E, Vlozni D, Inscore SC, Schramm CM: Expiratory volume clamping: A new method to assess respiratory mechanics in sedated infants. J Appl Physiol 1987;62: 2107–2114.

69 Feher A, Castile R, Kisling J, Angelicchio C, Filbrun D, Flucke R, Tepper R: Flow limitation in normal infants: A new method for forced expiratory maneuvers from raised lung volumes. J Appl Physiol 1996;80:2019–2025.

70 Henschen M, Stocks J, Hoo AF, Dixon P: Analysis of forced expiratory maneuvers from raised lung volumes in preterm infants. J Appl Physiol 1998;85:1989–1997.

71 Castile R, Filbrun D, Flucke R, Franklin W, McCoy K: Adult-type pulmonary function tests in infants without respiratory disease. Pediatr Pulmonol 2000;30:215–227.

72 Jones M, Castile R, Davis S, Kisling J, Filbrun D, Flucke R, Goldstein A, Emsley C, Ambrosius W, Tepper RS: Forced expiratory flows and volumes in infants. Am J Respir Crit Care Med 2000;161:353–359.

73 Lum S, Hoo AF, Stocks J: Effect of airway inflation pressure on forced expiratory maneuvers from raised lung volume in infants. Pediatr Pulmonol 2002;33:130–134.

74 Ranganathan SC, Hoo AF, Lum SY, Goetz I, Castle RA, Stocks J: Exploring the relationship between forced maximal flow at functional residual capacity and parameters of forced expiration from raised lung volume in healthy infants. Pediatr Pulmonol 2002;33: 419–428.

75 Hayden MJ, Sly PD, Devadason G, Gurrin LC, Wildhaber JH, LeSouef PN: Influence of driving pressure on raised-volume forced expiration in infants. Am J Respir Crit Care Med 1997;156:1876–1883.

76 Lum S, Hoo AF, Dezateux C, Goetz I, Wade A, DeRooy L, Costeloe K, Stocks J: The association between birthweight, sex, and airway function in infants of nonsmoking mothers. Am J Respir Crit Care Med 2001;164: 2078–2084.

77 Lum S, Hoo AF, Stocks J: Influence of jacket tightness and pressure on raised lung volume forced expiratory maneuvers in infants. Pediatr Pulmonol 2002;34:361–368.

78 Allen J, Gappa M: The raised volume rapid thoracoabdominal compression technique. The Joint American Thoracic Society/European Respiratory Society Working Group on Infant Lung Function. Am J Respir Crit Care Med 2000;161:1760–1762.

79 Jones MH, Howard J, Davis S, Kisling J, Tepper RS: Sensitivity of spirometric measurements to detect airway obstruction in infants. Am J Respir Crit Care Med 2003;167:1283–1286.

80 Turner DJ, Lanteri CJ, LeSouef PN, Sly PD: Pressure transmission across the respiratory system at raised lung volumes in infants. J Appl Physiol 1994;77:1015–1020.

81 Hoo AF, Lum S, Goetz I, Dezateux CA, Stocks J: Influence of jacket placement on respiratory compliance during raised lung volume measurements in infants. Pediatr Pulmonol 2001;31:51–58.

82 Turner DJ, Lanteri CJ, LeSouef PN, Sly PD: Improved detection of abnormal respiratory function using forced expiration from raised lung volume in infants with cystic fibrosis. Eur Respir J 1994;7:1995–1999.

83 Ranganathan S, Dezateux CA, Bush A, Carr SB, Castle R, Madge L, Price JF, Stroobant J, Wade AM, Wallis CE, Stocks J: Airway function in infants newly diagnosed with cystic fibrosis. Lancet 2001;358:1964–1965.

84 Ranganathan SC, Bush A, Dezateux C, Carr SB, Hoo AF, Lum S, Madge S, Price J, Stroobant J, Wade A, Wallis C, Wyatt H, Stocks J: Relative ability of full and partial forced expiratory maneuvers to identify diminished airway function in infants with cystic fibrosis. Am J Respir Crit Care Med 2002;166:1350–1357.

85 Turner DJ, Sly PD, LeSouef PN: Assessment of forced expiratory volume-time parameters in detecting histamine-induced bronchoconstriction in wheezy infants. Pediatr Pulmonol 1993;15:220–224.

86 Hammer J, Newth CJL: Effect of lung volume on forced expiratory flows during rapid thoracoabdominal compression in infants. J Appl Physiol 1995;78:1993–1997.

87 Hammer J, Sivan Y, Deakers TW, Newth CJL: Flow limitation in anesthetized rhesus monkeys: A comparison of rapid thoracoabdominal compression and forced deflation techniques. Pediatr Res 1996;39:539–546.

88 Hayden MJ, Devadason SG, Sly PD, Wildhaber JH, LeSouef PN: Methacholine responsiveness using the raised volume forced expiration technique in infants. Am J Respir Crit Care Med 1997;155:1670–1675.

89 Hall GL, Hantos Z, Wildhaber JH, Petak F, Sly PD: Methacholine responsiveness in infants assessed with low frequency forced oscillation and forced expiration techniques. Thorax 2001;56:42–47.

90 Goldstein AB, Castile RG, Davis SD, Filbrun DA, Flucke RL, McCoy KS, Tepper RS: Bronchodilator responsiveness in normal infants and young children. Am J Respir Crit Care Med 2001;164:447–454.

91 Hayden MJ, Wildhaber JH, LeSouef PN: Bronchodilator responsiveness testing using raised volume forced expiration in recurrently wheezing infants. Pediatr Pulmonol 1998;26: 35–41.

Manfred Modl, MD.,
Klinische Abteilung für Pädiatrische Pulmonologie/Allergologie
Univ. Klinik für Kinder- und Jugendheilkunde Auenbruggerplatz 30
AT–8036 Graz (Austria)
Tel. +43 316 385 2620
Fax +43 316 385 3276
E-Mail manfred.modl@klinikum-graz.at

Hammer J, Eber E (eds): Paediatric Pulmonary Function Testing.
Prog Respir Res. Basel, Karger, 2005, vol 33, pp 44–53

....

Infant Whole-Body Plethysmography

Monika Gappa[a]   Georg Hülskamp[b]

[a]Paediatric Pulmonology and Neonatology, Medizinische Hochschule Hannover, Hannover, and
[b]Department of Paediatrics, Universitätsklinikum Münster, Westfälische Wilhelms-Universität,
Münster, Germany

Abstract

Measurement of lung volume is an important part of infant lung function testing both for assessing growth and development of the lungs in health and disease, and for interpretation of volume-dependent lung function parameters such as respiratory mechanics including airway resistance and forced expiratory flows. The only static lung volume that can be readily assessed in non-co-operative infants and very young children is functional residual capacity. Whole-body plethysmography assessment of functional residual capacity is simple to apply, rapid and reproducible. In addition, with adaptation of the equipment, simultaneous measurements of airway resistance may be obtained. Following the publication of recommendations for both equipment and methodology by an international task force, a new generation of infant whole-body plethysmographs has become available. Although standardization of the equipment has facilitated the application of whole-body plethysmography, its use for routine physiological and clinically orientated measurements is still limited by the lack of appropriate reference data. Recent evidence suggests that with modern equipment new reference data will have to be established to avoid misinterpretation of test results. Airway resistance measurements, which used to be dependent on heated rebreathing bags, could potentially be facilitated by electronic compensation for BTPS conditions; these algorithms, however, have not yet been validated. The aim of this chapter is to describe whole-body plethysmography in infants and very young children, explain the most commonly measured indices of lung function using this technique and discuss their potential clinical value, describe changes in these parameters expected in paediatric respiratory disease, discuss the availability of normal reference values, and give advice for interpretation of test results.

Introduction

An infant whole-body plethysmograph is a valuable tool for obtaining simultaneous measurements of lung volume and airway resistance. Functional residual capacity (FRC) is the volume remaining in the lung at end-tidal expiration and is the only lung volume that can be measured routinely in infants and very young children. It is important for interpreting volume-dependent pulmonary mechanics such as forced expiratory flows and airway resistance, and for assessing lung growth and development both in health and disease. FRC can be assessed either by using whole-body plethysmography (FRC_{pleth} or FRC_p), or by gas dilution techniques ($FRC_{gaswashout}$) [1]. Assessment of FRC_{pleth} is rapid and reproducible, but, as the equipment has been complex and required considerable operator training, has generally been restricted to specialized centres [2]. More recently, following the publication of recommendations regarding equipment and methodology for infant whole-body plethysmography [3], a new generation of infant whole-body plethysmographs has become commercially available, potentially allowing a more widespread application of this technique [3, 4].

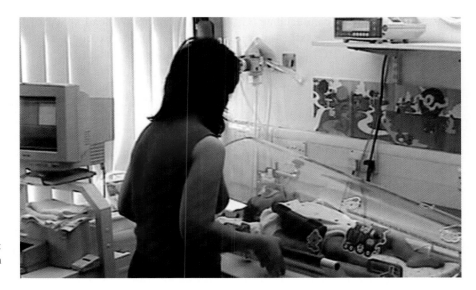

Fig. 1. Infant whole-body plethysmography: setting within an infant lung function laboratory.

Whole-body plethysmography was first described by DuBois et al. [5, 6] in 1956 and has since been adapted for use in infants. In contrast to adults and co-operative children, infants are measured in a supine position lying within a rigid, closed container, the plethysmograph (fig. 1). Tidal flow (and, by integration, volume) is recorded from a flowmeter through which the infant is breathing via a facemask. Assessment of intrathoracic lung volume (FRC_{pleth}) is based on Boyle's law, which states that under isothermal conditions the product of pressure and volume of a fixed mass of gas will be constant. This translates to infant whole-body plethysmography as follows. During occlusion at the airway opening, which is usually performed by a remotely controlled shutter to hold the lung at a constant volume, the infant makes respiratory efforts against this occlusion which lead to compression and rarefaction of the intrathoracic lung volume. The resultant changes in alveolar pressure are reflected at the airway opening during periods where there is no airflow with equilibration of pressures throughout the respiratory system. The alveolar pressure changes can then be related to changes in alveolar volume, which are reflected by changes in plethysmographic volume (or pressure) to calculate lung volume during the occlusion. By subtracting the dead space of the apparatus and any tidal volume (Vt) above end-expiration at the moment of occlusion, FRC_{pleth} can be calculated.

Under certain conditions, airway resistance can be measured at the same test occasion with the infant breathing spontaneously within the closed plethysmograph [2, 3].

Terminology and Definitions

The primary lung function parameters assessed during whole-body plethysmography are FRC_{pleth} and airway resistance (R_{aw}). FRC_{pleth} is the volume remaining within the thorax at end-tidal expiration, including any areas of gas trapped behind obstructed airways. The term 'airway resistance' should be reserved for plethysmographic measurements where changes in alveolar pressure are related to changes in airflow. In contrast, pulmonary resistance as assessed from changes in transpulmonary (oesophageal) pressure includes airway and lung tissue resistance, and finally, the resistance of the respiratory system as assessed by single or multiple occlusion techniques includes airway, lung tissue and chest wall resistance.

R_{aw} is the pressure difference that must be applied between alveoli and the external atmosphere to produce a gas flow of 1 litre/s at the airway opening. However, in- and expired gas has to be kept fully saturated with water vapour and at body temperature [body temperature, pressure, and saturated (BTPS) conditions], or thermal changes occurring during in- and expiration have to be adequately corrected electronically. Then, pressure changes within the plethysmograph and alveolar pressure are inversely proportional such that R_{aw} can be calculated from changes in plethysmographic pressure and flow. The advantage of plethysmographic assessment of airway resistance is that it can be measured throughout the respiratory cycle and thus reflects dynamic conditions. Several other lung function parameters can be derived from these measurements: airway conductance (G_{aw}) is the reciprocal of R_{aw}; specific resistance (sR_{aw}) is the product of R_{aw} and FRC ($sR_{aw} = R_{aw} \cdot FRC$) and can be obtained during normal tidal breathing without the need for airway occlusions, and specific conductance (sG_{aw}) is G_{aw} in relation to FRC ($sG_{aw} = G_{aw}/FRC$).

Equipment

Detailed information regarding recommendations for equipment when using an infant whole-body plethysmograph can be found in several documents published by a joint European Respiratory Society/American Thoracic Society Task Force on Standards for Infant Respiratory Function Tests [3, 7].

The volume of the plethysmograph should be 70–100 litres to allow measurements in infants up to 15 kg and a length of approximately 85 cm. It should be noted that the smaller the lungs in relation to the volume of the box, the smaller the box signal. For example, if the actual FRC = 100 ml, and $\Delta P_{alv} = \pm 2$ kPa during an airway occlusion at end-inspiration (i.e. 2% of the ambient pressure which is approximately 100 kPa), ΔV_{pleth} will be 2 ml only. In a volume-constant infant whole-body plethysmograph with a box volume of 100 litres, this 2-ml change in volume will cause a box pressure change of $\sim 100 \cdot 2/100,000$ kPa or 2 Pa! This illustrates, why an infant lung function laboratory should be in a quiet environment where the doors can stay closed during the entire measurement procedure.

The lid of the box should be designed to allow observation of the infant during the entire measurement procedure and to allow rapid access to the child at any time. Within the box, compressible objects such as cushions and foam mattresses should be kept to a minimum. The combined time constant of the equipment should approximate 10–14 s. The box signal should respond in a linear fashion to known inputs over an appropriate range of breathing frequencies (e.g. 20–100 breaths/min) taking into account that the changes in plethysmographic pressure may be as small as 1–2 ml during assessment of FRC and may be even smaller during assessment of airway resistance. Manufacturers for each individual system should provide the exact specifications.

The flowmeter must be linear over the range of flows encountered. This applies to both heated and unheated systems. The shutter should be automated and remotely controlled with a default to the open position in case of software or hardware failure. Occlusion should be possible both at end-inspiration and end-expiration. The combined dead space of the flowmeter and the shutter should not exceed $2 \, \text{ml} \cdot \text{kg}^{-1}$. The combined apparatus resistance should be less than 20% of the infant's intrinsic resistance. The linearity of the flowmeter should not be altered by the introduction of the shutter into the system. The face mask used with the flowmeter and the shutter should have the lowest possible dead space (effective dead space of the mask can be estimated as 50% of the water displacement volume) [8], should be transparent and firm, and be sealed with a rim of therapeutic putty to achieve an airtight seal.

Conventionally, airway resistance used to be measured using a heated rebreathing system to allow respired gases to reach BTPS conditions [9, 10]. However, as such systems are highly complex to construct and to operate, attempts have been made to electronically compensate for thermal changes in modern commercially available whole-body plethysmographs. As this electronic compensation has not been validated yet, recommendations for airway resistance measurements cannot be given in this review. Preliminary data suggest that values of airway resistance obtained with electronic compensation differ from those obtained using the old-fashioned heated rebreathing systems [9, 11]. They do, however, appear to reflect baseline airway resistance and bronchial responsiveness in children and adults [12, 13]. Perhaps most interesting is the assessment of specific resistance [14] because it can be calculated from unoccluded tidal breathing only, making it feasible to obtain data in unsedated infants and young children.

Data Collection

When performing whole-body plethysmography in infants and very young children, measurement conditions including recommendations regarding sedation, posture, monitoring, recent respiratory tract infections, and recording of the actual weight and length are similar to the ones for other methods for assessing infant lung function. Details have been published elsewhere [15].

For assessment of both FRC_{pleth} and R_{aw}, the recommended sampling rate is 200 Hz.

For safety reasons the infant should be monitored (pulse oximetry) throughout the measurement and tidal flow (volume) and pressure at the airway opening (P_{ao}) should be displayed continuously on the monitor whenever mask and apparatus are connected. When measurements of forced expiratory flows using the 'squeeze' technique are intended during the same test occasion, the 'squeeze' jacket should not be tightened as it may influence tidal breathing, lung volume and pulmonary mechanics [16]. Similarly, the

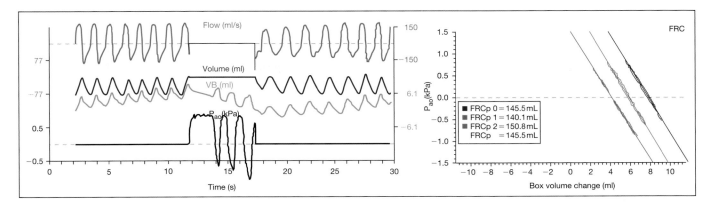

Fig. 2. Time-based plot of signals recorded during plethysmographic assessment of FRC: flow, volume, box volume (VB), airway opening pressure (P_{ao}) (note: no evidence of leak, 2 complete efforts against the occlusion). x-y plot of pressure at the airway opening versus changes in box volume (note: good phase relation, no 'looping').

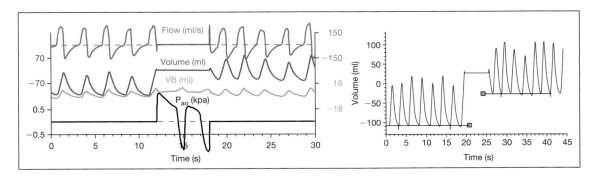

Fig. 3. Significant leak with 'step-up' in EEL post occlusion. Decay in airway opening pressure (P_{ao}) during occlusion. Change in EEL = 70%. Data not acceptable.

measurement protocol should be such that all tidal breathing measurements including plethysmographic assessment of FRC and R_{aw} are performed prior to the forced expiratory manoeuvres as results may be influenced by the order in which the measurements are performed [17].

Once the mask is applied and the apparatus is attached, an occlusion should be performed to ensure a leak-free seal. Only then, may the box lid be closed and is tidal breathing monitored. Thermal equilibration within the plethysmograph can be assessed by observing the time-based trace of the plethysmographic pressure (volume) signal. When there is no significant drift of the box pressure signal, tidal breathing may be recorded for the calculation of airway resistance. With the infant breathing regularly in quiet sleep with a stable end-expiratory level (EEL), an airway occlusion is performed at end-inspiration. The shutter

is released after at least two complete respiratory efforts against the occlusion have been recorded (fig. 2).

Post occlusion, the EEL is checked, with a marked step-up usually indicating a leak (fig. 3). In the absence of an obvious leak, the phase relationship of P_{ao} and the box pressure signal is visually inspected from an x-y plot (fig. 2). This manoeuvre is repeated until at least three satisfactory manoeuvres have been obtained [18].

To allow adequate assessment of data quality both during actual data collection and immediately following each individual manoeuvre, the monitor display should be set up to include time-based traces of flow, volume, P_{ao} and box pressure, an x-y plot of P_{ao} versus box volume during the occlusion (fig. 2); for resistance measurements, x-y plots of flow versus box volume should be displayed in addition to the time-based traces (fig. 5).

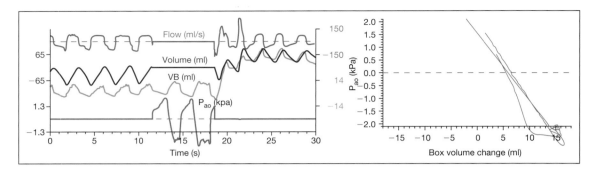

Fig. 4. Unacceptable data: Severe phase lag ('looping'), distorted box volume and Vt.

Calculation of FRC_pleth

The total occluded gas volume (TOGV, i.e. FRC_{pleth} plus apparatus dead space including face mask plus any volume occluded above the previously established EEL) is determined from the ratio of change in box volume to the pressure at the airway opening during respiratory efforts against the closed shutter ($\Delta V_{pleth}:\Delta P_{ao}$). Prior to all calculations, Vt has to be converted to BTPS conditions and corrected for any remaining drift. The EEL has to be calculated from at least six end-expiratory points following BTPS and drift correction. The volume occluded above this EEL (V_{occ}) has to be calculated to allow subsequent subtraction from the TOGV. Drift correction of the box signal is performed as follows. By definition, V_{pleth} should be 'zero' at points where P_{ao} is 'zero'. The change in V_{pleth} from one such transition point to the next can then be subtracted from the value recorded by applying a linear drift correction in time. The P_{ao} and V_{pleth} signals are then evaluated further during that part of the respiratory effort where there are rapid changes in P_{ao} (to improve the signal to noise ratio). To do this, the signal trace is separated into single respiratory efforts, each consisting of an 'inspiratory' (decreasing P_{ao}) and an 'expiratory' (increasing P_{ao}) effort against the occlusion. The slopes of the ratio $V_{pleth}:P_{ao}$ are then calculated by regression of V_{pleth} and P_{ao} through all data points excluding the final 5% in order to truncate peaks and troughs where the noise of the box signal will be greatest. An average slope is calculated from a combined inspiratory and subsequent expiratory effort. TOGV is then calculated from these average slopes. Satisfactory slopes for each occlusion manoeuvre are then averaged to give a single result for that manoeuvre:

$$TOGV = \text{average slope } (\Delta V_{pleth}:\Delta P_{ao}) \cdot (P_{amb} - P_{H_2O})$$
$$\cdot \, [(V_{pleth} - V_{infant})/V_{pleth}]$$

where P_{amb} is the ambient barometric pressure, P_{H_2O} is the water vapour pressure at 37°C (i.e. 6.25 kPa), and V_{infant} is the infant's volume in litres (calculated from the weight, i.e. 1 kg body weight equals 1 litre volume displacement).

To obtain FRC_{pleth}, apparatus dead space (ds_{app}) and volume occluded above the EEL (V_{occ}) have to be subtracted from TOGV:

$$FRC_{pleth} = TOGV - V_{dsapp} - V_{occ}.$$

As final result, the mean (and SD) of five (minimum three) satisfactory occlusions is reported.

Criteria for Acceptable Data

Only data where there has been a stable EEL before and after occlusion should be accepted. During the occlusion, flow has to be 'zero' and changes in box pressure and P_{ao} should be in phase with no evidence of glottic closure or leak (see above and table 1 for quality criteria).

Assumptions and Limitations

For the assessment of FRC_{pleth}, the occlusion is usually performed at end-inspiration. Historically, occlusions were usually performed at end-expiration. However, occlusion at end-inspiration is generally less disturbing to the infant as the Hering-Breuer reflex is more active at higher lung volumes and glottic closure is less likely to occur. Even after correctly subtracting the actual Vt above FRC from TOGV the resultant FRC_{pleth} calculated from occlusions at end-inspiration may be slightly higher (around 1 ml/kg) as compared to data calculated from end-expiration [19].

Because the airways are more distended at end-inspiration, airway resistance is lower and equilibration of pressures throughout the respiratory system is more readily achieved. For valid results to be obtained, during the occlusion when

Table 1. Summary of criteria for technical acceptability of FRC_{pleth} data

Subject in quiet sleep prior to and during measurement	
Stable EEL: variability (SD) of EEL of the last 5 breaths prior to occlusion <5 (10)% of mean Vt of these breaths	
No evidence of leak during occlusion: no decay of pressure plateau during end-inspiratory pause; no flow through the pneumotachometer during occlusion; no significant change in EEL after release of occlusion [difference in EEL prior to and after occlusion <15 (25)% of the mean Vt]	Fig. 3
At least two complete respiratory efforts against the occlusion: essential for adequate correction of the drift of V_{pleth} during airway occlusions	Fig. 2
No phase lag or 'looping' between V_{pleth} and P_{ao}; no signs of glottic closure or permanent of intermittent airway obstruction precluding rapid and adequate equilibration of alveolar and mouth pressures (x-y plot at appropriate magnification with a minimal angle of ~30° recommended to ascertain such signal quality)	Fig. 4
Reported results based on 3 acceptable occlusions: mean, SD and/or coefficient of variation (CV; CV = SD · mean^{-1} · 100) to be reported. CV <10% between results from the 3 acceptable occlusions	
Cross-check of results by an independent expert observer if possible	

there is no flow (absence of leak, no resistive pressure losses) complete equilibration between pressures in the alveoli and the airway opening must be assured. For pressures to equilibrate it is assumed that pressure changes applied to the lung are evenly distributed and that pressure-volume changes are limited to gas within the thorax. Furthermore, changes in volume and pressure are assumed to be isothermal.

Clinical Applications

Whole-body plethysmography measures all gas within the thorax (in contrast, gas dilution techniques only measure gas communicating readily with the large airways). In the presence of intrathoracic airway obstruction, FRC_{pleth} may be increased and thus may be a sensitive index of obstructive airway disease primarily involving more peripheral airways such as bronchiolitis or cystic fibrosis [20].

Low FRC_{pleth} may be detected if alveolar development is abnormal, e.g. following premature delivery, if there is marked atelectasis, or in lung diseases with reduced lung compliance, e.g. interstitial lung disease.

Table 2 summarizes a selection of studies to illustrate the broad spectrum of possible applications of FRC_{pleth} measurements in: (1) the assessment of normal growth and development of the lungs and factors affecting them, (2) the use of FRC as a reference lung volume to interpret volume-dependent mechanical characteristics of the lungs, (3) the assessment of severity of lung disease, and (4) determining

the degree of gas trapping (difference between simultaneous assessments of FRC_{pleth} and $FRC_{gas-washout}$. Most of these studies provide both FRC_{pleth} and R_{aw} data (table 2).

Appropriate reference data are essential if a misinterpretation of the results obtained is to be avoided. The inappropriate use of reference values may lead to a failure to identify true lung disease or may misclassify test results as abnormal. It is essential that only reference values are used that are obtained in a similar population, using the same technique with the same protocol and equipment. For FRC_{pleth}, a prediction equation with confidence limits was proposed in 1995 by Stocks and Quanjer [29] as part of an ATS Task Force on lung volumes:

$$FRC_{pleth}\text{-predicted} = 2.36 \cdot length(cm)^{0.75} \cdot weight(kg)^{0.63}.$$

However, when data were collated for developing this prediction equation it became apparent that there was a trend for values of FRC_{pleth} to become lower with time. This phenomenon was recently explored by one of us (GH) [18] and we observed a progressive decline in plethysmographic lung volumes in infants, with the lowest values obtained with the new generation of infant whole-body plethysmographs, which have been developed following the publication of recommendations for standardization of equipment, data collection, and analysis. The mean difference in FRC_{pleth} obtained in healthy infants to predicted values in this most recent study amounted to 7 ml/kg body weight, a difference which is both statistically significant and clinically relevant. The observed differences could be related to differences in the

Table 2. Application of FRC_{pleth} measurements

Stocks, 1977 [21]	Assessment of the functional growth and development of the lungs during the first year of life
Stocks and Godfrey, 1977 [22]	Assessment of sG_{aw} in relation to postconceptional age during infancy
Kraemer and Schoni, 1990 [23]	Assessment of FRC_{pleth} and R_{aw} in wheezy infants treated with inhaled β_2-agonists
Wauer et al., 1998 [24]	Comparison of FRC_{pleth} and $FRC_{gas-washout}$ in infants with and without chronic neonatal lung disease
Milner et al., 1999 [25]	Assessment of effects of smoking during pregnancy on neonatal lung function
Dezateux et al., 1999 [26]	Characterization of impaired airway function and wheezing in infancy (the influence of maternal smoking and a genetic predisposition to asthma)
Ljungberg et al., 2002 [20]	Assessment of trapped gas in infants with cystic fibrosis as indicator of early small airway involvement
Castile et al., 2004 [27]	Assessment of gas trapping in normal infants and those with cystic fibrosis
Robin et al., 2004 [28]	Comparison of pulmonary function between infants with bronchopulmonary dysplasia and normal subjects

study populations, changes in the protocols for data acquisition, analysis and quality control, or to differences in equipment. It had to be concluded that the published reference data [29] cannot be used for interpretation of results obtained with new equipment. This has several implications: there is an urgent need to develop new reference data from collaborative studies using the same equipment and standardized protocols. Furthermore, the relationship between lung volumes measured by infant plethysmography and gas dilution techniques will have to be re-evaluated. It may well be that the physiological difference in infants is much lower than previously assumed and in fact very similar to that found in healthy adults and older children [20].

Thus, based on this very recent evidence, currently no recommendations can be given as to which reference data should be used for interpreting FRC_{pleth} in infants. If modern equipment is used, the 'old' equation certainly should not be used as misinterpretation of data is likely. Normal values appear to be similar to those expected from the gas dilution techniques and are likely to fall within the range of 13–26 ml/kg body weight.

Calculation of Airway Resistance

As mentioned above, the traditional method to measure airway resistance has been to use a heated rebreathing bag for maintaining respired gas at BTPS conditions. However, there is no commercial system offering this approach.

Instead, electronic compensation for thermal changes has been introduced by the manufacturers. However, this approach still needs to be validated, values obtained are not the same as those from a heated rebreathing system, and recent evidence suggests that considerable validation work will be necessary before these new systems can be used with confidence [11].

Thus, only a broad overview for the calculation of airway resistance data will be given in this paper. The essential quality criterion for assessing plethysmographic R_{aw} is that there is a good phase relationship between pressure (the box volume or pressure signal) and flow (fig. 5).

As for FRC_{pleth}, prior to any calculations, V_{pleth} must be drift corrected. Breaths should not be used for analysis if the drift is very marked. Note that in healthy infants the signal to noise ratio may be a considerable problem as plethysmographic pressure changes are very small in healthy infants with a low resistance. From the total R_{aw} calculated, apparatus resistance (R_{app}; usually shutter and flowmeter) must be subtracted.

Because airway resistance is highly dependent on lung volume, with an increase in lung volume due to growth or as an effect of disease resulting in an increase in airway calibre and, therefore, decrease in resistance, it is important to relate R_{aw} to FRC, i.e. calculate specific R_{aw}: $sR_{aw} = FRC \cdot R_{aw}$.

Specific airway resistance can also be calculated directly from the relationship of change in V_{pleth} to change in flow prior to any airway occlusion provided that there are no artefacts due to changes in humidity and temperature of the

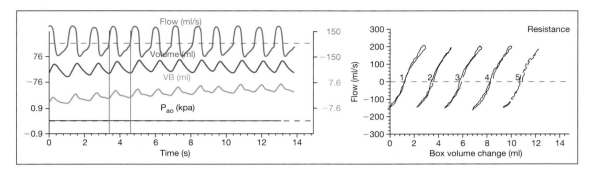

Fig. 5. Assessment of sR$_{aw}$ during quiet tidal breathing in the closed plethysmograph. Note: good phase relationship between pressure (box volume or pressure signal) and flow.

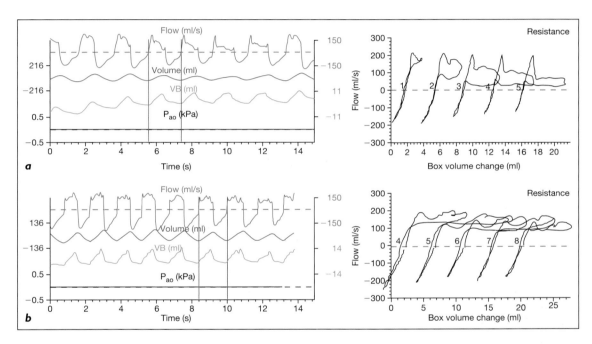

Fig. 6. Examples of severely distorted flow volume relationships due to intermittent (*a*) and permanent (*b*) upper airway obstruction.

respired gas (illustrating how crucial valid algorithms for electronic compensation are):

$$sR_{aw} = (\Delta V_{pleth}/\Delta flow) \cdot (P_{amb} - P_{H_2O}) \cdot (V_{pleth} - V_{infant})/V_{pleth} - sR_{app}$$

where sR$_{app}$ is the specific resistance of the apparatus (sR$_{app}$ = R$_{app}$ · FRC$_{pleth}$). If FRC$_{pleth}$ is not available, a predicted value of 22 ml/kg can be substituted.

If valid FRC$_{pleth}$ measurements have been obtained, R$_{aw}$ can be calculated for the exact lung volume at which it has been measured: R$_{aw}$ = sR$_{aw}$/FRC. This allows calculation

of conductance (G$_{aw}$ = 1/R$_{aw}$) and specific G$_{aw}$ (sG$_{aw}$ = 1/sR$_{aw}$).

When results are reported, a minimum of five breaths should be used to calculate the mean (SD). In addition, a typical pressure-flow loop should be part of the result reported.

As resistance varies throughout the breath, several different resistance values reflecting different parts of the tidal respiratory effort may be calculated. Various approaches have been described. Perhaps the most robust approach if electronic compensation is used will be to calculate effective resistance (R_{eff}) which is total resistance using all sample points throughout the breath.

However, changes in resistance through single breaths may provide important information. For example, an infant with upper airway obstruction will have an elevated inspiratory resistance; in contrast, an infant with small airway obstruction will have an elevated expiratory resistance depending on severity and localization of the underlying changes (see fig. 6 for examples of severe upper airway obstruction). The technique is highly sensitive, and hence measurements are likely to be affected by minimal changes in the patency of the upper airways, which may even occur during quiet sleep.

Conclusions

Infant whole-body plethysmography remains an invaluable tool when assessing infant lung function. Within minutes of starting the measurement, information regarding lung volume and airway function may be obtained.

For assessment of FRC modern equipment has become available that complies with recent recommendations regarding equipment, data collection and analysis. However, it appears as if existing reference data will not be useful for interpretation of data obtained with this equipment.

For assessment of airway resistance, electronic compensation may become a convenient way to facilitate the actual measurements. At present, however, this approach is not validated at all. Furthermore, there is no consensus yet, which is the best way of analyzing R_{aw} data. Probably, more than one parameter will have to be used if R_{aw} is to be described adequately. A promising approach is to assess sR_{aw} without performing any airway occlusion. However, further validation is required before these data can be used with confidence.

Although the actual measurements have been greatly facilitated by modern equipment, interpretation of data obtained is currently very difficult as new ways of data transformation will still have to be fully validated and appropriate reference data are lacking for both FRC_{pleth} and $(s)R_{aw}$.

References

1 Morris MG, Gustafsson P, Tepper R, Gappa M, Stocks J: The bias flow nitrogen washout technique for measuring the functional residual capacity in infants. ERS/ATS Task Force on Standards for Infant Respiratory Function Testing. Eur Respir J 2001;17: 529–536.

2 Stocks J, Marchal F, Kraemer R, Gutkowski P, Bar-Yishay E, Godfrey S: Plethysmographic assessment of functional residual capacity and airway resistance; in Stocks J, Sly PD, Tepper RS, Morgan WJ: Infant Respiratory Function Testing, ed 1. New York, Wiley, 1996, pp 191–239.

3 Stocks J, Godfrey S, Beardsmore C, Bar-Yishay E, Castile R: Standards for infant respiratory function testing: Plethysmographic measurements of lung volume and airway resistance. Eur Respir J 2001;17:302–312.

4 Reinmann B, Stocks J, Frey U: Assessment of an infant whole-body plethysmograph using an infant lung function model. Eur Respir J 2001;17:765–772.

5 DuBois AB, Botelho SY, Comroe JH: A new method of measuring airway resistance in man using a body plethysmograph. J Clin Invest 1956;35:327–334.

6 DuBois AB, Botelho SY, Bedell GN, Marshall R, Comroe JH: A rapid plethysmographic method for measuring TGV. J Clin Invest 1956;35:322–326.

7 Frey U, Stocks J, Coates A, Sly P, Bates J: Standards for infant respiratory function testing: Specifications for equipment used for infant pulmonary function testing. Eur Respir J 2000;16:731–740.

8 Morris MG: A simple new technique to measure the effective dead space of the face mask with a water volumeter in infants. Eur Respir J 1999;14:1163–1166.

9 Stocks J, Godfrey S: Specific airway conductance in relation to postconceptional age during infancy. J Appl Physiol 1977;43:144–154.

10 Stocks J, Levy NM, Godfrey S: A new apparatus for the accurate measurement of airway resistance in infancy. J Appl Physiol 1977; 43:155–159.

11 Subbarao P, Hulskamp G, Stocks J: Limitations of electronic compensation for measuring airway resistance in infants. Am J Respir Crit Care Med 2004;169;A488.

12 Peslin R, Duvivier C, Malvestio P, Benis AR, Polu JM: Frequency dependence of specific airway resistance in a commercialized plethysmograph. Eur Respir J 1996;9:1747–1750.

13 Klug B, Bisgaard H: Measurement of the specific airway resistance by plethysmography in young children accompanied by an adult. Eur Respir J 1997;10:1599–1605.

14 Dab I, Alexander F: A simplified approach to the measurement of specific airway resistance. Pediatr Res 1976;10:996–999.

15 Gaultier C, Fletcher M, Beardsmore C, Motoyama E, Stocks J: Measurement conditions; in Stocks J, Sly PD, Tepper RS, Morgan WJ (eds): Infant Respiratory Function Testing, ed 1. New York, Wiley, 1996, pp 29–44.

16 Hoo A-F, Lum S, Goetz I, Dezateux CA, Stocks J: Influence of jacket placement on respiratory compliance during raised lung volume measurements in infants. Pediatr Pulmonol 2001;31:51–58.

17 Lum S, Hulskamp G, Hoo AF, Ljungberg H, Stocks J: Effect of the raised lung volume technique on subsequent measures of V'maxFRC in infants. Pediatr Pulmonol 2004;38:146–154.

18 Hulskamp G, Hoo AF, Ljungberg H, Lum S, Pillow JJ, Stocks J: Progressive decline in plethysmographic lung volumes in infants: Physiology or technology? Am J Respir Crit Care Med 2003;168:1003–1009.

19 McCoy KS, Castile RG, Allen ED, Filbrun DA, Flucke RL, Bar-Yishay E: Functional residual capacity (FRC) measurements by plethysmography and helium dilution in normal infants. Pediatr Pulmonol 1995;19: 282–290.

20 Ljungberg H, Hulskamp G, Hoo A-F, Pillow JJ, Lum S, Gustafsson P, Stocks J: Estimates of plethysmographic FRC exceed those by gas dilution in infants with cystic fibrosis (CF) but not in healthy controls. Thorax 2002;57(suppl 3):iii23.

21 Stocks J: The functional growth and development of the lung during the first year of life. Early Hum Dev 1977;1:285–309.

22 Stocks J, Godfrey S: Specific airway conductance in relation to postconceptional age during infancy. J Appl Physiol 1977;43: 144–154.

23 Kraemer R, Schoni MH: Improvement from pulmonary hyperinflation and bronchial obstruction following sympathomimetics systemically given in infants with bronchopulmonary diseases. Z Erkr Atmungsorgane 1990;174:85–96.

24 Wauer RR, Maurer T, Nowotny T, Schmalisch G: Assessment of functional residual capacity using nitrogen washout and plethysmographic techniques in infants with and without bronchopulmonary dysplasia. Intensive Care Med 1998;24:469–475.
25 Milner AD, Marsh MJ, Ingram DM, Fox GF, Susiva C: Effects of smoking in pregnancy on neonatal lung function. Arch Dis Child Fetal Neonatal Ed 1999;80:F8–14.
26 Dezateux C, Stocks J, Dundas I, Fletcher ME: Impaired airway function and wheezing in infancy. The influence of maternal smoking and a genetic predisposition to asthma. Am J Respir Crit Care Med 1999;159:403–410.

27 Castile RG, Iram D, McCoy KS: Gas trapping in normal infants and in infants with cystic fibrosis. Pediatr Pulmonol 2004;37: 461–469.
28 Robin B, Kim YJ, Huth J, Klocksieben J, Torres M, Tepper RS, Castile RG, Solway J, Hershenson MB, Goldstein-Filbrun A: Pulmonary function in bronchopulmonary dysplasia. Pediatr Pulmonol 2004;37:236–242.
29 Stocks J, Quanjer PH: Reference values for residual volume, functional residual capacity and total lung capacity. Eur Respir J 1995;8: 492–506.

Prof. Dr. med. Monika Gappa
Paediatric Pulmonology and Neonatology
Medizinische Hochschule Hannover
Carl-Neuberg-Strasse 1, DE–30625
Hannover (Germany)
Tel. +49 511 532 9137
Fax +49 511 532 9125
E-Mail gappa.monika@mh-hannover.de

Hammer J, Eber E (eds): Paediatric Pulmonary Function Testing.
Prog Respir Res. Basel, Karger, 2005, vol 33, pp 54–65

....

Measurement of Functional Residual Capacity and Ventilation Inhomogeneity by Gas Dilution Techniques

P.M. Gustafsson[a]   H. Ljungberg[b]

[a]Department of Paediatric Clinical Physiology, Queen Silvia Children's Hospital, Göteborg, and
[b]Sachs Children's Hospital, Karolinska Institute, Stockholm, Sweden

Abstract

The functional residual capacity (FRC) is the only static lung volume measured routinely in infants. It can be measured using infant whole body plethysmography or one of several gas dilution tests. While plethysmography measures all compressible gas within the thorax, the gas dilution methods measure the volumes readily communicating with the central airways. Normative data have been published on FRC in infants both with gas dilution methods and plethysmography. A correct measure of FRC is important when interpreting other lung function test findings. An abnormally raised FRC suggests hyperinflation and low values suggest a restrictive disorder. A markedly higher FRC with plethysmography versus gas dilution suggests the presence of marked gas trapping. Several gas dilution methods can be used in infants, but newer methods based on breath-by-breath recordings have the advantage of providing data on the overall efficiency of gas mixing, i.e. on inhomogeneity of ventilation distribution. Simple indices of impaired gas mixing are sensitive indicators of peripheral airway obstruction and may be of particular importance for early detection of lung involvement in chronic lung disorders such as cystic fibrosis. New methods for analyzing washout recordings may provide further information on the mechanisms behind the impaired gas mixing.

Introduction

The functional residual capacity (FRC) is the volume of gas remaining in the lungs after a tidal expiration. Currently it is the only static lung volume measured routinely in infants [1]. In the older child and in the adult the FRC is the result of a balance between the expanding elastic forces of the chest wall and the inward recoil of the lung. Because the chest wall of the infant is more compliant than in older subjects, the infant has to actively 'protect' its FRC. This is undertaken autonomously by closing the glottis and activating inspiratory muscles during expiration, and by starting inspiration before the mechanical balance point has been reached [2]. In a sense the FRC is therefore a dynamically controlled lung volume in the infant. Like all other lung volumes the FRC is presented at body temperature, pressure, and saturation conditions. The infant is investigated during quiet sleep, generally after sedation with chloral hydrate or triclofos sodium, and the same measurement conditions as for other infant lung function tests should be adhered to [3].

A correct measure of FRC is needed when estimating lung size and lung growth in the infant, and it is essential when interpreting other, volume-dependent, measures of lung function such as forced expiratory flows or measures of lung mechanics. The FRC may be pathologically raised as a result of hyperinflation in obstructive airway disorders and reduced in restrictive conditions.

The design of the airway tree with dichotomous branching of the conducting and the intra-acinar airways allows for optimal mixing of the resident gas in the lungs with fresh inspired air. This is essential for matching of the ventilation to perfusion in the lungs and for efficient gas exchange. Generalized or focal obstruction of the airways, particularly of the peripheral airways (arbitrarily defined as airway

Table 1. Methods of measuring FRC in infants

Infant whole-body plethysmography
Gas dilution methods
   Closed-circuit helium dilution
   Open-circuit N_2 washout (bypass flow method)
   Breath-by-breath inert gas washout techniques
      e.g. N_2 MBW (multiple-breath washout)
      e.g. SF_6 MBW

Table 2. Inert marker gases that may be used for measuring FRC in infants and recording techniques

Inert gas	Measuring techniques
Ar	Mass spectrometry
CH_4 (methane)	IR detector
He	He catharometer; mass spectrometry
N_2	Nitrogen analyzer (emission spectrophotometry); mass spectrometry
SF_6	Mass spectrometry; IR detector; ultrasound technique (molar mass measurements)

generation ≥ 8), will result in uneven distribution of ventilation, reduced efficiency of gas mixing, and gas trapping. Such abnormalities may be early signs of conditions known to affect the peripheral airways in infants, e.g. cystic fibrosis (CF). Data obtained when measuring FRC by some gas dilution methods can be used to assess the degree of non-uniformity of ventilation distribution. Some information can also be obtained about the mechanisms causing ventilation inhomogeneity and where along the airway tree the disease process is taking place. Furthermore, the presence or extent of gas trapping can be assessed in conjunction with FRC measurements. The peripheral airways have been called the 'silent zone of the lung' because other methods of assessing lung function are in principal insensitive to obstruction in these pathways [4] in infants as well as in older children and adults. Measuring FRC using methods giving additional data on ventilation distribution and gas trapping may consequently provide the clinician and the researcher with unique and relevant information about the pathological processes resulting in dysfunction of the peripheral airways.

Methods

FRC may be measured using infant whole-body plethysmography [5–7] or gas dilution techniques [8] (table 1).

The gas dilution methods use inert marker gases to measure the lung volume that readily communicates with the central airways during tidal breathing and therefore do not include volumes that are closed off or ventilated extremely slowly. Plethysmography, on the other hand, measures all compressible intrathoracic gas volume, including noncommunicating regions. These may include gas-filled cysts, emphysematous bullae, air beyond closed off or obstructed airways or other volumes of gas in the thorax such as in the digestive tract. The difference in FRC obtained with the two techniques will therefore represent any such volumes, and is sometimes referred to as 'trapped gas'. Infant whole body plethysmography is covered in detail in the chapter of Gappa and Hülskamp [9].

Gas Dilution Methods

The marker gas used for these tests is a so-called inert gas, i.e. a gas that does not participate in gas exchange and has minimal or low solubility in blood and body tissue. Table 2 shows examples of inert marker gases that can be used for measuring FRC and ventilation inhomogeneity, and techniques that can be used to measure these gases. All gas dilution methods will underestimate true FRC in the presence of significant airway closure during tidal breathing. The gas dilution techniques used to measure FRC in infants are generally performed during tidal breathing, and include the closed-circuit helium dilution technique [10, 11] and open-circuit techniques (table 1).

Closed-Circuit Helium Dilution

When measuring FRC by the helium dilution technique, the infant is connected to a spirometer or a rebreathing bag containing a known helium concentration (fig. 1). Rebreathing continues until the helium concentration within the apparatus and the infant's lung have become equilibrated. CO_2 produced by the infant is continuously absorbed from the circuit and O_2 is added to the system, ideally at the same rate as it is consumed. In the ideal situation, the apparatus and the infant's lung are of similar volumes as this provides the largest changes in helium concentrations and minimizes errors in measurements. Assuming mass balance, FRC is calculated from the initial and the final helium concentrations and the known volume of the spirometer. The helium dilution technique is not as suitable for assessing ventilation inhomogeneity as open-circuit systems are. The time needed for achieving equilibration of helium concentration depends not only on the infant's condition but also to a large degree on the size and construction of the apparatus connected to the infant. To our knowledge, there are no helium dilution systems commercially available.

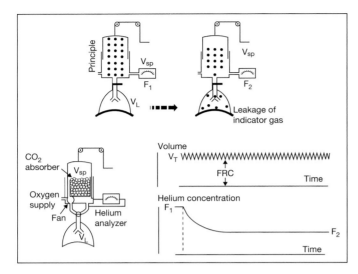

Fig. 1. Schematic illustration of FRC measurement using the closed-circuit helium dilution method. V_L = Infant's lung volume (FRC); V_{sp} = volume of the spirometer; F_1 = initial helium concentration; F_2 = final helium concentration, when equilibration between the reservoirs and the infant's lung has occurred [from 11, with permission].

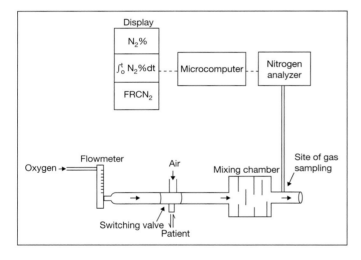

Fig. 2. Schematic illustration of FRC measurement using the N_2 bias flow system [from 10, with permission].

Bias Flow Nitrogen Washout

The first open-circuit system for FRC determination was the rather simple but robust system first described by Gerhardt et al. [12]. European Respiratory Society(ERS)/ American Thoracic Society (ATS) standards for the bias flow system have recently been published [8]. A schematic illustration of the method is given in figure 2. Via a sealed

face mask the infant is connected to a three-way valve allowing him to breathe either room air or 100% O_2 from a bias flow set above the infant's inspiratory flow rate, generally in the range of 5–10 litres/min for an infant of 5 kg body weight. At the end of an ordinary expiration the infant is switched from breathing room air to breathing pure oxygen from the bias flow. Expired gas is led to a mixing chamber. N_2 concentrations are continuously measured at the outlet port of the mixing chamber. The infant breathes pure oxygen until the reading is less than 0.5%. The system is calibrated using syringes containing given volumes of room air. The syringe is attached to the three-way valve, and pumped at similar tidal volumes (VT) and rates as the infant is thought to breathe with. The N_2 concentration integrated over time gives the amount of N_2 expired at a fixed bias flow from which the FRC is calculated [8, 12]. The bias flow N_2 washout method does not provide indices of ventilation inhomogeneity. Although robust in principal, this method has several potential sources of error [8]. One is the problem of connecting the infant at end expiration, which is difficult at high respiratory rates. A pneumotachometer may, however, be inserted between the face mask and the three-way valve to facilitate correct timing of infant connection. Another problem is the non-linearity of N_2 analyzers [13], which is difficult to account for with the original setup of this system. The bias flow N_2 washout system was marketed as part of the SensorMedics 2600 infant lung function testing system during the 1980s and early 1990s. To our knowledge, this system is not commercially available today.

Breath-by-Breath Washout Methods

In principal, breath-by-breath washout systems consist of a gas analyzer and a flow meter, recording marker gas concentrations and gas flow, respectively, close to the mouth, plus a device for delivering gas. A schematic illustration of such a system is given in figure 3a and b. The amount of inert gas inspired and expired is calculated by integration of gas concentration over volume [14]. FRC can be calculated from the cumulative expired volume of tracer gas divided by the difference in end-tidal concentrations at the start and end of the washout [14], and almost any index of ventilation inhomogeneity can be derived [15]. The challenges with the method are to be able to record gas concentrations accurately at a high respiratory rate with minimal sample volume, and to correctly align each gas sample with the corresponding flow sample. Furthermore, when using a pneumotachometer the dynamic viscosity of each gas sample needs to be accounted for before using the flow signal [13]. Keeping the external dead space (face mask plus flowmeter and adaptors) to a minimum is also

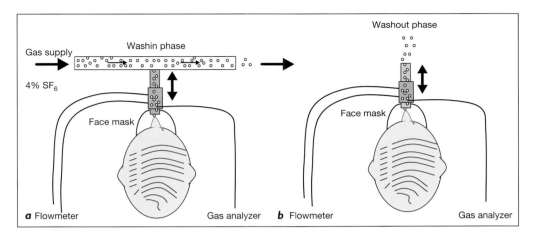

Fig. 3. *a*, *b* Schematic illustration of setup of a system for breath-by-breath measurements of FRC and ventilation inhomogeneity in infants using SF_6 as the inert marker gas, and a gas mixture containing 4% SF_6 for washin (see text for further explanations).

essential, not only for safety reasons but also to obtain representative information on ventilation inhomogeneity. No standards for this technique, when used in infants, have been published so far. Ideally, the external dead space volume should be less than 1 ml/kg body weight and the gas sample flow rates should be less than 10 ml/min. The gas analyzer should be linear in the range of concentrations measured, have a 10–90% response time less than 50 ms, and should update the signal by at least 50 Hz. The flowmeter should also be able to correctly record the breath signals, which means that it should have a flat dynamic response curve up to at least 10 Hz. Further information on general requirements for infant lung function testing is given in published ERS/ATS standards documents [16, 17]. Methods for correctly aligning gas concentration and flow signals in time have been described previously [18].

A new and exciting method of performing inert gas washout is the use of an ultrasonic device, which can measure both respiratory flows and molar mass of the gas samples at a high rate (200 Hz) [19]. A foreign inert marker gas with a molecular mass differing greatly from that of air, such as sulphur hexafluoride (SF_6), is used with this method. The method has the potential to circumvent many of the technical problems with conventional techniques. It is not the actual concentration of the particular inert gas that is measured, however, but the composition of the gas sample as a whole.

Several papers have been published using breath-by-breath inert gas washout in infants [14, 19–21]. Either a resident inert marker gas (N_2) has been washed out using pure oxygen [21], or a foreign inert gas, such as SF_6, has been washed in and washed out [14, 19, 20]. Different kinds of gas analyzers can be used for measuring various inert marker gases (table 2). The cheapest is the N_2 analyzer, which is still commercially available. It is rapidly responding but may need linearization to improve accuracy at low concentrations [13]. The mass spectrometer is the most versatile device. It is linear and can in principle measure any gas but it is rather expensive to buy and maintain. Analyzers based on infrared (IR) technology can measure marker gases, which absorb light in the IR range, such as SF_6 and CH_4. Both mainstream and sidestream devices can be used.

The advantage of doing an N_2 washout is that no foreign gases are needed and 100% O_2 for the washout is always available in a hospital setting. Commonly a breath-by-breath washout is continued until the end-tidal N_2 concentration is 2%, i.e. 1/40 of the initial concentration. This conventional limit comes from the fact that the first N_2 analyzers produced in the 1950s were unable to correctly record lower concentrations. One disadvantage with N_2 washout with oxygen is that the administration of pure O_2 may affect the infant's breathing pattern. We have frequently seen that the infant may reduce his VT markedly over 5–10 breaths when suddenly exposed to 100% O_2 [22]. The FRC obtained by N_2 washout should theoretically be greater than that measured using foreign marker gases because N_2 from other tissues is washed into the lungs via the blood during washout of the lungs.

A non-resident inert marker gas may instead be used, but this requires a washin phase before washout. On the

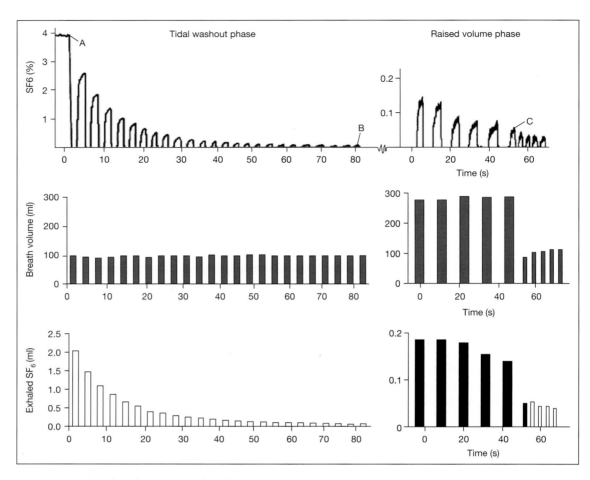

Fig. 4. Examples of washout tracings from breath-by-breath measurements of FRC and ventilation inhomogeneity in infants using SF_6 as the inert marker gas, and a gas mixture containing 4% SF_6 for washin. Data from the tidal phase are used for calculation of FRC, LCI and other indices of ventilation inhomogeneity. Data from the raised volume phase are used to calculate the volume of trapped gas. See text for further explanations. 'A' denotes end-tidal SF_6 concentration immediately before the start of washout; 'B' denotes end-tidal SF_6 concentration at end of tidal washout, and 'C' denotes end-tidal SF_6 concentration at end of raised volume phase [from 14, with permission].

other hand, the washin phase may also be used to calculate FRC and assess ventilation inhomogeneity [20]. FRC measurements in infants using an IR SF_6 detector have been described by Vilstrup et al. [20]. In our laboratory we use a gas mixture containing 4% SF_6 and 4% helium as a standard washin gas for various purposes. When doing breath-by-breath washouts in infants, the SF_6 signal but not the helium signal is used for calculation of FRC or indices of ventilation inhomogeneity, but both are utilized when doing single-breath tests in older subjects [23, 24]. During the washin phase the subject breathes the gas mixture containing 4% SF_6, 4% He, 21% O_2 and balance N_2 until equilibration of SF_6 is achieved throughout the lungs plus another 30 s [14]. For the washout phase, the

gas supply is then disconnected during expiration and the subject breathes room air, which continues until the end-tidal SF_6 concentration is below 0.1% (i.e. 1/40 of the starting concentration). The gas concentration is measured at the mouth opening using, for example, a respiratory mass spectrometer and the inspiratory and expiratory flows are measured with a flowmeter, for example a pneumotachometer. From such a washout (fig. 4), the FRC may be calculated and various indices of ventilation inhomogeneity are derived [14, 25].

Indices of Ventilation Inhomogeneity

While there are a number of publications reporting indices of ventilation inhomogeneity in children and

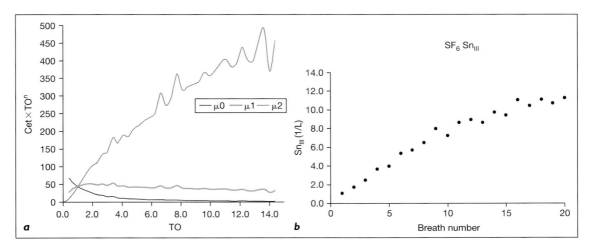

Fig. 5. Examples of curves extracted from a tidal washout using the technique described in figure 3 in a patient (JC) with CF [male, age 26 months, body weight 12.5 kg, diagnosis: CF colonized with *Pseudomonas aeruginosa*, FRC 344 ml, LCI 13.0 (+19.7 SD)]. SD denotes standard deviations above predicted mean. **a** Moment analysis curves. Cet = End-tidal inert gas concentration, normalized so that initial concentration corresponds to 100; TO = lung volume turnover number; n = 0, 1 or 2, which are the numbers used when calculating $\mu 0$, $\mu 1$ and $\mu 2$, respectively. See text for further explanations. **b** Sn_{III} for each breath during SF_6 washout plotted against breath number. This plot is used for delineation of the mechanisms behind ventilation inhomogeneity. In this subject Sn_{III} increases all through the washout suggesting inhomogeneity in the conducting airways, well proximal to the gas exchange zone. See text for further explanations.

adults, there are only a few studies available in infants [14, 19, 21]. In older children and adults increased ventilation inhomogeneity has been reported in diseases affecting the peripheral airways such as CF [26–31], asthma [13, 32–34], obliterative bronchiolitis [35], and chronic obstructive pulmonary disease [36]. In infants, increased ventilation inhomogeneity has been observed in subjects with CF, bronchopulmonary dysplasia, and wheezing bronchitis [14, 37–39]. Ventilation inhomogeneity seems to be a far more sensitive measure of lung involvement in subjects with CF than conventional spirometry or body plethysmography [31]. A distinct advantage of the breath-by-breath washout is that this tidal breathing test requires little cooperation, and is therefore one of the few lung function tests that can be performed throughout life, from infancy to adulthood [31, 39, 40]. In addition, though some conflicting reports exist (which may in part be due to methodological differences), indices of ventilation inhomogeneity, such as the lung clearance index (LCI), appear to change little with age or growth in health [31, 40]. That these parameters should be unaffected by age, puberty, lung size, or gender over a large age range is possibly unique for a biological marker, and would greatly facilitate interpretation and the future establishment of reference values.

Conventional Indices of Overall Ventilation Inhomogeneity. Several indices of overall ventilation inhomogeneity have been published [15]. The lung clearance index (LCI) is calculated as the cumulative expired volume needed to lower the end-tidal marker gas concentration to 1/40 of the starting concentration divided by FRC, i.e. the number of lung volume turnovers (TO) needed to clear the lungs from the marker gas. The mixing ratio (MR) is calculated as the ratio between the actual and the ideal number of breaths needed to lower the end-tidal tracer gas concentration to 1/40 of the starting values [41]. The ideal number of breaths is calculated from the ratio between the logarithm for the end-tidal marker gas concentration at end washout and the logarithm for the FRC/(FRC + alveolar VT) ratio. The alveolar VT is calculated as average VT during the multiple-breath washout (MBW) minus the predicted airway dead space (Vdaw = body weight × 2 ml).

A technique called moment analysis can be used to quantify the degree of inhomogeneity of ventilation distribution as described by the inert gas washout curve [15]. The 1st and 2nd moments (μ_1 and μ_2) give more weight to the later part of the washout curve, which means that the higher these indices are, the more skewed is the washout curve (fig. 5a, 6a). This in turn indicates that a greater portion of the lungs is slowly ventilated. A brief explanation

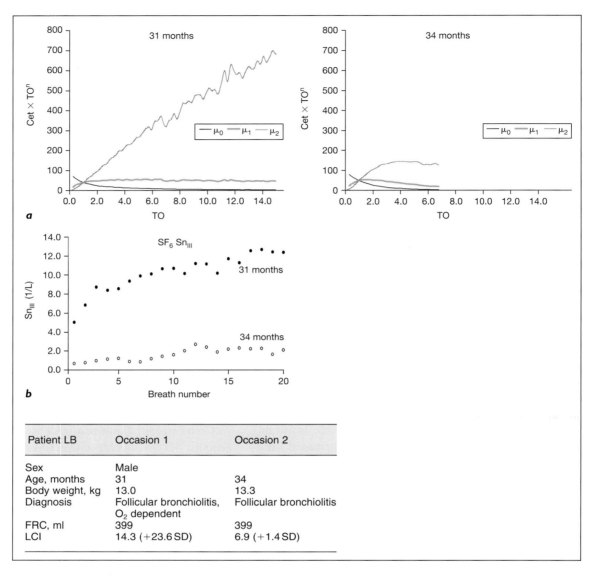

Patient LB	Occasion 1	Occasion 2
Sex	Male	
Age, months	31	34
Body weight, kg	13.0	13.3
Diagnosis	Follicular bronchiolitis, O_2 dependent	Follicular bronchiolitis
FRC, ml	399	399
LCI	14.3 (+23.6 SD)	6.9 (+1.4 SD)

Fig. 6. Examples of curves extracted from a tidal washout using the technique described in figure 3 in a patient with biopsy-verified follicular bronchiolitis before and after treatment with methotrexate. SD denotes standard deviations above predicted mean. *a* Moment analysis curves. Cet = End-tidal inert gas concentration, normalized so that initial concentration corresponds to 100; TO = lung volume turnover number; n = 0, 1 or 2, which are the numbers used when calculating μ_0, μ_1, and μ_2, respectively. See text for further explanations. *b* Sn_{III} for each breath during SF_6 washout plotted against breath number. This plot is used for delineation of the mechanisms behind ventilation inhomogeneity. In this subject Sn_{III} is high already from the start of washout and tends to reach an asymptote after breath 5 approximately, suggesting inhomogeneity in distal airways close to the gas exchange zone. See text for further explanations.

is given of how the moment ratios can be calculated: first the end-tidal gas concentration is plotted as a function of TO (fig. 5a, 6a). The area under this curve is denoted the 0th moment (μ_0). Then each end-tidal gas concentration value is multiplied with the corresponding TO value, and this new parameter is plotted as a function of TO. The area under this curve is denoted the 1st moment (μ_1). In the next step the end-tidal marker gas concentration value is multiplied with the square of the corresponding TO value (i.e. TO × TO). Again this new parameter is plotted as a function of TO. The area under this curve is denoted the 2nd moment (μ_2). The ratios between the 1st and 0th

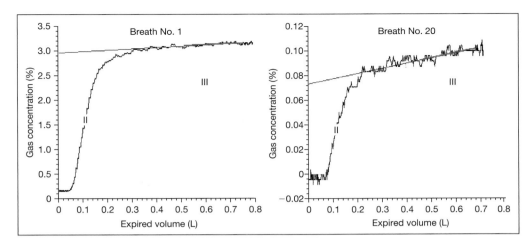

Fig. 7. Plots of inert gas concentration versus expired volume in breaths number 1 and 20 using the technique described in figure 3. The phase III slope is calculated over the last third of the breath by linear regression. Sn_{III} can further be calculated by dividing the phase III slope with the mean gas concentration over the regressed portion. It is obvious that the Sn_{III} is greater in breath No. 20 than in breath No. 1. See text for further explanations.

moments (μ_1/μ_0), and between the 2nd and 0th moments (μ_2/μ_0) are then calculated over the whole washout or over an arbitrary number of TO, e.g. the first eight TO. Although the moment analysis may seem to be a more sophisticated way of describing ventilation inhomogeneity, we have not found it to be more sensitive than simpler indices such as the LCI, either in clinical routine testing or in some studies [25]. Furthermore, the LCI can be intuitively understood by the referring physician and the parent: the sicker the child is, the more air it must breathe to clear the lungs. Further refinements of the MR and moment analysis can be achieved if the airway dead space is actually measured and accounted for. This can be done by calculating the Fowler airway dead space, i.e. using gas concentration plotted versus expired volume for each breath in the washout [42].

The described indices of overall ventilation inhomogeneity are sensitive to differences in specific ventilation between lung regions. This means that if one or several regions of the lungs obtain a smaller percentage of the VT, in proportion to their volume, compared to the rest of the lung, then these regions will be cleared more slowly. Consequently, the LCI will become higher as the lungs must be ventilated for a longer time, and the moment ratios become higher as more of the marker gas leaves the lungs late during washout. Although these simple tests are highly sensitive to airway pathology [31], particularly obstruction of the peripheral airways, they do not give any information about the mechanisms behind inhomogeneity or where along the airway tree obstruction has occurred.

Sn_{III} Analysis. New, alternative approaches to analyzing inert gas washout data may provide such additional information. A new technique, often called concentration-normalized phase III slope (Sn_{III}) analysis, takes into account both the convective and diffusive mixing of the marker gas [36, 43]. Sn_{III} analysis acknowledges that the phase III slope (alveolar plateau; fig. 7) of an expired inert marker gas has two components. One is due to convection-dependent inhomogeneity occurring in the conducting airways as a result from differences in specific ventilation between parallel lung units, which fill and empty in sequence, and which have their branch point well proximal to the diffusion-convection front for the tracer gas used [43]. This front is situated in the vicinity of the terminal bronchioles for most marker gases, in the healthy adult during resting breathing. The other mechanism is interaction between diffusive and convective gas mixing, which occurs in the zone of the diffusion-convection front. The reader is referred to original work by Paiva and Engel [43] to obtain an in-depth description of this theory. When doing an Sn_{III} analysis, a gas concentration versus expired volume plot is first made for each breath during the washout (fig. 7). The slope of the alveolar plateau (phase III) is calculated by linear regression, and this slope is then normalized by dividing with the mean gas concentration over the slope. This results in an Sn_{III}. The Sn_{III} is

calculated for the first 20 or 25 breaths of the washout, and these are plotted against breath number or TO. In subjects with marked inhomogeneity occurring as a result of convection-dependent mechanisms the Sn_{III} will increase steadily during the washout, as seen in a boy with CF (fig. 5b). This is the result of uneven ventilation distribution among the conducting airways, possibly as a result of one or several focal lesions. In subjects with marked inhomogeneity occurring more peripherally, in the vicinity of the diffusion-convection front, Sn_{III} will be high already at the first breath and reach an asymptote after approximately 5 breaths. Figure 6a and b shows recordings in a young boy who presented with tachypnoea and hypoxemia at the age of 3 months and in whom an open lung biopsy at 2.5 years of age showed a follicular bronchiolitis. A recording done at 31 months of age showed a high LCI and abnormal moment analysis, and the Sn_{III} progression indicated a marked component of diffusion-convection-dependent inhomogeneity, although there also is a component of convection-dependent inhomogeneity (fig. 6b). After 2 months of treatment with methotrexate the patient had improved markedly clinically and did not need O_2 therapy. Overall ventilation inhomogeneity as measured by LCI was then normalized, and moment analysis and Sn_{III} progression were also normalized (fig. 6 and b). These cases illustrate the potential usefulness of this technique but much remains to be done before it can be used as a clinical tool.

Unfortunately, there is currently no system commercially available for breath-by-breath washout except for the new ultrasound device from Ecomedics (Exhalyzer D, fig. 8). Because this system measures molar mass and not the concentration of a particular gas, it remains to be established whether this method can be used for Sn_{III} analysis.

Gas Trapping

Trapped gas volumes, i.e. lung volumes that do not or only very slowly communicate with the central airways during normal breathing, are characteristic findings in obstructive airway disease, particularly when obstruction is severe [13, 33]. As whole body plethysmography measures all gas in the thorax, and gas dilution methods measure only lung volumes communicating with the central airways, the difference between these FRC assessments can be used as an indicator of the trapped gas volume [44, 45]. This approach may be prone to errors because the plethysmographically determined FRC may be overestimated under certain circumstances [46, 47]. Furthermore, both the plethysmographically assessed FRC and the FRC measured by gas

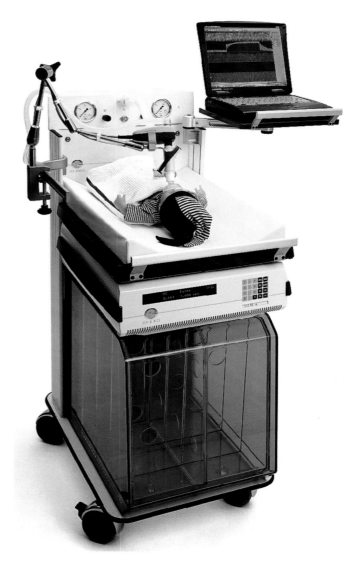

Fig. 8. The Exhalyzer D system for inert gas washout and other infant lung function tests, marketed by EcoMedics (used with permission).

dilution have some variability, and by subtracting one from the other this error may increase. Another approach is to obtain an index of gas trapping by forcing the subject to take 3–5 large breaths after the inert gas washout. The marker gas then mobilized can serve as an indicator of the degree of gas trapping [13, 14, 33]. When using a foreign inert marker gas, then several large breaths must be taken during the washin, before the start of washout. This approach is feasible also in infants and appears to be a sensitive marker of airway disease in infants [14] as well as in older children [13, 33]. It is, however, likely that gas trapping is underestimated by this method.

Normative Data for FRC and Ventilation Inhomogeneity

It is essential to use appropriate normative data to meaningfully interpret lung function parameters, and to avail oneself of the possibility to characterize and monitor disease severity. The choice of reference equations must be appropriate for the age, body size, gender and ethnic origin of the person or population that is investigated, and for the measurement technique that is used. Ideally, reference values used should have been collected with the same method and using the same protocol as used when testing patients. In scientific studies a group of patients should be compared with an appropriately chosen control group [48]. While reference equations for FRC in infants have been published [48], no such data is available for ventilation distribution. Reference equations for FRC are prone to secular trends, emphasized after recent standardization work of the ATS/ ERS that has led to alterations and developments in equipment and protocol [7]. While both the nitrogen washout method and the helium dilution technique appear to yield reproducible FRC values in healthy infants and in those with respiratory disease [10], these values may not be appropriate for measurements using the SF_6 MBW washout. Most of the published values of plethysmographically determined FRC are distinctly higher than those derived from gas dilution techniques [48], but recent data [7] compared with a summary of published values of plethysmographically assessed FRC over the last 35 years suggest that diminished values in healthy infants primarily reflect gradual technologic advances and refinements in protocols. This is in agreement with recent findings comparing plethysmographically determined FRC and FRC measured by gas dilution, where no [44] or only small [45] differences between FRC values assessed by both techniques were seen in health.

A workshop report and official statement of the ERS [48] summarizes previously published FRC values attained using both gas dilution and plethysmographic techniques. FRC has often been expressed as millilitres per kilogram body weight during the first month of life, but this approach is not valid in older infants where distribution of lung volumes is non-linear with growth, and is heteroscedastic. In the ERS statement, an attempt at producing more reliable reference values was made by including data from several centres. For studies to be included, all raw data had to be available and studies had to include at least 25 healthy Caucasian infants. Separate equations were calculated for FRC measured by helium dilution and plethysmography. Data on FRC derived from helium dilution was available from 378 infants from four studies, and the resulting prediction equation is given by Stocks and Quanjer [48]:

$$FRC_{He} = 0.0036 \cdot length^{2.531} \text{ (with a residual standard}$$
deviation of 0.177). FRC is given in millilitres and length in centimetres.

This equation may be used to calculate the number of standard deviations that a measured value deviates from the mean FRC of the populations included in the studies. It should, however, be emphasized that the equation must be validated by testing a representative sample of a healthy population locally.

Unfortunately there are, as yet, no reference values that describe ventilation inhomogeneity in healthy infants, and standards for calculating and presenting such data are lacking. While there is a paucity of studies describing parameters of gas mixing in healthy infants, there is another obstacle in that no official consensus has been reached as to which index of the many available ones [15] should be presented. While the current authors have found LCI and to a lesser extent the MR to be easy to use and intuitive to grasp, there are almost as many indices used as publications of indices of ventilation inhomogeneity in healthy infants available [14, 19, 38, 39, 49]. More data are available in older children and adults, and may help the future establishment of reference values as our own initial data suggest that ventilation distribution is unchanged from infancy to adulthood [40], and that there is optimal gas mixing in the human lung in health throughout most, except the extremes, of life. The constancy and homoscedasticity that were found also help the establishment of reference values, and as a guideline we have found a mean LCI of 6.56 (standard deviation 0.34) in healthy infants, irrespective of length, weight or gender. These values are very close to those found in older healthy Swedish children (mean 6.33; standard deviation 0.43) [31].

Clinical Role of Measuring Lung Volumes and Ventilation Inhomogeneity in Infants

There are now a number of techniques available for measuring infant lung function. Methods that have been designed for following lung growth and development are not necessarily suitable for clinical use. Often, the availability of a specific test at a centre has determined which test or tests are performed, rather than the appropriate tests needed to answer a specific clinical or even research question. Recent development and standardization of infant lung function testing techniques are, however, likely to lead to a clearer role in clinical management.

Measurements of Lung Volume

Measuring FRC is necessary for interpreting measurements of lung mechanics and tidal forced expiratory flows. Increased FRC may be seen in obstructive lung disease, but it should be remembered that measurements achieved using gas dilution techniques may underestimate lung volume, especially hyperinflation due to severe obstruction. In contrast, plethysmographically determined FRC will then be more sensitive, but may overestimate actual lung volume. Ideally, both techniques should be used and compared to estimate the amount of trapped gas [44, 45]. Reduced FRC can be seen in conditions of restrictive lung disease or impaired lung development. If possible, a measurement of FRC should be included in the clinical evaluation of an infant with suspected respiratory disease. One should keep in mind, however, that there is a wide range of FRC values that would be considered 'normal' in infancy, and therefore it may be difficult to draw conclusions from a single measurement. Longitudinal evaluations in a patient are more likely to be clinically useful.

Measurements of Ventilation Inhomogeneity

Obstructive airway disorders generally result in asymmetrical narrowing of the intrapulmonary airways. This leads to differences in ventilation distribution among different lung units, but gas trapping commonly occurs also. Ventilation inhomogeneity and gas trapping can be measured in infants with patient-friendly methods. Measurements of ventilation inhomogeneity and gas trapping are clearly useful for demonstrating and quantifying lung diseases characterized by peripheral airway obstruction, which include a wide range of common and rare conditions. These tests may prove to be of particular importance when managing early CF lung disease in the infant and young child.

References

1 Stocks J, Sly PD, Morris MG, Frey U: Standards for infant respiratory function testing: What(ever) next? Eur Respir J 2000;16: 581–584.

2 Taussig LM, Helms PJ: Introduction; in Stocks J, Sly PD, Tepper RS, Morgan WJ (eds): Infant Respiratory Function Testing. New York, Wiley-Liss, 1996, pp 1–18.

3 Gaultier C, Fletcher ME, Beardsmore C, England S, Motoyama E: Respiratory function measurements infants: Measurement conditions. Working Group of the European Respiratory Society and the American Thoracic Society. Eur Respir J 1995;8:1057–66.

4 Macklem PT: The physiology of the small airways. Am J Respir Crit Care Med 1998;157: S181–S183.

5 Stocks J, Godfrey S, Beardsmore C, Bar-Yishay E, Castile R: Plethysmographic-measurements of lung volume and airway resistance. ERS/ATS Task Force on Standards for Infant Respiratory Function Testing. European Respiratory Society/American Thoracic Society. Eur Respir J 2001;17:302–312.

6 Stocks J, Marchal F, Kraemer R, Gutkowksi P, Bar Yishay E, Godfrey S: Plethysmographic assessment of functional residual capacity and airway resistance; in Stocks J, Sly PD, Tepper RS, Morgan WJ (eds): Infant Respiratory Function Testing. New York, Wiley-Liss, 1996, pp 191–239.

7 Hülskamp G, Hoo A, Ljungberg H, Lum S, Pillow JJ, Stocks J: Progressive decline in plethysmographic lung volumes in infants: Physiology or technology? Am J Respir Crit Care Med 2003;168:1003–1009.

8 Morris MG, Gustafsson P, Tepper R, Gappa M, Stocks J: ERS/ATS Task Force on Standards for Infant Respiratory Function Testing. The bias flow nitrogen washout technique for measuring the functional residual capacity in infants. ERS/ATS Task Force on Standards for Infant Respiratory Function Testing. Eur Respir J 2001;17:529–536.

9 Gappa M, Hülskamp G: Infant whole-body plethysmography; in Hammer J, Eber E (eds): Paediatric Pulmonary Function Testing. Prog Respir Res. Basel, Karger, 2005, vol 33, pp 44–53.

10 Tepper RS, Asdell S: Comparison of helium dilution and nitrogen washout measurements of functional residual capacity in infants and very young children. Pediatr Pulmonol 1992; 13:250–254.

11 Merth IT: Pulmonary Function Testing in Newborns and Infants; thesis University of Leiden, 1996.

12 Gerhardt T, Hehre D, Bancalari E, Watson H: A simple method for measuring functional residual capacity by N_2 washout in small animals and newborn infants. Pediatr Res 1985;19: 1165–1169.

13 Gustafsson PM, Johansson HJ, Dahlback GO: Pneumotachographic nitrogen washout method for measurement of the volume of trapped gas in the lungs. Pediatr Pulmonol 1994;17: 258–268.

14 Gustafsson PM, Kallman S, Ljungberg H, Lindblad A: Method for assessment of volume of trapped gas in infants during multiple-breath inert gas washout. Pediatr Pulmonol 2003;35:42–49.

15 Larsson A, Jonmarker C, Werner O: Ventilation inhomogeneity during controlled ventilation. Which index should be used? J Appl Physiol 1988;65:2030–2039.

16 Frey U, Stocks J, Sly P, Bates J: Specification for signal processing and data handling used for infant pulmonary function testing. ERS/ATS Task Force on Standards for Infant Respiratory Function Testing. European Respiratory Society/American Thoracic Society. Eur Respir J 2000;16:1016–1022.

17 Frey U, Stocks J, Coates A, Sly P, Bates J: Specifications for equipment used for infant pulmonary function testing. ERS/ATS Task Force on Standards for Infant Respiratory Function Testing. European Respiratory Society/American Thoracic Society. Eur Respir J 2000;16:731–740.

18 Brunner JX, Wolff G, Cumming G, Langenstein H: Accurate measurement of N_2 volumes during N_2 washout requires dynamic adjustment of delay time. J Appl Physiol 1985;59: 1008–1012.

19 Schibler A, Hall GL, Businger F, Reinmann B, Wildhaber JH, Cernelc M, Frey U: Measurement of lung volume and ventilation distribution with an ultrasonic flow meter in healthy infants. Eur Repir J 2002;20:912–918.

20 Vilstrup CT, Bjorklund LJ, Larsson A, Lachmann B, Werner O: Functional residual capacity and ventilation homogeneity in mechanically ventilated small neonates. J Appl Physiol 1992;73:276–283.

21 Hjalmarson O, Sandberg K: Abnormal lung function in healthy preterm infants. Am J Respir Crit Care Med 2002;165:83–87.

22 Gustafsson PM, Källman S, Bhiladvala M, Fletcher ME: N_2-washout with pure oxygen reduces tidal volumes markedly in sedated infants. Eur Respir J 1997;10:165s.

23 Ljungberg HK, Gustafsson PM: Peripheral airway function in childhood asthma, assessed by single-breath He and SF_6 washout. Pediatr Pulmonol 2003;36:339–347.

24 Gustafsson PM, Ljungberg HK, Kjellman B: Peripheral airway involvement in asthma assessed by single-breath SF_6 and He washout. Eur Respir J 2003;21:1033–1039.

25 Gronkvist M, Bergsten E, Eiken O, Gustafsson PM: Inter- and intraregional ventilation inhomogeneity in hypergravity and after pressurization of an anti-G suit. J Appl Physiol 2003; 94:1353–1364.

26 Kraemer R, Meister B: Fast real-time moment-ratio analysis of multibreath nitrogen washout in children. J Appl Physiol 1985;59:1137–1144.

27 Wall MA: Moment analysis of multibreath nitrogen washout in young children. J Appl Physiol 1985;59:274–279.

28 Lutchen KR, Habib RH, Dorkin HL, Wall MA: Respiratory impedance and multibreath N_2 washout in healthy, asthmatic, and cystic fibrosis subjects. J Appl Physiol 1990;68: 2139–2149.

29 Gozal D, Bailey SL, Keens TG: Evolution of pulmonary function during an acute exacerbation in hospitalized patients with cystic fibrosis. Pediatr Pulmonol 1993;16:347–353.

30 Van Muylem A, Baran D: Overall and peripheral inhomogeneity of ventilation in patients with stable cystic fibrosis. Pediatr Pulmonol 2000;30:3–9.

31 Gustafsson PM, Aurora P, Lindblad A: Evaluation of ventilation maldistribution as an early indicator of lung disease in children with cystic fibrosis. Eur Respir J 2003;22:972–979.

32 Kraemer R, Pacozzi S, Casaulta Aebischer C: Assessment of intrapulmonary ventilation disorders in children with bronchial asthma using the nitrogen elimination technique. Pneumologie 1994;48:704–710.

33 Strömberg NOT, Gustafsson PM: Ventilation inhomogeneity assessed by nitrogen washout and ventilation-perfusion mismatch by capnography in stable and induced airway obstruction. Pediatr Pulmonol 2000;29:94–102.

34 Wall MA, Misley MC, Brown AC, Vollmer WM, Buist AS: Relationship between maldistribution of ventilation and airway obstruction in children with asthma. Respir Physiol 1987; 69:287–297.

35 Estenne M, Van Muylem A, Knoop C, Antoine M: Detection of obliterative bronchiolitis after lung transplantation by indexes of ventilation distribution. Am J Respir Crit Care Med 2000; 162:1047–1051.

36 Verbanck S, Schuermans D, Van Muylem A, Melot C, Noppen M, Vincken W, Paiva M: Conductive and acinar lung-zone contributions to ventilation inhomogeneity in COPD. Am J Respir Crit Care Med 1998;157:1573–1577.

37 Schibler A, Schneider M, Frey U, Kraemer R: Moment ratio analysis of multiple breath nitrogen washout in infants with lung disease. Eur Respir J 2000;15:1094–1101.

38 Shao H, Sandberg K, Hjalmarson O: Impaired gas mixing and low lung volume in preterm infants with mild chronic lung disease. Pediatr Res 1998;43:536–541.

39 Ljungberg H, Gustafsson P, Hülskamp G, Hoo A-F, Pillow J, Stocks J: Increased ventilation inhomogeneity in infants with cystic fibrosis (CF). Eur Respir J 2002;20:209s.

40 Ljungberg H, Aurora P, Oliver C, Hulskamp G, Hoo A, Lum S, Pillow J, Gustafsson P, Stocks J; LCCFS: Assessments of ventilation inhomogeneity throughout childhood in healthy subjects and those with cystic fibrosis (CF) lung disease. Am J Respir Crit Care Med 2003;167:A921.

41 Edelman NH, Mittman C, Norris AH, Shock NW: Effects of respiratory pattern on age differences in ventilation uniformity. J Appl Physiol 1968;24:49–53.

42 Fowler WS: Lung function studies. II. The respiratory dead space. Am J Physiol 1948; 154:405–416.

43 Paiva M, Engel LA: Gas mixing in the lung periphery; in Chang HK, Paiva M (eds): Respiratory Physiology. An Analytical Approach. New York, Dekker, 1989, vol 40, pp 245–276.

44 Ljungberg H, Hulskamp G, Hoo AF, Pillow JJ, Lum S, Gustafsson P, Stocks J: Estimates of plethysmographic FRC exceed those by gas dilution in infants with cystic fibrosis but not in healthy controls. Thorax 2002;57(suppl 3):23.

45 Castile RG, Iram D, McCoy K: Gas trapping in normal infants and in infants with cystic fibrosis. Pediatr Pulmonol 2004;37:461–469.

46 Stanescu DC, Rodenstein DO, Cauberghs M, Van de Woestijne KP: Failure of body plethysmography in bronchial asthma. J Appl Physiol Respir Environ Exerc Physiol 1982;52: 939–948.

47 Rodenstein D, Stanescu DC: Elastic properties of the lung in acute induced asthma. J Appl Physiol 1983;54:152–158.

48 Stocks J, Quanjer PH: Reference values for residual volume, functional residual capacity and total lung capacity. ATS Workshop on Lung Volume Measurements. Official statement of the European Respiratory Society. Eur Respir J 1995;8:492–506.

49 Bolton DP: Diffusional inhomogeneity: Gas mixing efficiency in the new-born lung. J Physiol 1979;286:447–455.

Per M. Gustafsson, MD
Assistant Professor of Paediatrics
Department of Paediatric Clinical Physiology
Queen Silvia Children's Hospital
SE–416 85 Göteborg (Sweden)
Tel. +46 31 343 45 74, Fax +46 31 84 16 05
E-Mail per.gustafsson@vgregion.se

Hammer J, Eber E (eds): Paediatric Pulmonary Function Testing.
Prog Respir Res. Basel, Karger, 2005, vol 33, pp 66–77

· ·

Techniques for the Measurement of Lung Function in Toddlers and Preschool Children

Graham L. Hall[a, b]   Isobel M. Brookes[c]

[a]Respiratory Medicine, Princess Margaret Hospital for Children and [b]School for Paediatric and Child Health, University of Western Australia, Perth, Australia; [c]Department of Child Health, University of Leicester, Leicester, UK

Abstract

The application of lung function testing to the preschool age group is difficult due to the limited cooperation that can be obtained in this group. The advent of commercially available equipment for a number of techniques has allowed more widespread use and an increase in the knowledge of the practicalities of these tests. This chapter covers two of the major techniques utilized in 2- to 5-year-old children, the interrupter and forced oscillation techniques. An overview for each method is given, including recommended measurement protocols, and a summary of available reference data and differences associated with respiratory disease. The future and limitations of these techniques are also discussed.

Measurement of Respiratory Function in Children 2–5 Years of Age

To accurately quantify the mechanical properties of the respiratory system in young children has remained a significant challenge for those working in the field of respiratory physiology. In recent years rapid advances in technology have allowed the use of lung function testing in preschool children to become more widespread. The increasing awareness of the impact of respiratory events in early life on significant respiratory disease in adulthood [1, 2] has added new impetus to the study of respiratory physiology and the factors influencing the development of respiratory disease in infancy and early childhood.

Historically the techniques for the measurement of lung function in infancy have been restricted to individual research units with locally made equipment. While the knowledge obtained from these units has greatly advanced our understanding of the growth and development of the respiratory system and the precedents of respiratory disease, the 'isolation' of these centres made direct comparisons of studies difficult. The recent efforts of the American Thoracic Society/European Respiratory Society Working Group on Infant and Young Children Pulmonary Function Testing have resulted in a number of standardization papers for the majority of lung function tests used in infants [3–8].

Lung function testing in the preschool child has lagged behind that of infants, older children and adults. The majority of lung function tests used in routine clinical laboratories require active subject cooperation and have limited application in those children younger than 5 years. While a number of studies have reported the use of standard lung function tests in this age group (spirometry for example [9]; see also chapter by Eber and Zach [10]), generally the success rates are low. Thus the measurement of respiratory function in those children unable to actively cooperate with testing procedures and too old to sedate for lung function testing form a unique challenge for scientists and clinicians in the field of paediatric respiratory medicine [11–13].

The development or application of specific lung function tests in the preschool age group has rapidly expanded in recent years. This development of 'preschool' lung function tests has come about from two separate streams. One stream has seen the translation of existing passive techniques into the preschool age group. These tests generally have been limited to clinical and physiological research and are not used in routine clinical assessment of respiratory function. Examples of these methods are the forced oscillation technique (FOT), the interrupter technique, and assessment of tidal breathing parameters. The second stream of studies has been driven by the innovative application of tests used in the routine assessment of lung function to the preschool age group. These include spirometry, body plethysmography, and gas dilution techniques. In general, the applications of this second stream of techniques mimic those in older children and are reviewed elsewhere in this book.

The interrupter technique and FOT were originally described in the early half of the 1900s and have been extensively applied in both animal and human studies. However, it is only the advent of computerization of techniques that has allowed the widespread use of these methods. The remainder of this chapter describes the application of the interrupter and FOT in preschool children, specifically children 2–5 years of age.

Interrupter Technique

Background and Development of the Technique

In the face of a lack of simple techniques for measurement of lung function in preschool children, resistance by airflow interruption (R_{int}) has several practical advantages; it is measured during tidal breathing using portable equipment, and it is a non-invasive, effort-independent technique, which requires minimal subject cooperation.

R_{int} is obtained by measuring pressure and flow at the airway opening and using a shutter device to bring about a brief interruption to airflow. The technique was first described in 1927 by von Neergard and Wirz [14], but fell from favour due to theoretical reservations. Modern computers have enabled a thorough examination of the technique and led to a greater understanding of exactly what it measures, and the potential pitfalls for users [15–20]. As a result, interest in the technique has increased, especially in those measuring preschool lung function.

Overview

R_{int} is an estimate of airway resistance (R_{aw}), which requires a brief interruption to expiratory flow, during which flow (V'_{ao}) and pressure at the airway opening (P_{ao}) are recorded. The change in P_{ao} occurring during the interruption is used to estimate the driving pressure across the airway that was present at the moment of interruption [15].

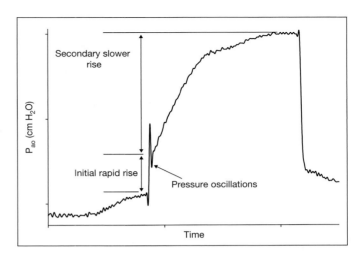

Fig. 1. Schematic representation of changes in P_{ao} following a brief interruption to flow at the mouth. The initial rapid rise relates to the flow-dependent resistance drop across the airway tree with the secondary slower rise relating to the visco-elastic properties of the respiratory tissues. The pressure oscillations following the initial rapid rise are due to the inertive properties of the gas column in the large central airways.

The technique relies on the assumptions that (1) the valve or shutter closes instantaneously and (2) is followed by an instantaneous equilibration of P_{ao} with alveolar pressure (P_{alv}; i.e. the driving pressure) during the period of interruption. Estimates of actual P_{alv} at the point of interruption are made by various back-extrapolation procedures on the P_{ao} trace after interruption, which are required because the initial change in pressure is obscured by oscillations (see below). This is then related to flow at the point of interruption to obtain a value for resistance. R_{int} is not a 'physiological' resistance because no single value for P_{alv} exists, but is a representation of resistance to flow within the airways.

There are two distinct phases in the P_{ao} trace following interruption, an initial rapid jump accompanied by pressure oscillations, and a second slow rise to a plateau (fig. 1). Work in animal models has helped elucidate the meaning of these changes [16, 17]. In open-chested anaesthetized dogs where P_{alv} could be directly measured, the initial rise in P_{ao} after interruption reflected R_{aw} (with the surrounding oscillations being related to the inertia of the gas in the airway tree and the compliance of the airway walls) and the second slow rise stress relaxation of the respiratory tissues and movement of air between lung units after interruption ('pendelluft') [16]. Under conditions of airway obstruction after inhalation of histamine, despite increased heterogeneity of P_{alv}, R_{aw} could still be accurately estimated using the interrupter technique [17]. Lastly, the interrupter resistance also contains elements of chest wall and pulmonary resistance, and R_{int} values are generally higher than plethysmographically determined R_{aw} when both are measured in the same individuals [21–24].

Technical Aspects of the Method

Several commercially available devices, suitable for use in settings such as outpatient departments, are now available to measure R_{int}. There are several important equipment issues that must be considered.

Ideally shutter closure time should be minimized (probably within 10–20 ms), if the effect on the resulting data is to be insignificant [19]. The shutter is required to be completely airtight, as leakage of air during the interruption around the closed shutter will decrease the measured P_{ao}. These physical characteristics are contradictory; thus, a compromise must be made [25].

The choice of a facemask or a mouthpiece and nose clip will influence the value of resistance, as R_{int} includes the resistance of the equipment proximal to the shutter, as well as that of the upper airways. In the preschool child, this issue is particularly relevant as the choice of facemask over mouthpiece is highly dependent on the developmental stage of the child, as well as the skill of the operator in dealing with young children. Ideally, a mouthpiece (which is non-compressible and of known dead space and resistance) should be used, with a nose clip to ensure mouth breathing. Younger children may struggle to maintain an adequate seal around a mouthpiece and measurements have been shown to be feasible in only 56% of 2- to 3-year-olds [26], and 55% of 1- to 2-year-olds [27] for these reasons. Facemasks have been used to increase the feasibility of the test, however this results in increased values of R_{int} when compared to those obtained using a mouthpiece [28].

Other technical issues to consider include the flow at which the interruption is triggered, and the length of the interruption. Most studies measure R_{int} at peak tidal expiratory flow. The interruption therefore occurs at or near mid-expiration, minimizing breath-to-breath variation in inflation level and R_{aw}. There is some evidence that expiratory R_{int} is slightly more sensitive in detecting (subclinical) differences in airway calibre within and between subjects than R_{int} measured during inspiration [27]. Ideally tidal expiratory flow should be premeasured and the device programmed to interrupt at this flow. Generally, an interruption of 100 ms duration is performed, although in unsedated sleeping infants a longer interruption has been used [29].

Practical Aspects of Measurement

Measurement Environment

Personnel skilled in dealing with preschool children, and persuading them to accept the mouthpiece and tolerate measurements are vital. Because the technique requires 'passive cooperation', distraction with children's videos are often used [27, 30].

Collection of R_{int} Data

The child should be seated upright with the head slightly extended, and instructed to breathe quietly. An adequate seal of the child's lips around the mouthpiece is important. Breathing pattern should be observed for irregularities due to tongue movements, swallowing or sucking.

Many investigators will recommend standing behind the child with hands placed over the cheeks and/or neck to support the upper airway. The impact of cheek support has been found to have no effect on R_{int} in one study [31], but other studies in older children have found the reverse [32, 33]. In those studies, as expected, R_{int} values obtained with cheek support were significantly higher than those without, presumably due to decreased compliance of the upper airway.

Once the child is comfortable, before actual measurements are made, he or she should be familiarized with the sensation and sound of the shutter closure. Most investigators will record 10 measurements, with the aim of acquiring at least 5 technically acceptable measurements (see section below).

Data Analysis and Interpretation

Quality Control

Raw data should be examined before analysis to exclude data affected by leak, variable glottic closure, or active breathing against the shutter, which all result in a variable or falling P_{ao} trace during the interruption. The ideal P_{ao} trace (in expiration, for example) should rise rapidly to initial oscillations and then be followed by a smooth rise during the remainder of the interruption.

Analysis Method

Once acceptable data have been identified, a method of estimating P_{alv} from the P_{ao} trace should be chosen. Four methods have been described, (1) a curvilinear back extrapolation, (2) a two-point linear back extrapolation, (3) end oscillatory pressure, and (4) end interruption pressure. When the ability of the different methods to detect a change in R_{int} after inhaled methacholine challenge was compared, the linear back-extrapolation method was found to be most sensitive [34]. In 1997, it was proposed that a linear back

Table 1. Reference data for the interrupter technique in young children

Reference	Equation	R^2	RSD	n	Age range, years
McKenzie et al. [40]	$\log_{10}R_{int} = 0.528 - 0.00569 \times Ht$	–	0.104	~180	2–10
Merkus et al. [27]	$R_{int} = 2.61 - 0.016 \times Ht$	0.41	0.13	~40	2–7
Lombardi et al. [31]	$R_{int} = 2.127 - 0.01254 \times Ht$	0.141	–	~255	3.0–6.4
Klug and Bisgaard [41]	$R_{int} = 0.97 - 0.0067 \times (Ht - 112.3)$	0.21	0.166	~80	2–7

R_{int} = Interrupter resistance (expressed in $kPa \cdot L^{-1} \cdot s$); Ht = height (cm); R^2 = square of the coefficient of correlation; RSD = residual standard deviation; n = estimated number of children ≤ 120 cm body height; age range = range of the original study group.

extrapolation be used in order to standardize data analysis [35], and subsequent reports have generally used this method. Not only the method of extrapolation, but the point to which the extrapolation is extended must be clearly defined. Generally, this has been the onset of shutter closure as defined as 25% of the first upstroke of the pressure oscillations [36], or an arbitrary time (15 ms) after closure. A recent report found that baseline R_{int} values differ significantly depending on both the algorithm used for back extrapolation and the choice of the point to which the extrapolation is extended [37]. Measurements of change following bronchodilator did not differ consistently with algorithm, but baseline differences mean that the same algorithm should be used for longitudinal purposes. As well as estimating the pressure change during the interruption, the flow at the point of interruption is also required to calculate resistance.

Reproducibility

Two recent studies of short- and long-term repeatability found the limits of agreement for within-occasion repeatability to be similar (approximately 20% of baseline values) [27, 30, 38], and this value was unaffected by age or health status. This means that, in the populations studied using the same methodology, a change after short-term intervention (such as inhaled bronchodilator) greater than 20% can be considered 'real'. For long-term variability (weeks rather than minutes) the situation is different, with values for repeatability in unselected healthy children of 26% [30] and 32% [38], and in children with cough or asthma of around 50% [38]. As the hallmark of asthma is variable airway calibre, it is to be expected that variability over weeks will be greater than that between measurements repeated on the same day. Repeated measurements over time that fall outside the expected variability in normal children could help in the diagnosis of asthma.

Reporting of Data

Once values for R_{int} are available, they should be summarized. One group found that the mean or median values are not significantly different [39], but another suggested the median as a more correct statistic, as values of R_{int} are not normally distributed [27].

Reference Data

R_{int} has been measured in groups of children from age 2 years upwards, using several different types of equipment and data analysis; as a result equipment-specific reference values are required. Several reports containing reference values have recently been published [27, 31, 40, 41]. Current published reference values are summarized in table 1 and plotted against height in figure 2. The majority of studies have found standing height to be the best predictor of R_{int} in a linear model, with age and weight not contributing significantly to the model. Similar to other lung function techniques used in young children significant effects of gender on R_{int} were not noted.

Reference values are population, equipment, and analysis specific, and further standardization of the technique is required before interlaboratory comparisons can be made. Otherwise each centre employing the technique is required to record data on a large local 'unselected population' in order to generate their own specific reference values.

Clinical Applications

The exact clinical role of R_{int} in the future has been subject to debate and remains controversial [42, 43]. Further standardization of the technique is required to accurately assess its value in research and clinical applications.

Baseline Airway Obstruction

Several studies have demonstrated that baseline R_{int} measurements are higher in young asthmatic children

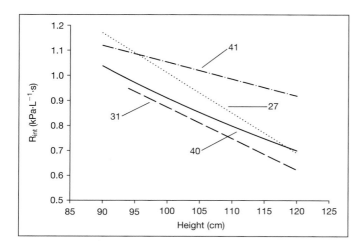

Fig. 2. Regression curves of R_{int} versus height in those studies reporting significant numbers of healthy preschool-aged subjects [27, 31, 40, 41].

[44, 45], children with a history of wheeze [46], and preschool children with cystic fibrosis [47] compared with healthy children. As a group, children with persistent wheeze were shown to have higher R_{int} values than those with transient or no previous wheeze, but an overlap in R_{int} values between the three groups means R_{int} alone cannot be used in individuals to predict outcome [48].

Assessment of Airway Responsiveness

R_{int} has been shown to be capable of detecting changes after inhaled bronchodilator in a number of studies of wheezy preschool children [26, 36]. Children with frequent cough have an intermediate response to bronchodilator, as measured by R_{int} [46, 49]. Healthy children also respond with a decrease in R_{int} after inhaled bronchodilator, but to a lesser degree than those with asthma [45, 50].

R_{int} has been used to assess the response to bronchial challenge testing with methacholine in young children [36, 51, 52] but was a relatively insensitive measurement of response compared with transcutaneous oxygen tension. R_{aw} rather than R_{int} or resistance of the respiratory system (R_{rs}) best assessed the response to cold air challenge in preschool children by impulse oscillation [53], but plethysmography requires much more complex equipment and more patient cooperation than R_{int}. Using R_{int} the test was positive in 12/38 asthmatics, and only 1/29 healthy controls. After a free running exercise test in fifty 5- to 15-year-old children, a significant change in forced expiratory volume in 1 s (FEV_1) was detected in 32% of subjects as opposed to 20% with R_{int} [54]. Because of the lack of simple lung function testing in preschool children, the clinical value (i.e. the ability of the result to aid management of individual patients) of assessing bronchial responsiveness in this age group remains unclear.

Two studies investigating the changes in R_{int} in children with a history of recurrent wheeze or asthma due to inhaled corticosteroids reported only small decreases in R_{int} (<25%) [55, 56] and well within the reported reproducibility (~50%) of the technique in this disease group [38].

Forced Oscillation Technique

The FOT was developed in 1956 by DuBois et al. [57], and described the application of a series of sinusoidal pressure waves of varying frequencies to the airway opening. This technique has gone from the gross clinical tool described by DuBois et al. to one able to provide specific insight into the physiology and mechanical behaviour of the respiratory system [58]. The development of the FOT has expanded exponentially in recent years to the point that commercial equipment based on standardized approaches is now available.

In contrast to spirometry which requires high levels of subject effort the FOT requires no more than quiet tidal breathing for short periods of time. This requirement makes it an ideal lung function test for use in young children in whom active cooperation is difficult to achieve. This section covers the basic concepts of the FOT, and focuses on the application of the FOT to preschool-aged children, specifically those 2–5 years old.

Overview

The underlying principle of the FOT is the application of an external signal to the respiratory system and the derivation of the mechanical response of the system to the applied signal. This response is termed the respiratory system impedance (Z_{rs}), and is the frequency-dependent relationship between pressure (P) and flow (V'). Impedance is a generalization of resistance, but whereas resistance describes only resistive (or frictional) induced pressure differences, impedance describes pressure differences across resistive, elastic or inertive elements [59]. The Z_{rs} can be divided into its real (resistive, R_{rs}) and imaginary (reactive, X_{rs}) components such that:

$$Z_{rs} = P/V' = R_{rs} + jX_{rs} \quad \text{where } j = \sqrt{(-1)}.$$

The resistive component is that portion of the impedance in which pressure changes are in phase with changes in flow, whereas the reactive component is the part of the impedance in which pressure changes are out of phase with changes in flow.

Z_{rs} can be determined in two ways. For measurement of input impedance, oscillations are applied and pressure and flow at the airway opening are measured. With the other method, transfer impedance applies oscillations to the body surface and the impedance is calculated from the pressure surrounding the chest wall and airway opening flows. The most commonly employed method is the measurement of the input impedance and the remainder of the discussion will centre on the measurement of input impedance alone.

The advantages of the FOT are that the technique provides a non-invasive way to evaluate the respiratory system, and that the ability to apply either a single frequency or a band of frequencies can provide useful information about the respiratory structures. The disadvantages are that information is provided about all respiratory structures, of which only the lung and chest wall are of primary interest, and that interpretation of the information is frequency dependent [58]. The use of selected frequencies can overcome some problems, as can the selective use of models of the respiratory system to partition the respiratory structures allowing those of interest to be further studied.

The upper airways act as a shunt impedance and absorb a certain amount of the applied oscillatory signal. This impedance falls significantly with increasing frequency and is more pronounced in children and infants than in older subjects [60]. Firm support of the cheeks and floor of the mouth will reduce, but not eliminate this effect. The use of the head generator technique, which applies the oscillatory signal around the head and at the mouth, significantly reduces the motion of the cheeks [61], however the technique has limited use in young children [62–65]. Mazurek et al. [62] suggested X_{rs} obtained using the standard technique may have improved diagnostic value compared to X_{rs} from the head generator technique while the reverse was true for R_{rs}. The use of the inverse of impedance (admittance) has also been shown to improve the diagnostic capacity of the standard technique [64].

Technical Aspects of the Method

Due to the flow and volume dependence of the respiratory tissues and airways [66–70], the construction of the oscillatory signal is of crucial importance. The simplest way of determining the respiratory impedance is the successive application of sinusoids of different frequencies. However, this is a time-consuming procedure susceptible to changes in patient condition. The use of composite signals

and appropriate signal processing allows simultaneous determination of Zrs across a defined frequency range. These composite signals can take three forms: (1) random noise, (2) a train of impulses, and (3) pseudorandom noise. Random noise is impractical due to respiratory system 'noise' (e.g. spontaneous breathing or inadequate respiratory muscle relaxation), hence resulting in a low signal to noise ratio. Impulses or square wave signals (such as in the impulse oscillatory systems) allow a broad band of frequencies to be applied but do not allow the optimization of the amplitude and energy content of the signal at differing frequencies. Pseudorandom signals allow the total signal energy to be maximized for a given amplitude limit and for the signal to noise ratio to be optimal across the whole frequency range [71]. This optimized signal can then be applied to spontaneously breathing patients without discomfort [71]. The range of signal frequencies used allows differing information to be obtained regarding the structural and mechanical properties of the respiratory system. Zrs obtained using oscillatory signals encompassing the spontaneous breathing rate (<1 Hz) exhibits a frequency-dependent behaviour of R_{rs} and X_{rs} related to the mechanical properties of the respiratory tissues [58]. This method allows the use of modelling [72] to simultaneously assess the mechanical properties of the respiratory tissues and airways [73–77]. However, the requirement to perform measurements during an apnoeic period limits the application of this adaptation of the FOT. The use of oscillatory frequencies above 100 Hz is dominated by the acoustic properties of the airway tree and has been suggested to reflect airway wall compliance [78–81]. The most routine-used oscillatory signals range from approximately 2 to 50 Hz. The advantage of these 'mid-range' frequencies is that the oscillatory signal can be superimposed over the spontaneous breathing of the subject, and hence provides a broader application. The disadvantage is that model-based approaches cannot easily be applied, and thus limit the amount of information on separate airway and respiratory tissue mechanics that can be obtained.

The use of low- and high-frequency oscillatory signals is not widespread and is limited to a few research centres. The most applicable oscillatory signal for use in the preschool child is the mid-range signal, and the remainder of the discussion will be limited to that method.

Practical Aspects of Measurement
Equipment

The advent of commercial FOT equipment has resulted in the FOT being available to a wider audience and an increase of its use in preschool-aged children. In general,

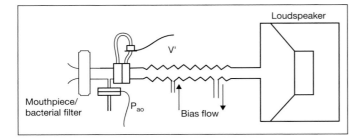

Fig. 3. Schematic representation of the equipment setup used in the FOT.

the equipment includes a computer-controlled loudspeaker to generate the oscillatory signal; pressure and flow are measured at the airway opening with the subject being connected to the system via a mouthpiece. A bias flow arrangement is used to minimize the dead space and to provide a shunt pathway for the subject's spontaneous breathing (fig. 3). The majority of commercial equipment is portable or can be placed on a trolley for ease of movement, allowing studies to be performed in the standard lung function laboratory, at the bedside, in the ward environment, or in the field.

Measurement Environment

Forced oscillatory equipment needs sufficient time to stabilize in the environment the measurements are to be collected in, as the performance of the measurement transducers will be affected by temperature, humidity, and barometric pressure.

As young children are likely to be intimidated or distracted by unfamiliar environments, measurements are best performed in a quiet area, usually with the parent/s present. A period of training should be used in all children to ensure that subsequent measurements are performed with consistent tidal breathing, and to minimize potential alterations of lung volumes. Feasibility and success rates of the FOT are age dependent with success rates of approximately 60% in 2- to 3-year-old healthy children [41] and <20% in 2- to 3-year-old children with acute asthma [82]. These success rates increase to 83–100% of older, acute asthmatic or healthy children, respectively. The technician-child interaction is the most important factor influencing the practical implementation of routine testing in preschool children. The technician must be able to identify measurements influenced by artefact (see below) and to encourage the subjects to maximize their cooperation.

Collection of Impedance Data

Measurements are performed with the child seated comfortably with a straight back and the head in the neutral position or slightly extended; they are predominantly performed with a mouthpiece, usually incorporated into a bacterial filter, and a nose clip. Some investigators [41, 83] routinely use a facemask that incorporates a mouthpiece. The cheeks and floor of the mouth of the child must be firmly supported by a technician or parent to minimize the influence of the upper airways on the measurements. The use of a technician is preferred to allow accurate feedback on patient behaviour that may influence measurement quality, such as jaw movements, leak around the mouthpiece, or swallowing. Sufficient measurements to allow the calculation of the intrasubject variability must be performed, usually between three and five technically acceptable measurements.

Data Analysis and Interpretation
Quality Control

The identification of technically substandard data is essential; ideally this should include the real-time display of flow or volume, P_{ao} and R_{rs}. Patient artefact such as leak, incomplete expiration, glottic closure, or swallowing may all be identified in this manner. Accurate feedback from the technician supporting the cheeks is also invaluable.

Reproducibility

Within- and between-test reproducibility has been assessed in some studies. The within-test variation of R_{rs} has been reported to be between 6.2 and 11.2% [41, 83–86]. The reproducibility of X_{rs} is not well documented. Klug and Bisgaard [83, 84] have reported within-test variation of Xrs between 16 and 17%. Few studies have assessed between-test reproducibility in young children with one report of similar within- and between-test repeatability of approximately 6% [85]. Further research is required to accurately assess the between-test variability of the FOT in young children, in whom lower reproducibility compared to school-aged children and adults might be expected. Day-to-day and weekly reproducibility in older children appears to be similar with values of approximately 16–17% [87, 88]. Information on the reproducibility of respiratory admittance may also improve the understanding of the technique [64].

Reporting of Data

Z_{rs} data should be reported as the mean and standard deviation (SD) of R_{rs} and/or X_{rs} at specific frequencies or

92 Delacourt C, Lorino H, Fuhrman C, Herve-Guillot M, Reinert P, Harf A, Housset B: Comparison of the forced oscillation technique and the interrupter technique for assessing airway obstruction and its reversibility in children. Am J Respir Crit Care Med 2001; 164:965–972.

93 Delacourt C, Lorino H, Herve-Guillot M, Reinert P, Harf A, Housset B: Use of the forced oscillation technique to assess airway obstruction and reversibility in children. Am J Respir Crit Care Med 2000;161:730–736.

94 Konig P, Gayer D, Kantak A, Kreutz C, Douglass B, Hordvik NL: A trial of metaproterenol by metered-dose inhaler and two spacers in preschool asthmatics. Pediatr Pulmonol 1988;5:247–251.

95 Nussbaum E, Eyzaguirre M, Galant SP: Dose-response relationship of inhaled metaproterenol sulfate in preschool children with mild asthma. Pediatrics 1990;85:1072–1075.

96 Pauwels JH, Desager KN, Creten WL, Van der Veken J, Van Bever HP: Study of the bronchodilating effect of three doses of nebulized oxitropium bromide in asthmatic preschool children using the forced oscillation technique. Eur J Pediatr 1997;156:329–332.

97 Groggins RC, Milner AD, Stokes GM: Bronchodilator effects of clemastine, ipratropium, bromide, and salbutamol in preschool children with asthma. Arch Dis Child 1981;56:342–344.

98 Hellinckx J, De Boeck K, Demedts M: No paradoxical bronchodilator response with forced oscillation technique in children with cystic fibrosis. Chest 1998;113:55–59.

99 Klug B, Bisgaard H: Repeatability of methacholine challenges in 2- to 4-year-old children with asthma, using a new technique for quantitative delivery of aerosol. Pediatr Pulmonol 1997;23:278–286.

100 Wilson NM, Bridge P, Phagoo SB, Silverman M: The measurement of methacholine responsiveness in 5 year old children: Three methods compared. Eur Respir J 1995;8:364–370.

101 Lenney W, Milner AD: Recurrent wheezing in the preschool child. Arch Dis Child 1978; 53:468–473.

102 Ducharme FM, Davis GM, Ducharme GR: Pediatric reference values for respiratory resistance measured by forced oscillation. Chest 1998;113:1322–1328.

103 Hordvik NL, Konig P, Morris DA, Kreutz C, Pimmel RL: Normal values for forced oscilliatory respiratory resistance in children. Pediatr Pulmonol 1985;1:145–148.

104 Hantos Z, Daroczy B, Gyurkovits K: Total respiratory impedance in healthy children. Pediatr Pulmonol 1985;1:91–98.

105 Lebecque P, Desmond K, Swartebroeckx Y, Dubois P, Lulling J, Coates A: Measurement of respiratory system resistance by forced oscillation in normal children: A comparison with spirometric values. Pediatr Pulmonol 1991;10:117–122.

106 Solymar L, Aronsson PH, Bake B, Bjure J: Respiratory resistance and impedance magnitude in healthy children aged 2–18 years. Pediatr Pulmonol 1985;1:134–140.

107 Stanescu D, Moavero NE, Veriter C, Brasseur L: Frequency dependence of respiratory resistance in healthy children. J Appl Physiol 1979;47:268–272.

108 Mazurek H, Willim G, Marchal F, Haluszka J, Tomalak W: Input respiratory impedance measured by head generator in preschool children. Pediatr Pulmonol 2000;30:47–55.

Dr. Graham Hall
Respiratory Medicine
Princess Margaret Hospital for Children
GPO Box D184, Perth 6840 (Australia)
Tel. +61 8 9340 8830
Fax +61 8 9340 8181
E-Mail graham.hall@health.wa.gov.au

Hammer J, Eber E (eds): Paediatric Pulmonary Function Testing.
Prog Respir Res. Basel, Karger, 2005, vol 33, pp 78–91

Applications and Future Directions of Infant Pulmonary Function Testing

Janet Stocks   Sooky Lum

Portex Anaesthesia, Intensive Therapy and Respiratory Medicine Unit, Institute of Child Health,
London, UK

Abstract

During the past 20 years there has been enormous progress
in the field of infant lung function testing, with respect to the
range of tests and equipment now available, their applications in
research and clinical studies, and the degree of national and
international collaboration. The major role for lung function
testing in infants remains firmly within the research arena, where
it has been extensively used to examine the early determinants
of airway function and to investigate underlying pathophysiology
and response to therapeutic interventions in a variety of respiratory diseases during early life. During recent years there has
been increasing emphasis on developing techniques that can be
used in unsedated infants and for those requiring ventilatory
support. Future strategies need to encompass a multicenter,
multidisciplinary, collaborative approach, with results from infant
pulmonary function tests being integrated with those from
other disciplines, including imaging, genetics, inflammation and
immunology. The aims of this chapter are to (1) provide an
overview of the extent to which infant lung function tests have
been used in clinical and epidemiological research in the past,
(2) describe some of the recently developed techniques that
may have increasing application in future years and (3) consider
potential future contributions of infant pulmonary function
testing in the management of respiratory disease during infancy.

Introduction

As will be evident from the previous chapters, accurate assessment of lung function in infants is no mean

undertaking – requiring not only the highest specifications
from equipment in terms of frequency response, safety and
minimization of both dead space and resistance, but
infinite patience and meticulous attention to detail from
the operators. The specialized nature of the equipment and
time-consuming nature of the tests, which usually require
the presence of at least two highly skilled individuals for
several hours, means that these tests are far more expensive to perform than those available for older cooperative
children. In addition, the information gained from these
studies may be limited by lack of appropriate reference
data with which to separate the effects of lung disease
from those of growth and development, and the need for
sedation beyond the neonatal period, which limits study
duration, the frequency with which assessments can be
undertaken and the acceptability of these tests to many
parents.

Despite all these problems, interest in assessing lung
function during early life continues to increase. The reasons for this are manifold, but include the fact that it is now
realized that much of the burden of respiratory disease in
childhood and later life has its origins in infancy and early
childhood. Indeed, there is increasing evidence that insults
to the developing lung may have lifelong effects, due to the
phenomenon of fetal programming, and that remarkable
'tracking' of lung function occurs from infancy throughout
life. This has emphasized the need to prevent lung injury
both before and after delivery when lung growth is so rapid.
In addition, despite recent advances in molecular biology, it
is becoming increasingly evident that the effects of new
diagnostic and therapeutic advances will still need to be

evaluated in vivo by employing objective physiological outcome measures in order to better understand the implications of genetics and gene-environment interactions for normal lung growth and development, as well as interpreting the effects of various disease states and response to therapeutic interventions. Furthermore, medical and technological advances have led to increased survival of extremely preterm infants but no reduction in the prevalence of chronic lung disease. This has increased awareness of the need for a better understanding, both of lung growth and development, and the effect of different ventilatory strategies, in order to minimize lung injury during this critical period.

The need to meet this increased demand and overcome at least some of the barriers to obtaining accurate and relevant information in this age group was recognized by the formation of the joint American Thoracic Society/European Respiratory Society (ATS/ERS) Task Force. This international task force has been extremely active in this field for the past 10 years, organizing regular workshops and postgraduate courses, and publishing a textbook and series of manuscripts to provide guidelines for developing more standardized equipment and techniques. Nevertheless, as will be discussed below, the clinical usefulness of these tests within individual infants remains far more limited than in older subjects.

The aims of this chapter are to (1) provide an overview of the extent to which infant lung function tests have been used in clinical and epidemiological research in the past, (2) describe briefly some of the lesser-known recently developed techniques that may have increasing application in future years and (3) consider potential future contributions of infant pulmonary function tests (PFTs) in the management of respiratory disease during infancy, including what would be required before infant PFTs could play a significant role in the clinical management of individual infants; in other words, what we know, what we need to know and what the future challenges are.

Previous Applications of Infant PFTs

Introduction
The major role for lung function testing in infants remains firmly within the research arena, where it has been extensively used to examine the early determinants of airway function and to investigate underlying pathophysiology and response to therapeutic interventions in a variety of respiratory diseases during early life. An impressive array of tests is now available for use in infants, allowing

accurate assessment of lung volumes, respiratory mechanics and control of breathing by those with the necessary skills and patience to apply them. The most commonly used tests have been those of forced expiration, passive respiratory mechanics and measurements of lung volume by inert gas dilution or whole body plethysmography. Application of these tests in clinical research studies has furthered our knowledge with respect to (1) the early determinants of airway function, including the adverse effect of preterm delivery, intrauterine growth retardation and pre- and postnatal exposure to tobacco smoke, (2) natural history of diseases such as cystic fibrosis (CF), chronic lung disease and wheezing illnesses (which affect up to 40% infants in first year of life), (3) bronchial responsiveness in early life and (4) lung growth and development following neonatal lung disease.

Some of the more recent applications and findings are summarized below.

Applications of Infant Lung Function Testing in Epidemiological Research
Early Determinants of Respiratory Function
Numerous studies have shown that the sex of an infant has a marked effect on airway function, as reflected by the lower maximal expiratory flows observed in boys compared with girls at any given height both during infancy [1–5] and later childhood. This may contribute to the increased prevalence of wheezing in boys at all ages to puberty. Although this male disadvantage disappears after puberty, the increased perinatal mortality and respiratory morbidity among boys suggest a broader vulnerability to early life events in young males. It is therefore important to use sex-specific reference data when predicting 'normal ranges' of airway function [6], to avoid underestimating the degree of any impairment in girls, or overestimating it in boys. Although less is known about the impact of ethnic group on lung function during early life, both nasal and airway resistance have been shown to be lower in Afro-Caribbean than Caucasian infants. Significant differences in breathing pattern and forced expired flows between these two groups have also been reported in those delivered prematurely [2, 7] suggesting either that the respiratory system is more mature, or that lung and airway function are relatively enhanced in Afro-Caribbean infants delivered prematurely.

During the last few years, there has been increasing evidence of the adverse effects of maternal smoking on infant lung function [5, 8–10]. This effect is apparent at least 7 weeks prior to the expected date of delivery [7], and is independent of any postnatal exposure, as demonstrated by studies that have assessed lung function in healthy infants prior to discharge from the neonatal unit [7, 11, 12]. A recent review of the literature found that, while there is no convincing evidence from studies in human infants that smoking during pregnancy is associated with increased airway responsiveness at birth, many studies have demonstrated a reduction in baseline forced expiratory flows (by an average of around 20%), as well as increases in both airway and total resistance [13]. In addition, there is substantial evidence regarding the adverse effect of maternal smoking during pregnancy on postnatal control of breathing, particularly with respect to a blunted response to hypoxia, hypercapnia and arousal stimuli [14, 15]. In infants born to atopic mothers, exhaled nitric oxide levels are increased shortly after birth in those exposed to maternal smoking, while the reverse appears to be true amongst those delivered to nonatopic mothers [16]. This underlines the complex interactions of maternal and environmental factors on the development of airway disease. While maternal smoking during pregnancy remains the most significant source of early life exposure to tobacco products and is likely to be largely responsible for diminished airway function in the first few years of life, continuing postnatal tobacco smoke exposure from either parent will increase the risk of respiratory infections, wheezing illnesses and diminished lung function throughout childhood [13]. The effect of parental smoking has an equally adverse effect on infants with lung disease [17], thereby necessitating careful recording of such exposures if results from either clinical or research studies are to be interpreted correctly.

A family history of atopy, particularly maternal asthma, has also been shown to be associated with diminished airway function and increased airway responsiveness during the first years of life [1, 4, 8, 9, 18–21]. Despite increasing emphasis on the potential effect of intrauterine growth retardation on subsequent health throughout life [22–24], relatively little was known until recently about the impact of being born 'small for gestational age' on lung function during infancy. During the past few years, a study has been undertaken in which over 200 healthy infants were recruited to address this issue. After adjusting for all known confounders, including age, sex and current body size, timed forced expiratory volumes from raised lung volume were found to be significantly lower in infants born small for gestational age than in appropriately grown controls, with a similar tendency for forced expired flows [19], these changes persisting throughout the first year of life [20]. This study also highlighted the complex interactions between birth weight, socioeconomic status, family history of atopy, parental smoking and airway function in infants, and emphasized the need for large numbers of infants to be recruited to studies such as these if meaningful conclusions are to be reached.

Infant Lung Function as a Predictor of Subsequent Respiratory Morbidity?

The Tucson Children Respiratory Study was the first longitudinal assessment of the natural history of asthma that included infant lung function tests [25]. Over 1,200 children were enrolled at birth. Eight hundred of these were still participating at 13 years of age [26], although only 10% of these subjects had had lung function measured in the first few months of life. This study was the first to provide evidence that diminished airway function precedes wheezing illness, in that the tidal breathing ratio (t_{PTEF}:t_E) was significantly lower in boys (though not in girls) who subsequently wheezed with a lower respiratory illness (LRI) in the first year of life. Although there was no significant difference in V'_{maxFRC} between those who did and did not wheeze when follow-up was limited to the first year of life, subsequent follow-up revealed a diminution of V'_{maxFRC} shortly after birth in those who wheezed during the first year and who had had at least one additional wheezing LRI by 3 years of age [26]. Similar findings were reported from the Boston study [10] (who also used V'_{maxFRC} as an outcome measure) and in the London study, which found elevated premorbid values of airway resistance in those who subsequently wheezed in the first year [9]. By contrast, the Perth longitudinal study suggested that reduced airway function in early life was associated with persistent wheeze at 11 years but not with transient wheeze [27]. Discrepancies between results may reflect differences in techniques, methods of statistical analysis, population and environment as well as the fact that, although a large number of children may be recruited to longitudinal studies during infancy, the number in whom repeated lung function measures can be made on all test occasions may be relatively small due to the inherent difficulties in conducting such studies. Nevertheless, despite the wide range of techniques used, all of these studies have provided evidence of diminished premorbid lung function shortly after birth amongst those with subsequent wheezing illness.

While one of the major aims of these epidemiological studies, namely to predict which infants who wheeze are likely to progress to asthma in later life, has not yet been realized, considerable knowledge has been gleaned regarding the range of different wheezing phenotypes. It is now generally acknowledged that those with very early onset of wheeze (first year of life), whose mothers smoke and in whom there is no family history of asthma or atopy have a relatively low risk for asthma. By contrast, those in whom

Stocks/Lum

onset of wheeze occurs later and/or in the absence of any significant exposure to pre- or postnatal tobacco smoke, where there is a maternal history of asthma, persistent personal atopy (initially to food and later to inhaled allergens) and an increased bronchial responsiveness (with or without diminished flows) in infancy, will have a much higher risk for subsequent asthma [26].

Serial measurements of lung function from cohort studies have also revealed considerable tracking of lung function (i.e. those with the lowest levels of airway function initially tend to retain this position throughout life). This has been demonstrated in healthy term [20] and preterm [28] infants, in infants and young children with CF [29, 30] and between infancy and school age in those with bronchopulmonary dysplasia [31]. There is thus increasing evidence that some infants are born more susceptible to respiratory problems and that lung function during later life may be largely determined by factors occurring before or shortly after birth.

Problems in Assessing Lung Function in Infants with Respiratory Disease

Despite numerous attempts to monitor changes in lung function as a means of identifying early onset of pulmonary disease during the first year of life, the natural course of pulmonary involvement in infants with respiratory disorders remains relatively poorly understood [32, 33]. Problems encountered include: (1) contraindication of sedation in the presence of acute respiratory disease [34], (2) difficulties in repeating measurements frequently enough, (3) difficulties in distinguishing the effects of disease from those of growth and development, in the absence of a control group or appropriate reference data, (4) confounding of measurements by developmental changes in chest wall compliance and/or the dominance of the upper airways when measuring airway or total respiratory resistance [35], and (5) increased within-subject variability of measurements among infants with respiratory disease [36, 37].

Further difficulties in interpreting results from clinical studies – whether in an individual infant or within the context of a research study – arise from the fact that many of the assumptions underlying measurements of lung volumes and mechanics, such as rapid equilibration of pressures throughout the respiratory system (as required for accurate measures of lung volumes by plethysmography or passive respiratory mechanics using airway occlusion techniques), or the presence of a single time constant during passive lung emptying (single breath technique), may be violated in the presence of severe airway obstruction. Similarly, the choice of method used to assess lung volumes may be critical, with

any gas trapped behind closed or slowly ventilating areas secondary to airway obstruction being detectable by plethysmographic but not gas dilution techniques.

Applications of Infant Lung Function Testing in Clinical Research Studies

Despite these problems there is a vast literature describing the application of infant lung function tests in clinical research: the rapid thoracoabdominal compression technique for measuring V'_{maxFRC} being the most commonly used method for assessing airway function in this age group.

Baseline Lung Function in Infants with Respiratory Disease

V'_{maxFRC} has been shown to be lower in infants with recurrent wheeze [26], bronchiolitis [38], tracheomalacia [39] and those with history of life-threatening events [40]. Application of these tests in infants with CF has been summarized recently [41, 42]. Most studies have reported diminished lung and airway function in symptomatic infants [42–47]. It has recently been shown that airway function is reduced at an early stage in infants with CF, even in the absence of clinically recognized LRI [48] and that this does not catch up during infancy and early childhood [29]. These findings have important potential implications for early interventions in CF. While several reports have suggested that the raised volume technique may be a more sensitive means of discriminating changes in lung function in infants with respiratory disease than either tidal breathing parameters [49] or V'_{maxFRC} [17, 50], it should be remembered that this technique is more complex to apply and that guidelines to standardize data collection and analysis are only just beginning to emerge [51, 52].

Response to Therapeutic Interventions

Several studies have been designed wherein results from lung function tests have been used to assess response to therapeutic interventions, such as antibiotic treatment or administration of corticosteroids [43, 44, 47]. The varying conclusions from such studies may be partially attributable to the heterogeneous nature of both disease severity and individual response to therapy among the infants studied, but may also reflect the relatively small number of subjects within each of these studies, with inevitable consequences with respect to potential sampling bias and power of study.

Bronchial Responsiveness

One of the most extensively studied clinical research areas in which infant lung function tests have been applied is that of bronchial responsiveness using both bronchial challenge and bronchodilation [36, 53–59]. There is currently no standardized approach to performing either type of intervention, with respect to agent used, dosage, mode of delivery, outcome measures or methods of analyzing and reporting results. This has resulted in considerable difficulties when attempting to elucidate age-related changes in airway responsiveness during early life [60, 61].

Measurements of resistance and forced expiratory flows have been the two most commonly used methods for assessing change in airway function during such studies, although recent work has suggested that assessment of tissue mechanics may also be valuable [54]. Although resistance is a direct assessment of airway caliber, airway or pulmonary resistance may be dominated by the caliber of extrathoracic nose breathing in infants. Forced expiratory flows should provide a better reflection of changes in intrathoracic airway caliber, but are themselves highly dependent on lung volume and airway tone, both of which may change in response to the intervention, resulting in an underestimation of the degree of airway responsiveness. Interpretation of these studies is further complicated by the lack of information regarding intra-subject, between-test repeatability on the same occasion [36, 53, 62].

Despite the generally poor response to bronchodilators in early life, there is convincing evidence that the airways are fully innervated and capable of responding to a range of challenges during both fetal and early postnatal life (56, 63). The effectiveness of bronchodilators in wheezy infants remains controversial [59, 64], reflecting the fact that, in many infants who wheeze, the reduction in baseline airway function is not due to reversible bronchoconstriction, but transient conditions associated with diminished airway patency [65].

Applications during and following Intensive Care

Numerous studies have attempted to use parameters derived from infant lung function tests to assess the effects of preterm delivery, neonatal lung disease and ventilatory support [15, 66–75]. The most commonly used approaches in recent years have been assessments of passive respiratory mechanics and lung volumes [66, 67, 76]. The only volume that has been routinely measured in infants during mechanical ventilation has been that at end expiration with or without positive end-expiratory pressure [67, 70, 77–79], although determination of lung volumes over an extended volume range using the negative deflation technique has also been described in specialized centers [80, 81].

Specific difficulties in undertaking and interpreting measurements of infant lung function during intensive care (over and above those encountered when assessing spontaneously breathing infants) have been reviewed previously [74, 76, 82, 83] and arise from factors including the following:

1. Relative invasiveness of these techniques in clinically unstable infants.
2. Insensitivity of the test to changes in respiratory mechanics within individuals due, for example, to the relative magnitude of resistance of the tracheal tube [84, 85] or the underlying pathophysiology.
3. Inaccuracies in displayed values of tidal volume [86].
4. Confounding of results due to interactions between the ventilator and spontaneous breathing activity [76].
5. Leaks around the tracheal tube [87], which may invalidate attempts to assess lung function in intubated infants and yet remain difficult to eliminate due to widespread use of uncuffed tubes in this age group. Recent evidence suggesting that, at least beyond the neonatal period, cuffed tubes may not be associated with an increased risk of upper airway trauma and may facilitate ventilatory management in those with severe respiratory problems [88, 89] may reduce such problems in the future.
6. Heterogeneous nature of the population with respect to maturity, body size and clinical severity.
7. Multitude of possible treatment modalities that infants may be exposed to.
8. Fact that results are frequently corrected for body size simply by expressing data as a ratio (per kilogram body weight or, even worse, per centimeter body length). Unless it can be shown that there is a linear relationship between the selected lung function parameter and body size, with no intercept on extrapolation (which is unlikely to be the case following preterm delivery) the use of such ratios may severely distort comparisons between infants of differing body size and maturity, and hence the effect of any disease process, its resolution or treatment. In such circumstances the use of multivariate analysis is likely to be the preferred option, but demands substantial sample size to achieve adequate power of study.

Although several studies have suggested that measurements of respiratory mechanics may be predictive of subsequent bronchopulmonary dysplasia (BPD) [72, 90, 91], this was not confirmed in a randomized controlled study of mechanically ventilated neonates who were assigned to conventional management with or without daily assessments of lung mechanics [92]. Post hoc analysis did, however, show that survivors in whom such measurements had been performed were ventilated for a significantly shorter period (median 3 vs. 5 days) compared with controls. The authors also calculated that a much larger sample size would be required to achieve adequate power of study for their original study aim.

It is becoming increasingly evident that preterm delivery, even in the absence of any initial respiratory disease may have an adverse effect on subsequent lung growth and development [93–95] which persists and may even worsen throughout the first years of life [28, 96, 97]. Most studies in infants with BPD or chronic lung disease of infancy have suggested that lung volumes are low early in infancy but subsequently become normal or elevated [66]. This has been attributed to the fact that, over time, pulmonary fibrosis may become less important relative to airway disease and that lung volumes may, therefore, increase disproportionately with growth. Studies of infants with BPD/chronic lung disease of infancy have also reported reduced compliance [90, 91, 98] and increased resistance [90, 91] during the first year of life. As mentioned above, some caution may be required when interpreting these results, depending on the methods used to express pulmonary function in relation to body size. Lung function tests have also been used as objective outcome measures to assess the effect of different types of ventilatory support, including extra-corporeal membrane oxygenation and high frequency oscillation, during the neonatal period on subsequent lung growth and development [71, 97, 99–103].

New Approaches to Assessing Respiratory Function in Infants

The expanding role of infant lung function testing in both clinical and research studies has been accompanied in recent years by the development of new approaches to assessing lung function during early life as well as further modification of well-established techniques. While their use is not yet widespread and commercially available equipment is scarce, several of these techniques have considerable future potential for clinical measurements and are therefore reviewed briefly below.

Beyond the neonatal period, wheezing disorders of either a transient or persistent pattern tend to dominate most of the respiratory problems encountered in infants and young children, as reflected by the emphasis placed on assessment of airway function in this age group. Nevertheless there is increasing awareness that airway resistance and forced expired flows are determined not only by the caliber of the airways, but by the compliance of the airway wall and recoil of the surrounding parenchyma, leading to the search for suitable parameters that will reflect these characteristics and hence improve interpretation of results.

Recent modifications of the long-established forced oscillation technique, in which respiratory impedance (Z_{rs}) is measured by superimposing small amplitude pressure oscillations on the respiratory system and measuring the resultant oscillatory flow [104], have met with remarkable success in this area. One of the advantages of this technique is that it can be applied during spontaneous tidal breathing and requires no special maneuvers, making it potentially applicable in young and unsedated infants. Depending on the frequency of the applied pressure wave, the resultant impedance will contain different mechanical information. The response to very slow pressure oscillations (<2 Hz), during what is commonly referred to as the low-frequency forced oscillation technique (LFOT), allows the noninvasive partitioning of lung function into airway and tissue parameters [73, 105, 106]. By contrast, at very high frequencies, using a technique that has come to be known as the 'high frequency interrupter technique' or HIT, the information derived is primarily related to airway wall mechanics, which is particularly important in wheezing disorders [107]. Impedance measurements should only be used if measured signals are of high quality since large errors and misinterpretation of data can occur with poor quality signals. The key advantage of both the HIT and LFOT is that they can be applied during relatively brief interruptions to the normal breathing pattern during spontaneous quiet sleep, even in rapidly breathing infants. The major limitation of the LFOT is the requirement for apnea during the external oscillations, since the small amplitude oscillatory signal does not contain sufficient power to suppress the influence of the higher harmonics of spontaneous breathing. This is usually achieved by administering several augmented breaths (2 kPa) and holding the lung at raised lung volume to invoke the Hering-Breuer reflex and hence a respiratory pause before applying the oscillations. Development of a monitoring technique that provides information on tissue mechanics is of particular interest for studies in preterm infants, where parenchymal disease is a major component of acute respiratory illness, and in whom failure of alveolarization has been targeted as a major feature of subsequent chronic lung disease [66]. In addition to monitoring lung growth and development, the LFOT has the potential for estimating the mechanically optimal lung volume in intubated infants during high-frequency oscillatory ventilation, as recently shown in the preterm lung model [108].

Although initially described many years ago, the multiple breath inert gas washout technique has only been used intermittently in infants and young children [94, 109], possibly reflecting the complexity of data analysis and the lack of commercially available equipment and software. During recent years, technological advances combined with increasing awareness that indices of ventilation inhomogeneity, such as the lung clearance index (cumulative expired volume/FRC), provide a sensitive measure of small airway disease [110, 111] and that conventional measures of airway function may not detect early changes in peripheral airway function until lung disease is well-established [111] have led to a resurgence of interest in this field. The multiple breath gas mixing technique has great potential as measurements are performed during spontaneous breathing, making it applicable to subjects of all ages, including unsedated infants. A further advantage of this approach is that, in health, gas mixing efficiency remains remarkably stable throughout life, enabling the effects of disease to be distinguished from those of growth and development with far greater confidence than when dealing with most parameters of lung function which are highly dependent on age and body size. Recent work has demonstrated that the multiple breath inert gas washout technique is a far more sensitive method of detecting early changes in lung function amongst infants and children with CF than more conventional measures of forced expired flows and volumes [111, 112]. Recent development and ongoing validation of the ultrasonic flowmeter may mean that, in the future, reliable measurements will be available not only in unsedated preterm and newborn infants, but on the intensive care unit (ICU) [74, 113].

Recent refinements of the noninvasive imaging method of electrical impedance tomography to assess spatial distribution of ventilation and its application in both ventilated and spontaneously breathing infants also bode well for the future use of this method, both during and following pediatric intensive care. Serial measurements using electrical impedance tomography in ventilated infants were able to identify the redistribution of lung ventilation and changes in the magnitude of regional ventilation in response to alterations in ventilator settings, surfactant instillation and changes in posture [114, 115]. Provided further adaptations of hardware and software can be implemented to improve practical handling and facilitate stable and undisturbed measurements in the ICU, this noninvasive method could become a useful bedside monitoring tool of regional lung ventilation in critically ill infants, with important implications for optimizing lung volume and minimizing lung injury.

A relatively neglected area of investigation that has received more attention recently has been that relating to chest wall mechanics and the respiratory muscles [116]. Dysfunction of the respiratory muscles may not only result in disease, but render an infant unable to compensate for the effects of such disease, with the underlying cause of ventilatory failure in approximately 50% preterm infants being attributed to respiratory muscle failure. Knowledge relating to the strength of the respiratory muscles may be potentially useful in a number of clinical situations, including whether or not to wean an infant from the ventilator and when assessing recovery from acute infections [116]. Methods of assessing respiratory muscle strength include the determination of maximal inspired and expired pressures during respiratory efforts against brief airway occlusions [117], although the marked within- and between-subject variability of this measure may limit its clinical usefulness. Furthermore, simple assessment of respiratory muscle strength does not reflect either endurance or susceptibility to fatigue. Work is currently being undertaken to evaluate the discriminative ability of alternative indices, such as the tension time index of the respiratory muscles. The latter has several advantages in that it is completely noninvasive, does not require placement of gastric or esophageal pressure transducers and assesses muscle fatigue in all the respiratory muscles – not simply the diaphragm. Its potential usefulness has, however, still to be evaluated in infants [116].

Esophageal manometry was once commonplace during assessments of lung function in infants [118], but nowadays its use has generally been replaced by the assessment of passive respiratory mechanics using one of the occlusion techniques [119], except in ventilated or preterm infants who may already be receiving regular nasogastric feeds. In situations where esophageal manometry is still required, the use of esophageal balloons and water-filled catheters has largely been replaced by catheter tip transducers [120].

The need to assess not only respiratory mechanics but gas exchange and control of breathing when assessing infants with respiratory disease, particularly in those delivered prematurely or requiring ventilatory support, has been recognized in several recent publications [14, 15, 66, 121–125]. Similarly, despite recognized difficulties in accurately interpreting measures of exhaled nitric oxide as a noninvasive marker of airway inflammation in infants, due to the influence of nasal breathing and the marked flow dependency of such measures, there have been some interesting reports describing their potential utility in both clinical and epidemiological studies, which warrant further investigation [16, 126–128]. Although further refinement and standardization of the technique are required, bedside equipment for evaluation of such markers is now available for use in infants.

Requirements for noninvasive methods of assessing lung function during natural sleep or during prolonged periods of monitoring have resulted in persistent efforts to analyze tidal breathing parameters, whether derived from changes in flow and volume at the airway opening or from body surface measurements [129]. Following initial reports regarding the potential predictive value of the time to peak expiratory flow as a ratio of total expiratory time (t_{PTEF}:t_E) [25], a plethora of publications was followed by a degree of disillusionment as it became obvious that the prime role of such indices would be in large epidemiological studies of newborn infants, rather than any clinical application within individuals [130–134]. Nevertheless the potential for such noninvasive methods has inspired several groups to continue the search for improved methods of analyzing and reporting such data [135]. Frey et al. [136] have proposed that tidal flow is an integrated output of the neural respiratory oscillator in the brainstem, which in turn reflects the processing of interacting chemo- and stretch receptor feedback mechanisms as well as passive mechanics of the lung and chest wall. They subsequently quantified the harmonic content of the tidal flow wave form, arguing that such complex neuromechanical respiratory control would be better characterized by considering the entire periodic tidal flow waveform rather than simple indices derived from a limited number of points, as is the case when simply reporting t_{PTEF}:t_E. Not only does this approach have exciting potential in terms of increasing and integrating our understanding of respiratory mechanics and control of breathing during early life, but it has been recently adapted for use in the clinical scenario. Habib et al. [137] recently extended this approach by analyzing the tidal flow waveform derived from respiratory inductance plethysmography in spontaneously breathing preterm infants and reported that the harmonic content of tidal flow in such infants is characterized by a power law functional form power spectrum. They were also able to demonstrate that essentially equivalent flow spectra and corresponding shape indices could be attained from direct measurements at the mouth or indirect distant flows measured at the chest wall. Providing this can be confirmed by other groups, this is an important finding, given the desirable nonintrusive nature of body surface measurements, which can potentially: (1) avoid errors arising either from leaks around the face mask or from the adverse effects of apparatus dead space and resistance when recording breathing patterns at the airway opening in very small infants [138, 139], (2) facilitate measurements over longer time periods and (3) allow delivery of treatments such as nasal continuous positive airway pressure and inspired oxygen during the measurement period.

The potential limitations of deriving either qualitative or quantitative assessments of flow and volume from body surface recordings, particularly in the presence of any marked asynchrony between chest wall and abdominal movements [140, 141] must, however, be borne in mind when attempting such measurements.

What Is the Potential Contribution of Infant PFTs to Future Management of Respiratory Disease during Early Life?

Infant lung function tests could potentially be used for early diagnosis and monitoring of lung disease, assessment of the therapeutic interventions and evaluation of disease outcome. While there is little doubt about the potential value of infant lung function tests as a means of providing objective outcome measures in clinical or epidemiological research studies, their potential usefulness with respect to influencing clinical management within an individual infant remains far more debatable, as reviewed in several recent publications [32, 33, 74, 142–145].

Lung function tests at any age are rarely performed for diagnostic purposes, but rather to monitor the nature and severity of respiratory disease or to assess the response to treatment [146]. The clinical usefulness of any technique depends not only on its ability to measure parameters that are relevant to the underlying pathophysiology and to discriminate between health and disease, but on within-subject repeatability both within and between test occasions. As discussed above, whilst highly reproducible measurements of lung function can be made in infants during the same test occasion, little is yet known about the 'between-test repeatability'. For spontaneously breathing infants, this lack of data relates primarily to factors such as difficulties of repeat sedation, and the time constraints of working parents to bring infants for repeat measurements at intervals less than 4–6 monthly. By contrast, the ability to assess repeatability in the intubated inpatient is limited more by factors such as clinical instability, or problems in maintaining stable measurement conditions between such repeat measures. Considerable effort will be required to collect data in this field if we are to distinguish what constitutes a clinically significant change within an individual infant as a result of disease progression or response to treatment.

Similar problems arise with respect to distinguishing the effects of disease from those of growth and development

[147]. The need for sedation limits the numbers of healthy infants that can be studied during spontaneous breathing, while relatively few truly 'normal' infants are anesthetized or ventilated and hence available to provide representative values under these particular circumstances. Some limited attempts have been made to establish reference data for intubated infants and children but far more work will be required in this field if newly developed techniques are to be fully utilized.

Recent international collaborative efforts have led to the publication of sex-specific reference data for V'_{maxFRC} during infancy [6]. The development of more standardized equipment and techniques for infant lung function testing will hopefully encourage and facilitate similar initiatives in the future, so that appropriate regression equations, which can take into account important determinants such as length, body weight, age, maturity, sex and ethnic group, can be developed. It is important to realize that much of the older published literature, frequently quoted when interpreting data from infants with respiratory disease, may no longer be appropriate due to the technological advances in both equipment and methodology that have occurred during recent years [148]. It is therefore imperative that, as with measurements in older children [149, 150], infant lung function results are interpreted with great caution unless the operators can verify the validity of their chosen reference data.

If appropriate equipment was to be miniaturized and/or incorporated into the ventilatory circuit, so that continuous online monitoring of appropriate parameters could be undertaken, the major area in which infant lung function tests could influence clinical management in the future probably lies in the neonatal and pediatric ICU. Given the current rate of technological development, this is certainly feasible, but will demand a major commitment by all concerned, plus the recognition that most of the tests used in the past are too complex and/or too insensitive to provide the clinician with reliable and relevant information with which to guide treatment. Techniques that should be targeted include those that measure absolute, and changes in, lung volume, tissue mechanics, distribution of ventilation, gas mixing efficiency, oxygen consumption, control of breathing and respiratory muscle function, with results being carefully integrated with other relevant outputs, including blood gases, ventilator settings and direct or non-invasive markers of inflammation. Many of these measurements will require not only the presence of leak-free tracheal tubes in infants who are intubated, but a much improved knowledge of respiratory physiology amongst pediatricians and intensivists if the information provided is

to be utilized in a meaningful fashion. Interpretation of results will also depend on knowledge of growth and development of the lung, particularly after extremely preterm delivery, and more sophisticated adjustment for body size than simply dividing by weight or length as is all too common at present. The latter is particularly critical in the presence of somatic growth retardation.

Other areas where there may be a real role for infant lung function testing are with respect to longitudinal measurements from birth and throughout the preschool years in high risk groups – such as those with persistent wheezing, CF and chronic lung disease. The potential prognostic value of such tests within individual subjects is as yet unknown, since it is only during the last few years that more routine assessments of lung function have been possible throughout the preschool years [151–154], but such studies are currently being undertaken. Interpretation of such data will require similar longitudinal measurements to be performed among healthy children from birth to school age.

Within an individual infant, the clinical usefulness of any lung function test will always be enhanced if serial measures can be undertaken rather than a single assessment, and if the choice of test is based on the question to be answered, clinical reasoning and a knowledge of the suspected underlying pathophysiology, rather than simply on the equipment that happens to be available in any given center. Thus if bronchial responsiveness is to be assessed using either a bronchodilator or bronchial challenge, the selected test should: (1) have low intrasubject variability (which should ideally be assessed on the same occasion, and under similar measurement conditions), (2) be sensitive to the physiological changes that are likely to occur during the challenge, and (3) remain valid in the presence of alterations of airway mechanics.

Similarly, while assessment of respiratory compliance may be relevant in a newborn infant receiving surfactant (provided it is combined with measures of lung volume), it is unlikely to provide much insight into the effects of treatment in a wheezy toddler. The choice of technique will also very much depend on the setting, with many of the currently available tests such as the raised volume technique requiring highly trained staff and sophisticated equipment.

It is generally agreed that no single lung function test will ever provide the answer, and that a combination of tests is required, the results of which should be interpreted in the light of other information regarding present clinical status and prior medical and social history. Given the marked influence of factors such as preterm delivery, intrauterine growth retardation, sex and maternal smoking during pregnancy, it is particularly important to take a careful history from the parents when performing such tests. Accurate measures of weight and length (using a calibrated stadiometer and 2 trained individuals [34]) is also essential – as is taking into account the potential influence of failure to thrive on the results obtained. Thus in a child with CF whose weight is below the 3rd centile for age, expression of lung volume per kilogram body weight will tend to overestimate the presence of any hyperinflation, while the reverse will be true in an obese young child with recurrent wheezing.

The largest groups of infants with respiratory problems are those with wheezing disorders, infants with chronic lung disease or respiratory failure during the neonatal period, who may suffer from combined obstructive and restrictive lung disease, and those with chronic progressive diseases such as CF. If more information were available regarding within-subject, within- and between-occasion repeatability of selected measurements together with appropriate reference data, any of these infants could potentially benefit from serial measurements to assess disease progression and possibly to determine appropriate therapeutic strategies. This possibility would be enhanced if more sensitive techniques were developed – including assessments of alveolar surface area, pulmonary capillary blood flow and tissue mechanics for those recovering for chronic lung disease. By contrast, while respiratory infections are common in infancy, assessments of lung function are unlikely to have any impact on their management.

In a recent review, Godfrey et al. [144] concluded that the only infants in whom assessments of lung function should be performed for purely clinical reasons were: (1) those who present with unexplained tachypnea, hypoxia, cough or respiratory distress in whom a definitive diagnosis is not apparent from physical examination and other investigations, (2) infants with severe, continuous, chronic obstructive lung disease who do not respond to an adequate clinical trial of combined corticosteroid and bronchodilator therapy or (3) infants with known respiratory disease of uncertain severity in whom there is a need to justify management decisions.

Whether or not these criteria will be extended in the future, if improved noninvasive methods of studying unsedated infants or those receiving ventilatory support are developed, remains to be seen.

It is not yet known whether serial assessment of lung function in infants with CF, chronic lung disease or persistent wheeze will alter their clinical management. To some extent this will depend on the prognostic value of assessments of lung function during the first year of life, information that will only become available once serial lung function measurements from diagnosis to school age become available.

Conclusions

During the past 20 years there have been major advances in the field of infant lung function testing, with respect to the quality of equipment now available, the range of tests applicable in this age range and the degree of national and international collaboration and standardization. Challenging areas in which infant lung function tests could usefully be employed in the future include: (1) elucidation of the mechanisms by which insults to the developing lung contribute to respiratory disease, (2) identification of which of the many infants who wheeze in the first year of life go on to develop asthma, (3) determination of the most beneficial treatments for various lung diseases, (4) preservation of lung function in infants with progressive lung diseases such as CF by detection of, and appropriate interventions for, early changes in lung function, (5) identification of factors that contribute to the development of chronic lung disease of prematurity so that alternative, improved strategies of both antenatal and postnatal management can be developed, (6) continuous on-line, noninvasive monitoring of appropriate respiratory parameters in ventilated infants for individual optimization of ventilatory support, and (7) longitudinal studies of lung growth and development in health and disease from birth to school age, taking advantage of recent developments in the field of preschool testing.

Future strategies need to encompass a multicenter, multidisciplinary, collaborative approach, whereby there are increasing links between structure and function (particularly with respect to some of the exciting developments in the field of noninvasive imaging) and between physiology, epidemiology, genetics, inflammation and immunology. Ultimately the aim should be to further develop and validate infant respiratory function tests so that they can be used as objective and reliable outcome measures both in individual infants and in multicenter clinical trials, thereby strengthening the scientific basis for the prevention and treatment of respiratory disease in early life, as well as providing insights into the mysteries of the developing lung.

References

1 Clarke JR, Salmon B, Silverman M: Bronchial responsiveness in the neonatal period as a risk factor for wheezing in infancy. Am J Respir Crit Care Med 1995;151:1434–1440.

2 Stocks J, Henschen M, Hoo A-F, Costeloe KC, Dezateux CA: Influence of ethnicity and gender on airway function in preterm infants. Am J Respir Crit Care Med 1997;156:1855–1862.

3 Jones M, Castile R, Davis S, Kisling J, Filbrun D, Flucke R, Goldstein A, Emsley C, Ambrosius W, Tepper RS: Forced expiratory flows and volumes in infants. Am J Respir Crit Care Med 2000;161:353–359.

4 Lum S, Hoo AF, Dezateux C, Goetz I, Wade A, DeRooy L, Costeloe K, Stocks J: The association between birthweight, sex, and airway function in infants of nonsmoking mothers. Am J Respir Crit Care Med 2001;164:2078–2084.

5 Young S, Sherrill DL, Arnott J, Diepeveen D, Le Souëf PN, Landau LI: Parental factors affecting respiratory function during the first year of life. Pediatr Pulmonol 2000;29:331–340.

6 Hoo AF, Dezateux C, Hanrahan J, Cole TJ, Tepper R, Stocks J: Sex-specific prediction equations for V′maxFRC in infancy: A multi-center collaborative study. Am J Respir Crit Care Med 2002;165:1084–1092.

7 Hoo A-F, Henschen M, Dezateux CA, Costeloe KC, Stocks J: Respiratory function among preterm infants whose mothers smoked during pregnancy. Am J Respir Crit Care Med 1998;158:700–705.

8 Dezateux C, Stocks J, Dundas I, Fletcher ME: Impaired airway function and wheezing in infancy. The influence of maternal smoking and a genetic predisposition to asthma. Am J Respir Crit Care Med 1999;159:403–410.

9 Dezateux C, Stocks J, Wade AM, Dundas I, Fletcher ME: Airway function at one year: Association with premorbid airway function, wheezing and maternal smoking. Thorax 2001;56:680–686.

10 Tager IB, Hanrahan JP, Tosteson TD, Castile RG, Brown RW, Weiss ST, Speizer FE: Lung function, pre- and post-natal smoke exposure, and wheezing in the first year of life. Am Rev Respir Dis 1993;147:811–817.

11 Lodrup Carlsen KC, Jaakkola JJK, Nafstad P, Carlsen KH: In utero exposure to cigarette smoking influences lung function at birth. Eur Respir J 1997;10:1774–1779.

12 Stick SM, Burton PR, Gurrin L, Sly PD: Effects of maternal smoking during pregnancy and a family history of asthma on respiratory function in newborn infants. Lancet 1996;348:1060–1064.

13 Stocks J, Dezateux C: The effect of parental smoking on lung function and development during infancy. Respirology 2003;8:266–285.

14 Chang AB, Wilson SJ, Masters IB, Yuill M, Williams J, Williams G, Hubbard M: Altered arousal response in infants exposed to cigarette smoke. Arch Dis Child 2003;88:30–33.

15 Sawnani H, Jackson T, Murphy T, Beckerman R, Simakajornboon N: The effect of maternal smoking on respiratory and arousal patterns in preterm infants during sleep. Am J Respir Crit Care Med 2004;169:733–738.

16 Frey U, Kuehni C, Roiha H, Cernelc M, Reinmann B, Wildhaber JH, et al: Maternal atopic disease modifies effects of prenatal risk factors on exhaled nitric oxide in infants. Am J Respir Crit Care Med 2004;170:260–265.

17 Ranganathan SC, Bush A, Dezateux C, Carr SB, Hoo AF, Lum S, Madge S, Price J, Stroobant J, Wade A, Wallis C, Wyatt H: Relative ability of full and partial forced expiratory maneuvers to identify diminished airway function in infants with cystic fibrosis. Am J Respir Crit Care Med 2002;166:1350–1357.

18 Sheikh S, Goldsmith LJ, Howell L, Parry L, Eid N: Comparison of lung function in infants exposed to maternal smoking and in infants with a family history of asthma. Chest 1999;116:52–58.

19 Dezateux C, Lum S, Hoo AF, Hawdon J, Costeloe K, Stocks J: Low birth weight for gestation and airway function in infancy: Exploring the fetal origins hypothesis. Thorax 2004;59:60–66.

20 Hoo A-F, Stocks J, Lum S, Wade AM, Castle RA, Costeloe KL, et al: Development of lung function in early life: Influence of birthweight in infants of non-smokers. Am J Respir Crit Care Med, in press.

21 Murray CS, Pipis SD, McArdle EC, Lowe LA, Custovic A, Woodcock A: Lung function at one month of age as a risk factor for infant respiratory symptoms in a high risk population. Thorax 2002;57:388–392.

22 Godfrey KM, Barker DJ: Fetal programming and adult health. Public Health Nutr 2001;4:611–624.

23 Osmond C, Barker DJ: Fetal, infant, and childhood growth are predictors of coronary heart disease, diabetes, and hypertension in adult men and women. Environ Health Perspect 2000;108(suppl 3):545–553.

24 Stein CE, Kumaran K, Fall CHD, Shaheen SO, Osmond C, Barker DJP: Relation of fetal growth to adult lung function in South India. Thorax 1997;52:895–899.

25 Martinez FD, Morgan WJ, Wright AL, Holberg CJ, Taussig LM: Diminished lung function as a predisposing factor for wheezing respiratory illness in infants. N Engl J Med 1988;319:1112–1117.

26 Taussig LM, Wright AL, Holberg CJ, Halonen M, Morgan WJ, Martinez FD: Tucson Children's Respiratory Study: 1980 to present. J Allergy Clin Immunol 2003;111:661–675.

27 Turner SW, Palmer LJ, Rye PJ, Gibson NA, Judge PK, Cox M, Young S, Goldblatt J, Landau LI, Le Souef PN: The relationship between infant airway function, childhood airway responsiveness, and asthma. Am J Respir Crit Care Med 2004;169:921–927.

28 Hoo AF, Dezateux C, Henschen M, Costeloe K, Stocks J: Development of airway function in infancy after preterm delivery. J Pediatr 2002;141:652–658.

29 Ranganathan SC, Stocks J, Dezateux C, Bush A, Wade A, Carr S, Castle R, Dinwiddie R, Hoo AF, Lum S, Price J, Stroobant J: The evolution of airway function in early childhood following clinical diagnosis of cystic fibrosis. Am J Respir Crit Care Med 2004;169:928–933.

30 Marostica PJ, Weist AD, Eigen H, Angelicchio C, Christoph K, Savage J, Grant D, Tepper RS: Spirometry in 3- to 6-year-old children with cystic fibrosis. Am J Respir Crit Care Med 2002;166:67–71.

31 Filippone M, Sartor M, Zacchello F, Baraldi E: Flow limitation in infants with bronchopulmonary dysplasia and respiratory function at school age. Lancet 2003;361:753–754.

32 Dezateux CA, Wade AM, Schmalisch G, Landau L: Maximizing effective research in infant respiratory function; in Stocks J, Sly PD, Tepper RS, Morgan WJ (eds): Infant Respiratory Function Testing. New York, Wiley, 1996, pp 521–550.

33 Frey U: Clinical applications of infant lung function testing: Does it contribute to clinical decision making? Paediatr Respir Rev 2001;2:126–130.

34 Gaultier C, Fletcher M, Beardsmore C, Motoyama E, Stocks J: Measurement conditions; in Stocks J, Sly PD, Tepper RS, Morgan WJ (eds): Infant Respiratory Function Testing. New York, Wiley, 1996, pp 29–44.

35 Stocks J: Developmental physiology and methodology. Am J Respir Crit Care Med 1995;151:S15–S17.

36 Lagerstrand L, Ingemansson M, Bergstrom SE, Lidberg K, Hedlin G: Tidal volume forced expiration in asthmatic infants: Reproducibility and reversibility tests. Respiration 2002;69:389–396.

37 Malmberg LP, Pelkonen A, Hakulinen A, Hero M, Pohjavuori M, Skytta J, Turpeinen M: Intraindividual variability of infant whole-body plethysmographic measurements: Effects of age and disease. Pediatr Pulmonol 1999;28:356–362.

38 Modl M, Eber E, Weinhandl E, Gruber W, Zach MS: Assessment of bronchodilator responsiveness in infants with bronchiolitis. A comparison of the tital and the raised volume rapid thoracoabdominal compression technique. Am J Respir Crit Care Med 2000;161:763–768.

39 Davis S, Jones M, Kisling J, Angelicchio C, Tepper RS: Effect of continuous positive airway pressure on forced expiratory flows in infants with tracheomalacia. Am J Respir Crit Care Med 1998;158:148–152.

40 Hartmann H, Seidenberg J, Noyes JP, O'Brien L, Poets CF, Samuels MP, Southall DP: Small airway patency in infants with apparent life-threatening events. Eur J Pediatr 1998;157:71–74.

41 Gappa M, Ranganathan S, Stocks J: Lung function testing in infants with cystic fibrosis: Lessons from the past and future directions. Pediatr Pulmonol 2001;32:228–245.

42 Gappa M: The infant with cystic fibrosis: Lung function. Paediatr Respir Rev 2004; 5(suppl 1):S361–S364.

43 Beardsmore CS, Thompson JR, Williams A, Mcardle EK, Gregory GA, Weaver LT, Simpson H: Pulmonary function in infants with cystic fibrosis: The effect of antibiotic treatment. Arch Dis Child 1994;71:133–137.

44 Clayton RG Sr, Diaz CE, Bashir NS, Panitch HB, Schidlow DV, Allen JL: Pulmonary function in hospitalized infants and toddlers with cystic fibrosis. J Pediatr 1998;132:405–408.

45 Dakin CJ, Numa AH, Wang H, Morton JR, Vertzyas CC, Henry RL: Inflammation, infection, and pulmonary function in infants and young children with cystic fibrosis. Am J Respir Crit Care Med 2002;165:904–910.

46 Nixon GM, Armstrong DS, Carzino R, Carlin JB, Olinsky A, Robertson CF, Grimwood K: Early airway infection, inflammation, and lung function in cystic fibrosis. Arch Dis Child 2002;87:306–311.

47 Tepper RS, Eigen H, Stevens J, Angelicchio C, Kisling J, Ambrosius W, Heilman D: Lower respiratory illness in infants and young children with cystic fibrosis: Evaluation of treatment with intravenous hydrocortisone. Pediatr Pulmonol 1997;24:48–51.

48 Ranganathan S, Dezateux CA, Bush A, Carr SB, Castle R, Madge SL, Price JF, Stroobant J, Wade AM, Wallis CE, Stocks J: Airway function in infants newly diagnosed with cystic fibrosis. Lancet 2001;358:1964–1965.

49 Ranganathan SC, Goetz I, Hoo AF, Lum S, Castle R, Stocks J: Assessment of tidal breathing parameters in infants with cystic fibrosis. Eur Respir J 2003;22:761–766.

50 Jones MH, Howard J, Davis S, Kisling J, Tepper RS: Sensitivity of spirometric measurements to detect airway obstruction in infants. Am J Respir Crit Care Med 2003; 167:1283–1286.

51 ATS-ERS consensus statement: Raised volume forced expirations in infants: Guidelines for current practice. Am J Respir Crit Care Med, in press.

52 Lum S, Hulskamp G, Hoo AF, Ljungberg H, Stocks J: Effect of the raised lung volume technique on subsequent measures of V'maxFRC in infants. Pediatr Pulmonol 2004;38:146–154.

53 Goldstein AB, Castle RG, Davis SD, Filbrun DA, Flucke RL, McCoy KS, Tepper RS: Bronchodilator responsiveness in normal infants and young children. Am J Respir Crit Care Med 2001;164:447–454.

54 Hall GL, Hantos Z, Wildhaber JH, Petak F, Sly PD: Methacholine responsiveness in infants assessed with low frequency forced oscillation and forced expiration techniques. Thorax 2001;56:42–47.

55 Hayden MJ, Devadason SG, Sly PD, Wildhaber JH, Le Souëf PN: Methacholine responsiveness using the raised volume forced expiration technique in infants. Am J Respir Crit Care Med 1997;155:1670–1675.

56 Weist A, Williams T, Kisling J, Clem C, Tepper RS: Volume history and effect on airway reactivity in infants and adults. J Appl Physiol 2002;93:1069–1074.

57 Palmer LJ, Rye PJ, Gibson NA, Burton PR, Landau LI, Le Souëf PN: Airway responsiveness in early infancy predicts asthma, lung function, and respiratory symptoms by school age. Am J Respir Crit Care Med 2001; 163:37–42.

58 Young S, Arnott J, O'Keeffe PT, Le Souëf PN, Landau LI: The association between early life lung function and wheezing during the first 2 years of life. Eur Respir J 2000;15:151–157.

59 Modl M, Eber E, Weinhandl E, Gruber W, Zach MS: Assessment of bronchodilator responsiveness in infants with bronchiolitis. A comparison of the tidal and the raised volume rapid thoracoabdominal compression technique. Am J Respir Crit Care Med 2000; 161:763–768.

60 Collis GG, Cole CH, Le Souëf PN: Dilution of nebulised aerosols by air entrainment in children. Lancet 1990;336:341–343.

61 Le Souëf PN, Sears MR, Sherrill D: The effect of size and age of subject on airway responsiveness in children. Am J Respir Crit Care Med 1995;152:576–579.

62 Lum S, Stocks J: Reproducibility and reversibility of tidal forced expirations. Respiration 2003;70:556.

63 Hislop A: Fetal and postnatal anatomical development; in Greenough A, Roberton NRC, Milner AD (eds): Neonatal Respiratory Disorders. London, Arnold, 1995, pp 3–12.

64 Stick SM, Arnott J, Turner DJ, Young S, Landau LI, Le Souëf PN: Bronchial responsiveness and lung function in recurrently wheezy infants. Am Rev Respir Dis 1991; 144:1012–1015.

65 Hofhuis W, van der Wiel EC, Tiddens HA, Brinkhorst G, Holland WP, de Jongste JC, Merkus PJ: Bronchodilation in infants with malacia or recurrent wheeze. Arch Dis Child 2003;88:246–249.

66 Allen J, Zwerdling R, Ehrenkranz R, Gaultier C, Geggel R, Greenough A, Kleinman R, Klijanowicz A, Martinez F, Ozdemir A, Panitch HB, Nickerson B: Statement on the care of the child with chronic lung disease of infancy and childhood. Am J Respir Crit Care Med 2003;168:356–396.

67 Bhat RY, Leipala JA, Singh NR, Rafferty GF, Hannam S, Greenough A: Effect of posture on oxygenation, lung volume, and respiratory mechanics in premature infants studied before discharge. Pediatrics 2003; 112:29–32.

68 Choukroun ML, Tayara N, Fayon M, Demarquez JL: Early respiratory system mechanics and the prediction of chronic lung disease in ventilated preterm neonates requiring surfactant treatment. Biol Neonate 2003; 83:30–35.

69 Dimitriou G, Cheeseman P, Greenough A: Lung volume and the response to high volume strategy, high frequency oscillation. Acta Paediatr 2004;93:613–617.

70 Dinger J, Topfer A, Schaller P, Schwarze R: Functional residual capacity and compliance of the respiratory system after surfactant treatment in premature infants with severe respiratory distress syndrome. Eur J Pediatr 2002;161:485–490.

71 Dobyns EL, Griebel J, Kinsella JP, Abman SH, Accurso FJ: Infant lung function after inhaled nitric oxide therapy for persistent pulmonary hypertension of the newborn. Pediatr Pulmonol 1999;28:24–30.

72 Kavvadia V, Greenough A, Dimitriou G: Early prediction of chronic oxygen dependency by lung function test results. Pediatr Pulmonol 2000;29:19–26.

73 Petak F, Babik B, Asztalos T, Hall GL, Deak ZI, Sly PD, Hantos Z: Airway and tissue mechanics in anesthetized paralyzed children. Pediatr Pulmonol 2003;35:169–176.

74 Schibler A, Frey U: Role of lung function testing in the management of mechanically ventilated infants. Arch Dis Child Fetal Neonatal Ed 2002;87:F7–F10.

75 Seddon PC, Davis GM: Validity of esophageal pressure measurements with positive end-expiratory pressure in preterm infants. Pediatr Pulmonol 2003;36:216–222.

76 Sly PD, Lanteri C, Nicolai T: Measurement of respiratory function in the intensive care unit; in Stocks J, Sly PD, Tepper RS, Morgan WJ (eds): Infant Respiratory Function Testing. New York, Wiley, 1996, pp 445–484.

77 Dinger J, Topfer A, Schaller P, Schwarze R: Effect of positive end expiratory pressure on functional residual capacity and compliance in surfactant-treated preterm infants. J Perinat Med 2001;29:137–143.

78 McEvoy C, Bowling S, Williamson K, Stewart M, Durand M: Functional residual capacity and passive compliance measurements after antenatal steroid therapy in preterm infants. Pediatr Pulmonol 2001;31:425–430.

79 Schibler A, Henning R: Positive end-expiratory pressure and ventilation inhomogeneity in mechanically ventilated children. Pediatr Crit Care Med 2002;3:124–128.

80 Hammer J, Numa A, Newth CJ: Total lung capacity by N_2 washout from high and low lung volumes in ventilated infants and children. Am J Respir Crit Care Med 1998;158: 526–531.

81 Hammer J, Patel N, Newth CJ: Effect of forced deflation maneuvers upon measurements of respiratory mechanics in ventilated infants. Intensive Care Med 2003;29:2004–2008.

82 Hjalmarson O: Lung function testing – Useless in ventilated newborns? Eur J Pediatr 1994;153:S22–S26.

83 Stocks J: Infant respiratory function testing: Is it worth all the effort? Paediatr Anaesth 2004;14:537–540.

84 Keidan I, Fine GF, Kagawa T, Schneck FX, Motoyama EK: Work of breathing during spontaneous ventilation in anesthetized children: A comparative study among the face mask, laryngeal mask airway and endotracheal tube. Anesth Analg 2000;91:1381–1388.

85 Manczur T, Greenough A, Nicholson GP, Rafferty GF: Resistance of pediatric and neonatal endotracheal tubes: Influence of flow rate, size, and shape. Crit Care Med 2000;28:1595–1598.

86 Castle RA, Dunne CJ, Mok Q, Wade AM, Stocks J: Accuracy of displayed values of tidal volume in the pediatric intensive care unit. Crit Care Med 2002;30:2566–2574.

87 Main E, Castle R, Stocks J, James IG, Hatch DJ: The influence of endotracheal tube leak on the assessment of respiratory function in ventilated children. Intensive Care Med 2001;27:1788–1797.

88 James I: Cuffed tubes in children. Paediatr Anaesth 2001;11:259–263.

89 Newth CJ, Rachman B, Patel N, Hammer J: The use of cuffed versus uncuffed endotracheal tubes in pediatric intensive care. J Pediatr 2004;144:333–337.

90 Lui K, Lloyd J, Ang E, Rynn M, Gupta JM: Early changes in respiratory compliance and resistance during the development of bronchopulmonary dysplasia in the era of surfactant therapy. Pediatr Pulmonol 2000; 30:282–290.

91 Tortorolo L, Vento G, Matassa PG, Zecca E, Romagnoli C: Early changes of pulmonary mechanics to predict the severity of bronchopulmonary dysplasia in ventilated preterm infants. J Matern Fetal Neonatal Med 2002; 12:332–337.

92 Stenson BJ, Glover RM, Wilkie RA, Laing IA, Tarnow-Mordi WO: Randomised controlled trial of respiratory system compliance measurements in mechanically ventilated neonates. Arch Dis Child 1998;78:F15–F19.

93 Gappa M, Stocks J, Merkus P: Lung growth and development after preterm birth: Further evidence. Am J Respir Crit Care Med 2003; 168:399.

94 Hjalmarson O, Sandberg K: Abnormal lung function in healthy preterm infants. Am J Respir Crit Care Med 2002;165: 83–87.

95 Jobe AH: An unknown: Lung growth and development after very preterm birth. Am J Respir Crit Care Med 2002;166: 1529–1530.

96 Talmaciu I, Ren CL, Kolb SM, Hickey E, Panitch HB: Pulmonary function in technology-dependent children 2 years and older with bronchopulmonary dysplasia. Pediatr Pulmonol 2002;33:181–188.

97 Hofhuis W, Huysman MW, van der Wiel EC, Holland WP, Hop WC, Brinkhorst G, de Jongste JC, Merkus PJ: Worsening of V'maxFRC in infants with chronic lung disease in the first year of life: A more favorable outcome after high-frequency oscillation ventilation. Am J Respir Crit Care Med 2002; 166:1539–1543.

98 Baraldi E, Filippone M, Trevisanuto D, Zanardo V, Zacchello F: Pulmonary function until two years of life in infants with bronchopulmonary dysplasia. Am J Respir Crit Care Med 1997;155:149–155.

99 Beardsmore C, Dundas I, Poole K, Enock K, Stocks J: Respiratory function in survivors of the United Kingdom Extracorporeal Membrane Oxygenation Trial. Am J Respir Crit Care Med 2000;161:1129–1135.

100 Dundas I, Beardsmore CS, Wellman T, Stocks J: A Collaborative study of infant respiratory function testing. Eur Respir J 1998; 12:944–953.

101 Donn SM, Sinha SK: Can mechanical ventilation strategies reduce chronic lung disease? Semin Neonatol 2003;8:441–448.

102 Habib RH, Pyon KH, Courtney SE: Optimal high-frequency oscillatory ventilation settings by nonlinear lung mechanics analysis. Am J Respir Crit Care Med 2002;166:950–953.

103 Thomas MR, Rafferty GF, Limb ES, Peacock JL, Calvert SA, Marlow N, Milner AD, Greenough A: Pulmonary function at follow-up of very preterm infants from the United Kingdom oscillation study. Am J Respir Crit Care Med 2004;169:868–872.

104 Oostveen E, MacLeod D, Lorino H, Farre R, Hantos Z, Desager K, Marchal F: The forced oscillation technique in clinical practice: Methodology, recommendations and future developments. Eur Respir J 2003;22: 1026–1041.

105 Hall GL, Hantos Z, Sly PD: Altered respiratory tissue mechanics in asymptomatic wheezy infants. Am J Respir Crit Care Med 2001;164:1387–1391.

106 Pillow JJ, Hall GL, Willett KE, Jobe AH, Hantos Z, Sly PD: Effects of gestation and antenatal steroid on airway and tissue mechanics in newborn lambs. Am J Respir Crit Care Med 2001;163:1158–1163.

107 Frey U, Makkonen K, Wellman T, Beardsmore C, Silverman M: Alterations in airway wall properties in infants with a history of wheezing disorders. Am J Respir Crit Care Med 2000;161:1825–1829.

108 Pillow JJ, Sly PD, Hantos Z: Monitoring of lung volume recruitment and derecruitment using oscillatory mechanics during high-frequency oscillatory ventilation in the preterm lamb. Pediatr Crit Care Med 2004; 5:172–180.

109 Shao H, Sandberg K, Hjalmarson O: Impaired gas mixing and low lung volume in preterm infants with mild chronic lung disease. Pediatr Res 1998;43:536–541.

110 Coates AL: Classical respiratory physiology – Gone the way of the dinosaurs? Do we need a jurassic park? Pediatr Pulmonol 2000;30:1–2.

111 Gustafsson PM, Aurora P, Lindblad A: Evaluation of ventilation maldistribution as an early indicator of lung disease in children with cystic fibrosis. Eur Respir J 2003;22: 972–979.

112 Ljungberg H, Hulskamp G, Hoo AF, Lum S, Pillow JJ, Aurora P, Gustafsson P, Stocks J: Abnormal lung clearance index (LCI) is more common than reduced $FEV_{0.5}$ in infants with CF. Am J Respir Crit Care Med 2003; 167:A41.

113 Schibler A, Hall GL, Businger F, Reinmann B, Wildhaber JH, Cernelc M, Frey U: Measurement of lung volume and ventilation distribution with an ultrasonic flow meter in healthy infants. Eur Respir J 2002;20: 912–918.

114 Frerichs I, Schiffmann H, Oehler R, Dudykevych T, Hahn G, Hinz J, Hellige G: Distribution of lung ventilation in spontaneously breathing neonates lying in different body positions. Intensive Care Med 2003; 29:787–794.

115 Frerichs I: Electrical impedance tomography (EIT) in applications related to lung and ventilation: A review of experimental and clinical activities. Physiol Meas 2000;21:R1–21.

116 Traeger N, Panitch HB: Tests of respiratory muscle strength in neonates. Neo Rev 2004;5:e208–e214.

117 Manczur TI, Greenough A, Pryor D, Rafferty GF: Assessment of respiratory drive and muscle function in the pediatric intensive care unit and prediction of extubation failure. Pediatr Crit Care Med 2000;1:124–126.

118 Coates AL, Stocks J, Gerhardt T: Esophageal manometry; in Stocks J, Sly PD, Tepper RS, Morgan WJ (eds): Infant Respiratory Function Testing. New York, Wiley, 1996, pp 241–258.

119 Gappa M, Colin AA, Goetz I, Stocks J: Passive respiratory mechanics: The occlusion techniques. Eur Respir J 2001;17: 141–148.

120 Gappa M, Jackson EA, Pilgrim L, Costeloe KC, Stocks J: A new microtransducer catheter for measuring esophageal pressure in infants. Pediatr Pulmonol 1996;22:117–124.

121 Katz-Salamon M: Delayed chemoreceptor responses in infants with apnoea. Arch Dis Child 2004;89:261–266.

122 Galland BC, Taylor BJ, Bolton DP, Sayers RM: Respiratory responses to hypoxia/hypercapnia in small for gestational age infants influenced by maternal smoking. Arch Dis Child Fetal Neonatal Ed 2003;88:F217–F222.

123 Schulze A, Abubakar K, Gill G, Way RC, Sinclair JC: Pulmonary oxygen consumption: A hypothesis to explain the increase in oxygen consumption of low birth weight infants with lung disease. Intensive Care Med 2001;27:1636–1642.

124 Thach B: Fast breaths, slow breaths, small breaths, big breaths: Importance of vagal innervation in the newborn lung. J Appl Physiol 2001;91:2298–2300.

125 Tirosh E, Bilker A, Bader D, Cohen A: Capnography in spontaneously breathing preterm and term infants. Clin Physiol 2001;21:150–154.

126 Williams O, Bhat RY, Cheeseman P, Rafferty GF, Hannam S, Greenough A: Exhaled nitric oxide in chronically ventilated preterm infants. Arch Dis Child Fetal Neonatal Ed 2004;89:F88–F89.

127 Franklin PJ, Turner SW, Mutch RC, Stick SM: Measuring exhaled nitric oxide in infants during tidal breathing: Methodological issues. Pediatr Pulmonol 2004;37:24–30.

128 Leipala JA, Williams O, Sreekumar S, Cheeseman P, Rafferty GF, Hannam S, Milner A, Greenough A: Exhaled nitric oxide levels in infants with chronic lung disease. Eur J Pediatr, in press.

129 Bates J, Schmalisch G, Filbrun D, Stocks J: Tidal breath analysis for infant pulmonary function testing. Eur Respir J 2000;16: 1180–1192.

130 Stocks J, Dezateux CA, Jackson EA, Hoo A-F, Costeloe KL, Wade AM: Analysis of tidal breathing parameters in infancy. How variable is tPTEF:tE. Am J Respir Crit Care Med 1994;150:1347–1354.

131 Aston H, Clarke J, Silverman M: Are tidal breathing indices useful in infant bronchial challenge tests? Pediatr Pulmonol 1994;17: 225–230.

132 Mikkilineni S, England S: On tidal expiratory flow measurements in infants. Pediatr Pulmonol 1994;18:71–72.

133 Rusconi F, Gagliardi L, Aston H, Silverman M: Changes in respiratory rate affect tidal expiratory flow indices in infants with airway obstruction. Pediatr Pulmonol 1996; 21:236–240.

134 Seddon PC, Davis GM, Coates AL: Do tidal expiratory flow patterns reflect lung mechanics in infants. Am J Respir Crit Care Med 1996;153:1248–1252.

135 Suki B: Fluctuations and power laws in pulmonary physiology. Am J Respir Crit Care Med 2002;166:133–137.

136 Frey U, Silverman M, Suki B: Analysis of the harmonic content of the tidal flow waveforms in infants. J Appl Physiol 2001;91:1687–1693.

137 Habib RH, Pyon KH, Courtney SE, Aghai ZH: Spectral characteristics of airway opening and chest wall tidal flows in spontaneously breathing preterm infants. J Appl Physiol 2003;94:1933–1940.

138 Schmalisch G, Foitzik B, Wauer RR, Stocks J: Effect of apparatus deadspace on tidal breathing parameters in newborns: Comparison of the 'flow-through' and conventional techniques. Eur Respir J 2000;17:108–114.

139 Schmalisch G, Schmidt M, Foitzik B: Novel technique to average breathing loops for infant respiratory function testing. Med Biol Eng Comput 2001;39: 688–693.

140 Brown K, Aun C, Jackson EA, Mackersie AM, Hatch DJ, Stocks J: Validation of respiratory inductive plethysmography using the qualitative diagnostic calibration method in anaesthetized infants. Eur Respir J 1998;12: 935–943.

141 Jackson EA, Stocks J, Pilgrim L, Dundas I, Dezateux CA: A critical assessment of uncalibrated respiratory inductance plethysmography for the measurement of tidal breathing parameters in newborns and infants. Pediatr Pulmonol 1995;20:119–124.

142 Colin AA: Infant pulmonary testing – Techniques, physiological perspectives and clinical applications. Paediatr Respir Rev 2004;5(suppl 1):S73–S76.

143 Davis SD: Neonatal and pediatric respiratory diagnostics. Respir Care 2003;48:367–384.

144 Godfrey S, Bar-Yishay E, Avital A, Springer C: What is the role of tests of lung function in the management of infants with lung disease? Pediatr Pulmonol 2003;36:1–9.

145 Hanrahan J, Silverman M, Tepper R: Clinical epidemiology and future directions; in Stocks J, Sly PD, Tepper RS, Morgan WJ (eds): Infant Respiratory Function Testing. New York, Wiley, 1996, pp 551–562.

146 Castile RG: Pulmonary function testing in children; in Chernick V, Boat TF, Kendig EL (eds): Kendig's Disorders of the Respiratory Tract in Children. Philadelphia, Saunders, 1998, pp 196–214.

147 Stocks J, Quanjer PH: Reference values for residual volume, functional residual capacity and total lung capacity. Eur Respir J 1995;8: 492–506.

148 Hulskamp G, Hoo AF, Ljungberg H, Lum S, Pillow JJ, Stocks J: Progressive decline in plethysmographic lung volumes in infants: Physiology or technology? Am J Respir Crit Care Med 2003;168:1003–1009.

149 Merkus PJ, Tiddens HA, de Jongste JC: Annual lung function changes in young patients with chronic lung disease. Eur Respir J 2002;19:886–891.

150 Subbarao P, Lebecque P, Corey M, Coates AL: Comparison of spirometric reference values. Pediatr Pulmonol 2004;37:515–522.

151 Aurora P, Stocks J, Oliver C, Saunders C, Castle R, Chaziparasidis G, Bush A; London Cystic Fibrosis Collaboration: Quality control for spirometry in preschool children with and without lung disease. Am J Respir Crit Care Med 2004;169:1152–1159.

152 Nielsen KG, Bisgaard H: Discriminative capacity of bronchodilator response measured with three different lung function techniques in asthmatic and healthy children aged 2 to 5 years. Am J Respir Crit Care Med 2001;164:554–559.

153 Nielsen KG, Pressler T, Klug B, Koch C, Bisgaard H: Serial lung function and responsiveness in cystic fibrosis during early childhood. Am J Respir Crit Care Med 2004; 169:1209–1216.

154 ATS-ERS consensus statement, Sly P, Beydon N, Davies S, Gaultier C, Lombardi E, et al: Lung function testing in preschool children: The next frontier. Am J Respir Crit Care Med, in press.

Janet Stocks, PhD
Professor of Respiratory Physiology
Portex Anaesthesia, Intensive Therapy and
Respiratory Medicine Unit
Institute of Child Health
30 Guilford St, London, WC1N 1EH (UK)
Tel. +44 20 7905 2382
Fax +44 20 7829 8634
E-Mail j.stocks@ich.ucl.ac.uk

Measurements of Pulmonary Function in Cooperative Children

Hammer J, Eber E (eds): Paediatric Pulmonary Function Testing.
Prog Respir Res. Basel, Karger, 2005, vol 33, pp 94–102

....

Spirometry: Volume-Time and Flow-Volume Curves

Ernst Eber   Maximilian S. Zach

Respiratory and Allergic Disease Division, Paediatric Department,
Medical University of Graz, Austria

Abstract

In cooperative children, spirometry is the most commonly used pulmonary function test. Because the test is simple and reproducible, it plays a key role in the assessment and management of respiratory diseases in this age group. However, the age at which a child develops the ability to perform forced ventilatory maneuvers reliably varies widely, and especially in young children the interaction with a well-trained technician is most important. Visual incentives or interactive computer-animated systems may be helpful in obtaining reliable results even in preschool children. The American Thoracic Society (ATS) and the European Respiratory Society (ERS) defined criteria for acceptability as well as reproducibility of spirometric measurements. These standards are based almost exclusively on the studies of adults. However, many of these criteria were shown to be age and height dependent, and therefore are often not met when testing children. Thus, a reevaluation of international standards for forced expiratory maneuvers in children seems appropriate. Despite these limitations, most volume-time and flow-volume curves of cooperative children are useful for interpretation. The shape of the curve may allow to derive diagnostic clues from forced ventilatory maneuvers even in semicooperative children. Furthermore, spirometry is the most widely accepted method for assessing airway responses to bronchodilators as well as bronchoconstrictors.

Introduction

Static lung volumes, measured by registration of slow respiratory maneuvers, are distinguished from dynamic lung volumes which, together with forced inspiratory and expiratory flows, are derived from registration of forced ventilatory maneuvers. During forced ventilatory maneuvers, with maximal effort being applied throughout inspiration and/or expiration, volume or flow is measured at the airway opening. The results of these maneuvers are expressed as the relationship of inspired or expired volume to time (volume-time curve) or as the relationship of maximal flow to lung volume (flow-volume curve). After having been introduced as a valuable diagnostic tool almost 60 years ago, forced expiratory vital capacity (EVC) maneuvers have become the cornerstone of pulmonary function testing (PFT), and usually constitute the first stage in the clinical assessment of respiratory function. In addition, forced ventilatory maneuvers are also frequently used in research settings. Thus, the indications for registration of these maneuvers are manifold and can hardly be standardized. One of the most important areas is the long-term monitoring of patients with chronic lung diseases such as cystic fibrosis or asthma. In these patients, spirometry is an indispensable tool for assessing therapeutic interventions as well as monitoring the severity and progression of the disease. Forced ventilatory maneuvers, however, require a high degree of cooperation from the investigated subjects. Particularly young children often lack the necessary coordination and cooperation.

The aim of this chapter is to review the methodology with special emphasis on its use and usefulness in young children, and to discuss the limitations of accepted international standards that were designed for adults. Reference values, i.e. the estimates of normal lung function, and problems related to reference equations will be dealt with in another chapter of this book.

Equipment

Spirometer

Spirometers measure in- and expired volumes at the airway opening and are the instruments of choice for measuring vital capacity (VC) and its subdivisions [1]. Wet-type spirometers (such as the classical bell spirometer with a water seal) are simple and accurate but are no longer in use as they have a hygiene problem; they are distinguished from dry-type spirometers (e.g., bellows or piston spirometer). In a closed system, spirometers also allow assessment of functional residual capacity by gas dilution methods (e.g., helium equilibration) [2]. For this purpose, the spirometer must be equipped with facilities for carbon dioxide adsorption and oxygen supply.

Pneumotachometer

Pneumotachometers measure gas flow at the airway opening and are the most widely used devices for registration of forced expiratory maneuvers. They are coupled with a differential pressure transducer, an amplifier, and an integrator to derive volume from flow over time. Usually the pneumotachometers are heated to reduce variations in resistance to gas flow due to condensation and evaporation of water. The most important prerequisites for an accurate measurement of lung volume are linearity (consistent measurements of a fixed volume of gas administered from a calibrated syringe at varying flows) and stability (only minimal and constant drift of the volume signal which to some extent is unavoidable) [1].

Hot-Wire Anemometer

Alternatively, hot-wire anemometers may be used for measuring gas flow, and have been shown to satisfy demands as to accuracy, response time and temperature variations. Recently, a new infant hot-wire anemometer and monitoring system was demonstrated to provide reliable measurements of tidal volume even during high-frequency oscillatory ventilation [3].

Ultrasonic Flowmeter

The ultrasonic flowmeter is based on the principle that sound traveling through a streaming medium is accelerated or slowed by the movement of the medium, causing changes in transit times for a fixed distance across the medium. With the ultrasonic flowmeter, flow (and hence

Table 1. Accuracy of measurements: minimum requirements for spirometers and pneumotachometers [based on 1]

Signal	Minimum requirement
Volume	
Range	0–8 liters
Accuracy	±3% or ±50 ml, whichever is greater
Resolution (detectable change)	25 ml
Time	
Duration (for forced maneuver)	15 s
Accuracy	±1%
Flow	
Range	0–15 liters/s
Accuracy	±3.5% or 0.07 liter/s, whichever is greater
Driving pressure	<0.03 kPa
Mouth pressure	<0.6 kPa

volume) and molar mass of the mainstream gas can be measured at the same time. As this technique also offers potential advantages in terms of hygiene, it appears to be an attractive alternative to other methods for measuring lung volumes. However, apart from in vitro and animal work, at present there is only little clinical experience with this technique. Functional residual capacity measurement by the ultrasonic flowmeter was shown to be accurate and simple to use in ventilated children [4].

Accuracy, Precision, and Variability of Measurements

Spirometric measurements may be subject to errors of accuracy and precision. An error of accuracy consists in a systematic difference between the true and the measured value, an error of precision in the difference between successive measurements. The accuracy of flow and volume measurements with spirometers and pneumotachometers was subject of several standardization efforts, and recommendations for technical standards were published by the European Respiratory Society (ERS) and the American Thoracic Society (ATS) [1, 5]. The accuracy of a spirometry system depends on a number of factors including the resolution (i.e., the minimal detectable volume or flow) and linearity of the entire system. Thus, errors at any step in the process can affect the quality of the results. Table 1 summarizes the minimum requirements for spirometers and pneumotachometers, as based on ERS recommendations. In some aspects these recommendations differ slightly from the ATS statements on standardization of spirometry (e.g., flow range and accuracy). In addition to errors of accuracy and precision, measurements are subject to observer errors and biological variability. The latter is independent of errors attributable to equipment or operator, but rather relates to factors such as time and circumstances of the test, instruction and cooperation of the tested subject, and training of personnel.

Calibration, Equipment Quality Control

Frequent calibration of all spirometry equipment is part of the standardization of measurements and procedures and aims at improvement of accuracy. Spirometers should be calibrated for volume at least once daily with an airtight 3-liter calibrated syringe which should be accurate within 25 ml. The linearity of the system should be tested by injecting the volume from the 3-liter syringe with several different flows (the measured volume should be independent of flow). Closed system spirometers should be tested for leaks daily (ATS) or at least weekly (ERS). Time scale accuracy of mechanical recorders must be checked with a stopwatch at least quarterly and be accurate within 1% [1, 5].

Standard Conditions

Volume measurements should refer to conditions in the lung, i.e. body temperature, pressure, saturated with water vapor (BTPS); thus, correction factors are needed for spirometers as well as pneumotachometers. For spirometers it is recommended that gas temperatures within the instrument should be between 17 and 40°C. Corrections for pneumotachometers are much more complex than for simple volume-type devices; the condition of the gas depends on a number of factors such as how the instrument is heated, how close it is to the mouth, and whether the gas is inspired or expired. Thus, the method used to calculate or estimate the BTPS factor can potentially introduce a significant error [1, 5]. Primary data should be available in order to allow manipulation of uncorrected values by the user.

Display

The entire ventilatory maneuver should be displayed and recorded to facilitate quality control [1, 5]. Requirements with regard to the display include an appropriate size of the diagram (e.g., 1 liter corresponding to 2 cm), one or (maximal) two scales, and fixed proportions between the flow and volume scales (e.g., a flow of 2 liters/s and a volume of 1 liter correspond to 2 cm on the y- and x-axis, respectively). For optimal quality control, both volume-time and flow-volume displays are useful. By expanding the terminal portions of the forced VC (FVC) maneuver, a display in form of a volume-time curve allows to assess the duration of effort and whether a plateau is

achieved or not. A display of the flow-volume graph, by expanding the initial portion of the FVC maneuver, is useful in assessing the magnitude of effort. Usually, experienced investigators may derive the most important diagnostic information from analysis of the shape of the displayed graphs only. The numerical data then serve as additional quantification.

Infection Control

Hygienic measures have to be part of the daily routine in lung function laboratories. Recommendations about cleaning and disinfection as provided by the manufacturers of the different components of the equipment must be followed strictly. Generally, bacteria as well as fungi thrive in a moist environment. Thus, equipment should be kept dry, and secretions should be trapped and disposed of. When feasible disposable articles should be used. Bacterial filters may be effective in preventing contamination of equipment; however, significant differences exist in the ability to remove bacteria between different filters [6]. Usually these filters do not affect the mechanical characteristics of the measuring device to a clinically relevant degree [7].

Personnel, Environment

Apart from trained subjects/patients, well-trained personnel experienced in measuring pulmonary function in children and a pleasant environment are essential for obtaining reliable measurements. As forced expiratory (and inspiratory) maneuvers are highly effort-dependent, the interaction between technician and tested subject/patient is most important. Especially young children have a very limited attention span; thus, distractions must be avoided.

Registration

Prior to the test, the subject/patient should be at rest for at least 15 min. Especially with inexperienced children, the procedure should be carefully described, and the maneuver subsequently demonstrated and trained. In young children, the use of either computerized visual incentives (e.g., burning candles) that stimulate either a rapid and forced start of a maximal expiration or a long forced expiration time, or interactive computer-animated systems may be helpful [8, 9]. The mouthpiece should be inserted between the teeth and held by the lips; according to ERS and ATS

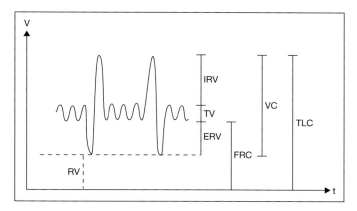

Fig. 1. Schematic illustration of static lung volumes and capacities of a healthy subject. An IVC maneuver is followed by an EVC maneuver. IRV = Inspiratory reserve volume; TV = tidal volume; ERV = expiratory reserve volume; FRC = functional residual capacity.

recommendations, a noseclip should be used in any case [1, 5]. This, however, is somewhat controversial. In a recent study, measurements made with and without noseclips were compared in children and adolescents with asthma or cystic fibrosis [10]. While variability was found to be decreased when wearing noseclips, no systematic difference between the measurements could be demonstrated. Thus, it was suggested that in clinical practice the optimal technique for the individual subject should be used consistently. Nevertheless, research protocols using current reference values should continue to include the use of noseclips. The measurements are performed with the subject seated upright, so that the head is not tilted. Tight clothing should be loosened to avoid any compression of neck, thorax, or abdomen.

The registration of static lung volumes begins with tidal breathing. For the VC maneuver the subject should either inhale completely from a position of full expiration (inspiratory vital capacity, IVC), or exhale completely from a position of full inspiration (EVC). A slow or relaxed VC maneuver may yield a more accurate determination of VC than forced maneuvers. Especially in subjects with airway obstruction the FVC tends to be lower than the VC obtained with a relaxed maneuver. Similarly, in this situation the IVC may be higher than the EVC; thus, the IVC is preferably used to calculate total lung capacity (TLC) [1]. A typical volume-time curve for registration of static lung volumes is shown in figure 1. The smallest units are denoted 'volumes', and totals of volumes are characterized as 'capacities'.

The registration of forced expiratory VC maneuvers also begins with tidal breathing. Then, after a maximal inhalation and a pause of approximately 2 s at TLC, a forced exhalation to residual volume (RV) follows. Throughout the maneuver, the subject should be coached enthusiastically and encouraged to exhale fully. Observing both subject and display of the maneuver during the test helps to ensure maximal effort. After a short pause in maximal expiration a forced inspiratory VC maneuver may follow. Typical volume-time and flow-volume curves of forced expiratory (and inspiratory) VC maneuvers are shown in figure 2. A number of common problems that may be encountered in the registration of ventilatory maneuvers are listed in table 2.

A minimum of three acceptable FVC maneuvers have to be performed. Acceptability and reproducibility must be determined during or immediately after these maneuvers by both analysis of the shape of the curves and objective criteria (see below). Ventilatory maneuvers with submaximal effort are rarely reproduced exactly. In case of large variability, up to eight maneuvers may be carried out [1, 5]. As in adults, obtaining three acceptable curves seems sufficient, and continuing PFT after eight attempts is hardly useful in children [1].

In order to reduce intraindividual variability, serial measurements should be performed at the same time of the day, under the same environmental conditions, and preferably with the same technician and equipment [1].

Acceptability and Reproducibility

Criteria for acceptability, as defined by the ATS, include a satisfactory start of the test, a minimum exhalation time, and meeting end-of-test criteria [5]. To determine the start of the test (zero point of time and volume), the back extrapolation method, tracing back from the steepest slope of the volume-time curve (manual measurement) or using the largest slope averaged over an 80-ms period (computerized measurement), is recommended. In order to ensure that the measured parameters stem from a maximal effort maneuver, according to ATS standards the extrapolated volume must be less than 5% of the FVC or 0.15 liter, whichever is greater. In contrast, the ERS recommends a volume of less than 5% of the FVC or 0.1 liter, whichever is greater [1]. In accordance with standards issued by the ATS, the duration of maximal expiratory effort should be at least 6 s, unless there is an obvious plateau in the volume-time curve [5]. However, it is also stated in these standards that in some instances (e.g., the testing of children and young adults) shorter exhalation times are often acceptable, but the recommendations are not specific in this regard. In

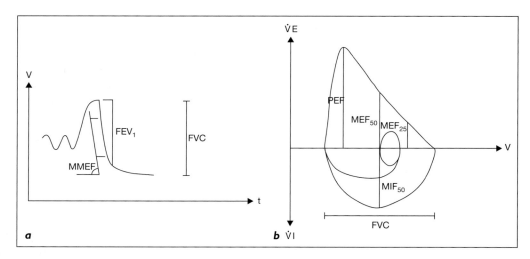

Fig. 2. *a, b* Schematic illustration of a volume-time (*a*) and a flow-volume (*b*) curve of forced EVC (and IVC) maneuvers of a healthy subject. MMEF = Maximal mid-expiratory flow; MIF_{50} = maximal inspiratory flow at 50% FVC.

Table 2. Common problems in the registration of ventilatory (in particular forced expiratory) maneuvers

---

Leak between lips and mouthpiece
Occlusion of the mouthpiece by the tongue
Obstruction of the mouthpiece by pursing the lips or closing the teeth
Incomplete inspiration
No pause at or near TLC
Hesitant start of the forced expiratory maneuver
Glottis closure during the forced expiratory maneuver
Expiration not maximally forced/with variable effort
Incomplete expiration
Cough during the forced expiratory maneuver

---

contrast, ERS recommendations do not include a minimum duration of the forced expiration. ATS-recommended end-of-test criteria are: (1) exhaustion of the subject, or (2) a plateau in the volume-time curve (no change in volume for at least 1s) after an exhalation time of at least 6 s, or (3) an exhalation of reasonable duration (up to 15 or 20 s).

Subsequent to acceptability criteria, reproducibility criteria have to be applied. According to the ATS, the largest VC (FVC) and second largest VC (FVC) from acceptable maneuvers must not vary by more than 0.2 liter. In addition, the largest and second largest forced expiratory volume in 1 s (FEV_1) also must not vary by more than 0.2 liter [5]. The ERS recommends that the highest FVC or FEV_1 should not exceed the next highest one by more than 5% or 0.1 liter, whichever is greater [1].

Schoolchildren

Particularly end-of-test criteria, which are based almost exclusively on studies of adults, in reality are often not met when testing children. Recently, several authors evaluated the applicability of ATS criteria [12, 13], and one group the applicability of ATS as well as ERS criteria [8] for spirometry in schoolchildren, and also sought to develop new criteria. Overall, while the strict criteria for acceptability were frequently not met, most of the tests did meet the criteria for reproducibility [8, 12, 13]. Desmond et al. [12] reported that in a cross-sectional analysis of patients (age 5–18 years) referred for pediatric PFT, only 19% met current ATS end-of-test criteria, while 91% met the reproducibility criteria for both FVC and FEV_1. By using exponential curve fitting techniques they determined the theoretical full FVC for the individual patient and suggested to use 95% of the full FVC as end-of-test criterion, which was reached by 90% of the children. While 37% of children ≤7 years of age still failed to reach this criterion, only 4% of the older children failed to do so. As can be expected, most of the children who did not reach this end-of-test criterion showed a wide variability in effort. Enright et al. [13] in a large field study investigated somewhat older children and adolescents (age 9–18 years) and concluded that subjects of this age group can meet each of the ATS criteria about 95% of the time. However, about 35% of their subjects had an exhalation time <6 s during their best maneuvers. As only 5% exhaled for less than 4 s and healthy children often reach a plateau in <3 s, the authors suggested to use 4 s as acceptability criterion for spirometry in children. In contrast to studies in adults, they found that children with a history of asthma or wheeze performed better quality spirometry than did others. Finally, Arets et al. [8] investigated children and adolescents (age 5–19 years) who had extensive experience in maximal expiratory maneuvers. In this study, the majority of children could perform acceptable forced expiratory maneuvers according to ATS and ERS start-of-test criteria; although the curves were judged to have been acceptably performed, however, only a minority of the children (15%) exhaled as long as required by ATS criteria. Most importantly, many of the acceptability and reproducibility criteria were shown to be age and height dependent. Thus, these absolute criteria, which were designed for use in adults, were considered to be less suitable in children. Based on the intention that at least 90% of the children reach the respective acceptability and reproducibility criteria, the authors suggested the following minimum criteria: (1) an extrapolated volume <0.12 liter for children <15 years and <0.15 liter for those >15 years; (2) an exhalation time >2 s in children >8 years and >1 s in those <8 years, provided that a gradual, asymptotic approach of the flow-volume curve to the volume axis is seen, and (3) a difference <5% between the two highest FVC and FEV_1 values.

Preschool Children

Several authors evaluated spirometric measurements in preschool children [14–18]. Two groups investigated children with a variety of respiratory disorders (age 3–5 years) who carried out spirometric tests for the first time [14, 15]. Kanengiser and Dozor [14] reported that nearly 60% of the patients performed maximal efforts resulting in a reproducible and reliable FVC before and after bronchodilator. However, only 32% performed reproducible sets of FEV_1. Thus, they concluded that reliability cannot be assumed in this age group. Similarly, Crenesse et al. [15] reported that 55% of their study population performed reliable forced expiratory maneuvers provided that they were supervised by trained medical staff. The mean forced expiratory time of only 1.7 s is consistent with the fact that young children may empty their lungs within 1–2 s. Thus, in this age group FEV_1 does not appear to be a useful parameter; as a consequence, forced expiratory volume in 0.5 s ($FEV_{0.5}$) and particularly forced expiratory volume in 0.75 s ($FEV_{0.75}$) are believed to be more appropriate parameters for the quantification of airway obstruction [14, 15]. Two other groups investigated healthy preschool children (age 3–6 years) who also were naïve to PFT [16, 18]. In these somewhat older study

populations, the authors found that 60–80% were able to perform technically acceptable and reproducible maneuvers; thus, they could derive reference values for their respective populations. In addition, a significant decrease in the ratio FEV_1/FVC was documented with increasing height (e.g., a mean predicted FEV_1/FVC of 0.97 at 90 cm height, and of 0.89 at 125 cm height, respectively) [16]. Finally, one group also investigated preschool children (age 3–6 years) who performed spirometry for the first time; these children were in part healthy, in part had a history of asthmatic symptoms [17]. Again, many of the studied children achieved acceptable and reproducible maneuvers.

In summary, although many volume-time and flow-volume curves of children do not meet ATS and/or ERS criteria most of them are useful for interpretation. Thus, a reevaluation of international criteria for forced expiratory maneuvers in children seems indicated.

Even rudimentary forced expiratory maneuvers in young, semicooperative children may be useful in many instances, as they at least allow a shape analysis of the registered tracings.

Interpretation and Reporting of Forced Expiratory Maneuvers

According to ATS and ERS criteria, the largest FVC and the largest FEV_1 should be reported after examining the data from acceptable and reproducible curves, even if they do not stem from the same curve [1, 5]. Other parameters from the volume-time curve should be derived from a single acceptable curve that gives the largest sum of FVC plus FEV_1. When repeated forced expiratory maneuvers cause bronchoconstriction so that consecutive measurements become less, the curve with the largest FVC should be analyzed.

Longitudinal measurements, taking the individual subject as its own reference, can detect progressive deviation from normal, and thus are much more useful than cross-sectional measurements.

It is common practice to report maximal mid-expiratory flow which is obtained by measuring the slope of the middle half of the volume-time curve, as well as maximal expiratory flow at 50% remaining FVC (MEF_{50}) from forced expiratory maneuvers. Both measures are considered to be more sensitive in detecting small airway dysfunction (which is an early feature of many obstructive lung diseases such as asthma and cystic fibrosis) than FEV_1 [19, 20]. In a recent study, investigating children with a broad range of pulmonary abnormalities, the two parameters were shown to be highly correlated with a fairly constant ratio of the two even in severe airway obstruction [21]. Thus, the practice of reporting both measures appears to be unnecessary, and MEF_{50} seems to be the preferable parameter because it is directly measured rather than calculated.

Maximal Expiratory Flow-Volume Curve

In comparison to a volume-time curve, the instantaneous plot of maximal expiratory flow against lung volume allows a more detailed analysis of lung function and is a very sensitive method of detecting minor airway obstruction or loss of elastic recoil [22]. In a healthy child, the curve, after rapidly achieving a high peak expiratory flow (PEF), is convex or straight until the point RV on the x-axis is reached (fig. 2b).

The three best out of a series of maximal expiratory flow-volume (MEFV) curves may be analyzed in different ways. With the envelope method, the curves are superimposed from TLC to form a composite maximal curve [1]. Then, the largest FVC is used to measure the highest instantaneous flows at specified lung volumes. Alternatively, the respective highest instantaneous flows from the three best curves are taken as the results.

The determinants of expiratory flow during a forced expiration are complex. After a brief effort-dependent phase (approximately the first quarter of FVC) that includes PEF, forced expiratory flows are determined by airway mechanics (dynamically compressed airways act as flow-limiting segments), and thus are effort-independent. It follows that PEF shows a higher variability than other forced expiratory flows; consequently, its significance is limited to a rough assessment of the caliber of central airways [1]. In contrast, MEF_{50} and particularly maximal expiratory flow at 25% remaining FVC (MEF_{25}) are representative for the function of the smaller intrathoracic airways. Compared to FEV_1 (which will not detect minor obstruction in the smaller airways), however, these measures are of only moderate reproducibility [23]. Flows near RV may be effort-dependent, because expiratory muscle contraction may not be able to provide sufficiently high intrathoracic pressures to maintain flow limitation at very low lung volume.

In addition to obtaining numerical data for the quantification of lung function, a visual analysis of the MEFV curve is important. Increased airway resistance is reflected in the shape of the MEFV curve. With increasing peripheral airway obstruction the MEFV curve becomes more and more concave with an only slightly decreased PEF and a profoundly decreased MEF_{25} (fig. 3). On the other hand,

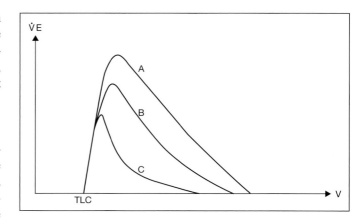

Fig. 3. Schematic illustration of typical MEFV curves in healthy children and in children with peripheral airway obstruction: curve from a healthy child (**A**), curve from a child with mild airway obstruction (**B**), and curve from a child with severe airway obstruction (**C**).

obstruction of the intrathoracic part of the trachea as well as a fixed obstruction of the extrathoracic airway result in massive flow limitation, thereby causing a plateau in the MEFV curve (fig. 4). In patients with restrictive dysfunction, the MEFV curve is smaller in all dimensions but its shape is normal. To clearly differentiate restrictive dysfunction from airway obstruction with hyperinflation, TLC and thus RV must be determined by plethysmography or gas dilution methods.

By recording a maximal forced expiration and a maximal forced inspiration as a continuous maneuver, a flow-volume loop is obtained. In contrast to forced expiration, airway-effected flow limitation does not occur during forced inspiration in healthy subjects. Usually, maximal inspiratory flow at 50% FVC is about the same as MEF_{50} (fig. 2b). Forced inspiratory maneuvers are useful in diagnosing and monitoring flow-limiting upper (extrathoracic) airway obstruction which causes a plateau in the maximal inspiratory flow-volume (MIFV) curve. For this purpose, a visual analysis of the shape of the MIFV curve is essential. A complete flow-volume loop allows to distinguish a variable from a fixed stenosis. A variable intrathoracic stenosis (e.g., tracheomalacia) results in a plateau in the MEFV curve and in a normal MIFV curve, a variable extrathoracic stenosis (e.g., vocal cord dysfunction) in a plateau in the MIFV curve and in a normal or near normal MEFV curve, and a fixed stenosis (e.g., glottic stenosis) in a box-like loop with plateaus in both the MIFV and MEFV curves, respectively (fig. 4).

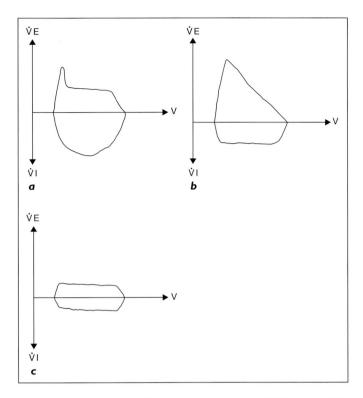

Fig. 4. *a–c* Schematic illustration of typical MEFV and MIFV curves in children with central airway obstruction: curve from a child with double aortic arch and tracheomalacia (***a***), curve from a child with vocal cord dysfunction (***b***), and curve from a child with glottic stenosis (***c***) (for details see text).

Assessment of Bronchial Reactivity to Bronchodilators and Bronchoconstrictors

Airway responses to bronchodilators are frequently assessed to quantify reversibility of airway obstruction and thus help to confirm a diagnosis of asthma. These responses are usually assessed as change in FEV_1, an index considered to be the most relevant parameter in this respect due to its good reproducibility [1]. When interpreting responses to bronchodilators (and bronchoconstrictors) by changes in flow parameters (maximal mid-expiratory flow, MEF_{50}, and MEF_{25}) it must be taken into account that lung volume may change during the assessment. Such a shift of the volume landmark of the measurement, resulting in a change of the static-elastic recoil pressure, makes comparisons between measurements before and after an intervention physiologically questionable. Consequently, the latter parameters are not suitable for monitoring induced changes, as long as they are not related to the absolute lung volume that was used for the initial measurements, a feature usually not included in standard software packages. For a bronchodilator response to be clinically meaningful it should exceed spontaneous intraindividual variability, and to be unambiguous it should exceed the bronchodilator response in healthy subjects. In healthy adults, the upper 95% confidence limit of the change in FEV_1 has been reported to be 7.7–10.5% of the initial value [1]. The ERS standardization paper calls for an unambiguous bronchodilator response in FEV_1 to be both larger than 12% of the predicted value and exceed 200 ml [1]. Similarly, in healthy children the upper 95% confidence limit of the bronchodilator response in FEV_1 has been reported to be 9.0–11.0% predicted [24, 25]. Expressing the bronchodilator-induced change in FEV_1 relative to the initial value has the disadvantage that the response is dependent on the baseline value of FEV_1. In addition, in children the absolute change in FEV_1 is related to both stature and age. Thus, it was suggested that the bronchodilator response in children should be expressed in percent predicted, similar to the recommendations in adults [26]. However, when characterizing individual measurements in relation to reference values, using standardized deviation scores (Z scores) may be advantageous (for details see chapter on reference equations in this book).

The demonstration of increased bronchial responsiveness to various challenges may also play a role in the diagnosis of asthma; measurements of bronchial responsiveness with direct and indirect airway challenge tests are detailed in another chapter of this book. For these tests, the primary outcome measure is also the change in FEV_1. In asthmatic subjects, forced expiration maneuvers have been reported to have bronchoconstrictor as well as bronchodilator effects [1]. After induced bronchoconstriction, a deep inspiration is usually followed by a bronchodilator response. Thus, the recording of FEV_1 is flawed by the preceding deep inspiration which may affect the degree of obstruction; nevertheless, it leads to more reproducible results than other measurements without a preceding deep inspiration (e.g., specific airway conductance) [27].

References

1 Quanjer PH, Tammeling GJ, Cotes JE, Pedersen OF, Peslin R, Yernault JC: Lung volumes and forced ventilatory flows. Report Working Party Standardization of Lung Function Tests, European Community for Steel and Coal. Official Statement of the European Respiratory Society. Eur Respir J Suppl 1993;16:5–40.

2 Hathirat S, Mitchell M, Renzetti AD Jr: Measurement of the total lung capacity by helium dilution in a constant volume system. Am Rev Respir Dis 1970;102:760–770.

3 Scalfaro P, Pillow JJ, Sly PD, Cotting J: Reliable tidal volume estimates at the airway opening with an infant monitor during high-frequency oscillatory ventilation. Crit Care Med 2001;29:1925–1930.

4 Schibler A, Henning R: Measurement of functional residual capacity in rabbits and children using an ultrasonic flow meter. Pediatr Res 2001;49:581–588.

5 American Thoracic Society: Standardization of spirometry. 1994 update. Am Rev Respir Dis 1995;152:1107–1136.

6 Canakis AM, Ho B, Ho S, Kovach D, Matlow A, Coates AL: Do in-line respiratory filters protect patients? Comparing bacterial removal efficiency of six filters. Pediatr Pulmonol 2002;34:336–341.

7 Kamps AW, Vermeer K, Roorda RJ, Brand PL: Effect of bacterial filters on spirometry measurements. Arch Dis Child 2001;85:346–347.

8 Arets HG, Brackel HJ, van der Ent CK: Forced expiratory manoeuvres in children: Do they meet ATS and ERS criteria for spirometry? Eur Respir J 2001;18:655–660.

9 Vilozni D, Barker M, Jellouschek H, Heimann G, Blau H: An interactive computer-animated system (SpiroGame) facilitates spirometry in preschool children. Am J Respir Crit Care Med 2001;164:2200–2205.

10 Chavasse R, Johnson P, Francis J, Balfour-Lynn I, Rosenthal M, Bush A: To clip or not to clip? Noseclips for spirometry. Eur Respir J 2003;21:876–878.

11 Houthuijs D, Remijn B, Brunekreef B, de Koning R: Estimation of maximum expiratory flow-volume variables in children. Pediatr Pulmonol 1989;6:127–132.

12 Desmond KJ, Allen PD, Demizio DL, Kovesi T, Coates AL: Redefining end of test (EOT) criteria for pulmonary function testing in children. Am J Respir Crit Care Med 1997;156:542–545.

13 Enright PL, Linn WS, Avol EL, Margolis HG, Gong H Jr, Peters JM: Quality of spirometry test performance in children and adolescents: Experience in a large field study. Chest 2000;118:665–671.

14 Kanengiser S, Dozor AJ: Forced expiratory maneuvers in children aged 3 to 5 years. Pediatr Pulmonol 1994;18:144–149.

15 Crenesse D, Berlioz M, Bourrier T, Albertini M: Spirometry in children aged 3 to 5 years: Reliability of forced expiratory maneuvers. Pediatr Pulmonol 2001;32:56–61.

16 Eigen H, Bieler H, Grant D, Christoph K, Terrill D, Heilman DK, Ambrosius WT, Tepper RS: Spirometric pulmonary function in healthy preschool children. Am J Respir Crit Care Med 2001;163:619–623.

17 Nystad W, Samuelsen SO, Nafstad P, Edvardsen E, Stensrud T, Jaakkola JJ: Feasibility of measuring lung function in preschool children. Thorax 2002;57:1021–1027.

18 Zapletal A, Chalupová J: Forced expiratory parameters in healthy preschool children (3–6 years of age). Pediatr Pulmonol 2003;35:200–207.

19 McFadden ER Jr, Linden DA: A reduction in maximum mid-expiratory flow rate. A spirographic manifestation of small airway disease. Am J Med 1972;52:725–737.

20 Lebecque P, Kiakulanda P, Coates AL: Spirometry in the asthmatic child: Is FEF25–75 a more sensitive test than FEV1/FVC? Pediatr Pulmonol 1993;16:19–22.

21 Bar-Yishay E, Amirav I, Goldberg S: Comparison of maximal midexpiratory flow rate and forced expiratory flow at 50% of vital capacity in children. Chest 2003;123:731–735.

22 Zapletal A, Motoyama EK, Van De Woestijne KP, Hunt VR, Bouhuys A: Maximum expiratory flow-volume curves and airway conductance in children and adolescents. J Appl Physiol 1969;26:308–316.

23 Hutchison AA, Erben A, McLennan LA, Landau LI, Phelan PD: Intrasubject variability of pulmonary function testing in healthy children. Thorax 1981;36:370–377.

24 Casan P, Roca J, Sanchis J: Spirometric response to a bronchodilator. Reference values for healthy children and adolescents. Bull Eur Physiopathol Respir 1983;19:567–569.

25 Dales RE, Spitzer WO, Tousignant P, Schechter M, Suissa S: Clinical interpretation of airway response to a bronchodilator. Epidemiologic considerations. Am Rev Respir Dis 1988;138:317–320.

26 Waalkens HJ, Merkus PJ, van Essen-Zandvliet EE, Brand PL, Gerritsen J, Duiverman EJ, Kerrebijn KF, Knol KK, Quanjer PH: Assessment of bronchodilator response in children with asthma. Dutch CNSLD Study Group. Eur Respir J 1993;6:645–651.

27 Sterk PJ, Fabbri LM, Quanjer PH, Cockcroft DW, O'Byrne PM, Anderson SD, Juniper EF, Malo JL: Airway responsiveness. Standardised challenge testing with pharmacological, physical and sensitizing stimuli in adults. Report Working Party Standardization of Lung Function Tests. European Community for Steel and Coal. Official Statement of the European Respiratory Society. Eur Respir J Suppl 1993;16:53–83.

Prof. Dr. Ernst Eber
Klinische Abteilung für
Pulmonologie/Allergologie
Univ.-Klinik für Kinder- und Jugendheilkunde
Auenbruggerplatz 30
AT–8036 Graz (Austria)
Tel. +43 316 385 2620
Fax +43 316 385 4621
E-Mail ernst.eber@meduni-graz.at

Hammer J, Eber E (eds): Paediatric Pulmonary Function Testing.
Prog Respir Res. Basel, Karger, 2005, vol 33, pp 103–117

....

Plethysmography and Gas Dilution Techniques

François Marchal   Cyril Schweitzer

Service d'Explorations Fonctionnelles Pédiatriques, Hôpital d'Enfants, Vandoeuvre, France

Abstract

Measurement of static lung volumes – i.e., total lung capacity (TLC), functional residual capacity, and residual volume (RV) – has undergone significant progress in its routine application in paediatrics over the last decade. In addition to providing an index of lung size and growth, many techniques are able to explore uneven ventilation and air trapping. Body plethysmography – by either variable pressure or volume displacement – offers the possibility to measure both thoracic gas volume and airway resistance, and is the gold standard to study these two parameters. Specific airway resistance – the product of airway resistance and thoracic gas volume – is increasingly measured in preschool children. It appears to be useful in the assessment of responses to bronchodilators but requires careful and critical methodological evaluation when performed during tidal breathing. Gas dilution techniques are widely used in children employing multiple-breath or single-breath techniques. The wash-in helium dilution technique is easy to perform even in preschool children, and results may be compared to thoracic gas volume determined by body plethysmography to estimate the volume of trapped air in the lungs. Nitrogen wash-out techniques may also provide indices of ventilation inhomogeneity. Asthma, cystic fibrosis, and chronic lung disease of prematurity represent the main chronic obstructive disorders in childhood. The measurement of static lung volumes is of help in interpreting spirometry, and may document hyperinflation as well as provide indices of uneven ventilation. The simple index RV/TLC is a robust indicator of lung hyperinflation and trapped air. In addition, body

plethysmography offers the unique opportunity to assess the effects of volume history on lung function, which deserves further evaluation in childhood. In the next decade, optical reflectance motion analysis and magnetic resonance functional imaging may provide further insight into the physiological mechanisms that control lung volume and a more precise assessment of uneven ventilation.

Introduction

While principle and methodology of most lung function measurements have been described as early as the mid of the 20th century, their routine application in paediatrics has increased dramatically during the past 20 years. Measuring equipment has become more stable, accurate and readily available, and computerization has greatly facilitated its handling. The development of easy-to-use computer-assisted systems has resulted in the need to standardize measurement procedures and to provide recommendations and guidelines.

In paediatrics, most efforts in the past 20 years have aimed at developing equipment, technique, procedure, and methodology of lung function tests applicable to the unco-operative child. These issues have received much less attention in school children, because the technology is usually identical to that used in adults and assumed to be validated. Specially adapted reference values, however, are required for the interpretation of lung function data during growth, as described in the chapter by Merkus [1].

Static lung volumes are residual volume (RV), functional residual capacity (FRC), and total lung capacity (TLC) [see fig. 1 in 2]. RV is the volume of gas present in the lung at the end of a complete expiration; FRC is the lung volume at the end of a tidal expiration, and usually corresponds to the equilibrium between chest wall and lung elastic recoils; TLC is the maximum volume of gas that can be inspired. Breathing may thus mobilize these volumes only partially (TLC and FRC) or not at all (RV). Therefore, indirect methods are needed for their measurement. Body plethysmography takes advantage of gas compression properties, and dilution techniques are based on the mass conservation principle.

This chapter presents methods to measure static lung volumes – also frequently referred to as absolute lung volumes – in cooperative children and points to their clinical usefulness.

Methodology

Body Plethysmography

This technique used to measure lung volumes and airway resistance (R_{aw}) is increasingly applied in young children. The principle and methodology summarized below have previously been reviewed in detail elsewhere [3–6].

Principle
Thoracic Gas Volume
Compression or decompression of a gas in a rigid container (DP) at constant temperature from initial pressure P and volume V produces a volume change (ΔV) given by Boyle's law:

$$P \cdot V = (P + \Delta P) \cdot (V + \Delta V) \qquad (1)$$

It is common practice to neglect the small product $\Delta P \cdot \Delta V$ so that:

$$\Delta V / \Delta P = -V/P \qquad (2)$$

$\Delta V / \Delta P$ is gas compressibility or compliance (Cg). Hence, whenever Boyle's law applies:

$$Cg = -V/P \qquad (3)$$

Boyle's law applies only if compression occurs slowly enough for temperature within the container to remain constant, i.e., if there is sufficient time for the heat generated by compression to be dissipated across the wall. These conditions are called isothermal, meaning that heat exchange between the container and its environment is fast relative to the rate of gas compression. The rate of thermal exchange between the container and its surroundings is characterized by a thermal time constant which depends on ratio of container gas volume to total wall area. Isothermal conditions are satisfied when the thermal time constant is much shorter than the period – the reciprocal of frequency – of compression.

If gas is compressed rapidly relative to the thermal time constant of the container, not enough time is available for the heat to be dissipated through the wall. Thus, temperature rises during compression which is said to be adiabatic, and obeys Poisson's law:

$$Cg = -V/(\gamma \cdot P) \qquad (4)$$

where γ, the ratio of the specific heat of the gas at constant pressure and at constant volume, is 1.4 for air.

In conditions where the period of gas compression increases and approaches the thermal time constant, Cg becomes dependent on the frequency of gas compression, which is called polytropic. This situation is clearly to be avoided whenever the estimation of ΔV relies on the corresponding pressure change (see 'The Variable Pressure – Constant Volume or Barometric Plethysmograph' below).

At this stage, we may consider how these principles apply to the lung. The volume of gas of an individual alveolus is very small and the corresponding thermal time constant is expected to be very short. Hence, compression or decompression of the pooled alveolar volume – which represents most of the thoracic gas volume (TGV) – is assumed to occur under isothermal conditions. Therefore, applying equation 3 to TGV yields:

$$C_{TGV} = -TGV/(P_B - 47) \qquad (5)$$

where $P_B - 47$ (mm Hg), barometric pressure minus water pressure at body temperature, is the initial pressure applied to the initial volume of compressible gas in the lung.

Airway Resistance
When a subject breathes within a plethysmograph, there is some gas displacement or compression related to breathing and this ΔV has three origins [7, 8]. (1) A mechanical component is explained by compression/decompression of the alveolar gas (TGV) resulting from alveolar pressure (P_{alv}) – which depends on R_{aw} – and is in phase with airflow (V'). This is the component of interest when measuring R_{aw} and will be referred to as ΔV_{aw}. (2) A thermal component relates to the difference in temperature and humidity between inspired and expired gas and is mostly – but not entirely – in phase with volume. (3) A gas exchange

component is related to the fluctuation of the respiratory exchange ratio – mainly CO_2 output – along the breathing cycle. The third factor is usually neglected but the second is a major component of the signal and must be eliminated to study ΔV_{aw}.

Considering only the mechanical effect, ΔV_{aw} is related to P_{alv} as well as to the compressibility of alveolar volume (C_{TGV}). Indeed, the larger the TGV, the larger the C_{TGV} and therefore the larger the ΔV_{aw} which may thus be written:

$$\Delta V_{aw} = P_{alv} \cdot C_{TGV} \qquad (6)$$

P_{alv} may be expressed relative to P_B as a function of R_{aw} and V':

$$P_{alv} - P_B = R_{aw} \cdot V' \qquad (7)$$

Replacing C_{TGV} by equation 5 gives:

$$\Delta V_{aw} = V' \cdot R_{aw} \cdot TGV/(P_B - 47) \qquad (8)$$

The term $R_{aw} \cdot TGV$ is called specific airway resistance (sR_{aw}), i.e., the R_{aw} at a given volume of the lung. Airway conductance (G_{aw}) is the reciprocal of R_{aw}, and the specific airway conductance (sG_{aw}) is obtained by dividing G_{aw} by TGV.

Equipment and Types of Plethysmographs

The subject seated in a body plethysmograph compresses and decompresses his lung volume by performing expiratory and inspiratory efforts against an obstructed airway opening. This will be referred to as the TGV manoeuvre, during which pressure is assumed to be identical in the different parts of the lungs and airways, namely pressure at the mouth (P_m) is equal to P_{alv}. Expressing C_{TGV} (equation 5), TGV reads:

$$TGV = -(\Delta V_L/\Delta P_m) \cdot (P_B - 47) \qquad (9)$$

where ΔV_L is the change in lung volume and ΔP_m the corresponding change in mouth pressure, reflecting the change in P_{alv}. While ΔP_m is easily measured by a differential pressure transducer referenced to atmosphere, the main metrological issue of body plethysmography relates to the measurement of ΔV_L which is very small relative to TGV and to the volume of the plethysmograph. It may be obtained in two ways: indirectly, by the corresponding change in pressure within the body box, or directly as the volume being displaced from and into the body box.

The Variable Pressure – Constant Volume or Barometric Plethysmograph

In the variable pressure – constant volume or barometric plethysmograph [9], ΔV_L is estimated from the change in pressure within the body box (δP) when the subject is compressing/decompressing his alveolar gas. Once the door of the plethysmograph is closed, the heat produced by the subject induces a rise in box temperature leading to a drift in the δP signal. Therefore, the plethysmograph must have a small leak with a time constant of about 10–20 s to allow for thermal equilibration. δP is measured by a sensitive differential pressure transducer, the other side of which is referenced to a chamber with similar mechanical characteristics than the body box, so as to filter out extraneous noise (fig. 1a). The volume of the body box is such that the thermal time constant is long with reference to the usual frequency of gas compression manoeuvres adopted by the subject (around 1–2 Hz), so that δP occurs under adiabatic conditions [10]. This type of plethysmograph has the advantage of providing a comparatively stable signal, once the thermal drift has stabilized. On the other hand, the mechanical leak, together with the frequency dependence of the $\delta P - \Delta V_L$ relationship when compression becomes polytropic at lower frequencies, prevents studying slow events, such as vital capacity (VC) manoeuvres [6]. The upper frequency response of the system depends on the characteristics of the pressure transducers, usually flat up to 10–15 Hz.

The Volume Displacement Plethysmograph

In the original description of the volume displacement plethysmograph [11], ΔV_L was directly measured by a spirometer connected to the body box. Hence, during the TGV manoeuvre, the gas was displaced from the body box to the spirometer from which ΔV_L was read directly. The advantages are that the gas undergoes little compression/decompression and slow respiratory events may be studied. However, the difficulties inherent in the frequency response of this equipment have hampered its development in the routine laboratory. The second type of volume displacement plethysmograph or flow plethysmograph is a body box open to atmosphere through a wire mesh screen. During compression/decompression manoeuvres, gas flows through the screen across which the pressure drop is measured by a sensitive pressure transducer (fig. 1b). The flow signal is integrated (δV). During the manoeuvre, gas is also compressed within the box because of the screen resistance, and this effect is proportional to the product of the body box Cg and the screen resistance, i.e., the mechanical time constant of the flow plethysmograph. Once this has been determined, a correction may be used to calculate ΔV_L. The other side of the box transducer is referenced to a chamber with a similar mechanical time constant to eliminate external noise (fig. 1b). The flow plethysmograph combines some advantages of the volume and the pressure plethysmographs, namely

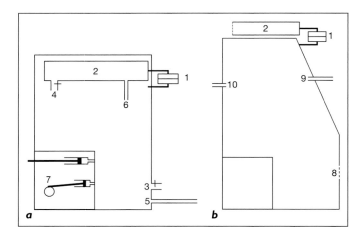

Fig. 1. Schematics of the commonly used plethysmographs: variable pressure plethysmograph (***a***) and volume displacement flow plethysmograph (***b***). Sensitive pressure transducer (1) connected to body box and reference chamber (2). Solenoid valves to vent the box to atmosphere (3), and to connect the reference chamber to the body box to avoid loading of the pressure transducer when manoeuvring the door (4). Mechanical leak to the outside (5). Long-time constant connection for faster thermal equilibration between chambers (6). Electrical pump for calibration and manually handled syringe for mechanical time constant determination (7). Wire mesh screen acting as a pneumotachograph (8). Port to connect subject to the outside (9). Port to circulate bias flow (10) [redrawn from 6, with permission].

(1) gas compression/decompression is small as in the volume plethysmograph, and slow respiratory events may be studied, (2) after correction for the mechanical time constant, the frequency response in the higher range, as in the pressure plethysmograph, is only limited by that of the pressure transducer, and (3) in addition, since the plethysmograph is open to atmosphere, a constant bias flow may be circulated to vent the box during long-lasting studies. The drawback is that ΔV_L is based on the integration of a small flow signal and is therefore subjected to significant drift, and the zero must be repeatedly adjusted.

Some commercially available plethysmographs may be operated in both the pressure and the flow mode. Thus, TGV is measured by the barometric method, taking advantage of the more stable signal, and VC by the volume displacement method, while the subject breathes in and out of the plethysmograph and box volume is displaced through a screen resistance.

A pneumotachograph with its own differential pressure transducer is necessary to obtain airway flow when measuring R_{aw}. Its integrated output allows to measure tidal volume and VC in the barometric plethysmograph.

Measurements

Measuring Conditions and Quality Check

A plethysmograph should be placed in a quiet room because the signal corresponding to gas compression is small and easily corrupted by external noise resulting from door slamming or air drafts, although these effects are minimized by the reference chamber.

Time Constants. The measurement of the thermal time constant requires complete air tightness and should be performed and specified by the manufacturer. The mechanical (leak) time constant of a barometric box may be checked by applying a step change in volume and calculating the time necessary for the pressure to decrease by 63%. It should be in the range of 10–20 s.

Calibration. Calibration should be performed daily. Usually, a reciprocating electrical pump compresses (δP) or displaces (δV) a known volume of gas, respectively, in the barometric or the flow plethysmograph. This procedure allows calibrating δP or δV in terms of ΔV_L. An important implication to avoid the effects of possible polytropic gas compression in a barometric box is that the TGV manoeuvre should be made at a frequency comparable to that of the calibration [10]. The pressure transducer measuring ΔP_m (equation 9) is calibrated with a water manometer.

Most commercialized plethysmographs are equipped for calibration as well as determination of leak time constant (fig. 1a).

Measuring TGV and R_{aw}

The child is seated inside the plethysmograph and the whole procedure is explained to him/her. While the door is still open, the child is trained to take the mouthpiece and put on the nose clip. Trials of shutter activations are useful to teach the child to perform inspiratory/expiratory efforts against closed airways at 1–2 Hz and to pant at about the same frequency for the measurement of sR_{aw}. The child should be asked to support his/her cheeks with both hands during the measurement and be told that he/she may take off the mouthpiece and nose clip in between measurements. A complete session will last up to 10 min in a cooperative child, but each measurement will take only a few seconds.

There are different ways to proceed. Whenever possible, measurements of TGV and sR_{aw} should be closely associated in time as both parameters are necessary to obtain R_{aw} (equation 8) and should therefore be measured under the same conditions. In the following description, sR_{aw} is measured before TGV. Indeed the latter is ended by a VC manoeuvre which should be avoided immediately prior to measuring sR_{aw}. When the door is closed, the ΔV signal drifts as heat builds up inside the body box of a barometric plethysmograph. After about a minute, the box pressure reaches a steady value. The subject is asked to connect to the mouthpiece, hold his cheeks firmly with both hands and breathe calmly. At the end of an expiration (at FRC), the child is asked to pant for 3–5 s while ΔV_{aw} and V′ are displayed as an X-Y plot on an oscilloscope or a computer screen. The shutter is then activated and the child continues to make inspiratory-expiratory efforts at about the same frequency for the same period of time. The child and the X-Y plot of $\Delta V_L - \Delta P_m$ are followed closely. The shutter is released and the child asked to take a maximal inspiration followed by a maximal expiration, so that not only FRC but also TLC and RV may be computed. The whole procedure should be repeated 3–5 times to assess the variability of the parameters.

Another method, increasingly used in the young child, cooperative enough to enter the body box, but unable to perform a proper TGV manoeuvre, consists in measuring only sR_{aw}, generally during tidal breathing [12]. The issues associated with this particular technique are detailed in the section 'Quality Control and Interpretation' below.

Data Analysis

A short description of the algorithms that may be used to solve the $\Delta V_L - \Delta P_m$ and the $\Delta V_{aw} - \Delta V'$ relationships is given here to emphasize the considerable progress in data processing associated with computerization. Formerly, the use of X-Y recorders with low frequency responses as well as the lack of digital processing could induce significant errors in the solving of equations 8 and 9 as there was only little opportunity for accurate drift correction. A number of algorithms may now be applied to the digitized $\Delta P_m - \Delta V_L$ relationship. For instance, a linear regression may be calculated between ΔP_m (y-axis) and ΔV_L (x-axis) where TGV is inversely proportional to the slope of the line, and the corresponding correlation coefficient may be used as an index of quality control. Even during valid manoeuvres, a drift on ΔV_L is frequent, particularly in the flow mode, and should be eliminated. If a regression analysis is used, a simple algorithm may efficiently eliminate a constant drift by optimizing the regression coefficient [13]. Alternatively – provided the manoeuvre is reasonably periodic – the Fourier coefficients may be extracted from the fundamentals of the ΔP_m and ΔV_L signals and allow calculating TGV, an elegant way to eliminate the drift [13]. Furthermore, the phase angle between P_m and ΔV_L may give some indication of the quality of the manoeuvre and/or of the subject's respiratory condition. To eliminate the drift, it has also been proposed to calculate TGV from the derivative of the signals [14].

Replacing ΔV_L and ΔP_m, respectively, by ΔV_{aw} and V′ allows the solving of equation 8 using similar algorithms.

Quality Control and Interpretation

The frequency of respiratory efforts may have critical effects on the measurement of both TGV and R_{aw}. It should, therefore, be either standardized or – at the very least – recorded for interpretation and comparison within a given subject or a patient population.

Thoracic Gas Volume

During the TGV manoeuvre, the $\Delta V_L - \Delta P_m$ plot of the signals should display a straight line. Deviation from a line may relate to methodological causes or to the disease itself.

Methodological causes include the following.

(1) A leaky body box, partial obstruction or leak at the connection of the mouth pressure transducer. These causes should easily be avoided by regular inspection of tubing connections and checking of the mechanical time constant.

(2) Poor connection of the subject to the shutter resulting in a leak at the mouthpiece or nose clip which should easily be detected by close observation of the child during the measurement.

(3) Improper manoeuvres that result in differences between P_{alv} and P_m, including glottis closure – a very frequent cause of data corruption in children – and excessive cheek motion.

(4) Examples of poor $\Delta V_L - P_m$ relationships are illustrated in figure 2. With computerized systems the numerical solving of equation 8 may provide objective quality control criteria (see 'Data Analysis'). Any measurement presenting a gross deviation from a line should be rejected.

The subject's condition itself may be responsible for a phase lag between ΔV_L and ΔP_m. Indeed, the measurement of TGV depends on a number of assumptions which, under certain pathological circumstances, are not satisfied anymore.

(1) The difference between P_B and P_{alv} that actually occurs during the TGV manoeuvre is neglected when using equation 9. This induces a small and systematic error, is minimized by limiting the excursion of P_m, and may be corrected for [15].

(2) It is assumed that the compressible gas is entirely represented by the alveolar gas, while compression also occurs in the conducting airways and in the abdomen. These volumes are reasonably small compared with the alveolar volume but their significance and the fact that gas compression may not be entirely isothermal have not been quantified in children.

(3) It is also necessary that pressure is uniform within the lung, and that gas motion is only related to compression.

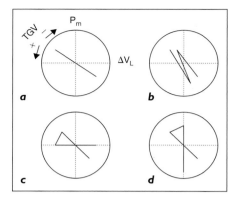

Fig. 2. Illustrations of patterns of $\Delta V_L - P_m$ relationships during measurement of TGV [redrawn from 127, with permission]. Correct manoeuvre: the slope of the line is inversely proportional to TGV, arrows indicate changes associated with larger $(+)$ or smaller $(-)$ TGV (**a**); drift of ΔV_L (**b**); change in ΔV_L not associated with change in P_m related to obstruction of the mouthpiece (**c**), and change in P_m without change in ΔV_L resulting from cheek motion without chest volume change (**d**). ΔV_L = Change in lung volume.

Compliant upper airway walls may induce a pressure difference between P_m and P_{alv}, the artefact being potentially more important in young children than in adults [16]. In addition, upper airway closure during an inspiratory manoeuvre against an occluded airway will result in a marked dissociation between P_m and P_{alv}, as shown in figure 2.

(4) Generally, any obstructive airway disease may contribute to gas flow in the occluded airways and amplify the effect of upper airway wall motion by (a) increasing the difference between P_m and P_{alv} as a result of increased R_{aw}, (b) increasing bronchial wall compliance, and (c) inducing regional inhomogeneities of ventilatory time constants and P_{alv}. In addition, gas flow in the airways will also be affected by chest distortion and uneven distribution of pleural pressure [17, 18], which may occur with significant airway disease.

(5) The effect of gas flow in the airways will be greater with increasing frequency. Although the figure may vary among subjects, a 20% overestimation of TGV may be expected in relation to these artefacts at a frequency of 2 Hz in the presence of airway obstruction [17–22].

(6) Should a spuriously high value be observed it may be worthwhile comparing measurements with airway occlusions at different lung volumes [23] or measuring oesophageal pressure instead of P_m [20]. It is worth noting that the sometimes considerable increase in TGV at FRC and RV in children with cystic fibrosis was reasonably matched by radiographic estimation of lung volume [24].

Airway Resistance

During the measurement of sR_{aw}, the $X - Y$ display of the signals depends on how the manoeuvre is performed. In fact, equation 8 may be studied only if ΔV related to the change in physical gas composition during breathing is eliminated. This may be achieved in three ways.

The most accurate but technically demanding, cumbersome, and possibly questionable from the point of view of hygiene [25] is the conditioning of inspired gas to body temperature, pressure, saturated with water vapour (BTPS) [4].

Panting of small tidal volumes through a dead space which should limit thermal exchanges with the gas in the plethysmograph [26] is the easiest way to eliminate the looping related to the thermal effect, whenever the child understands how to perform the manoeuvre. In addition, it is associated with widening of the larynx and a decrease in the contribution of upper R_{aw} as well as a decrease in tidal volume which minimize the effect of changes in volume history [23]. Another advantage is that the $X - Y$ plot of the $\Delta V - V'$ relationship during panting may bear some information regarding the physiological conditions of the airways [26]. The different patterns described below are illustrated in figure 3.

(1) Once the drift has stabilized, the normal representation is a slightly 'S'-shaped curve that flattens toward high inspiratory and expiratory flows, expressing the flow dependence of R_{aw} (fig. 3a). An increase in R_{aw} is associated with a decrease in slope, i.e., a larger change in ΔV_{aw} in a given range of V'.

(2) An exaggerated flattening of the 'S' suggests increased turbulent flow that may be expected during central airway obstruction such as tracheal stenosis (fig. 3b).

(3) A decrease in slope during expiration indicates a selective increase in expiratory resistance (fig. 3c).

(4) A clockwise looping during expiration indicates an increase in R_{aw} at end expiration, i.e., with decreasing lung volume (fig. 3d). The pattern has also been documented in young children [27].

(5) Complete clockwise looping of ΔV_{aw} and V' during the entire respiratory cycle suggests trapped air or delayed emptying or filling of lung regions: there is a phase lag between gas flow from/into that region and the corresponding pressure change (fig. 3e).

(6) In equation 8 it was assumed that ΔV_{aw} was entirely related to R_{aw}. Since gas must also be accelerated during breathing, a phase lag may occur between ΔV_{aw} and V' because of airway inertance, which normally is negligible. However, in a patient with significant central airway obstruction panting at frequencies around 2 Hz, the second term of the equation may become significant because

Marchal/Schweitzer

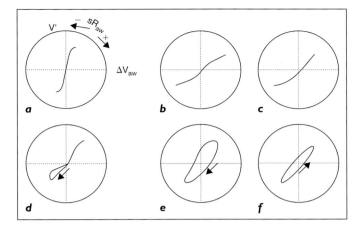

Fig 3. Some aspects of the $\Delta V_{aw} - V'$ relationship: normal pattern (**a**); increased upper airway (tracheal) resistance (**b**); increased expiratory resistance (**c**); increased end-expiratory resistance (**d**); air trapping and inhomogeneous ventilation [redrawn from 26] (**e**) and increased airway inertance [redrawn from 7] (**f**). ΔV_{aw} = Mechanical component of the change in volume; V' = airflow. sR_{aw} = specific airway resistance.

airway inertance is dependent on large airway dimensions. This induces a counterclockwise looping of the $\Delta V_{aw} - V'$ relationship (fig. 3f) [28].

An electronic compensation correcting for that part of the box signal in phase with volume has been proposed [28]. Indeed, during spontaneous tidal breathing without conditioning of the inspired gas to BTPS, gross looping occurs between the signals because of the thermal effect. This is usually the case when investigating young children, cooperative enough to enter the body box and breathe through a flowmeter, but unable to produce regular panting. The electronic compensation is based on the assumption that the thermal effect is entirely in phase with tidal volume, i.e., that thermal equilibration is instantaneous, which is not the case. As demonstrated by several analyses [8], thermal exchange occurs with a time constant, and part of the thermal effect is in phase with flow and not subtracted by the electronic compensation. The resulting frequency dependence of sR_{aw} (which decreases markedly as frequency decreases) was demonstrated with an experimental setup in healthy adults [29] but also with commercial equipment in young patients and adults [30]. This frequency dependence of sR_{aw} is far from negligible between spontaneous breathing and 2 Hz [29, 30]. At this frequency and above, sR_{aw} reaches a plateau, a reason explaining why looping disappears during panting [8]. Whenever sR_{aw} is measured during tidal breathing, the breathing frequency should be noted for further reference.

Relationship between R_{aw} and TGV

Body plethysmography is a unique tool to study the relationship between airway dimensions and volume history. The early measurements in adults have demonstrated that R_{aw} was exponentially decreasing, and G_{aw} linearly increasing with TGV, from RV to TLC [31]. This is explained by the attachment of lung parenchyma onto the conducting airway walls. As volume increases, the elastic recoil of lung tissue pulls on these airways. An interesting aspect is related to the fact that lung tissue and airway wall both are viscoelastic rather than purely elastic. With significant bronchoconstriction, alteration of the mechanical properties of the bronchial wall induces a significant change in the mechanical interdependence between conducting airways and lung parenchyma. Hence, a deep breath may induce significant and prolonged bronchodilation [32]. There are little data on these effects of volume history from body plethysmography in children, although R_{aw} or G_{aw} are particularly suited for such studies, as they are usually considered to characterize the more central – i.e., conducting – airways.

R_{aw} not only changes within an individual subject with lung volume but undergoes considerable reduction with growth, as the diameter of the airways increases. A recent evaluation of sR_{aw} in early childhood suggests this parameter to be constant from 2 up to 7 years [27].

Mass Conservation Principle

Gas dilution techniques are widely used for the determination of static lung volumes with a tracer gas. They may be divided into wash-in (usually helium: He) and wash-out (usually nitrogen: N_2) methods. None has specifically been developed for children, and the results need to be interpreted as a function of the child's cooperation.

Wash-In Methods
Multiple-Breath He Dilution
Principle. The use of a foreign gas to determine lung volumes was first described for hydrogen and was adapted in 1941 for safety reasons with He instead of hydrogen [33–35]. He is an inert, readily available and insoluble gas. Its concentration ([He]) is easily measured by a thermal conductivity analyzer because its thermal conductivity is very different from those of O_2 and N_2. Because it is insoluble, He will not diffuse into the blood during the time of the measurement. Therefore, the He quantity initially contained in a closed circuit, once connected to the subject's lung, will diffuse only in the airspaces and the same He quantity is recovered at the end of the measurement.

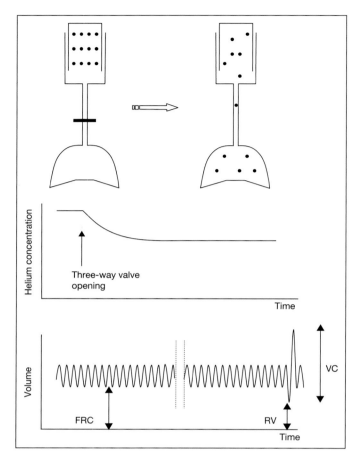

Fig. 4. Basic principles of functional residual capacity (FRC) and residual volume (RV) measurement by the multiple-breath closed-circuit helium dilution.

Measurement. The closed circuit includes a water-sealed or a rolling-sealed spirometer, a three-way valve and a He analyzer. CO_2 is absorbed by soda lime and O_2 continuously added so as to maintain constant the volume of the system. The volume of the spirometer (V_{sp}) must be known. Prior to measuring, He is introduced in the spirometer to achieve an initial concentration $[He]_1$, corresponding to the quantity $[He]_1 \cdot V_{sp}$. The subject is seated, wearing a nose clip and connected through a mouthpiece to the three-way valve, first quietly breathing room air. The valve is switched to the spirometer at the end of a normal expiration, i.e., at FRC, and the subject continues to breathe normally. The mixing of gases from the spirometer and the lung is followed by a decrease in [He], until a stable value is recorded $[He]_2$ (fig. 4) The final He quantity is equal to the initial one so that:

$$(FRC + Vsp) \cdot [He]_2 = Vsp \cdot [He]_1 \qquad (10)$$

and

$$FRC = V_{sp} \cdot ([He]_1 - [He]_2)/[He]_2 \qquad (11)$$

Recommendations have been published for the routine application of this method [5, 36]. Equilibration is defined as a difference lower than 0.02% between two successive [He] measured 15 s apart. The average equilibration time is about 5 min and is age dependent, being shorter in smaller children. It may be markedly elevated in severe airway obstruction. Current guidelines indicate the duration of the measurement should not exceed 10 min [5], so that the method may underestimate FRC, which mainly happens in the presence of air-trapping or gross ventilation inhomogeneity. After 10 min a small amount of He may diffuse into the blood. Because the method requires little cooperation, it may easily be applied to preschool children.

Once equilibration has occurred, the child is asked to inspire maximally from FRC and then to expire fully. Inspiratory VC, TLC, and RV are derived from this manoeuvre which should be done before disconnection from the mouthpiece. The manoeuvre may be repeated and the largest value should be reported.

With irregular and/or fast breathing, it may be difficult for the technician to connect the child to the closed circuit exactly at the end of a tidal expiration, at the start of the measurement. This leads to an over- or underestimation of FRC. Current measuring systems are able to compensate for such errors by assessing FRC from several breathing cycles.

An imbalance between O_2 consumption and O_2 added to the spirometer will induce a drift in the tidal volume trace. Therefore, care should be taken to maintain a horizontal trace throughout. Again, a computer-assisted system will automatically adjust the oxygen supply.

Leaks may occur when the child does not place his/her lips tightly enough around the mouthpiece or when the nose clip is loose. He leak through perforated eardrums has been reported [37].

Single-Breath He Dilution
This method is performed in conjunction with the single-breath CO transfer factor for determination of alveolar volume. The subject takes a deep breath and holds it for 10–15 s. This measurement is not recommended to be used routinely for the sole determination of FRC in children since there is not enough time for He to diffuse into all airspaces [5].

Wash-Out Methods
Multiple-Breath N_2 Wash-Out
This technique was developed in the 1940s [38, 39] to avoid the difficulties of closed circuit techniques related to O_2 consumption. With this open circuit method N_2 is washed out of the lung by administration of pure O_2 via a

non-rebreathing valve. The system is initially flushed with O_2 and the subject switched from room air to pure O_2 at FRC. The expired gas is collected in a spirometer or a Douglas bag until N_2 concentration ($[N_2]$) falls below 0.02%. Thus, N_2 collected in the spirometer comes from the lung at FRC which may be calculated – similarly to equation 11 – from the increase of the spirometer volume and the final $[N_2]$, assuming an initial alveolar $[N_2]$ of 80%. An alternative procedure has been proposed based on the determination of expired volumes by integration of expiratory flow over a few breaths with simultaneous measurements of $[N_2]$ in the expired gas [40]. Such a determination requires a rapid N_2 analyzer, dynamic adjustments of flow and $[N_2]$ signals, and linearization of the analyzer [41]. N_2 wash-out exhibits a trend to overestimate FRC as N_2 is soluble in body fluids and lung tissues, but it has the valuable capability of assessing ventilation inhomogeneities (see 'Estimation of Air Trapping and Uneven Ventilation' below) [42].

Single-Breath Nitrogen Wash-Out

This technique may be used in cooperative children for assessing lung volumes and non-uniform gas distribution [43, 44]. A major advantage of the test is its short duration; thus, the method has been proposed for epidemiological studies [45, 46]. The subject first exhales to RV, then inhales slowly and evenly pure O_2 to TLC and exhales at a steady rate to RV. Inspiratory and expiratory flows are kept constant and lower than 0.5 litre·min^{-1} (see above) using a feedback device. Both changes in lung volumes and $[N_2]$ are continuously recorded and plotted against each other. $[N_2]$ needs to be monitored by a rapid analyzer. The reliability of the test is dependent on the subject's cooperation and technical aspects. For instance, the integration of the pneumotachograph signal is a convenient way to measure VC but the difference between inspired and expired gas viscosities may lead to significant errors. Conveniently, the pneumotachograph may be located in the wall of a bag-in-box system to avoid this effect [43].

A characteristic curve is presented in figure 5. Pure O_2 appears first, as dead space marker (phase I). A rapid rise in $[N_2]$ follows, corresponding to a mixture of dead space and alveolar gases (phase II). A quasi-linear slope corresponds to alveolar gas (phase III) and, in most subjects, a sharp rise in N_2 concentration marks the onset of the closing volume (phase IV). This pattern has been explained by inhomogeneity of the gas distribution within the lung. Single-breath N_2 wash-out allows the determination of TLC after calculation of the mean alveolar and expired $[N_2]$. The measurement of FRC, RV, or TLC is only part of the information provided by the single-breath N_2 wash-out

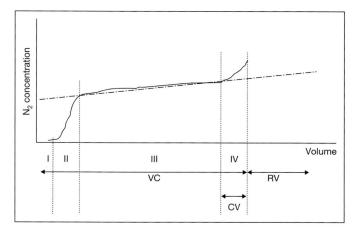

Fig 5. Continuous record of expired nitrogen concentration during exhalation (single breath) after inspiration of pure O_2. Phase I represents dead space gas, phase II a mixture of dead space gas and alveolar gas, phase III alveolar gas, and phase IV the gas issuing from the slow-emptying regions of the lung. The slope of phase III is determined by the best-fit line between the end of phase II and the onset of phase IV (– · –). CV = closing volume; VC = vital capacity; RV = residual volume.

which is mainly indicated to evaluate non-homogeneous ventilation (see 'Estimation of Air Trapping and Uneven Ventilation' below) [47].

Sulphur Hexafluoride (SF_6) Wash-Out

This method has been developed mainly for the assessment of lung volumes during mechanical ventilation [48] with good correlation to N_2 wash-out [see 49]. Recent applications have been described to assess distribution of ventilation in spontaneously breathing school and pre-school children [42, 50].

Estimation of Air Trapping and Uneven Ventilation

Air trapping and lung distension may occur in the course of an obstructive airway disease. The measurement of static lung volumes offers a unique opportunity to estimate such abnormalities. A simple way to estimate lung distension is to express RV as a function of TLC, obtained by either He wash-in or plethysmography, although the latter should theoretically be more accurate in identifying air trapping.

Techniques of N_2 wash-out allow different estimations of uneven ventilation and gas trapping. Closing volume may be derived from the single-breath N_2 wash-out. In normal subjects, there is a gravity-dependent, sequential opening of lung regions because the stretch of lower and upper zones is similar at TLC whereas lower zones are more compressed at

RV. Therefore, ventilation is larger in the lower (fast-emptying) zones than in the upper (slow-emptying) zones, and a maximal breath of pure O_2 dilutes the alveolar gas more in the lower than the upper zones. The positive slope of phase III is, therefore, related to the sequential emptying of, first, lower lung zones with lower $[N_2]$ and, second, upper lung zones with higher $[N_2]$. The onset of phase IV is a marker of the closing volume, i.e., the lung volume at which closure of fast-emptying regions occurs, while gas continues to flow out of slow-emptying regions. Closing volume is often expressed as a fraction of VC or TLC. The slope of phase III may be increased by any lung disorder increasing the mechanical heterogeneity of the lung. In obstructive airway diseases, slow-emptying compartments, i.e., regions with increased mechanical time constants, result from increased local R_{aw} and/or local lung compliance. The slope of phase III is determined by the best-fit line between the end of phase II and the onset of phase IV.

The volume of trapped air (V_{TA}) is an indicator of peripheral bronchial obstruction that may be derived from the multiple-breath N_2 wash-out [51]. V_{TA} is a compartment that communicates poorly or not at all with the airway opening during tidal breathing. To achieve the measurement of V_{TA} by nitrogen wash-out (V_{TA, N_2}) the subject performs five maximal inspirations once the N_2 concentration has fallen below 0.02%. The calculation of V_{TA, N_2} is based on the assumption that N_2 remaining in the lung at the end of the wash-out is mobilized by the deep inspirations and appears in the exhaled gas. V_{TA} may also be estimated from a double determination of FRC by He dilution before and after exposure of the respiratory system to a positive expiratory pressure [52].

With a body plethysmograph in the volume displacement mode and the subject breathing out of the box through a pneumotachograph, VC may be estimated both from the box volume signal and from the flow at the mouth. During a forced expiration, alveolar gas undergoes compression and some alveolar gas may be dynamically trapped upstream to the equal pressure point. This leads to a difference between the two estimates of VC. It is thus possible to estimate the volume difference related to gas compression [53], which may be markedly elevated in some airway diseases. The estimation of the volume difference related to gas compression was, however, found to be poorly reproducible in children [54].

Other approaches are based on different estimates of lung volumes. A classical index is based on the comparison between FRC measured by plethysmography and by He wash-in. Indeed, He dilution measures only ventilated areas while plethysmography estimates both ventilated

areas and trapped air. V_{TA} has been described as significant when the ratio of plethysmographic to He FRC is larger than 1.10 [55]. Most estimations of V_{TA} have been performed in children with asthma [56–58], cystic fibrosis [57, 59, 60], or scoliosis [61].

Variability of FRC Measurements

A mean coefficient of variation of 7 and 5%, respectively, was reported for FRC by helium dilution and body plethysmography in healthy children studied 6–7 times at hourly intervals [62]. In a population of asthmatic children aged 4–16 years, the short-term coefficient of variation, calculated from three consecutive measurements, was 8.8% for TGV and 9.3% for sR_{aw} [63]. In asthmatic preschool children, the coefficient of variation for sR_{aw} ranged from 8 to 11% [27]. In healthy adults, the short-term variability was minimized when the analysis of the $\Delta V_L - P_m$ relationship also eliminated the drift, particularly in flow mode plethysmography [13]. Comparatively larger coefficients of variation were reported in asthmatic adults using a non-computerized analysis for both TGV and R_{aw} [64]. In addition, the variability is likely to be larger for FRC than for TLC, since the end-expiratory level may vary with time and respiratory frequency. Furthermore, lung inhomogeneity in obstructive airway diseases is likely to be expressed to a greater extent at low lung volumes than at TLC.

Between-day repeatability of TGV and sR_{aw} was found to be less than 10% for TGV and about 20% for sR_{aw} in healthy adults [13].

When Should Static Lung Volumes Be Measured?

Static lung volumes are useful in evaluating and in understanding the mechanisms of chronic respiratory diseases such as asthma, cystic fibrosis, and chronic lung disease of prematurity. A key feature of the measurement of static lung volumes is the estimation of trapped air. In addition, static lung volumes are of importance whenever a restrictive lung defect is suspected.

Asthma [see 65]

In the majority of well-controlled asthmatic children, routine spirometry is adequate to the longitudinal evaluation of lung function. On the other hand, plethysmographic measurement of lung volumes may be of interest in difficult asthma, as it provides a fast assessment of the degree of lung distension/air trapping and its response to therapy [66].

FRC may be elevated due to airway closure and/or dynamically elevated with an increased expiratory time constant, in which case it is not only determined by the balance between the chest wall and the lung elastic recoil [67]. Such hyperinflation may be regarded as a compensatory mechanism that minimizes the increase in R_{aw} and the expiratory flow limitation in obstructive airway disease. Hence, at an early stage of the disease, FVC and forced expiratory volume in 1 s (FEV_1) may be normal, and an isolated increase in lung volume may be the sole functional abnormality [68, 69]. In asthmatic children, FRC is increased in those without treatment [70] and is more elevated in symptomatic than in asymptomatic children [71]. FRC may be reliably determined in preschool children, and is worth measuring whenever inhaled steroids are considered. This therapy is associated with reduced hyperinflation in young asthmatic children after 6 weeks of treatment [72]. FRC is known to decrease in patients becoming asymptomatic with steroid treatment [71]. In a recent study, FRC was similar in asthmatics on inhaled steroids and healthy controls [73]. Persistent hyperinflation in children after an acute asthma attack does not correlate necessarily with clinical asthma severity [74]. Hyperinflation as assessed by He dilution also occurs during methacholine challenge, but the large intersubject variability does not allow its use to assess bronchial responsiveness [75]. Bronchodilators were shown to decrease FRC in 80% of children aged 2–7 years, and the decrease was significantly correlated to baseline FRC. Some children exhibited an increase in FRC after bronchodilation when the baseline value was low [76]. FRC was found to decrease from the prone to the supine position in healthy and moderately severe asthmatic children but remained unchanged in severe asthmatic patients [77], while V_{TA} increased in the supine position [78]. The presence of trapped air is associated with hypoxaemia [56] and non-specific bronchial hyperreactivity [79], but correlates poorly with flow limitation, and may be lacking in patients with severe asthma [57]. A retrospective analysis suggested that gas trapping as estimated from RV/TLC by plethysmography was significantly associated with a methacholine $PC_{20} \leq 8$ mg/ml [79]. An increase of V_{TA} determined by N_2 wash-out [80] and a decrease in sG_{aw} [81] were found to be sensitive indices to detect exercise-induced bronchoconstriction, which may also be associated with a significant elevation of FRC in children [82].

Since the early description of sR_{aw} measurement [83], important developments have taken place regarding its application in young children. Recent data suggest that sR_{aw} is able to identify responses to bronchodilators [84], inhaled steroids [85], and airway challenge [86] in preschool children, and may also be of interest in epidemiological studies [87]. However, there is no established cutoff for sR_{aw} to separate healthy subjects from asthmatics. In addition, it should be kept in mind that sR_{aw} may be altered both by hyperinflation and decreased airway diameter, and the physiological meaning of the parameter is different from R_{aw} or from respiratory resistance. Again, particular care should be taken when measuring sR_{aw} during tidal breathing in small children because of the marked frequency dependence of the parameter [27, 29].

Cystic Fibrosis [see 88]

Lung distension may be demonstrated at different stages of cystic fibrosis lung disease [89–91], and RV/TLC has been suggested to be a sensitive index [92]. Digital clubbing has been shown to correlate with RV as well as with the slope of phase III N_2 wash-out [93]. It is worth noting that large discrepancies between techniques may be found in cystic fibrosis patients as a result of airway obstruction, trapped air, or ventilation inhomogeneities. He dilution tends to underestimate lung volumes [94], particularly when not enough time is allowed for equilibration. An estimate of V_{TA} – based on the difference between measurements by plethysmography and He dilution – was found to correlate with flow limitation [57] and daytime hypoxaemia [95] as well as lowest nocturnal oxygen saturation [60]. V_{TA} was also found to improve significantly with mucolytic agents [96]. Plethysmography has been used to assess the airway response to β-adrenergic drugs which may be paradoxical when evaluated by forced expiration in cystic fibrosis patients [90, 97]. This phenomenon was, however, unrelated to the degree of gas compression within the lung during forced expiration [57]. High-dose ipratropium bromide and salbutamol were reported to decrease R_{aw} with no change in TGV [98].

Multiple [99]- and single-breath [50, 100] N_2 wash-out has been used to describe lung inhomogeneities as an early index of lung function impairment. This appears to be of interest but experience is currently limited to a few laboratories [100]. The growing interest in these techniques will help determine their role in the routine management of cystic fibrosis patients. Some of the indices derived from these techniques have also been used in assessing acute rejection after lung transplant [101].

Outcome of Neonatal Disorders [see 102]

The outcome of prematurity in childhood and young adulthood is now being described in a number of studies. The issue is complex as it involves abnormal lung growth with premature delivery, lung injury with respiratory distress, and management that varies considerably with time and in different regions of the world. TLC and FRC are indicators of the alveolar number in the normal child [103]. However, such an interpretation is not possible in the outcome of neonatal respiratory disease, because of the frequent occurrence of emphysema [104]. The American Thoracic Society recently issued a document devoted to the caring of the child with chronic lung disease that included data on lung function outcome in childhood with bronchopulmonary dysplasia [104]. Static lung volumes after hyaline membrane disease without bronchopulmonary dysplasia were not altered at age 11 [105], and were not affected by antenatal dexamethasone at age 7–9 [106]. The longitudinal follow-up of very premature children at preschool age showed hyperinflation assessed by He dilution [107]. At school age, premature children with bronchopulmonary dysplasia were also found to have larger RV and RV/TLC [108, 109] and lower sG_{aw} [109] than healthy controls. Compared with matched premature children without bronchopulmonary dysplasia, they also showed more hyperinflation [108]. Progressive reduction in RV/TLC was suggested from childhood to adolescence in a longitudinal study [110]. On the other hand, adolescents and young adults with bronchopulmonary dysplasia were found to have a number of respiratory function abnormalities compared with age-matched controls, including airway hyperreactivity, fixed airway obstruction, and hyperinflation as indicated by an elevated RV/TLC [111]. Discrepancies among studies of long-term outcome may be explained by differences among cohorts in birth weight, severity of the disease, and early neonatal management. Nevertheless, hyperinflation as measured by He dilution or plethysmography is a consistent finding in children and young adults with a history of significant bronchopulmonary dysplasia. RV/TLC thus is considered a useful parameter in the assessment of air trapping in the long-term outcome of neonatal respiratory disorders. The diagnostic value of RV/TLC appears to differ from that of spirometry in some studies, perhaps because a consequence of lung distension is to minimize expiratory flow limitation.

Children born with congenital diaphragmatic hernia studied between 7 and 17 years were also found to have higher RV and RV/TLC than controls matched for age and gestational age [112]. Newborn infants with the meconium aspiration syndrome requiring only supplemental oxygen or ventilatory support <24 h showed no abnormalities in static lung volumes when examined at age 7 [113].

Identification of a Restrictive Syndrome

Restrictive lung disease was initially defined by a reduction of TLC below 80% predicted [55]. For convenience, with increasing use of spirometry, a reduction in VC of similar magnitude was also used to define restriction. It was, therefore, proposed to distinguish restrictive and hypodynamic syndromes in order to specify the origin of a decrease in VC [114]. A restrictive syndrome is characterized by a homogenous decrease in VC, RV, and TLC, such as seen after parenchymal amputation [115], in fibrosing alveolitis [116], or in various chest wall disorders [117]. A hypodynamic syndrome is characterized by normal TLC with increased RV and low VC, as in the early course of neuromuscular disorders. The decreases in TLC, VC, and FEV_1 are linked to the gradual worsening of respiratory muscle weakness [118]. An increase in RV and RV/TLC [119, 120] indicates the more prominent impairment of expiratory muscles [121]. Such a presentation has recently been described in detail in patients with Duchenne's muscular dystrophy [119]. These children may later exhibit chest wall deformities leading to a true restrictive syndrome. In diastrophic dysplasia, TLC was found to correlate inversely with the angle of thoracolumbar scoliosis [122]. In scoliosis, V_{TA} may be of clinical usefulness to detect airway obstruction not evidenced by spirometry alone [61].

Conclusions and Future Directions

Static lung volumes appear as useful lung function parameters to complement the physiological information of spirometry. These measurements are particularly helpful in the identification of trapped gas, poorly ventilated areas, and uneven ventilation. Different methodological approaches are possible, some of them appearing particularly promising in the evaluation of uneven ventilation at an early stage of obstructive airway diseases.

It has been possible to estimate mechanical properties of airway and respiratory tissue in children without overt airway obstruction by the use of non-invasive measurements of TGV and respiratory transfer impedance, and simple modelling [123]. Further developments of such approaches may improve the current knowledge of respiratory disorders in children and the role of lung inflation at an early stage of chronic airway obstruction [67]. In addition, the considerable and recent interest in assessing the effects of volume history in acute bronchoconstriction deserves further development of body plethysmography in children. Optical reflectance motion analysis has been successfully used for the dynamic assessment of lung volume [124]. There are few data in children but it is likely that this technique will provide important information in research studies on the control of lung volume during tidal breathing. Future directions of lung function testing in children may also involve functional imaging. Significant radiation dose limits the repeated use of computerized tomography in children [125].

Alternative techniques such as [3]He inhalation and magnetic resonance imaging have been developed [126] and appear powerful enough to demonstrate regional airflow limitation in asthma or cystic fibrosis, and to identify regional inhomogeneity and the response to treatment.

Acknowledgments

The authors thank Doctor René Peslin for evaluation of the manuscript; Noëlle Bertin and Elisabeth Gerhardt for secretarial assistance.

References

1 Merkus PJFM: Reference equations for ventilatory function measurements in children from 6 to 16 years; Hammer J, Eber E (eds): Paediatric Pulmonary Function Testing. Prog Respir Res. Basel, Karger, 2005, vol 33, pp 118–124.

2 Eber E, Zach MS: Spirometry: Volume-time and flow-volume curves; Hammer J, Eber E (eds): Paediatric Pulmonary Function Testing. Prog Respir Res. Basel, Karger, 2005, vol 33, pp 94–102.

3 British Thoracic Society: Guidelines for the measurement of respiratory function. Respir Med 1994;88:165–194.

4 DuBois AB, van de Woestijne KP: Body plethysmography; in DuBois AB, van de Woestijne K (eds): Progress in Respiration Research. Basel, Karger, 1969.

5 Quanjer PH, Tammeling GJ, Cotes JE, Pedersen OF, Peslin R, Yernault JC: Lung volumes and forced ventilatory flows. Report Working Party Standardization of Lung Function Tests, European Community for Steel and Coal. Official Statement of the European Respiratory Society. Eur Respir J Suppl 1993;16:5–40.

6 Peslin R: Body plethysmography; in Otis A (ed): Technique in the Life Science P4/II. Limerick, Elsevier Scientific Publications, 1984, pp 1–26.

7 Jaeger MJ, Bouhuys A: Loop formation in pressure vs flow diagrams obtained by body plethysmographic techniques; in DuBois AB, van de Woestijne KP (eds): Progress in Respiration Research. Basel, Karger, 1969, pp 116–130.

8 Peslin R, Duvivier C, Vassiliou M, Gallina C: Thermal artifacts in plethysmographic airway resistance measurements. J Appl Physiol 1995; 79:1958–1965.

9 DuBois AB, Bothelo SY, Bedell GN, Marshall R, Comroe JH Jr: A rapid plethysmographic method for measuring thoracic gas volume: A comparison with a nitrogen washout method for measuring functional residual capacity in normal subjects. J Clin Invest 1956;35:322–326.

10 Bargeton D, Barrès G: Time characteristics and frequency response of body plethysmograph; in DuBois AB, van de Woestijne K (eds): Progress in Respiration Research. Basel, Karger, 1969, pp 2–23.

11 Mead J: Volume displacement body plethysmograph for respiratory measurements in human subjects. J Appl Physiol 1960;15: 736–740.

12 Bisgaard H, Klug B: Lung function measurement in awake young children. Eur Respir J 1995;8:2067–2075.

13 Peslin R, Gallina C, Rotger M: Methodological factors in the variability of lung volume and specific airway resistance measured by body plethysmography. Bull Eur Physiopathol Respir 1987;23:323–327.

14 Lorino H, Harf A, Atlan G, Brault Y, Lorino AM, Laurent D: Computer determination of thoracic gas volume using plethysmographic 'thoracic flow'. J Appl Physiol 1980;48: 911–916.

15 Coates AL, Desmond KJ, Demizio DL: The simplified version of Boyle's law leads to errors in the measurement of thoracic gas volume. Am J Respir Crit Care Med 1995; 152:942–946.

16 Marchal F, Haouzi P, Peslin R, Duvivier C, Gallina C: Mechanical properties of the upper airway wall in children and their influence on respiratory impedance measurements. Pediatr Pulmonol 1992;13:28–33.

17 Godfrey S, Leventhal A, Weintraub Z, Katzenelson R, Connolly NM: Distortion of chest movement by increased airways resistance. Thorax 1972;27:148–155.

18 Marchal F, Duvivier C, Peslin R, Haouzi P, Crance JP: Thoracic gas volume at functional residual capacity measured with an integrated-flow plethysmograph in infants and young children. Eur Respir J 991;4:180–187.

19 Bohadana AB, Peslin R, Hannhart B, Teculescu D: Influence of panting frequency on plethysmographic measurements of thoracic gas volume. J Appl Physiol 1982;52: 739–747.

20 Stanescu D: Was it just our problem, or yours too? Errors in body plethysmography, in infants, children, and adults. Pediatr Pulmonol 1991;11:285–288.

21 Stanescu DC, Rodenstein D, Cauberghs M, van de Woestije KP: Failure of body plethysmography in bronchial asthma. J Appl Physiol 1982;52:939–948.

22 Rodenstein DO, Stanescu DC, Francis C: Demonstration of failure of body plethysmography in airway obstruction. J Appl Physiol 1982;52:949–954.

23 Stanescu DC, Clement J, Pattijn J, van de Woestijne KP: Glottis opening and airway resistance. J Appl Physiol 1972;32:460–466.

24 Marchant J, Hansell DM, Bush A: Assessment of hyperinflation in children with cystic fibrosis. Thorax 1994;49:1164–1166.

25 Clausen JL: Lung volume equipment and infection control. ERS/ATS Workshop Report Series. European Respiratory ociety/American Thoracic Society. Eur Respir J 1997;10:1928–1932.

26 DuBois A: Significance of measurement of airway resistance; in DuBois AB, van de Woestijne KP (eds): Progress in Respiration Research. Basel, Karger, 1969, pp 109–115.

27 Klug B, Bisgaard H: Specific airway resistance, interrupter resistance, and respiratory impedance in healthy children aged 2–7 years. Pediatr Pulmonol 1998;25:322–331.

28 Smidt U, Muysers K, Buchheim W: Electronic compensation of differences in temperature and water vapour between in- and expired air and other signal handling in body plethysmography; in DuBois AB, van de Woestijne KP: Progress in Respiration Research. Basel, Karger, 1969, pp 39–49.

29 Peslin R, Duvivier C, Malvestio P, Benis AR, Polu JM: Frequency dependence of specific airway resistance in a commercialized plethysmograph. Eur Respir J 1996;9:1747–1750.

30 Klug B, Bisgaard H: Measurement of the specific airway resistance by plethysmography in young children accompanied by an adult. Eur Respir J 1997;10:1599–1605.

31 DuBois AB, Bothelo SY, Comroe JH: A new method for measuring airway resistance in man using a body plethysmograph: Values in normal subjects and in patients with respiratory disease. J Clin Invest 1956; 35:327–335.

32 Pellegrino R, Sterk PJ, Sont JK, Brusasco V: Assessing the effect of deep inhalation on airway calibre: A novel approach to lung function in bronchial asthma and COPD. Eur Respir J 1998;12:1219–1227.

33 Meneely GR, Ball COT, Kory RC: A simplified closed-circuit helium dilution method for the determination of the residual volume of the lungs. Am J Med 1960;28:824–827.

34 Meneely GR, Kaltreider NL: Use of helium for determination of pulmonary capacity. Proc Soc Exp Biol Med 1941;46:266–267.

35 Meneely GR, Kaltreider NL: The volume of the lung determined by helium dilution. J Clin Invest 1949;28:129–139.

36 Kendrick AH: Comparison of methods of measuring static lung volumes. Monaldi Arch Chest Dis 1996;51:431–439.

37 Zarins LP: Closed circuit helium dilution method of lung volume measurement; in Clausen JL (ed): Pulmonary Function Testing, Guidelines and Controversies. New York, Academic Press, 1982, pp 129–140.

38 Darling RC, Cournand A, Richards DW: Studies on intrapulmonary mixture of gases. III. Open circuit methods for measuring residual air. J Clin Invest 1940;19:609–618.

39 Jalowayski AA, Dawson A: Measurement of lung volume: The multiple breath nitrogen method; in Clausen JL (ed): Pulmonary Function Testing, Guidelines and Controversies. New York, Academic Press, 1982, pp 115–127.

40 Gustafsson PM, Johansson HJ, Dahlback GO: Pneumotachographic nitrogen washout method for measurement of the volume of trapped gas in the lungs. Pediatr Pulmonol 1994;17:258–268.

41 Brunner JX, Wolff G, Cumming G, Langenstein H: Accurate measurement of N_2 volumes during N_2 washout requires dynamic adjustment of delay time. J Appl Physiol 1985;59:1008–1012.

42 Gustafsson PM, Ljungberg H: Measurement of functional residual capacity and ventilation inhomogeneity by gas dilution techniques; Hammer J, Eber E (eds): Paediatric Pulmonary Function Testing. Prog Respir Res. Basel, Karger, 2005, vol 33, pp 54–65.

43 Gold MD: Single breath nitrogen test: Closing volume and distribution of ventilation; in Clausen JL (ed): Pulmonary Function Testing, Guidelines and Controversies. New York, Academic Press, 1982, pp 105–114.

44 Sixt R: The single breath nitrogen washout test. Eur Respir J Suppl 1989;4:167S–170S.

45 Teculescu D, Damel MC, Benamghar L, Costantino E, Pham QT, Marchand M: Estimation of static lung volumes by nitrogen washout method. Single breath of oxygen. Rev Mal Respir 1994;11:393–401.

46 Sterk PJ, Quanjer PH, van Zomeren BC, Wise ME, van der Lende R: The single breath nitrogen test in epidemiological surveys; an appraisal. Bull Eur Physiopathol Respir 1981;17:381–397.

47 Buist AS, Ross BB: Quantitative analysis of the alveolar plateau in the diagnosis of early airway obstruction. Am Rev Respir Dis 1973;108:1078–1087.

48 Jonmarker C, Jansson L, Jonson B, Larsson A, Werner O: Measurement of functional residual capacity by sulfur hexafluoride washout. Anesthesiology 1985;63:89–95.

49 Hammer J, Newth CJL: Pulmonary function testing in the neonatal and paediatric intensive care unit; Hammer J, Eber E (eds): Paediatric Pulmonary Function Testing. Prog Respir Res. Basel, Karger, 2005, vol 33, pp 266–281.

50 Van Muylem A, Baran D: Overall and peripheral inhomogeneity of ventilation in patients with stable cystic fibrosis. Pediatr Pulmonol 2000;30:3–9.

51 Christensson P, Arborelius M Jr, Kautto R: Volume of trapped gas in lungs of healthy humans. J Appl Physiol 1981;51:172–175.

52 Motoyama EK, Hen J Jr, Tamas L, Dolan TF Jr: Spirometry with positive airway pressure. A simple method of evaluating obstructive lung disease in children. Am Rev Respir Dis 1982;126:766–770.

53 Coates AL, Desmond KJ, Demizio D, Allen P, Beaudry PH: Sources of error in flow-volume curves. Effect of expired volume measured at the mouth vs that measured in a body plethysmograph. Chest 1988;94:976–982.

54 Walamies MA: Thoracic gas compression profile during forced expiration in healthy and asthmatic schoolchildren. Respir Med 1998;92:173–177.

55 Lung function testing: Selection of reference values and interpretative strategies. American Thoracic Society. Am Rev Respir Dis 1991;144:1202–1218.

56 Wolf B, Gaultier C, Lopez C, Boule M, Girard F: Hypoxemia in attack free asthmatic children: Relationship with lung volumes and lung mechanics. Bull Eur Physiopathol Respir 1983;19:471–476.

57 Desmond KJ, Coates AL, Martin JG, Beaudry PH: Trapped gas and airflow limitation in children with cystic fibrosis and asthma. Pediatr Pulmonol 1986;2:128–134.

58 Hussein A, Harrie K, Kussau D: Effects of ipratropium bromide and salbutamol on isolated lung hyperinflation in symptom-free intervals in asthmatic children. Monatsschr Kinderheilkd 1990;138:135–140.

59 Haluszka J, Zebrak J: Failure of static pulmonary volume measurements in mucoviscidosis. Rev Mal Respir 1984;1:285–288.

60 Versteegh FG, Bogaard JM, Raatgever JW, Stam H, Neijens HJ, Kerrebijn KF: Relationship between airway obstruction, desaturation during exercise and nocturnal hypoxaemia in cystic fibrosis patients. Eur Respir J 1990; 3:68–73.

61 Boyer J, Amin N, Taddonio R, Dozor AJ: Evidence of airway obstruction in children with idiopathic scoliosis. Chest 1996;109: 1532–1535.

62 Cogswell JJ, Hull D, Milner AD, Norman AP, Taylor B: Lung function in childhood. 2. Thoracic gas volumes and helium functional residual capacity measurements in healthy children. Br J Dis Chest 1975;69:118–124.

63 Buhr W, Jorres R, Knapp M, Berdel D: Diagnostic value of body plethysmographic parameters in healthy and asthmatic young children is not influenced by breathing frequency. Pediatr Pulmonol 1990;8:23–28.

64 Bylin G, Lagerstrand L, Hedenstierna G, Wagner PD: Variability in airway conductance and lung volume in subjects with asthma. Clin Physiol 1995;15:207–218.

65 Basek P, Straub D, Wildhaber JH: Childhood asthma and wheezing disorders; Hammer J, Eber E (eds): Paediatric Pulmonary Function Testing. Prog Respir Res. Basel, Karger, 2005, vol 33, pp 204–214.

66 Jenkins HA, Cherniack R, Szefler SJ, Covar R, Gelfand EW, Spahn JD: A comparison of the clinical characteristics of children and adults with severe asthma. Chest 2003;124: 1318–1324.

67 Stanescu D: Small airways obstruction syndrome. Chest 1999;116:231–233.

68 Paton JY: A practical approach to the interpretation of lung function testing in children. Paediatr Respir Rev 2000;1:241–248.

69 Landau LI, Mellis CM, Phelan PD, Bristowe B, McLennan L: 'Small airways disease' in children: No test is best. Thorax 1979;34:217–223.

70 Greenough A, Loftus BG, Pool J, Price JF: Abnormalities of lung mechanics in young asthmatic children. Thorax 1987;42:500–505.

71 Pool JB, Greenough A, Price JF: Abnormalities of functional residual capacity in symptomatic and asymptomatic young asthmatics. Acta Paediatr Scand 1988;77:419–423.

72 Greenough A, Pool J, Gleeson JG, Price JF: Effect of budesonide on pulmonary hyperinflation in young asthmatic children. Thorax 1988;43:937–938.

73 Beydon N, Pin I, Matran R, Chaussain M, Boule M, Alain B, Bellet M, Amsallem F, Alberti C, Denjean A, Gaultier C: Pulmonary function tests in preschool children with asthma. Am J Respir Crit Care Med 2003; 168:640–644.

74 Pool JB, Greenough A, Gleeson JG, Price JF: Persistent lung hyperinflation in apparently asymptomatic asthmatic children. Respir Med 1989;83:433–436.

75 Wilts M, Hop WC, van der Heyden GH, Kerrebijn KF, de Jongste JC: Measurement of bronchial responsiveness in young children: Comparison of transcutaneous oxygen tension and functional residual capacity during induced bronchoconstriction and dilatation. Pediatr Pulmonol 1992;12:181–185.

76 Greenough A, Pool J, Price JF: Changes in functional residual capacity in response to bronchodilator therapy among young asthmatic children. Pediatr Pulmonol 1989;7:8–11.

77 Greenough A, Everett L, Pool J, Price JF: Relation between nocturnal symptoms and changes in lung function on lying down in asthmatic children. Thorax 1991;46:193–196.

78 Gustafsson PM: Pulmonary gas trapping increases in asthmatic children and adolescents in the supine position. Pediatr Pulmonol 2003;36:34–42.

79 Stanbrook MB, Chapman KR, Kesten S: Gas trapping as a predictor of positive methacholine challenge in patients with normal spirometry results. Chest 1995;107:992–995.

80 Svenonius E, Lecerof H, Lilja B, Arborelius M Jr, Kautto R: The volume of trapped gas: A new and sensitive test for the detection of exercise-induced bronchospasm in children. Acta Paediatr Scand 1978;67:583–589.

81 Buckley JM, Souhrada JF: A comparison of pulmonary function tests in detecting exercise-induced bronchoconstriction. Pediatrics 1975;56:883–889.

82 Anderson SD, McEvoy JD, Bianco S: Changes in lung volumes and airway resistance after exercise in asthmatic subjects. Am Rev Respir Dis 1972;106:30–37.

83 Dab I, Alexander F: A simplified approach to the measurement of specific airway resistance. Pediatr Res 1976;10:998–999.

84 Nielsen KG, Bisgaard H: Discriminative capacity of bronchodilator response measured with three different lung function techniques in asthmatic and healthy children aged 2 to 5 years. Am J Respir Crit Care Med 2001;164:554–559.

85 Nielsen KG, Bisgaard H: The effect of inhaled budesonide on symptoms, lung function, and cold air and methacholine responsiveness in 2- to 5-year-old asthmatic children. Am J Respir Crit Care Med 2000;162:1500–1506.

86 Nielsen KG, Bisgaard H: Lung function response to cold air challenge in asthmatic and healthy children of 2–5 years of age. Am J Respir Crit Care Med 2000;161:1805–1809.

87 Lowe L, Murray CS, Custovic A, Simpson BM, Kissen PM, Woodcock A: Specific airway resistance in 3-year-old children: A prospective cohort study. Lancet 2002;359:1904–1908.

88 Ratjen F, Grasemann H: Cystic fibrosis; Hammer J, Eber E (eds): Paediatric Pulmonary Function Testing. Prog Respir Res. Basel, Karger, 2005, vol 33, pp 213–221.

89 Baran D, Englert M: Pulmonary mechanics and diffusing capacity in cystic fibrosis. Helv Paediatr Acta 1973;28:175–183.

90 Hellinckx J, De Boeck K, Demedts M: No paradoxical bronchodilator response with forced oscillation technique in children with cystic fibrosis. Chest 1998;113:55–59.

91 Williams EM, Madgwick RG, Thomson AH, Morris MJ: Expiratory airflow patterns in children and adults with cystic fibrosis. Chest 2000;117:1078–1084.

92 Cooper DM, Mellins RB, Mansell AL: Changes in distribution of ventilation with lung growth. J Appl Physiol 1981;51:699–705.

93 Nakamura CT, Ng GY, Paton JY, Keens TG, Witmer JC, Bautista-Bolduc D, Woo MS: Correlation between digital clubbing and pulmonary function in cystic fibrosis. Pediatr Pulmonol 2002;33:332–338.

94 Cutrera R, Helms P: Retrospective estimation of values for total lung capacity by plethysmography, helium gas dilution, and chest radiography in patients with cystic fibrosis. Thorax 1988;43:931–932.

95 Kraemer R, Schoni MH: Ventilatory inequalities, pulmonary function and blood oxygenation in advanced states of cystic fibrosis. Respiration 1990;57:318–324.

96 Ratjen F, Wonne R, Posselt HG, Stover B, Hofmann D, Bender SW: A double-blind placebo controlled trial with oral ambroxol and N-acetylcysteine for mucolytic treatment in cystic fibrosis. Eur J Pediatr 1985;144:374–378.

97 Landau LI, Phelan PD: The variable effect of a bronchodilating agent on pulmonary function in cystic fibrosis. J Pediatr 1973;82:863–868.

98 Sanchez I, De Koster J, Holbrow J, Chernick V: The effect of high doses of inhaled salbutamol and ipratropium bromide in patients with stable cystic fibrosis. Chest 1993;104:842–846.

99 Lewis SM: Emptying patterns of the lung studied by multiple-breath N2 washout. J Appl Physiol 1978;44:424–430.

100 Gustafsson PM, Aurora P, Lindblad A: Evaluation of ventilation maldistribution as an early indicator of lung disease in children with cystic fibrosis. Eur Respir J 2003;22:972–979.

101 Badier M, Guillot C, Magnan A, Raynaud-Gaubert M, Thomas P, Dumon JF, Garbe L, Gaubert JY, Viard L, Metras D, et al: Lung transplantation and respiratory function tests. Functional outcome in the presence and absence of chronic rejection. Rev Mal Respir 1995;12:127–134.

102 Trachsel D, Coates AL: Long-term sequelae of neonatal lung disease; Hammer J, Eber E (eds): Paediatric Pulmonary Function Testing. Prog Respir Res. Basel, Karger, 2005, vol 33, pp 255–265.

103 Gaultier C, Boule M, Allaire Y, Clement A, Girard F: Growth of lung volumes during the first three years of life. Bull Eur Physiopathol Respir 1979;15:1103–1116.

104 Allen J, Zwerdling R, Ehrenkranz R, Gaultier C, Geggel R, Greenough A, Kleinman R, Klijanowicz A, Martinez F, Ozdemir A, Panitch HB, Nickerson B, Stein MT, Tomezsko J, Van Der Anker J: Statement on the care of the child with chronic lung disease of infancy and childhood. Am J Respir Crit Care Med 2003;168:356–396.

105 Cano A, Payo F: Lung function and airway responsiveness in children and adolescents after hyaline membrane disease: A matched cohort study. Eur Respir J 1997;10:880–885.

106 Wiebicke W, Poynter A, Chernick V: Normal lung growth following antenatal dexamethasone treatment for respiratory distress syndrome. Pediatr Pulmonol 1988;5:27–30.

107 Thompson PJ, Greenough A: Hyperinflation in premature infants at preschool age. Acta Paediatr 1992;81:307–310.

108 Malmberg LP, Mieskonen S, Pelkonen A, Kari A, Sovijarvi AR, Turpeinen M: Lung function measured by the oscillometric method in prematurely born children with chronic lung disease. Eur Respir J 2000;16:598–603.

109 Hakulinen AL, Heinonen K, Lansimies E, Kiekara O: Pulmonary function and respiratory morbidity in school-age children born prematurely and ventilated for neonatal respiratory insufficiency. Pediatr Pulmonol 1990;8:226–232.

110 Koumbourlis AC, Motoyama EK, Mutich RL, Mallory GB, Walczak SA, Fertal K: Longitudinal follow-up of lung function from childhood to adolescence in prematurely born patients with neonatal chronic lung disease. Pediatr Pulmonol 1996;21:28–34.

111 Northway WH Jr, Moss RB, Carlisle KB, Parker BR, Popp RL, Pitlick PT, Eichler I, Lamm RL, Brown BW Jr: Late pulmonary sequelae of bronchopulmonary dysplasia. N Engl J Med 1990;323:1793–1799.

112 Ijsselstijn H, Tibboel D, Hop WJ, Molenaar JC, de Jongste JC: Long-term pulmonary sequelae in children with congenital diaphragmatic hernia. Am J Respir Crit Care Med 1997;155:174–180.

113 Nusslein TG, Benzing M, Riedel F, Rieger CH: Meconium aspiration in the newborn infant – Lack of long-term pulmonary sequelae. Klin Pädiatr 1994;206:369–371.

114 Cotes JE: Lung function in disease. Lung Function. 3rd ed. Oxford, Blackwell scientific publications, 1975, pp 396–467.

115 Becker MD, Berkmen YM, Austin JH, Mun IK, Romney BM, Rozenshtein A, Jellen PA, Yip CK, Thomashow B, Ginsburg ME: Lung volumes before and after lung volume reduction surgery: Quantitative CT analysis. Am J Respir Crit Care Med 1998;157:1593–1599.

116 Lukina OF, Shiriaeva IS, Savel'ev BP, Konrad NO: Respiratory function in children with alveolitis. Pediatriia 1992;4–6:34–38.

117 Braun U, Munz E, Voigt E, Fassolt A: Lung function after thoracic trauma. A contribution to the assessment of late functional lesions. Anaesthesist 1981;30:595–601.

118 Gozal D: Pulmonary manifestations of neuromuscular disease with special reference to Duchenne muscular dystrophy and spinal muscular atrophy. Pediatr Pulmonol 2000;29:141–150.

119 Tangsrud S, Petersen IL, Lodrup Carlsen KC, Carlsen KH: Lung function in children with Duchenne's muscular dystrophy. Respir Med 2001;95:898–903.

120 Schweitzer C, Camoin-Schweitzer MC, Beltramo F, Polu E, Marchal F, Monin P: Domiciliary assisted ventilation in children. Rev Pneumol Clin 2002;58:139–144.

121 Wesseling G, Quaedvlieg FC, Wouters EF: Oscillatory mechanics of the respiratory system in neuromuscular disease. Chest 1992;102:1752–1757.

122 Remes V, Helenius I, Peltonen J, Poussa M, Sovijarvi A: Lung function in diastrophic dysplasia. Pediatr Pulmonol 2002;33:277–282.

123 Marchal F, Bouaziz N, Baeyert C, Gallina C, Duvivier C, Peslin R: Separation of airway and tissue properties by transfer respiratory impedance and thoracic gas volume in reversible airway obstruction. Eur Respir J 1996;9:253–261.

124 Cala SJ, Kenyon CM, Ferrigno G, Carnevali P, Aliverti A, Pedotti A, Macklem PT, Rochester DF: Chest wall and lung volume estimation by optical reflectance motion analysis. J Appl Physiol 1996;81:2680–2689.

125 Simon BA: Non-invasive imaging of regional lung function using x-ray computed tomography. J Clin Monit Comput 2000;16:433–442.

126 Altes TA, de Lange EE: Applications of hyperpolarized helium-3 gas magnetic resonance imaging in pediatric lung disease. Top Magn Reson Imaging 2003;14:231–236.

127 Brown RA: Derivation, application, and utility of static lung volume measurements. Respir Care Clin North Am 1997;3:183–220.

François Marchal
Laboratoire de Physiologie Faculté de Médecine
Université Henri Poincaré, Avenue de la Forêt de Haye BP 184
FR–54505 Vandoeuvre (France)
Tel. +33 383683745
Fax +33 383683739
E-Mail f.marchal@chu-nancy.fr

Hammer J, Eber E (eds): Paediatric Pulmonary Function Testing.
Prog Respir Res. Basel, Karger, 2005, vol 33, pp 118–124

Reference Equations for Ventilatory Function Measurements in Children from 6 to 16 Years

P.J.F.M. Merkus

Division of Respiratory Medicine, Department of Pediatrics, Sophia Children's Hospital, Erasmus University Medical Centre, Rotterdam, The Netherlands

Abstract

The choice of reference equations directly influences the interpretation of pediatric lung function data, and this has a significant impact on patient care and research. Secular trends exist in patients and in their reference populations, and changes take place in measurement protocols and in equipment as well. Therefore, regular updating of reference equations is needed. Furthermore, the choice of specific reference equations will depend on the ethnic group, gender and age distribution. The reference population should resemble the native general population as much as possible. Formal quality control of reference equations is desired but does not exist. Researchers and pediatricians should – preferably on a national level – collectively decide which reference equations to use. Various statistical issues may play a role here, and these are briefly discussed. There is no sound reason to use percent of predicted when expressing lung function parameters, and standardized deviation scores (SDS or Z scores) can (and should) be used for expressing all lung function parameters. Extrapolation or use of reference equations of poor quality may lead to an erroneous interpretation.

Introduction

Measuring lung function parameters remains an important tool in optimizing health of and care for patients. But even the most sophisticated lung function technique is of limited value when we are not informed about normative values. Lots of energy and time are devoted to developing techniques and measuring function, but the choice of reference values is often not evaluated critically. That this can lead to erroneous conclusions is illustrated in this chapter. There is an impressive number of publications devoted to reference values for lung function indices for children. A Medline search for 'healthy children – reference values – lung function' produced 251 publications, of which the large majority was published after the 1989 *European Respiratory Journal* supplement on reference values for children [1]. However, the quality of these reference equations may differ considerably.

The aim of this chapter is not to come up with recommendations for appropriate, specific reference equations, because the suitability of reference equations depends on too many factors, such as country, ethnic group, and birth cohort. The aim of this chapter is to discuss the relevant aspects of reference equations, and to provide the physician and researcher with tools and tricks to be able to make the right decisions in choosing specific reference equations that are the most appropriate for his/her population.

Why Do We Need Reference Equations?

For a meaningful interpretation of lung function indices we need reference equations for several reasons:

1. To express pulmonary function in relation to that which would be expected for healthy individuals of a similar

age, gender, body size and ethnic group. This applies for single and repeated measurements.

2. To characterize and monitor disease severity. Especially for this purpose, longitudinal comparisons with the reference population are required. Most of the reference equations are cross-sectionally obtained, while cohort effects may play a role. In that case, the analyses are complicated. Ideally, updated reference equations, or longitudinally obtained reference equations should be available.

3. To expand knowledge regarding growth and development. Lung function measurements are by far the most convenient and least invasive tools to study growth and development of lungs and airways longitudinally, albeit indirectly.

4. To study mechanisms of normal and abnormal function. There is still a lot unknown about the structure-function relationship of the airways.

5. To investigate the natural history and sequelae of diseases (similarly to studying normal growth and development).

6. To avoid the use of (false) ratios. In clinical care, physicians appreciate simple, one-dimensional data when describing functional characteristics. The interpretation of ratios is difficult because some information is masked, and the ratio may be based on assumptions that are not valid. An example is FEV_1/FVC as a measure of airway obstruction that is more or less constant in healthy children and adolescents. A pitfall in using this index is the case in which both FEV_1 and FVC are affected by disease, resulting in spurious normal results.

Requirements for a Normal Population and Suitability of Reference Equations

The definition of a 'normal reference population' for pediatric reference equations was first formulated by Taussig et al. [2]. Inclusion criteria were: no present acute or past or present chronic condition of the upper and lower respiratory tract, no major respiratory disease, no major systemic disease which directly or indirectly influences the respiratory tract, no more than incidental antenatal or postnatal smoking exposure, and appropriate growth pattern for gestational age and postnatal age.

Obviously, a reference population should be a representative sample of the general population, and not an ideal population, because this will limit the external validity of the equations. Furthermore, the definition of normal will vary with time, and new reference equations may therefore

be needed because of factors such as changing prevalence of obesity and passive smoking. When choosing reference equations one should compare and verify the following: the type of populations should be comparable, the same technique [e.g. airway resistance (R_{aw}) vs. respiratory system resistance (R_{rs})] should be used, the same protocol and equipment should be used, the same degree of accuracy and precision should be employed, and furthermore, the statistical analyses should be based on valid and biologically meaningful assumptions (see below), and values should not be extrapolated (predicted values should not be calculated outside the range of the reference population).

Limitations of Reference Equations and Interpretation of Lung Function

The validity of reference equations depends on statistical factors and on the choice and characteristics of the reference population (see below). Interpretation of lung function indices may go wrong when reference equations are not valid, out of date, or extrapolated. Possible consequences are that pathology is overlooked, or a value is misclassified as being (ab)normal. For longitudinal measurements, the validity of reference equations is crucial: The rate of decline of lung function or growth of the lung may be over- or underestimated simply because of the choice of reference equations (fig. 1) [3–7].

The Independent Variable(s)

Standing Height
As development of lung function is somehow proportional to the needs and size of the body, most studies use height as independent variable, and sometimes in addition variables such as weight and age. The addition of weight usually does not add much to the quality of the statistical fit, but may reduce the variance of the residuals. One could speculate that with changing body proportions in the western world (resulting in taller and relatively heavier children and adolescents), the relative contributions of height and weight may change, and that the effect of weight will become more visible. Future lung function studies should address this issue.

Age
The addition of age as second independent variable is especially required to optimize reference equations during the pubertal growth spurt. That including age improves the

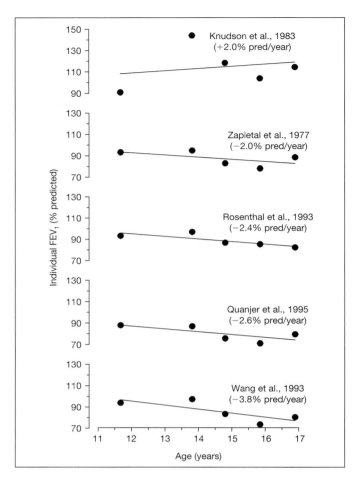

Fig. 1. Illustration of the effect of different reference equations on the estimated annual change of FEV_1 in a male adolescent with cystic fibrosis [modified from 7]. These reference equations are listed in [7].

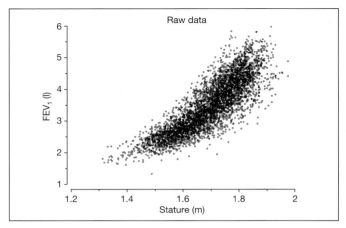

Fig. 2. Raw data of FEV_1 in 4,200 boys. Curvilinear relationship and heteroscedasticity between FEV_1 and stature.

quality of reference equations has been clearly demonstrated [6–9]. Ideally, one would like to incorporate the pubertal stage because of the considerable difference in the timing of the growth spurt but this has been proven highly unpractical [10]. Because in the western world puberty starts at an increasingly younger age [11], and final height increases as well [12, 13], regular updating of reference equations seems warranted.

Genetic Factors (Gender and Ethnic Group)

For the majority of lung function indices differences have been demonstrated that depend on ethnic group and gender. Therefore, most authors constructed gender-specific reference equations. In studies with relatively small numbers this distinction is not always made because the gender-related difference is not statistically significant due to the small

sample size. Numerous specific reference equations relating to ethnicity have been and will be published because it is obvious that these differ considerably [14, 15].

Alternative Measures of Body Size

A special category of patients are those in whom the measurement of length is not feasible, or highly demanding for the subjects. Examples are the children with progressive scoliosis and/or neuromuscular disease. Especially for these subgroups, separate reference equations have been published that are based on sitting height or arm span [16–19] or arm and ulna length [20, 21].

Statistical Issues of Reference Equations

When considering the use of specific reference equations, a critical evaluation of the statistical model is required. Preferably, the raw data are presented graphically in the original publication, to enable the reader to inspect the distribution, and to study the linearity and the distribution of the data, to look at outliers, and to consider the need for (log) transformation. The statistics should include an analysis of the added value of including more independent variables (often adding age next to height) and of interaction terms (fig. 2–4).

Homoscedasticity and Heteroscedasticity

For linear regression to be a valid means to describe reference data, the variability of the data should exhibit a more or less constant pattern around the mean regression line, i.e. should have homoscedasticity (fig. 2). If the

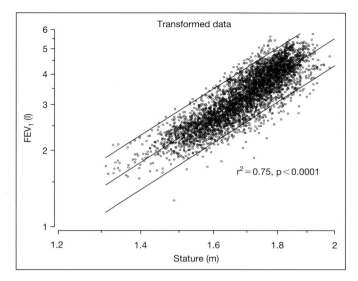

Fig. 3. Same data as in figure 2 after log-log transformation. Note homoscedasticity and close to linear relationship between FEV$_1$ and stature.

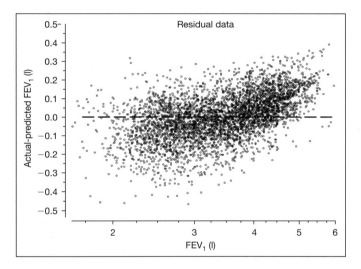

Fig. 4. Analysis of the residuals following linear regression (log-log model): trend towards overestimation of FEV$_1$ at both extremes and towards underestimation in the center of the measurement range (suboptimal model, requiring incorporation of other variables, e.g. age).

distribution of the residuals does not demonstrate a homoscedastic pattern, transformation is needed (fig. 3).

To proof that a model describes the reference data correctly, one should look for any possible (curvi)linear trend within the residuals (defined as the measured values − predicted values). If a symmetric and even distribution of the residuals around zero is lacking, more complex models are needed (fig. 4).

The use of a correlation coefficient as proof that the model is adequate is incorrect, as it largely depends on the range of the independent variable studied. So, the validity of reference equations may differ, and the estimated level and change of lung function over time in a particular patient depend on the choice of reference equations.

Secular Trends

Secular trends for lung function have been described in children and adults [3–5]. These are probably explained by changes in the age-height relationship [11–13], progressive earlier start of puberty in the younger cohorts, but also due to higher standards of living, improved vaccination status, and fewer airway infections in early childhood. In addition, secular trends in reference equations can also occur due to alterations in equipment and protocol. Hence, there are numerous reasons why reference equations may become out of date. Another example why cross-sectional reference equations may be unsuitable to study longitudinal changes within subjects is a lack of tracking. There is dispute as to whether tracking occurs during puberty [22, 23].

Expression of Lung Function Indices, Definitions of Abnormal

Disadvantages of Using Percent of Predicted

There is a strong – but irrational – tradition to use percent, or percent of predicted, in describing lung function parameters in relation to their reference population. This approach is only valid when the distribution, or biological variability, in the general population is proportional to the mean value. However, this is often not the case, certainly not in adults. For instance, the biological variability of volumes is more or less constant in absolute numbers across the height range. This means that a small subject may demonstrate a variability that is relatively large (in %) for his/her size. This results in difficulties in the interpretation. Furthermore, the variability of lung function indices in percent differs according to the parameter studied. For instance, a result of e.g. 70% of predicted may be well within the normal range for one lung function parameter, and way outside the normal range for another. Hence, the use of percent of predicted does not tell us if, and by how much, a lung function result is abnormal, because it is not related to the variability that is observed in the general population.

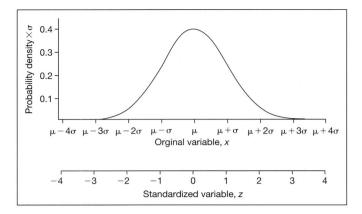

Fig. 5. The normal distribution described in original variables and in standardized variables.

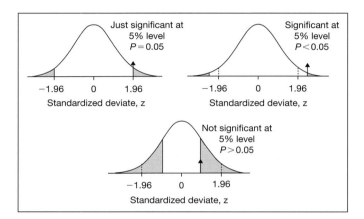

Fig. 6. The deviation from zero can be described in standardized deviation scores (or Z scores). This deviation is unusual at a population level when more than 1.96 standardized deviations away from zero (belonging to the upper or lower 2.5 percentiles).

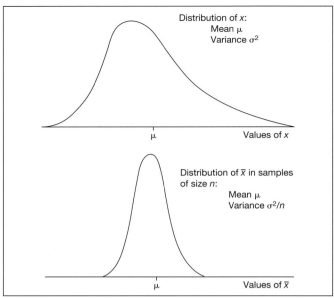

Fig. 7. When values are not normally distributed, (log) transformation is needed (e.g. FE_{NO}, PD_{20}).

1. Z scores indicate how likely a result is to occur within a 'normal population', and how far removed the result is from that predicted, having taken the natural variability of that parameter into account.
2. Z scores are useful for tracking changes in lung function with growth or treatment.
3. As Z scores are dimensionless (have no units), it is possible to compare various lung function results obtained with different techniques, e.g. to compare a resistance measure with an expiratory flow measure.

In general statistical terms, unusual values are found at both extremes of the spectrum of the data. Since most lung function data are normally distributed or transformed to a normal distribution, 90% of the normal values are found within the range -1.65 and $+1.65$ SD, and 95% of the normal values are found within the range -1.96 and $+1.96$ SD.

So, outside this range 'abnormal' or 'unusual' values are found. In general, and especially in pediatrics, lung function variables of healthy subjects and patients with respiratory symptoms and/or disease overlap to such an extent that a normal lung function parameter does not exclude disease. On the other hand, lung function parameters that are clearly abnormal will often – but not by definition – be associated with symptoms and disease.

Advantages of Using Z Scores

Z scores – or standardized deviation scores (SDS) – are defined as:

Z = (observed value − predicted value)/RSD, where RSD is the residual standard deviation in the reference population. Z scores from a healthy population are by definition normally distributed with a mean of 0 and an RSD of 1. Hence, the Z score indicates how many standardized deviations (SDs) an individual or group is below or above predicted for any given parameter (fig. 5, 6). Often, the raw data need to be log transformed to obtain a normal distribution, before Z scores can be calculated (fig. 7). Important advantages of Z scores are:

Requirements of Methods, Equipment and Protocols

Standardization of measurement protocols and equipment are of paramount importance when choosing the appropriate reference equations [24]. Subtle differences between populations may be explained by differences in the protocols (e.g. using inspiratory interruptions vs. expiratory interruptions for measurements of interrupter resistance, R_{int}). International ERS/ATS guidelines for measurement protocols for (pediatric) lung function testing exist [1, 25–28], but not for all techniques, and there are good arguments to reconsider some aspects of these guidelines, since they are not optimally designed for children [29]. For specific measurement protocols the reader is referred to the specific chapters in this book.

What to Do When Reference Equations Are Lacking?

For statistical reasons, the reliability of reference equations is best at the mean value of the independent variable; reliability is the least at both extremes of the independent variable range. Therefore, extrapolation is not advised since it may lead to wrong interpretations. Preferably, one should obtain reference equations for the age/height range studied. Often this is not possible or feasible. In those cases, only short-term interventions or changes can be studied within subjects, using absolute values; long-term studies will be hard to evaluate in the absence of reliable reference equations. The individual is often his/her own best reference when assessing change. In short-term (crossover) studies with minimal changes in height and weight, we can express a change in lung function as a relative or absolute change of baseline values. The clinical relevance of such changes can only be interpreted if within- and between-occasion repeatability is known.

Checklist for Choosing One's Own Reference Equations

The recommended procedure to choose appropriate reference equations [1] is the following:

1. Select a study in which the same technique and the same protocol were used, preferably according to the most recent guidelines.
2. Examine the characteristics of the population that was used to obtain the 'normal data': was it a sample from the general population, or from an ideal population? Is it comparable to the population (ethnicity, birth cohort, general health, distribution of age and gender) to be studied?
3. Are the numbers sufficient (>100 children per 10 cm height difference), are the height and age range appropriate (large ranges, e.g. 6–18 years), are the statistics transparent, and are raw data provided (graphically)? Are the residuals evenly distributed around zero?
4. Study a representative group of healthy native children and assess whether systematic differences exist between the native population and the predicted values of the chosen reference equations. If systematic – but constant – differences exist, consider: generating your own reference values, and calculating predicted values from those (disadvantage: less interstudy and international comparability) and proceeding to other reference equations.

It is of practical importance to agree on the choice of reference equations on a national level, and to aim for regular updated reference values for that specific population. Obtaining reference data, and choosing and updating reference equations may not be the most exciting aspect of pediatric pulmonology, and requires a significant investment. However, since evaluation of medical treatment and study results heavily depend on reference equations, we cannot afford to neglect this aspect.

References

1 Quanjer PH, Stocks J, Polgar G, Wise M, Karlberg J, Borsboom G: Compilation of reference values for lung function measurements in children. Eur Respir J Suppl 1989;4: 184S–261S.

2 Taussig LM, Chernick V, Wood R, Farrell P, Mellins RB: Standardization of lung function testing in children. Proceedings and Recommendations of the GAP Conference Committee, Cystic Fibrosis Foundation. J Pediatr 1980;97:668–676.

3 Glindmeyer HW, Diem JE, Jones RN, Weill H: Noncomparability of longitudinally and cross-sectionally determined annual change in spirometry. Am Rev Respir Dis 1982;125: 544–548.

4 van Pelt W, Borsboom GJ, Rijcken B, Schouten JP, van Zomeren BC, Quanjer PH: Discrepancies between longitudinal and cross-sectional change in ventilatory function in 12 years of follow-up. Am J Respir Crit Care Med 1994;149:1218–1226.

5 Pattishall EN, Helms RW, Strope GL: Noncomparability of cross-sectional and longitudinal estimates of lung growth in children. Pediatr Pulmonol 1989;7/1:22–28.

6 Rosenfeld M, Pepe MS, Longton G, Emerson J, FitzSimmons S, Morgan W: Effect of choice of reference equation on analysis of pulmonary function in cystic fibrosis patients. Pediatr Pulmonol 2001;31/3:227–237.

7 Merkus PJ, Tiddens HA, de Jongste JC: Annual lung function changes in young patients with chronic lung disease. Eur Respir J 2002;19: 886–891.

8 Nysom K, Ulrik CS, Hesse B, Dirksen A: Published models and local data can bridge the gap between reference values of lung function for children and adults. Eur Respir J 1997;10:1591–1598.

9 Sherrill DL, Lebowitz MD, Knudson RJ, Burrows B: Continuous longitudinal regression equations for pulmonary function measures. Eur Respir J 1992;5:452–462.

10 Rosenthal M, Bain SH, Cramer D, Helms P, Denison D, Bush A, Warner JO: Lung function in white children aged 4 to 19 years. I. Spirometry. Thorax 1993;48:794–802.

11 de Muinck Keizer SM, Mul D: Trends in pubertal development in Europe. Hum Reprod Update 2001;7:287–291.

12 Freedman DS, Khan LK, Serdula MK, Srinivasan SR, Berenson GS: Secular trends in height among children during 2 decades: The Bogalusa Heart Study. Arch Pediatr Adolesc Med 2000;154:155–161.

13 Fredriks AM, Van Buuren S, Burgmeijer RJF, Meulmeester JF, Beuker RJ, Brugman E, Roede MJ, Verloove-Vanhorick SP, Wit JM: Continuing positive secular growth change in the Netherlands 1955–1997. Pediatr Res 2000; 47:316–323.

14 Hellmann S, Goren AI: The necessity of building population specific prediction equations for clinical assessment of pulmonary function tests. Eur J Pediatr 1999;158:519–522.

15 Greenough A, Hird MF, Everett L, Price JF: Importance of using lung function regression equations appropriate for ethnic origin. Pediatr Pulmonol 1991;11:207–211.

16 Kivastik J, Kingisepp PH: Lung function in Estonian children: Effect of sitting height. Clin Physiol 1995;15:287–296.

17 Hibbert ME, Lanigan A, Raven J, Phelan PD: Relation of armspan to height and the prediction of lung function. Thorax 1988;43: 657–659.

18 Parker JM, Dillard TA, Phillips YY: Arm span-height relationships in patients referred for spirometry. Am J Respir Crit Care Med 1996;154:533–536.

19 Torres LA, Martinez FE, Manco JC: Correlation between standing height, sitting height, and arm span as an index of pulmonary function in 6–10-year-old children. Pediatr Pulmonol 2003;36:202–208.

20 Gauld LM, Kappers J, Carlin JB, Robertson CF: Prediction of childhood pulmonary function using ulna length. Am J Respir Crit Care Med 2003;168:804–809.

21 Jarzem PF, Gledhill RB: Predicting height from arm measurements. J Pediatr Orthop 1993;13:761–765.

22 Hibbert ME, Hudson IL, Lanigan A, Landau LI, Phelan PD: Tracking of lung function in healthy children and adolescents. Pediatr Pulmonol 1990;8:172–177.

23 Borsboom GJ, van Pelt W, Quanjer PH: Interindividual variation in pubertal growth patterns of ventilatory function, standing height, and weight. Am J Respir Crit Care Med 1996;153:1182–1186.

24 Hulskamp G, Hoo AF, Ljungberg H, Lum S, Pillow JJ, Stocks J: Progressive decline in plethysmographic lung volumes in infants: Physiology or technology? Am J Respir Crit Care Med 2003;168:1003–1009.

25 Clausen JL, Coates AL, Quanjer PH: Measurement of lung volumes in humans: Review and recommendations from an ATS/ERS workshop. Eur Respir J 1997;10: 1205–1206.

26 Quanjer PH, Sly PD, Stocks J: Uniform symbols, abbreviations, and units in pediatric pulmonary function testing. Pediatr Pulmonol 1997;24:2–11.

27 Quanjer PH, Tammeling GJ, Cotes JE, Pedersen OF, Peslin R, Yernault JC: Lung volumes and forced ventilatory flows. Report Working Party standardization of Lung Function Tests, European Community for Steel and Coal. Official Statement of the European Respiratory Society. Eur Respir J Suppl 1993;16:5–40.

28 Stocks J, Quanjer PH: Reference values for residual volume, functional residual capacity and total lung capacity. ATS Workshop on Lung Volume Measurements. Official Statement of the European Respiratory Society. Eur Respir J 1995;8:492–506.

29 Arets HG, Brackel HJ, van der Ent CK: Forced expiratory manoeuvres in children: Do they meet ATS and ERS criteria for spirometry? Eur Respir J 2001;18:655–660.

Peter J.F.M. Merkus, MD, PhD
Division of Respiratory Medicine
Department of Pediatrics
Sophia Children's Hospital
Erasmus University Medical Center
Rotterdam, PO Box 2060
NL–3000 CB Rotterdam (The Netherlands)
Tel. +31 10 4636295
Fax +31 10 4636772
E-Mail p.j.f.m.merkus@erasmusmc.nl

Hammer J, Eber E (eds): Paediatric Pulmonary Function Testing.
Prog Respir Res. Basel, Karger, 2005, vol 33, pp 125–136

Measurement of Bronchial Responsiveness in Children

Jürg Barben[a]   Josef Riedler[b]

[a]Paediatric Pulmonology and Allergology, Children's Hospital, St. Gallen, Switzerland;
[b]Paediatric Pulmonology and Allergology, Children's Hospital, Salzburg, Austria

Abstract

Bronchial hyperresponsiveness (BHR) is considered to be a complex system of various interactions between airway inflammation, airway smooth muscle function, and airway mechanics. Because BHR is still considered to be a key feature of asthma, measures of BHR are widely used for diagnosis and monitoring of asthma in clinical practice and for research. Bronchial provocation tests (BPT) provide additional and useful information, which is not always picked up by non-invasive markers of airway inflammation. Direct airway challenge tests (e.g. methacholine, histamine) cause airway narrowing by acting 'directly' on their respective receptors on bronchial smooth muscles. Indirect challenge tests (e.g. exercise, hypertonic saline, cold air, mannitol, adenosine monophosphate) induce airflow limitation by an action on cells other than smooth muscle cells, with a variety of cells, mediators and receptors being involved in this process. Due to the closer association with inflammation, indirect challenges seem to be more specific for current clinically relevant asthma, and changes in BHR after treatment with inhaled steroids are observed within days to weeks. While there are standardized protocols for BPT in adults and older children, BPT in preschool children and infants are still in the research domain.

Introduction

Bronchial hyperresponsiveness (BHR) is considered to be a characteristic pathophysiological feature of asthma in adults [1] and in children [2]. It is defined as an abnormal bronchoconstrictor response of the airways to a wide variety of specific and non-specific stimuli resulting in increased airflow limitation [3]. In addition, BHR in children is significantly determined by lung mechanics, and in particular smooth muscle mechanics (e.g. response to deep inhalation) [4]. BHR should be considered as a complex system of various interactions between airway inflammation, airway smooth muscle function, and airway mechanics [5, 6].

BHR may have a genetic background or be acquired as a result of acute (neonatal hyaline membrane disease or viral) or chronic (atopic or infective) inflammation of the airways with structural consequences [7]. The degree of BHR in asthma is usually higher than in other situations including children with very low birth weight [8] or bronchopulmonary dysplasia [9], cystic fibrosis [10], viral diseases [11], allergic rhinitis [12], tobacco smoking [13] or exposure to smoking [14] (fig. 1). However, BHR is only one element of asthma and it cannot be used as a synonym for asthma [15] (fig. 2). While the association between BHR and adult asthma is quite strong, it is less clear in children. Not all children with episodic wheeze have an increased bronchial response, and some children without any respiratory symptoms show BHR [16]. Although BHR is not specific for asthma in general, most patients with moderate to severe asthma have an increased airway responsiveness, which is more marked during symptomatic episodes [17] (fig. 3). The degree of BHR is more related to the severity of asthma than spirometry, and it often predicts the response to inhaled corticosteroids in adult

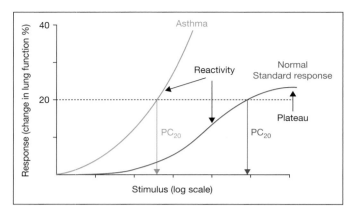

Fig. 1. Bronchial responsiveness: the concept from Beardsmore and Silverman [7].

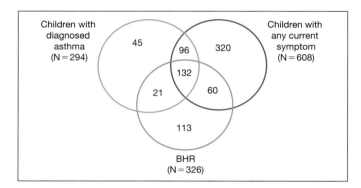

Fig. 2. BHR in 7- to 10-year-old New Zealand children with diagnosed asthma and with any current symptom (n = 2,053) [modified from 15].

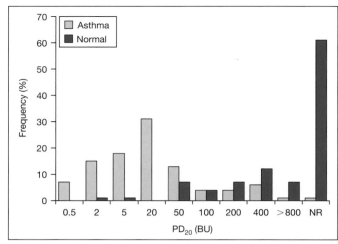

Fig. 3. Percent of normal and asthmatic children responding to methacholine challenge [modified from 17]. NR = No reaction; BU = breath units (1 BU of methacholine is equal to one inhalation of 1 mg/ml of methacholine).

carbachol), histamine, prostaglandin D_2, and leukotrienes $C_4/D_4/E_4$. These substances cause airflow limitation predominately via a direct effect on airway smooth muscles. Pharmacological challenges using methacholine and histamine are widely used and well standardized for adults and older children [1, 20]. For infants and toddlers, however, they are still in the research domain. A change of forced expiratory volume in 1 s (FEV_1) is the primary outcome measure whereby spirometry should meet American Thoracic Society (ATS) guidelines [22, for details and the limitations of the recommended criteria see 23]. For small children and infants, different techniques such as the rapid thoracic compression [24] or raised volume forced expiration technique [25], the measurement of transcutaneous oxygen tension [26, 27], the single breath occlusion method [28], an impedance technique [29], or whole body plethysmography [30] have been used to assess BHR; however, these are all not standardized.

Direct airway challenges depend much more on the inherent sensitivity of the airway smooth muscle to the respective agent than on the presence of airway inflammation, which is however a key feature of asthma. Because of this substantial limitation, the clinical utility of current direct airway challenges has been increasingly questioned.

Methacholine Challenge Test
Challenge tests using methacholine are well established and widely used bronchial provocation tests (BPT) [31]. Guidelines for methacholine challenge test (MCT) have

patients with asthma [18]. In epidemiological studies, BHR has a relatively poor sensitivity and specificity for wheeze, and changes in the degree of BHR do not correlate well with changes in the clinical expression of asthma over time [15, 19]. In addition, a lot of factors can temporarily increase and decrease BHR (tables 1, 2).

Different standardized protocols have been developed for bronchial challenges in adults and in children [1, 20, 21]. However, there are no standardized protocols for preschool children and infants. The indications for such challenges are summarized in table 3 and contraindications in table 4.

Direct Airway Challenge Tests

Direct airway challenge tests use pharmacological agents such as cholinergic agonists (methacholine, acetylcholine,

Table 1. Factors that increase bronchial responsiveness [modified from 20]

Factor	Duration of effect
Exposure to environmental antigens	1–3 weeks
Viral respiratory infection	3–6 weeks
Chemical irritants	days to months
Occupational sensitizers	months
Cigarette smoke	uncertain[a]

[a]Studies of the acute effects of smoking on BHR and methacholine challenge testing are not consistent. There is some evidence of a brief acute effect that can be avoided by asking subjects to refrain from smoking for a few hours before testing.

Table 2. Factors that decrease bronchial responsiveness [modified from 20]

Factor	Minimum time interval between last dose and study
Medications	
Short-acting β_2-agonists	8 h
Long-acting β_2-agonists	48 h
Ipratropium bromide	24 h
Liquid theophylline	12 h
Slow release theophylline	48 h
Cromolyn sodium	8 h
Nedocromil sodium	48 h
Antihistamines	72 h
Leukotriene antagonists	24 h
Foods	
Cola drinks, chocolate, tea, coffee	day of the study

Oral or inhaled corticosteroids are not routinely withheld before BHR testing but their anti-inflammatory effect may decrease BHR. Inhaled corticosteroids may need to be withheld depending on the question being asked.

Table 3. Indications for BPT in children

To rule out or confirm a diagnosis of asthma
To assess severity of asthma
To assess the effect of treatment
To monitor asthma
To determine and compare the duration of action of drugs
To help understand mechanisms of different airway diseases
To determine the prevalence of asthma in epidemiological surveys

Table 4. Contraindications for BPT in children [modified from 20]

Absolute
  Severe airflow limitation (FEV_1 <50% predicted or <1.0 litre)
  Uncontrolled hypertension
  Known aortic aneurysm
  Unstable cardiac ischaemia or malignant arrhythmias
Relative
  Moderate airflow limitation (FEV_1 <60% predicted or <1.5 litres)
  Inability to perform acceptable quality spirometry
  Acute viral infection of the upper and lower airways
  Current use of anti-asthmatic medications (see table 2)
  Current use of cholinesterase inhibitor medication (for myasthenia gravis)

recently been published by the ATS [20]. Responsiveness to methacholine is often measured in patients with a suspected diagnosis of asthma, especially if spirometry and bronchodilator response have been inconclusive. However, hyperresponsiveness to methacholine is not specific for asthma, since children with other chronic pulmonary diseases as well as children without any airway problem may show similar responses (fig. 3) [15, 17, 32]. An MCT is more useful in excluding asthma because its negative predictive value is greater than its positive predictive power. However, in schoolchildren with a history of breathlessness during or after exercise the diagnosis of exercise-induced asthma (EIA) cannot be excluded by a negative response to methacholine, and EIA cannot be established by the use of a direct airway challenge [20].

Equipment and Protocol
Methacholine (acetyl-β-methylcholine chloride) is available as dry crystalline powder (Provocholine®) as well as prepackaged, sealed vials. Sterile normal saline (0.9% sodium chloride) is used as the diluent of choice. Methacholine solution, mixed by a pharmacist or a well-trained person using a sterile technique, should be stored in a refrigerator at about 4°C which keeps it stable for 3 months. Since solution temperature affects nebulizer output, solutions should be warmed to room temperature approximately 30 min before use. Any unused methacholine solution remaining in a nebulizer should be discarded.

Many different dosing protocols have been used and each has advantages and disadvantages. There are two widely used techniques for administering methacholine: one of these methods, first described for histamine by Cockcroft et al. [33], involves tidal breathing of aerosol that is generated continuously by a nebulizer. The aerosol is delivered directly into a mouthpiece or a face mask, and little cooperation is required. The second method involves intermittent generation of aerosol by a nebulizer with a mouthpiece connected to a dosimeter that makes it possible to generate aerosol for a specified time interval. This method was first standardized by Chai et al. [34] in 1975 and later modified by Rosenthal [35]. The two proposed techniques appear to give similar results in both children and adults. Details about the protocols and the equipment needed have recently been published and are briefly outlined below [20]:

Two-Minute Tidal Breathing Protocol. After preparing 10 doubling concentrations of methacholine (from 0.03 to 16 mg/ml) 3 ml of each concentration is inhaled for 2 min via nebulizer. The nebulizer should produce an aerosol with a particle mass median diameter between 1.0 and 3.6 μm using compressed air; an exhalation filter is optional. The nebulizer is held upright and a mouthpiece with nose clip or a face mask is used. FEV_1 is measured in duplicate before the challenge as baseline, preferably after inhalation of the diluent (normal saline) and target FEV_1 that indicates a 20% fall in FEV_1 (baseline $FEV_1 \times 0.8$) is calculated. Thirty and 90 s after each challenge step, FEV_1 is measured and the highest FEV_1 from acceptable manoeuvres [22] is recorded. This should not take longer than 3 min to prevent wearing off the effect of methacholine. If FEV_1 falls by 20% or more, or the highest concentration is given, the challenge is terminated. Signs and symptoms are noted, inhaled salbutamol administered, and spirometry is repeated after 10 min. The 2-min tidal breathing protocol may be shortened by adjusting the starting concentration. However, small children with asthma symptoms are more likely than adults to have severe airway hyperresponsiveness, and more caution in increasing the concentration at each step is warranted. This increased sensitivity in children may reflect an increased dose per unit weight [36] but could also be partly explained by the dilution of nebulized aerosols by air entrainment which occurs when inspiratory flow exceeds nebulizer flow. This can cause an up to 5-fold dilution in inspired aerosol concentration in older children and adolescents as compared to infants [37].

Five-Breath Dosimeter Protocol. After preparing five concentrations of methacholine (e.g. 0.0625, 0.25, 1, 4, and 16 mg/ml), 2 ml of each concentration is inhaled via nebulizer. For research protocols, doubling concentrations are widely recommended because they give a more precise PC_{20} (provocative concentration causing a 20% fall in FEV_1) values. At end exhalation during tidal breathing, the subject inhales slowly and deeply from the nebulizer. The dosimeter is triggered (manually or automatically) soon after the inhalation begins, and the subject is encouraged to

Table 5. Assessment of bronchial responsiveness using the methacholine test [from 20]

PC_{20} mg/ml	Interpretation[a]
>16	normal bronchial responsiveness
4.0–16	borderline BHR
1.0–4.0	mild BHR (positive test)
<1.0	moderate to severe BHR

[a] Under condition that (1) baseline airway obstruction is absent, (2) spirometry quality is good and (3) there is substantial postchallenge FEV_1 recovery.

continue inhaling slowly and to hold the breath for another 5 s. This step is repeated for a total of five inspiratory capacity inhalations which should not take more than 2 min. The challenge is terminated when the FEV_1 falls by 20% or more, or the highest concentration is given (see above).

The results of an MCT are reported as percent decrease of FEV_1 from baseline, and PC_{20} is calculated. If FEV_1 does not fall by at least 20% after the highest concentration, then PC_{20} should be reported as >16 mg/ml. A general scheme for categorizing airway responsiveness using PC_{20} is given in table 5. In many studies, a PC_{20} <8 mg/ml is taken as a positive result for the diagnosis of BHR [20].

Histamine Challenge Test

Histamine is one of the major inflammatory mediators involved in asthma, producing airway obstruction by direct smooth muscle contraction. The protocols used for histamine challenge test are identical to those for MCT, and were described in detail for adults by Sterk et al. [1].

The Yan method [38] is frequently used for epidemiological surveys because it is a simple and rapid method for measuring BHR to inhaled histamine. It is a hand-operated method, delivering aerosols during inspiration only. Aerosols are generated by five calibrated DeVilbiss 40 glass, handheld bulb nebulizers. Saline and histamine in concentrations of 3.15, 6.25, 25 and 50 mg/ml are placed in the nebulizers. After assessment of baseline FEV_1, the saline nebulizer is placed between the teeth and the subject exhales to a maximum. At the beginning of an inspiratory capacity manoeuvre, the operator gives the nebulizer bulb one firm squeeze. The breath is held at maximum inspiration for at least 3 s, whereafter the subject exhales outside the nebulizer. This is repeated twice for saline but the number of breaths for each concentration of histamine varies according to the dose being administered, which ranges from 0.03 to 7.8 µmol histamine-di-phosphate, or greater if needed. FEV_1 is measured 60 s after each dose and the test is stopped when the FEV_1 has fallen by 20% or more from baseline (postsaline). Results are expressed as PD_{20} (cumulative dose causing a 20% fall in FEV_1). In contrast to methacholine, histamine is currently less commonly used because it is associated with more systemic side effects [31]. In addition, BHR measurements may be less reproducible when using histamine [39, 40]. Similar to the low specificity of the MCT for a diagnosis of asthma, histamine challenges have failed to identify current asthma as opposed to 'outgrown' or past asthma. In an Austrian study, 114 of 128 children with asthma met the criteria of hyper-responsiveness to histamine even though they had been free of symptoms for 18 months and medication free for 12 months. In contrast, only 52 of these 128 subjects were hyperresponsive to a cold air challenge [41].

Indirect Airway Challenge Tests

Indirect airway challenge tests include challenges with physical stimuli such as exercise, non-isotonic aerosols [hypertonic saline (HS), distilled water, mannitol], and cold dry air, and with pharmacological agents like adenosine monophosphate [42], sodium metabisulfite [43], tachykinin [44], and bradykinin [45]. These stimuli cause airway narrowing 'indirectly' by changing airway osmolarity due to altering fluid and salt homeostasis in the airways and releasing a variety of mediators from inflammatory cells, epithelial cells and nerves [3, 21, 46]. Due to the closer association with inflammation, indirect challenges seem to be more specific for current clinically relevant asthma, and changes in BHR are observed earlier after treatment with inhaled steroids than in direct airway challenges [45, 47, 48]. Late responses after indirect challenges are rare [49].

Exercise Testing

Exercise-induced bronchoconstriction (or EIA) occurs frequently in children with asthma during normal physical activities. Thus, the question 'When you run around, do you become wheezy and tight in the chest' is often asked by paediatricians to make the diagnosis of asthma in a clinical setting [7]. The close relation between exercise and airway narrowing in the majority of children with asthma has been used as a diagnostic tool for years, especially when the diagnosis of asthma is uncertain [50]. Hyperventilation resulting in increased airway osmolarity of the airway surface liquid is believed to be the exercise stimulus for bronchoconstriction [46]. The change of FEV_1 from baseline gives an index or degree of BHR, which reflects the severity of EIA.

Exercise provokes an asthma attack in 60–80% of the children with clinically recognized asthma [32, 51, 52]. Testing for EIA is not very sensitive, but highly specific for the diagnosis of asthma in children compared to direct airway challenge tests [20, 32, 42, 45, 53, 54]. A positive response to exercise identifies a child as having asthma, whereas a negative response does not rule out asthma. There is a wide range in sensitivity of exercise challenges to identify a child with asthma because of the differences in standardization of the exercise tests [53]. This is particularly important for field studies on asthma and BHR [55–58]. Some of these studies did not assess the workload or intensity of exercise throughout the challenge, and others did not take into account the humidity and temperature of the inspired air [46]. For example, the sensitivity of a free-running test developed by Haby et al. [57] to identify children with asthma was 52%. A similar test used by Williams et al. [58] had a sensitivity of only 30%, which is explained by the fact that temperature and air humidity were not measured, peak expiratory flow rate instead of FEV_1 was used, and the anti-asthma medication was not withheld from the children before exercise.

Most children with well-controlled asthma do not need medication before exercise [59]. Therefore EIA is often used as a marker of airway inflammation [60], and exercise testing is the preferred method to study the effectiveness and optimal dosage of new drugs and their protective effect against EIA [61–64], and to evaluate the long-term effects of preventive anti-inflammatory therapy [59, 65]. Exercise testing is also widely used in epidemiological surveys of asthma in children [55, 57, 66]. Further, exercise challenge tests are performed to investigate endurance of children with chronic obstructive disease (e.g. cystic fibrosis), to evaluate the fitness of a child, and occasionally to demonstrate to parents that obese children are able to perform sporting activities without getting at risk.

Equipment and Protocol

Exercise testing is usually done on a bicycle ergometer, on a treadmill, or as a free-running test. Free running is considered to be the most asthma-inducing exercise; however, exercise by cycling or running on a treadmill can be better standardized [20, 50, 67]. In contrast to laboratory studies using treadmills or bicycle ergometers, field workers mostly use free-running exercise tests for epidemiological surveys as they are easy to perform and do not have the disadvantage of needing sophisticated equipment [55, 57].

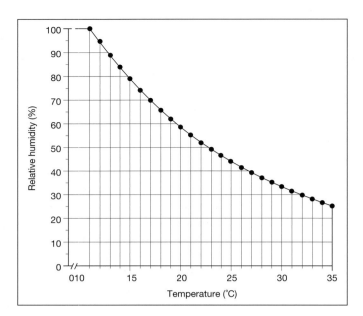

Fig. 4. Relationship between ambient temperature and relative humidity at an absolute water content of 10 mg H_2O/l air. The shaded area represents weather conditions which are suitable for exercise challenge [from 57, 68].

Free-running exercise tests, however, have the great disadvantage of depending on weather conditions; it is nearly impossible to reveal adequate results in countries with high humidity [46, 68] (fig. 4). In addition, continuous monitoring of the heart rate and oxygen saturation, or the maximum voluntary ventilation (MVV) as a measurement of the workload is hardly possible. At present, the preferred modes of exercise testing in the laboratory are the treadmill with adjustable speed and grade, or the electromagnetically braked cycle ergometer.

Guidelines for exercise challenge have been published by the European Respiratory Society (ERS) [1] and the ATS [20]. In brief, subjects perform a standardized exercise for 6–8 min inspiring dry air less than 25°C with a nose clip in place. This can be performed in an air-conditioned room (with a temperature of 20–25°C) with a relative humidity of less than 50% [49]. Inspired air temperature and humidity should be measured and recorded. Alternatively, the subject inspires air from a tank through a mouthpiece and a two-way breathing valve. Measuring pulmonary gas exchange during exercise is helpful, although not required. Heart rate and oxygen saturation should always be monitored by a pulse oxymeter, preferably with a forehead sensor. The total duration of exercise for adults and older children is usually 8 min, for children less than 12 years at least 6 min. Start is at low speed and grade, but

both are progressively advanced during the first 2–3 min until the heart rate is 80–90% of the predicted maximum (220 − age in years) which means a heart rate of >170–180/min. Ventilation should reach 40–60% of the predicted MVV (estimated as $FEV_1 \times 35$) [20]. For treadmills, a speed >4.5 km/h and a gradient >15%, or an oxygen consumption of >35 ml/min/kg will usually achieve the target heart rate or ventilation, which should be maintained for at least 4 min [50]. For children a slope of 10% and a speed of 5–8 km/h is often more suitable [69]. For bicycle ergometers, the target work load can be calculated with the following equation: watt = (measured $FEV_1 \times 53.76$) − 11.07. The starting workload is 60% of the target in the 1st minute, 75% in the 2nd minute, 90% in the 3rd minute, and 100% in the 4th minute which has to be sustained for at least 4 min. It is important to reach the target workload within 4 min because the rate of water loss is the determining factor for producing airway narrowing and refractoriness can develop if exercise is prolonged at submaximal work. The intensity of the exercise should be such that the child cannot exercise much beyond 6 or 8 min. If the subject can, it is unlikely that the workload was sufficient to provoke EIA. The ATS recommends a spirometry testing schedule of 5, 10, 15, 20 and 30 min after cessation of the exercise [20]. As most children have their nadir within 10–15 min, an alternative recommended spirometry testing scheme is 1, 3, 5, 7, 10 and 15 min after exercise [46]. Spirometry should be performed in duplicate using ATS guidelines [22] and the higher FEV_1 value should be recorded. If FEV_1 has returned from its nadir to the baseline level, spirometry testing may be terminated after 15–30 min. If there is no return to the baseline level after 30 min, a short-acting β_2-agonist (e.g. salbutamol 2–4 puffs via spacer) should be given to reverse the bronchoconstriction. The criterion for a positive response is still controversial. A fall of $FEV_1 \geq 10\%$ is considered to be abnormal; a fall of $\geq 15\%$ appears to be more diagnostic for EIA. There are no standardized cut-off levels for indices of small airway function (MEF_{25} or FEF_{75}). Around 50% of individuals with EIA are refractory to a second challenge within 1 h; most lose this refractory state within 2 h, but it can take as long as 4 h. As severe bronchoconstriction even during free running can occur [55], a doctor with adequate resuscitation equipment always needs to be present.

Cold Air Hyperventilation Challenge

The first protocols for cold air hyperventilation challenge (CACh) in children were published some 20 years ago [70, 71]. Zach et al. [70] used cooled room air (−15°C) for inhalation instead of dry air from a tank. Twenty-three children with asthma and 18 healthy children inhaled cold air for 4 min at 75% of their MVV. No overlapping in postchallenge lung function values between diseased and healthy children was seen. From then on, CACh and hyperventilation challenges incorporating dry but not necessarily cooled air have been used mainly for clinical purposes in children. CACh has been proven to be safe, and late asthmatic reactions are lacking [72, 73]. Most normo- and hyperresponsive individuals show a maximum reaction plateau which may contribute to the observed safety [74].

Equipment and Protocol

Most challenges in children have used a single step protocol [70, 71, 75, 76] since this technique has been shown to yield similar results as a multiple step CACh which is more time consuming [73]. Basically, by using this protocol, the child hyperventilates for a fixed time period at a fixed level of ventilation. In the protocol of Zach et al. [70], hyperventilation is performed at 75% of MVV which is calculated as prechallenge $FEV_1 \times 22.5$. The child inhales dry air at a temperature from -10 to $-15°C$ for 4 min via a special apparatus. To maintain the same level of ventilation, the child keeps a target balloon inflated during the challenge. A monitor analyzes expired CO_2 continuously throughout the challenge and CO_2 is added into the inspired air manually for keeping the subject eucapnic during the CACh. FEV_1 is measured before and 3 min after the challenge. The change in FEV_1 from baseline to postchallenge is expressed in percent baseline FEV_1. A change in FEV_1 of 9% or more defines BHR to CACh [70].

Other authors prefer a multiple step protocol using dry but not cooled air [1]. These protocols use increasing rates of ventilation for fixed time periods. The predicted MVV is calculated as $FEV_1 \times 35$ and ventilation rates used are from 20 to 90% of MVV, and MVV itself. Each level of ventilation is held for 3 min, and FEV_1 measured 3 min after each step. The individual response is usually expressed as percent fall in FEV_1 after each level of ventilation. A positive response is a 10% reduction in FEV_1, and a PD_{10} (provocative dose of ventilation causing a 10% fall in FEV_1) is calculated. Although CACh is a very elegant way of assessing BHR, it has the drawback of involving rather expensive and sophisticated equipment.

Hypertonic Saline Challenge

Several studies have shown that the hypertonic saline challenge (HSCh) is a useful, simple, and safe test in laboratory studies and epidemiological surveys of asthma in children [55]. Details about specifications of the equipment needed for use in children have been published [77, 78]. The

repeatability of the test has been assessed and shown to be good with the fold difference for PD_{15} (provocative dose to produce a 15% fall in FEV_1), over a 2-week period, being 1.70 for children in the age range of 10–14 years [79].

Equipment and Protocol

Ultrasonic nebulizers are used for HSCh because they produce denser aerosols and have a higher output than jet nebulizers. Age-related standardization regarding aerosol output and particle size exists [77]. These specifications are important and have to be assessed before a different nebulizer is used. A single concentration of 4.5% saline is recommended, and the dose of saline increased successively by doubling the inhalation time starting with 0.5, then 1, 2, 4 and 8 min with subjects inhaling at tidal volumes and wearing nose clips. In children, it is of critical importance to use non-rebreathing valves with an appropriately low dead space. FEV_1 is measured in duplicate before the challenge and 60 s after each challenge step. The challenge is terminated when the FEV_1 falls by 15% or more, or a cumulative inhalation time of 15.5 min has been achieved. The cut-off value of 15% has been derived from a population-based study in 393 children aged 13–15 years and represents the 95th percentile for percent change in FEV_1 in children without respiratory diseases [55].

Some children cough during the first 1–2 min of inhalation of HS and some children report nausea. However, this cough is transient and rarely leads to termination of the challenge. Only 6 of 393 children in an Australian study [55], and only 5 of 519 in an Austrian study on asthma were unwilling to complete the HSCh [80]. On the other hand, most children can be encouraged to cough up sputum that is induced by HS after 5–10 min of inhalation. Besides measurement of bronchial responsiveness, cell and mediator analysis from induced sputum might add valuable information on airway inflammation in a non-invasive way.

A dose-response curve is constructed by plotting the FEV_1 in litres on a linear scale against the cumulative dose of aerosol delivered, expressed in millilitres on a log scale for each inhalation period. A value for PD_{15} (provocative dose of HS causing a fall in FEV_1 of 15%) can be obtained by linear interpolation of the last two points. As PD_{15} values are log-normally distributed in the asthmatic population, these values need to be log-transformed prior to statistical analysis. For children who do not respond with a fall in FEV_1 of at least 15%, PD_{15} values cannot be calculated. In these children, the maximum percent fall in FEV_1 divided by the total dose of aerosol delivered is reported. This gives a response-dose ratio and the values can be compared with those obtained in healthy control subjects.

For comparison of children with different ages and sizes $PT_{15}sec$ (cumulative time of aerosol inhalation causing a fall in $FEV_1 \geq 15\%$) should be reported in addition to PD_{15} values. This is important to account for the fact that older children have bigger lung volumes than younger ones, and thus inhale more aerosol and have a greater PD_{15} even in the case of similar responsiveness. $PT_{15}sec$ gives a size-corrected value for the response to HS [79].

A challenge should not be performed in children with severe airflow limitation or those with a baseline FEV_1 less than 65% of predicted. After the challenge, children who feel discomfort or whose FEV_1 had fallen by more than 10% should inhale a bronchodilator. Children should never be left unattended and their airway narrowing should be reversed to within 90% of baseline before they are allowed to leave the office. To avoid very early reactions during the challenge in severely hyperresponsive children, the initial challenge period should only be 30 s. Although serious complications have not been seen, precautions set out by Sterk et al. [1] are recommended.

Ultrasonically Nebulized Distilled Water Challenge

As has been shown for hypertonic solutions, patients with asthma also respond to inhalation of hypotonic solutions with bronchoconstriction. Since the first description of ultrasonically nebulized distilled water challenge (UNDWCh) by Allegra and Bianco [81] in 1980, several modified challenge protocols have been developed for use in children [82–84]. Basically, these protocols involve inhalation of ultrasonically nebulized distilled (sometimes cooled) water in a single-step or in a multiple-step way.

Equipment and Protocol

Equipment and protocols are similar as for HSCh but exact standardization is lacking for UNDWCh. Not different to HS, mediator release from cells and stimulation of neurones are the main principles of mechanism by which distilled water leads to airway narrowing. Smith et al. [85] did not find a significant correlation between results from HSCh and UNDWCh in adults, whereas Wojnarowski et al. [86] reported a statistically significant negative correlation between log PD_{15} after HS and the maximum fall in FEV_1 after UNDWCh in 15 asthmatic children ($r_s = -0.63$; $p < 0.005$). The latter study confirmed earlier reports that UNDWCh is less sensitive than HSCh or exercise testing in identifying children with asthma [87].

Mannitol Dry Powder Challenge

In an effort to make an indirect airway challenge faster and needing fewer resources, Anderson et al. [88] have developed a dry powder of mannitol suitable for inhalation which provides the same hyperosmolar challenge as HS. Mannitol is a naturally occurring sugar alcohol ($C_6H_{14}O_6$) which is not absorbed by the gastro-intestinal tract. It is a stable substance, flows well when prepared as a dried powder spray, and retains its crystalline structure and resists moisture resorption at relatively high humidity. These characteristics make it an ideal substance to encapsulate for inhalation, and to use it in countries with high humidity or for epidemiological studies. Mannitol dry powder (MDP) preparation is standardized for the amount delivered and the particle size distribution – an advantage over the inconsistent delivery of many nebulizers. Mannitol dry powder challenge (MDPCh) is much easier and quicker to perform, better tolerated, and cheaper than the MCT or HSCh [88, 89]. The median time to complete an MDPCh is between 10 and 15 min [18, 89, 90].

BHR to MDP appears to be very specific for asthma, and has a similar sensitivity as HS, eucapnic hyperventilation and exercise testing [88, 89, 91, 92]; however, this has not been tested under conditions in the field such as those encountered in epidemiological studies. MDPCh demonstrates good repeatability of airway responsiveness in asthmatic patients under laboratory conditions in both adults [88, 93] and children [89, 90]. Healthy subjects with no current or past history of asthma and normal spirometry do not have any significant reduction in FEV_1 following an MDPCh [88, 89]. A retrospective analysis of MDPCh performed in 275 subjects (aged 13–70 years, mean 29 years) highlights some of the practical features of the procedure [18]. The median time to complete the test in asthmatic patients responsive to mannitol was 12 min (range: 3–27), and the median number of capsules administered was 6 (range: 1–18). Of all subjects responsive to mannitol, the geometric mean PD_{15} was 116 mg (95% CI: 99–135). Sixteen percent of the asthmatics were unresponsive to MDP, and the median time to administer the entire eighteen capsules was 20 min (range: 16–30 min) [18].

The only observed limitation of the MDPCh in children and adults is a transient cough after higher doses of MDP, which is common with osmotic stimuli. The cough is usually minor, lasting for only a few seconds, and does not substantially prolong the time to complete the challenge or lead to a termination of the test in children [89, 90].

Equipment and Protocol

So far, MDP capsules are not yet commercially available but an Australian company (Pharmaxis, Frenchs Forests, Australia) has started to produce them. The preparation of MDP has been described by Anderson et al. [88]. In brief,

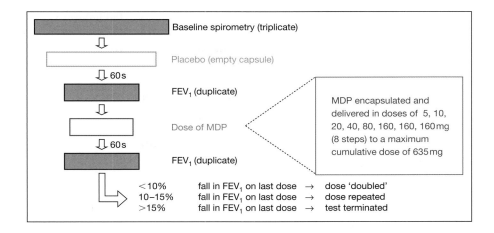

```
┌─────────────────────────────────┐
│ Baseline spirometry (triplicate)│
└─────────────────────────────────┘
           ⇩
┌─────────────────────────────────┐
│ Placebo (empty capsule)         │
└─────────────────────────────────┘
           ⇩ 60 s
┌─────────────────────────────────┐
│ FEV₁ (duplicate)                │
└─────────────────────────────────┘
           ⇩
┌─────────────────────────────────┐
│ Dose of MDP                     │
└─────────────────────────────────┘
           ⇩ 60 s
┌─────────────────────────────────┐
│ FEV₁ (duplicate)                │
└─────────────────────────────────┘
```

MDP encapsulated and delivered in doses of 5, 10, 20, 40, 80, 160, 160, 160 mg (8 steps) to a maximum cumulative dose of 635 mg

<10%   fall in FEV_1 on last dose → dose 'doubled'
10–15% fall in FEV_1 on last dose → dose repeated
>15%   fall in FEV_1 on last dose → test terminated

Fig. 5. MDP challenge [from 88, 90].

gelatine capsules are filled with 5, 10, 20 ($+/-.2$), and 40 ($+/-.5$) mg of MDP using an analytical balance. The filled capsules are stored under dry conditions. MDP is delivered in progressively increasing doses using a simple commercially available dry powder inhaler such as the Inhalator® (Boehringer Ingelheim). A minimum peak inspiratory flow of 30 litres/min is necessary. The test is a cumulative dose challenge that is performed by asking the subjects to inhale increasing doses of MDP through the delivery device. The following schedule is used: 0 mg (empty capsule acting as a placebo), 5, 10, 20, 40, 80, 160, 160 and 160 mg. The doses of 80 mg and above are achieved by administering multiples of 40-mg capsules (fig. 5). After inhalation of MDP from each capsule, subjects are instructed to perform a 5-second breath hold. Sixty seconds after the inhalation, spirometry is performed in duplicate according to ATS guidelines [22], and the higher FEV_1 value is recorded. The MDPCh is completed when a 15% fall in FEV_1 is documented, or a cumulative dose of 635 mg (in total 18 capsules) has been administered. Recovery to baseline lung function occurs spontaneously, usually within 15–30 min, but after a positive response to MDP, a standard dose of a short-acting β_2-agonist (e.g. salbutamol 2–4 puffs via spacer) should be given to reverse the bronchoconstriction. The results of an MDPCh are reported as a percent decrease of FEV_1 from baseline (measured after the 0-mg capsule), and the PD_{15} is calculated. A fall of $FEV_1 \geq 15\%$ with a cumulative dose ≤ 35 mg MDP is considered a severe, with a dose >35 mg and ≤ 155 mg a moderate, and with a dose >155 and <635 mg a mild response, respectively [49].

Adenosine Monophosphate Challenge

Adenosine 5′-monophosphate (AMP), a purine nucleoside, is a potent and specific bronchoconstrictor in adults [47, 94] and children with asthma [42, 95, 96]. It is assumed that AMP induces bronchoconstriction due to its releasing effect of mediators from mast cells and neuronal cells [3, 97, 98]. Inhaled AMP correlates closely to the airway response following inhaled mannitol [99]. However, AMP differs from mannitol in two ways: it is mediated via adenosine$_{2b}$ receptors and appears to be mostly mast-cell-specific rather than being a stimulus to all cells in the airways [49]. So far, adenosine 5′-monophosphate challenge (AMPCh) has been predominately used in research fields.

Equipment and Protocol

AMPCh involves similar equipment and a similar protocol as MCT or histamine challenge test [1]. Most studies with AMP in children [42, 51, 96] used the 2-min tidal breathing protocol, described by Cockcroft et al. [33]. AMP is prepared in doubling phosphate buffer solutions in a range from 3.125 to 400 mg/ml. Two millilitres of each concentration is inhaled for 2 min via nebulizer, and the challenge is terminated when the FEV_1 falls by 20% or more, or the highest concentration is given. The results of an AMPCh are reported as percent decrease of FEV_1 from baseline, and PC_{20} is calculated [49].

In a study with 135 asthmatic children, Avital et al. [51] using a cut-off limit of 200 mg/ml for the definition of BHR have found a sensitivity of the AMPCh of 96%, which is similar to the sensitivity of MCT (98%) with a cut-off limit of 8 mg/ml. Sensitivity of both tests was higher than that of exercise testing (65%). Specificity of AMPCh seems to be superior compared to MCT. The same research group has reported a very high specificity of AMPCh in differentiating children with asthma from controls and children with paediatric chronic obstructive pulmonary disease with an

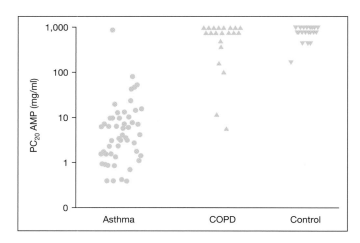

Fig. 6. PC$_{20}$ for AMP in children with asthma, paediatric chronic obstructive pulmonary disease (COPD), and control subjects [from 42].

explanation is that hyperresponsiveness to AMP is more affected by treatment with inhaled steroids [45, 47].

Unsolved Questions and Future Developments

Although there have been many studies strongly suggesting that indirect airway challenges are useful and objective tests for asthma with a closer relationship to airway inflammation than direct challenges, only limited data has been published on some of these stimuli such as AMP [45, 47] or mannitol [48, 100, 101] in children. More work needs to be performed to confirm the validity of this concept, and to identify the most suitable bronchial stimulus for the diagnosis of asthma and the most useful marker for monitoring asthma treatment. More field experience is necessary to validate the use of mannitol and AMP in epidemiological surveys. There is also a need for better standardization of some indirect pharmacological stimuli (e.g. bradykinin, tachykinin, metabisulfite). Future research directions should also focus on the application of BPT in preschool children. So far, it is unclear which endpoints should be used for measuring BHR in small children and infants where FEV$_1$ manoeuvres are not feasible. The interrupter technique for measuring airway resistance and the forced oscillation technique are potential candidates but have not yet been sufficiently standardized for bronchial challenge tests.

intersection point of sensitivity and specificity curves of 98% (210 mg/ml) and 90% (25 mg/ml), respectively (fig. 6) [42]. In contrast to MCT, AMPCh was less correlated with asthma severity [51]. This could be explained by the fact that methacholine acts directly on airway smooth muscles and nerve endings, and that in severe asthma the degree of mucosal inflammation and the number of denuded nerve endings are likely to be more pronounced, leading to higher responsiveness to methacholine. Another possible

References

1 Sterk PJ, Fabbri LM, Quanjer PH, Cockroft DW, O'Byrne PM, Anderson SD, Juniper EF, Malo JL: Airway responsiveness: Standardized challenge testing with pharmacological, physical and sensitizing stimuli in adults. Eur Respir J 1993;6(suppl 16):53–83.

2 Williams PV, Shapiro G: Inhalation bronchoprovocation in children; in Spector SL (ed): Provocation Testing in Clinical Practice. New York, Dekker, 1995, pp 451–478.

3 Van Schoor J, Joos GF, Pauwels RA: Indirect bronchial hyperresponsiveness in asthma: Mechanisms, pharmacology and implications for clinical research. Eur Respir J 2000;16: 514–533.

4 Marchal F, Schweitzer C, Moreau-Colson C: Respiratory impedance response to deep inhalation in children. Pediatr Pulmonol 2002; 33:418.

5 Brusasco V, Crimi E, Pellegrino R: Airway hyperresponsiveness in asthma: Not just a matter of airway inflammation. Thorax 1998; 53:992–998.

6 Frey U: Effects of deep inhalations on bronchial reactivity in pediatric asthma. Pediatr Pulmonol 2002;33:409–410.

7 Beardsmore C, Silverman M: Airway responses: Bronchoconstrictor responsiveness; in Silverman M, O'Callaghan CL (eds): Practical Paediatric Respiratory Medicine, ed 1. London, Arnold, 2001, pp 75–81.

8 Mai XM, Gaddlin PO, Nilsson L, Finnstrom O, Bjorksten B, Jenma MC, Leijon I: Asthma, lung function and allergy in 12-year-old children with very low birth weight: A prospective study. Pediatr Allergy Immunol 2003;14: 184–192.

9 Eber E, Zach MS: Long term sequelae of bronchopulmonary dysplasia (chronic lung disease of infancy). Thorax 2001;56: 317–323.

10 Sanchez I, Powell RE, Pasterkamp K: Wheezing and airflow obstruction during methacholine challenge in children with cystic fibrosis and in normal children. Am Rev Respir Dis 1993;147:705–709.

11 Sterk PJ: Virus-induced airway hyperresponsiveness. Eur Respir J 1993;6:894–902.

12 Cuttitta G, Cibella F, La Grutta S, Hopps MR, Bucchieri S, Passalacqua G, Bonsignore G: Non-specific bronchial hyper-responsiveness in children with allergic rhinitis: Relationship with the atopic status. Pediatr Allergy Immunol 2003;14: 458–463.

13 Hospers JJ, Postma DS, Rijcken B, Weiss ST, Schouten JP: Histamine airway hyperresponsiveness and mortality from chronic obstructive pulmonary disease: A cohort study. Lancet 2000;356:1313–1317.

14 Cook DG, Strachan DP: Parental smoking, bronchial reactivity and peak flow variability in children. Thorax 1998;53:295–301.

15 Pattemore PK, Asher MI, Harrison AC, Mitchell EA, Rea HH, Stewart AW: The interrelationship among bronchial hyperresponsiveness, the diagnosis of asthma, and asthma symptoms. Am Rev Respir Dis 1990;142: 549–554.

16 Hopp RJ, Robert G, Townley RG, Biven RE, Bewtra AK, Nair NM: The presence of airway reactivity before the development of asthma. Am Rev Respir Dis 1990;141:2–8.

17 Hopp RJ, Bewtra AK, Nair NM, Townley RG: Specificity and sensitivity of methacholine inhalation challenge in normal and asthmatic children. J Allergy Clin Immunol 1984;74: 154–158.

18 Leuppi JD, Brannan JD, Anderson SD: Bronchial provocation tests: The rationale for using inhaled mannitol as a test for airway hyperresponsiveness. Swiss Med Wkly 2002; 132:151–158.

19 Josephs LK, Gregg J, Muller MA, Holgate ST: Non-specific bronchial reactivity and its relationship to the clinical expression of asthma. Am Rev Respir Dis 1989;140:350–357.

20 American Thoracic Society: Guidelines for methacholine and exercise challenge testing – 1999. Am J Respir Crit Care Med 2000;161: 309–329.

21 Joos GF, O'Connor B; ERS Task Force: Indirect airway challenges. Eur Respir J 2003; 21:1050–1068.

22 American Thoracic Society and Medical Section of the American Lung Association: Standardization of spirometry – 1994 Update. Am J Respir Crit Care Med 1995;152: 1107–1136.

23 Eber E, Zach MS: Spirometry: Volume-time and flow-volume curves; Hammer J, Eber E (eds): Paediatric Pulmonary Function Testing. Prog Respir Res. Basel, Karger, 2005, vol 33, pp 94–102.

24 Clarke KR, Aston H, Silverman M: Delivery of salbutamol by metered dose inhaler and valved spacer to wheezy infants: Effect on bronchial responsiveness. Arch Dis Child 1993;69:125–129.

25 Hayden MJ, Devadason SG, Sly PD, Wildhaber JH, LeSouef PN: Methacholine responsiveness using the raised volume forced expiration technique in infants. Am J Respir Crit Care Med 1997;155: 1670–1675.

26 Phagoo SB, Wilson NM, Silverman M: Repeatability of methacholine challenge in asthmatic children measured by change in transcutaneus oxygen tension. Thorax 1992; 47:804–808.

27 Wilson NM, Bridge P, Phagoo SB, Silverman M: The measurement of methacholine responsiveness in 5 year old children: Three methods compared. Eur Respir J 1995;8: 364–370.

28 Bez C, Sach G, Jarisch A, Rosewich A, Reichenbach J, Zielen S: Safety and tolerability of methacholine challenge in infants with recurrent wheeze. J Asthma 2003;40: 795–802.

29 Frey U, Jackson AC, Silverman M: Differences in airway wall compliance as a possible mechanism for wheezing disorders in children. Eur Respir J 1998;12:136–142.

30 Klug B, Bisgaard H: Measurement of lung function in awake 2–4 year old asthmatic children during methacholine challenge and acute asthma: A comparison of the impulse oscillation technique, the interrupter technique and transcutaneous measurement versus whole-body plethysmography. Pediatr Pulmonol 1996;21:290–300.

31 Scott GC, Braun SR: A survey of the current use and methods of analysis of bronchoprovocational challenges. Chest 1991;100:322–328.

32 Godfrey S, Springer C, Noviski N, Maayan C, Avital A: Exercise but not methacholine differentiates asthma from chronic lung disease in children. Thorax 1991;46:488–492.

33 Cockcroft DW, Killian DN, Mellon JJA, Hargreave FE: Bronchial reactivity to inhaled histamine: A method and a clinical survey. Clin Allergy 1977;7:235–243.

34 Chai H, Farr RS, Froehlich LA, Mathison DA, MacLean JA, Rosenthal RR, Sheffer AL, Spector SL, Townley RG: Standardization of bronchial inhalation challenge procedures. J Allergy Clin Immunol 1975;56:323–327.

35 Rosenthal RR: Approved methodology for methacholine challenge. Allergy Proc 1989; 10:301–310.

36 LeSouef PN, Sears MR, Sherril D: The effect of size and age of subject on airway responsiveness in children. Am J Respir Crit Care Med 1995;152:576–579.

37 Collis GG, Cole CH, LeSouef PN: Dilution of nebulised aerosols by air entrainment in children. Lancet 1990;336:341–343.

38 Yan K, Salome C, Woolcock AJ: Rapid method for measurement of bronchial responsiveness. Thorax 1983;38:760–765.

39 Juniper EF, Frith PA, Dunnett C, Cockcroft DW, Hargreave FE: Reproducibility and comparison of responses to inhaled histamine and methacholine. Thorax 2004;33:705–710.

40 Higgins BG, Britton JR, Chinn S, Jones TD, Vathenen AS, Burney PGJ, Tattersfield AE: Comparison of histamine and methacholine for use in bronchial challenge tests in community studies. Thorax 1988;43:605–610.

41 Steinbrugger B, Eber E, Modl M, Weinhandl E, Zach MS: A comparison of a single-step cold-dry air challenge and a routine histamine provocation for the assessment of bronchial responsiveness in children and adolescents. Chest 1995;108:741–745.

42 Avital A, Springer C, Bar-Yishay E, Godfrey S: Adenosine, methacholine, and exercise challenge in children with asthma or paediatric chronic obstructive pulmonary disease. Thorax 1995;50:511–516.

43 Vandenbossche LE, Hop WC, de Jongste JC: Bronchial responsiveness to inhaled metabisulfite in asthmatic children increases with age. Pediatr Pulmonol 1993;16:236–242.

44 Van Schoor J, Joos GF, Chasson BL, Brourad RJ, Pauwels RA: The effect of the NK2 tachykinin receptor antagonist SR 48968 (saredutant) on neurokinin A-induced bronchoconstriction in asthmatics. Eur Respir J 1998;12:17–23.

45 Doull IJ, Sandall D, Smith S, Schreiber J, Freezer NJ, Holgate ST: Differential inhibitory effect of regular inhaled corticosteroid on airway responsiveness to adenosine 5' monophosphate, methacholine, and bradykinin in symptomatic children with recurrent wheeze. Pediatr Pulmonol 1997;23: 404–411.

46 Riedler J: Nonpharmacological challenges in the assessment of bronchial responsiveness. Eur Respir Mon 1997;5:115–135.

47 van den Berge M, Meijer RJ, Kerstjens HAM, Meijer RJ, de Reus DM, Koeter GH, Kauffman HF, Postma DS: Corticosteroid-induced improvement in the PC20 of adenosine monophosphate is more closely associated with reduction in airway inflammation than improvement in the PC20 of methacholine. Am J Respir Crit Care Med 2001;164:1127–1132.

48 Anderson SD, Brannan JD, Chan HK: Use of aerosols for bronchial provocation testing in the laboratory: Where we have been and where we are going. J Aerosol Med 2002;15: 313–324.

49 Anderson SD, Brannan JD: Methods for 'indirect' challenge testing including exercise, eucapnic voluntary hyperpnoea, and hypertonic aerosols. Clin Rev Allergy Immunol 2003;24:27–54.

50 Silverman M, Anderson SD: Standardization of exercise test in asthmatic children. Arch Dis Child 1972;47:882–889.

51 Avital A, Godfrey S, Springer C: Exercise, methacholine, and adenosine 5'-monophosphate challenges in children with asthma. Pediatr Pulmonol 2000;30:207–214.

52 Carlsen KH, Carlsen KCL: Exercise-induced asthma. Paediatr Respir Rev 2002;3:154–160.

53 Eliasson AH, Phillips YY, Rajagopal KR, Howard RS: Sensitivity and specificity of bronchial provocation testing. An evaluation of four techniques in exercise-induced bronchospasm. Chest 1992;102:347–355.

54 Godfrey S, Spirnger C, Bar-Yishay E, Avital A: Cut-off points defining normal and asthmatic bronchial reactivity to exercise and inhalation challenges in children and young adults. Eur Respir J 1999;14:659–668.

55 Riedler J, Reade T, Dalton M, Holst D, Robertson CF: Hypertonic saline challenge in an epidemiologic survey of asthma in children. Am J Respir Crit Care Med 1994;150: 1632–1639.

56 Haby MM, Peat JK, Mellis CM, Anderson SD: An exercise challenge for epidemiological studies of childhood asthma: Validity and repeatability. Eur Respir J 1995;8:729–736.

57 Haby MM, Anderson SD, Peat JK, Mellis CM, Toelle BG, Woolcock AJ: An exercise challenge protocol for epidemiological studies of asthma in children: Comparison with histamine challenge. Eur Respir J 1994;7:43–49.

58 Williams D, Bruton J, Wilson I: Screening a state middle school for asthma using the free running asthma screening test. Arch Dis Child 1993;69:667–669.

59 Jonasson G, Carlsen KH, Jonasson C, Mowinckel P: Low-dose inhaled budesonide once or twice daily for 27 months in children with mild asthma. Allergy 2000;55:740–748.

60 Anderson SD: Exercise-induced asthma in children: A marker of airway inflammation. Med J Aust 2002;177:S61–S63.

61 Silverman M, König P, Godfrey S: Use of serial exercise tests to assess the efficacy and duration of drugs for asthma. Thorax 1973;28:574–579.

62 Morton AR, Ogle SL, Fitch KD: Effects of nedocromil sodium, cromolyn sodium, and a placebo in exercise-induces asthma. Ann Allergy 1992;68:143–146.

63 Kemp JP, Dockhorn RJ, Shapiro GG, Nguyen HH, Reiss TF, Seidenberg BC, Knorr B: Montelukast once daily inhibits exercise-induced bronchoconstriction in 6–14-year-old children with asthma. J Pediatr 1998;133: 424–428.

64 Jonasson G, Carlsen KH, Hultquist C: Low-dose budesonide improves exercise-induced bronchospasm in schoolchildren. Pediatr Allergy Immunol 2000;11:120–125.

65 Pedersen S, Hansen OR: Budesonide treatment of moderate and severe asthma in children: A dose response study. J Allergy Clin Immunol 1995;95:29–33.

66 Peat JK, Salome CM, Sedgwick CS, Kerrebijn J, Woolcock AJ: A prospective study of bronchial hyperresponsiveness and respiratory symptoms in a population of Australian schoolchildren. Clin Exp Allergy 1989;19: 299–306.

67 Anderson SD, Connollly NM, Godfrey S: Comparison of bronchoconstriction induced by cycling and running. Thorax 1971;26: 396–401.

68 Anderson SD, Schoeffel RE, Black JL, Daviskas E: Airway cooling as the stimulus to exercise-induced asthma – A re-evaluation. Eur J Respir Dis 1985;67:20–30.

69 Godfrey S. Bronchial hyper-responsiveness in children. Paediatr Respir Rev 2000;1: 148–155.

70 Zach M, Polgar G, Kump H, Kroisel P: Cold air challenge of airway hyperreactivity in children: Practical application and theoretical aspects. Pediatr Res 1984;18:469–478.

71 Reisman J, Mappa L, De Benedicts F, McLaughlin J, Levison M: Cold air challenge in an epidemiological survey of asthma in children. Pediatr Pulmonol 1987;3:251–254.

72 Varga EM, Eber E, Zach MS: Cold air challenge for measuring airway reactivity in children: Lack of a late asthmatic reaction. Lung 1990;168:267–272.

73 Modl M, Eber E, Steinbrugger B, Weinhandl E, Zach MS: Comparing methods for assessing bronchial responsiveness in children: Single step cold air challenge, multiple step cold air challenge, and histamine provocation. Eur Respir J 1995;8:1742–1747.

74 Zach MS, Polgar G: Cold air challenge of airway hyperreactivity in children: Dose-response interrelation with a reaction plateau. J Allergy Clin Immunol 1987;80:9–17.

75 Nicolai T, Mutius EV, Reitmeir P, Wjst M: Reactivity to cold-air hyperventilation in normal and in asthmatic children in a survey of 5,697 schoolchildren in southern Bavaria. Am Rev Respir Dis 1993;147:565–572.

76 Eber E, Varga EM, Zach MS: Cold air challenge of airway reactivity in children: A correlation of transcutaneously measured oxygen tension and conventional lung functions. Pediatr Pulmonol 1991;10:273–277.

77 Riedler J, Robertson CF: Effect of tidal volume on the output and particle size distribution of hypertonic saline from an ultrasonic nebulizer. Eur Respir J 1994;7: 998–1002.

78 Anderson SD, Smith CM, Rodwell LT, du Toit JI, Riedler J, Robertson CF: The use of non-isotonic aerosols for evaluating bronchial hyperreponsiveness; in Spector SL (ed): Provocative Testing in Clinical Practice. New York, Dekker, 1994, pp 249–278.

79 Riedler J, Reade T, Robertson CF: Repeatability of response to hypertonic saline aerosol in children with mild to severe asthma. Pediatr Pulmonol 1994;18:330–336.

80 Riedler J, Gamper A, Eder W, Oberfeld G: Prevalence of bronchial hyperresponsiveness to 4.5% saline and its relation to asthma and allergy symptoms in Austrian children. Eur Respir J 1998;11:355–360.

81 Allegra L, Bianco S: Non-specific broncho-reactivity obtained with an ultrasonic aerosol of distilled water. Eur J Respir Dis 1980; 61(suppl 16):53–83.

82 Galdes-Sebalt M, McLaughlin FJ, Levison H: Comparison of cold air, ultrasonic mist and methacholine inhalations as tests of bronchial reactivity in normal and asthmatic children. J Pediatr 1985;107:526–530.

83 Eichler I, Götz M, Zarkovic J, Köfinger A: Distilled water challenges in asthmatic children. Chest 1992;102:753–758.

84 Frischer T, Studnicka M, Neumann M, Goetz M: Determinants of airway response to challenge with distilled water in a population sample of children aged 7 to 10 years old. Chest 1992;102:764–770.

85 Smith CM, Anderson SD: Inhalation challenge using hypertonic saline in asthmatic subjects: A comparison with response to hyperpnoea, methacholine, and water. EUR Respir J 1990; 3:144–151.

86 Wojnarowski C, Storm Van's Gravesande K, Riedler J, Eichler I, Gartner C, Frischer T: Comparison of bronchial challenge with ultra-sonic nebulized distilled water and hypertonic saline in children with mild to moderate asthma. Eur Respir J 1996;9:1896–1901.

87 Obata T, Iikura Y: Comparison of bronchial reactivity to ultrasonically nebulized distilled water, exercise and methacholine challenge test in asthmatic children. Ann Allergy 1994; 72:167–172.

88 Anderson SD, Brannan J, Spring J, Spalding N, Rodwell LT, Chan K, Gonda I, Walsh A, Clark AR: A new method for bronchial-provocating testing in asthmatic subjects using a dry powder of mannitol. Am J Respir Crit Care Med 1997;156:758–765.

89 Subbarao P, Brannan JD, Ho B, Anderson SD, Chan HK, Coates AL: Inhaled mannitol identifies methacholine-responsive children with asthma. Pediatr Pulmonol 2000;29:291–298.

90 Barben J, Roberts M, Chew N, Carlin JB, Robertson CF: Repeatabilty of bronchial responsiveness to mannitol dry powder in children with asthma. Pediatr Pulmonol 2003;36:490–494.

91 Brannan JD, Koskela H, Anderson SD, Chew N: Responsiveness to mannitol in asthmatic subjects with exercise- and hyperventilation-induced asthma. Am J Respir Crit Care Med 1998;158:1120–1126.

92 Brannan JD, Anderson SD, Freed R, Leuppi JD, Koskela H, Spring J, Spalding N, Rodwell LT, Chan HK: Bronchial provocation testing using inhaled mannitol: An analysis of the first 168 adult asthmatic subjects (abstract). Eur Respir J 1999;14:469s.

93 Brannan JD, Anderson SD, Gomes K, King GG, Chan HK: Fexofenadine decreases sensitivity to and montelukast improves recovery from inhaled mannitol. Am J Respir Crit Care Med 2001;163:1420–1425.

94 Cushley MJ, Tattersfield AE, Holgate ST: Inhaled adenosine and guanosine on airway resistance in normal and asthmatic subjects. Br J Clin Pharmacol 1983;15:161–165.

95 Benckhuijsen J, van den Bos JW, van Velzen E, de Bruijn R, Aalbers R: Differences in the effect of allergen avoidance on bronchial hyperresponsiveness as measured by methacholine, adenosine 5′-monophosphate, and exercise in asthmatic children. Pediatr Pulmonol 1996;22:147–153.

96 Avital A, Picard E, Uwyyed K, Springer C: Comparison of adenosine 5′-monophosphate and methacholine for the differentiation of asthma from chronic airway diseases with the use of the auscultative method in very young children. J Pediatr 1995;127:438–440.

97 Cushley MJ, Holgate ST: Adenosine-induced bronchoconstriction in asthma: Role of mast cell-mediator release. J Allergy Clin Immunol 1985;75:272–278.

98 Polosa R, Rorke S, Holgate ST: Evolving concepts on the value of adenosine hyperresponsiveness in asthma and chronic obstructive pulmonary disease. Thorax 2002;57:649–654.

99 Currie GP, Haggart K, Lee DK, Fowler SJ, Wilson AM, Brannan JD, Anderson SD, Lipworth BJ: Effects of mediator antagonism on mannitol and adenosine monophosphate challenge. Clin Exp Allergy 2003;33: 783–788.

100 Koskela HO, Hyvärinen L, Brannan JD, Chan HK, Anderson SD: Sensitivity and validity of three bronchial provocation tests to demonstrate the effect of inhaled corticosteroids in asthma. Chest 2003;124: 1341–1349.

101 Leuppi JD, Salome CM, Jenkins CR, Anderson SD, Xuan W, Marks GB, Koskela H, Brannan JD, Freed R, Andersson M, Chan HK, Woolcock AJ: Predictive markers of asthma exacerbation during stepwise dose reduction of inhaled corticosteroids. Am J Respir Crit Care Med 2001;163:406–412.

Dr. J. Barben
Paediatric Pulmonology
Ostschweizer Kinderspital
CH–9000 St. Gallen (Switzerland)
Tel. +41 71 243 71 11
Fax +41 71 243 76 99
E-Mail juerg.barben@gd-kispi.sg.ch

Extended Assessment of the Respiratory System in Paediatric Patients

Hammer J, Eber E (eds): Paediatric Pulmonary Function Testing.
Prog Respir Res. Basel, Karger, 2005, vol 33, pp 138–147

....

Measurements of Respiratory Muscle Function in Children

Brigitte Fauroux[a]   Frédéric Lofaso[b]

[a]Pediatric Pulmonology and INSERM E 213, Hôpital Armand Trousseau, Paris, and
[b]Physiology Department, Hôpital Raymond Poincaré, Garches, France

Abstract

The range of techniques available to assess respiratory muscle weakness has been greatly expanded over the last years. Respiratory muscle tests can be divided into non-invasive tests such as measurement of lung function parameters, maximal static pressures and sniff nasal pressures, and invasive tests such as measurement of transdiaphragmatic pressures during crying, sniff transdiaphragmatic pressures, and magnetic stimulation of the phrenic nerves. The measurement of sniff nasal pressures and magnetic stimulation of the phrenic nerves may be increasingly used in children in the coming years. The evaluation of respiratory muscle endurance is complementary to the assessment of respiratory muscle strength, but this test is not commonly performed in children. An evaluation of the respiratory muscles should be proposed not only in children with neuromuscular diseases but also in those with unexplained or disproportionate breathlessness. Moreover, recent research provides evidence that the impairment of respiratory muscles negatively affects the clinical outcome in chronic lung disease such as cystic fibrosis.

Introduction

Respiratory muscle testing is not routinely performed in children. However, it seems important that paediatricians, paediatric pulmonologists, intensivists and neurologists have some knowledge of respiratory muscle testing because respiratory muscle weakness can be a cause of respiratory failure. A dysfunction of the respiratory muscles can be difficult to detect clinically, justifying the importance of objective measures.

Children with clearly documented generalized neuromuscular disease usually also have respiratory muscle weakness. Treatment in the form of non-invasive positive pressure ventilation may be indicated for patients who present with alveolar hypoventilation. Pre-existing respiratory muscle weakness can precipitate respiratory distress during a respiratory exacerbation or an anaesthetic procedure. Indeed, it has been recently shown that diaphragmatic strength is reduced during the inhalation of nitrous oxide [1].

There is increased awareness that respiratory muscle weakness can be an important compounding factor in various other disease processes and situations such as malnutrition and during steroid therapy. Moreover, the respiratory muscles are the subject of intense research in chronic lung diseases such as chronic obstructive pulmonary disease (COPD) and cystic fibrosis [2, 3]. These studies show the negative impact of the impairment in respiratory muscle function on the clinical outcome of these patients.

For all these reasons, it seems important for the clinician to initiate and interpret respiratory muscle testing [4]. In this chapter, we differentiate between easy bedside tests and laboratory tests that can only be performed in specialized centres. Because of the paediatric aspect of this review, the different explorations vary according to the child's age [5].

Inspiratory Muscle Strength Evaluation

History and Clinical Assessment

The history of the patient is of major importance. A trauma history such as a difficult delivery with injury of the brachial plexus, thoracic surgery, or the presence of a neuromuscular disease are situations where a dysfunction of the respiratory muscles is highly probable. In generalized neuromuscular disorders, it is unusual for the respiratory muscles to be spared. The timing of the dysfunction and the type of muscles that will be affected vary according to the underlying disease. Classically, severe generalized respiratory muscle weakness causes breathlessness and tachypnoea but these symptoms and signs may be defaulted or difficult to detect in young children. When generalized weakness becomes sufficiently severe, nocturnal alveolar hypoventilation develops causing sleep disruption, daytime sleepiness and impaired intellectual function. Because of the insidious presentation of hypoventilation, however, the diagnosis is often delayed or made only during an acute respiratory exacerbation. This underlines the importance of subtle clinical symptoms that must be systematically and regularly looked for, such as breathlessness when supine, sitting, or standing in water. Frequent complications in patients with neuromuscular disease, such as aspiration and pneumonia, can be caused by weakness of bulbar and expiratory muscles [6].

On examination, the characteristic finding of profound bilateral diaphragm weakness or paralysis is paradoxical inward inspiratory abdominal motion, which is more obvious when the patient is supine. In case of diaphragm weakness, the abdominal muscles may be visibly recruited during expiration, serving to elevate the diaphragm and allowing subsequent descent during inspiration. But these clinical signs are seldom present until the strength of the diaphragm is reduced to about a quarter of normal; thus, substantial diaphragm weakness can be easily overlooked on clinical examination.

Non-Invasive Tests

Radiological Assessment

Conventional chest radiography plays a limited role in assessing respiratory muscle function. It can show an elevated hemidiaphragm in the case of hemidiaphragmatic paralysis. This, however, is a non-specific finding, since it can also occur in patients with other conditions, such as atelectasis or pneumonia. In addition, in the case of bilateral diaphragm weakness, the chest radiograph can even appear normal. These limitations underline the necessity of objective and reliable measures of respiratory muscle performance.

More recently, ultrasonography of the diaphragm has been used to evaluate diaphragmatic motion and structure. In 22 patients, aged from birth to 66 years, real-time ultrasonography proved feasible and useful in evaluating diaphragmatic motion [7]. Ultrasonography may also be used to measure the thickness of the diaphragm [8], but hypertrophy does not necessarily imply a better capacity to produce force, as dramatically exemplified in Duchenne muscular dystrophy [9]. Indeed, increased diaphragm mass inferred from imaging techniques may not be the result of muscle fibre hypertrophy but rather the expression of adipose and connective tissue deposition. Thus, ultrasonographic evaluation should be associated with a functional, and ideally, morphological and histological exploration of the diaphragm. However, ultrasonography has advantages over traditional fluoroscopy, including portability, lack of ionizing radiation, visualization of the thoracic bases and upper abdomen, and the ability to quantify diaphragmatic motion. The experience in paediatric patients is limited and further studies are warranted to include this technique into the routine battery of respiratory muscle testing in children.

Three-dimensional reconstruction of the diaphragm by spiral computed tomography has recently been evaluated in adult patients [10]. With this technique, total diaphragm length and surface area were measured, as well as the length and surface area of the dome, and the zone of apposition in patients with severe COPD and normal subjects [11]. Patients with COPD had significant reductions in the surface area of the diaphragm and the zone of apposition at functional residual capacity (FRC) but diaphragm dimensions were similar to those of normal subjects when compared at absolute volumes. Intersubject variability was explained by differences in body weight. Multiple trials were necessary for the patients to be able to breathe to different lung volumes, hold their breath, and relax against a closed airway. This technique would obviously be difficult to perform in children, and expose them to a relatively large dose of radiation. A routine use of this radiological technique does thus not seem appropriate for paediatric patients.

Lung Function Parameters

The association of a low vital capacity (VC) with a reduced total lung capacity and a preserved residual volume (RV) is the most characteristic abnormality of inspiratory muscle weakness. Measurement of VC is a simple and valuable test. But it has to be known that, based on the shape of the normal pressure-volume curve, one would expect a considerable loss of inspiratory muscle strength before observing a fall of VC [12]. In clinical practice, patients with neuromuscular disorders display a greater than expected loss in VC. This is due to the associated decrease in lung compliance (diffuse microatelectasis) and in chest wall compliance (ankylosis of joints and scoliosis associated with muscular dysfunction). In subjects with diaphragm weakness, VC falls when the patient is supine, although this fall must exceed 25% to be unequivocally abnormal. Indeed, the supine fall in VC has been shown to be associated with diaphragmatic weakness in 24 patients with generalized neuromuscular disease [13]. The regular monitoring of VC is of great value in patients at risk of rapidly progressive muscle weakness or paralysis. A major limitation of the measurement of VC is that it is volitional and depends on the patient's motivation, cooperation and ability. VC can thus only be measured in cooperative children, usually older than 6 years. In children who cannot use a mouthpiece, VC can be measured via a tight-fitting facemask. Finally, a decrease in VC is not specific, because it can be reduced by factors other than muscle weakness. A fall in VC must thus be interpreted together with the clinical history of the patient.

Inspiratory Mouth Pressure

The most widely applied test of global inspiratory strength is the maximal static inspiratory pressure (Pimax) measured at the mouth. When the airway is occluded and the glottis open, mouth pressure equals alveolar pressure. Pressure is measured with the child seated and wearing a noseclip. A cylindrical mouthpiece is recommended. A small leak, created by the placement of a needle in the mouthpiece, is necessary to eliminate glottic closure and artificially high maximal pressure values. Normally, maximal pressure is measured with a mouthpiece but some patients with orofacial muscle weakness may have difficulties in forming an airtight seal around either type of mouthpiece, which leads to an underestimation of static pressures. Conventionally, Pimax is measured from RV [14], which seems to be easier than from FRC. However, at RV the measured Pimax is the sum of the pressure developed by the inspiratory muscles and the outward recoil pressure of the respiratory system present at this lung volume (normally equal to $30 \text{ cm H}_2\text{O}$), whereas Pimax measured at FRC strictly represents the inspiratory muscles. Thus, simultaneous measurement of the lung volume at which maximal pressure is generated is recommended [15]. Each effort should be maintained for at least 1 s. In routine practice, it is recommended to perform five measurements or more until two reproducible maximal values are obtained. But the minimal number of recommended measurements, according to the underlying disease, has not

Table 1. Normal values of Pimax at residual volume and Pemax at total lung capacity in healthy children [from 13–16]

Age years	Pimax, cm H_2O		Pemax, cm H_2O	
	male	female	male	female
8	77 ± 24	71 ± 29	99 ± 23	74 ± 25
10	105 ± 27	71 ± 29	123 ± 27	74 ± 25
11–13	114 ± 27	108 ± 29	161 ± 37	126 ± 32
13–17	126 ± 22	109 ± 21	166 ± 44	135 ± 29

been validated in children. Because Pimax is a volitional maximal test, the best value is retained.

This test has the main advantage that it is non-invasive, and that normal values have been established in quite large series of children of different ethnicities (table 1) [14–17]. Maximal pressures generated by infants and children are surprisingly high compared with adults. This seems to be related to the small radius of the curvature of the rib cage, diaphragm, and abdomen, which, according to the Laplace relationship, converts small tensions into relatively high pressures [18]. In children, Pimax increases with age, and, as in adults, is greater in males than in females even prior to puberty [15]. By 11–12 years of age, adult values of Pimax are attained in both females and males. One major problem with static pressures is that they are volitional and thus impossible to be reliably obtained in young children. It is generally assumed that if three equal maximal efforts are obtained, the subject is supposed to have realized a maximal effort. But it has been shown that reproducibility does not ensure maximality. Moreover, many other factors such as a training effect, chest wall configuration and stabilization during manoeuvres may contribute to the range of pressures observed in normal children.

In infants, mouth pressures generated during crying efforts may provide an index of global respiratory muscle strength [19]. The firm application of a rubber cushion mask against the face of an infant is generally sufficient to elicit crying efforts. An artificial leak in the mask prevents glottic closure. Airway occlusions are performed at the end of a crying effort to measure crying Pimax. Only peak crying Pimax without a pressure plateau is available during crying. Normal mean peak crying Pimax was $118 \pm 21 \text{ cm}$ H_2O in a large group of healthy infants between the age of 1 month and 2 years and was independent of age and sex [19]. The main advantage of this test is simplicity, and its value has been proven in children with neuromuscular disease [20].

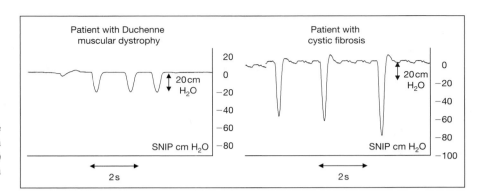

Fig. 1. Sniff nasal inspiratory pressure (SNIP) measurement in a patient with Duchenne muscular dystrophy (23 cm H_2O) and a patient with cystic fibrosis (85 cm H_2O).

Sniff Nasal Pressure

The sniff is a natural manoeuvre which many children find much easier to perform than Pimax. In normal subjects, the pressure measured in the mouth, nasopharynx and the nose during a sniff is closely related to that in the oesophagus [21, 22]. The sniff nasal inspiratory pressure (SNIP) involves measuring nasal pressure in an occluded nostril during a maximal sniff performed through the contralateral nostril from FRC (fig. 1). Transmission of the oesophageal pressure (Poes) to the nose is obtained considering that a transnasal pressure of 10–15 cm H_2O makes it possible to obtain a collapse of the unplugged nostril valve.

The best value obtained with this voluntary manoeuvre is considered. SNIP provides a reasonable estimate of the inspiratory muscle strength both in normal subjects and in patients with inspiratory muscle weakness. Normal values for SNIP have been established for children and for adults [22–25]. Values in healthy children aged 6–17 years are similar to those measured in healthy adults with a mean SNIP of 104 ± 26 cm H_2O in boys and 93 ± 23 cm H_2O in girls [23]. SNIP correlates with age, weight, and height in boys, but not in girls.

The measurement of mouth pressure during a sniff manoeuvre (PmoSniff) has been proposed as an alternative to Pimax in patients with neurological and neuromuscular diseases [26]. Indeed, Pimax can underestimate the inspiratory muscle strength, due to facial muscle weakness and the consequent difficulty in gripping the mouthpiece. The conclusions of a study performed in 30 patients and 41 control subjects were that (1) PmoSniff did not overcome the limitations of Pimax measurement, (2) the two manoeuvres were not interchangeable but rather complementary, and (3) PmoSniff may underestimate inspiratory muscle strength as assessed by Pimax in patients with severe respiratory muscle weakness [26].

The SNIP, unlike the Pimax, may underestimate inspiratory muscle strength because the short manoeuvre can be associated with dampening of the transmission of the pressure response from the oesophagus to the mouth and nose in patients with obstructive lung disease, such as cystic fibrosis [27]. A recent report comparing Pimax and SNIP in 241 patients with neuromuscular disease found that the value of Pimax was at least the same or even greater than the SNIP, particularly in patients with severe ventilatory restriction [28]. This can be explained by the fact that patients with severe neuromuscular disorders may not be able to perform a rapid sniff manoeuvre owing to significant muscle atrophy. Both tests should thus be considered, in combination with the measurement of VC, in patients with neuromuscular disease. The limit of the SNIP is that it is also a volitional test. However, it represents a valuable, easy, and non-invasive assessment of inspiratory muscle strength in patients without significant upper and lower airway disease.

Invasive Tests

In young children, simple non-invasive tests cannot be done or are unreliable. Also, in some patients it may be necessary to establish precisely the kind and the level of respiratory muscle weakness in order to make decisions about their management. In this situation, both diaphragmatic evaluation and non-volitional tests are required, which need the placement of oesophageal and gastric (for diaphragmatic evaluation) balloons or pressure transducers. Classically, latex balloons (Mercat, France or P.K. Morgan, Gillingham, UK) placed in the mid-oesophagus and stomach are used [29]. But Poes and gastric pressure (Pgas) can also be measured using a 2.1-mm-external-diameter catheter mounted pressure transducer system with two integral transducers mounted 5 and 35 cm from the distal tip (Gaeltec, Dunvegan, Isle of Skye, UK), inserted pernasally after local anaesthesia [30]. This catheter is very well tolerated, even in young children [31]. Simultaneous measurements of Poes and Pgas allow the calculation of transdiaphragmatic pressure (Pdi) with Pdi = Pgas − Poes. Measurement of Pdi is especially helpful for the diagnosis of diaphragmatic dysfunction. However, a considerable variability in the Pdi measurements makes it necessary to pay particular attention to the methods.

Spontaneous Breathing

During normal quiet breathing, contractions of the diaphragm and inspiratory muscles produce a positive change in Pgas and a negative change in Poes. Since in healthy subjects the magnitude of the increase in Pgas is greater than the decrease in Poes, the ratio of the Pgas change to the Poes change is less than −1. During total diaphragmatic paralysis this ratio will be +1. Therefore, the ΔPgas/ΔPoes ratio reflects the relative contributions of the diaphragm and the other respiratory muscles to quiet breathing.

Sniff Pdi and Poes

The majority of children after the age of 4 years are able to perform maximum sniff efforts. In normal subjects, the sniff Pdi change has a narrower normal range and a lower variability than the Pdi pressure change during the Pimax manoeuvre. Since the diaphragm is normally the most important single muscle of inspiration, it is not surprising that sniff Poes is closely related to sniff Pdi. In clinical practice, sniff Poes and sniff Pdi are the most accurate and reproducible volitional tests available to assess global inspiratory and diaphragmatic strength in cooperative children over 6–8 years of age.

Crying Pdi

Crying Pdi measurements allow the assessment of diaphragm muscle strength during inspiratory crying efforts in awake infants. Crying Pdi is ~60 cm H_2O at 1 month postnatal age, which is much lower than the reported crying Pimax values [19]. Crying Pdi increases with postconceptional age [32]. Pdi is specific for diaphragm contraction. Its limitations relate to the need for accurate measurement and the variability of lung volume.

Twitch Pressures

Even if sniff manoeuvres are more accurate and reproducible than isometric manoeuvres of Pimax, these tests still require the understanding and the cooperation of the patient. Electrical and magnetic stimulation of the phrenic nerves are the only tests that require no cooperation of the patient. Electrical stimulation of the phrenic nerve has been developed first. Many of the problems associated with electrical stimulation have been overcome by the

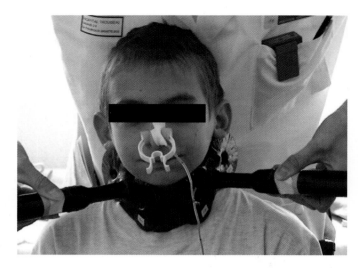

Fig. 2. Bilateral anterior magnetic stimulation of the phrenic nerves in a child with cystic fibrosis.

introduction of magnetic stimulation of the phrenic nerves. By discharging a magnetic field, it is possible to create a pulsed magnetic field which causes current to flow to nervous tissue within the field, which in turn causes muscles to contract. Supramaximal bilateral phrenic nerve stimulation may be achieved using a circular coil placed over the cervical phrenic nerve roots or a figure-of-eight coil placed bilaterally on the two phrenic nerves on the anterior part of the neck (fig. 2) [3, 33]. Magnetic stimulation will also induce current in metallic structures and is contraindicated in the presence of implanted devices such as cardiac pacemarkers, which is less common in children than in adult patients. Unilateral stimulation of the phrenic nerve is possible [34]. Magnetic stimulation has the main advantage that it is much less uncomfortable than electrical stimulation. The mean of at least five reproducible twitches at maximal output is calculated after a 20-min period of rest to avoid twitch potentiation.

Experience with magnetic phrenic nerve stimulation in paediatric patients is scarce. This technique has proved its usefulness in assessing diaphragm function in children following liver transplantation [35]. Indeed, in 3 of 8 patients studied, there was a >50% difference between the Pdi generated after left and right unilateral magnetic stimulation, and a complete right hemidiaphragm paralysis was diagnosed with this technique in one child. The same authors also used magnetic stimulation to assess diaphragm function in neonates but a high power magnetic stimulator is warranted to obtain a pressure response in such young children [29, 36]. In our experience, the measurement of

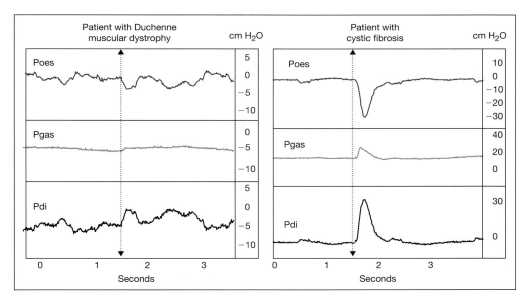

Fig. 3. Twitch transdiaphragmatic pressure obtained by bilateral anterior magnetic stimulation of the phrenic nerves (indicated by vertical dotted line) in a patient with Duchenne muscular dystrophy (5 cm H_2O) and a patient with cystic fibrosis (37 cm H_2O).

twitch transdiaphragmatic pressure (TwPdi) is well accepted and tolerated in children, and is useful to assess diaphragmatic strength in patients with cystic fibrosis [3] and neuromuscular disease (fig. 3). The use of this simple, reliable and non-volitional test to assess diaphragm strength and occurrence of diaphragmatic fatigue [37, 38] will probably increase over the coming years, a fortiori if the measurement of airway pressure can replace Poes [39, 40]. Indeed, it is possible to measure mouth twitch pressure, but the limit is the frequent upper airway or glottic closure during this manoeuvre, which, in this case, does not permit to approximate the alveolar pressure change [39].

Other Inspiratory Muscle Evaluation Methods
Surface Electromyography of the Inspiratory Muscles
Surface electromyography (EMG) of the respiratory muscles has been used in several research and clinical studies to monitor the activity of the diaphragm and the intercostal muscles. Compact, portable measurement apparatus have been developed, which allow the acquisition of electrical signals by electrodes placed on the thorax. With this technique, Sprikkelman et al. [41] observed a correlation between the increase in the electrical activity of the diaphragm (EMGdi) and the intercostal muscles and the fall in the forced expiratory volume in 1 s (FEV_1) in asthmatic children. The same group demonstrated a good reproducibility of the EMGdi and the EMG of the intercostal

muscles in adults, school children, and preschool children during tidal breathing [42]. The limitations of these surface EMG measurements are their alteration by body posture, by the activity of other inspiratory muscles for EMGdi, and by the variation in electrode positioning. However, this technique could be interesting in young children who are not able to perform adequate and reliable forced breathing manoeuvres.

Phrenic Nerve Conduction
Electrical and magnetic stimulations also allow the measurement of the EMG signal and, thus, the nerve conduction time. Phrenic nerve conduction time is measured as the time from stimulus artefact to the onset of the diaphragmatic action potential. For this purpose, the stimuli do not need to be at supramaximal intensity. Normal phrenic nerve latency is in the order of 6–8 ms at birth and decreases to about 5 ms at the age of 1 year despite an increase in conduction distance [43]. Phrenic nerve latency time diminishes slightly with age, by 0.5–1 ms between birth and 10 years of age, with a mean phrenic nerve latency in the order of 4.5–6.5 ms in children [44]. But a precise electrode placement is difficult and the stimulation is painful. For these reasons, this technique remains limited to assess phrenic nerve damage, e.g. in newborns with paralysis of the brachial plexus and patients recovering from cardiac surgery.

Tests of Inspiratory Muscle Endurance

Muscle endurance is the ability to sustain a specific muscular task over time. This highly integrated and complex quality of a muscle or a group of muscles is related to its resistance to fatigue. Any measurement of endurance is task specific. Task failure is an event defined by the inability to continue performing the required task. Although respiratory muscle strength and endurance appear to be closely linked in many conditions, there are numerous examples in which endurance would not be accurately predicted from estimates of maximum pressures or maximum ventilatory capacity. Also, for a given muscle, endurance changes with training, disuse and drug treatment.

A wide variety of techniques have been applied, and some are difficult to use for young patients [45]. A simple way is to assess the maximal time a subject can tolerate a threshold load fixed at a percentage of the individual Pimax [46]. This test has proved its feasibility and simplicity in patients with neuromuscular disease, in whom the threshold was fixed at 35% of Pimax [46]. In healthy children, a load corresponding to more than 50% of Pimax was necessary to induce fatigue and task failure. The threshold level should thus be adapted to the disease and the particular group of patients that will be evaluated [46].

A new test to evaluate inspiratory muscle endurance that overcomes several limitations of the previously described techniques has been developed recently in adult patients [47]. This test is based on the popular pressure-time index concept that describes the load seen by the respiratory chest wall muscles. The hypothesis is that the variation in endurance time could be predicted during the loading task by normalizing the oesophageal pressure time product (PTPoes) for the maximal negative Poes, this relationship being termed the respiratory load/capacity ratio. This test is thus able to quantify the respiratory 'work capacity' corrected for the individual's spontaneous breathing pattern, making it unnecessary to control the breathing rhythm rigidly. With this novel technique, it was possible to show that patients with interstitial lung disease had normal respiratory muscle strength but a reduction in inspiratory muscle endurance [47].

Unfortunately, these tests of respiratory muscle endurance are not widely used in clinical practice. Ideally, they should complete tests of respiratory muscle strength in children.

Expiratory Muscle Strength Evaluation

History and Clinical Assessment

A simple but not a sensitive test to detect expiratory muscle weakness is to ask the patient to perform cough manoeuvres. Indeed, ineffective cough impairs the clearance of bronchial secretions and represents a risk factor for recurrent bronchitis, pneumonia and atelectasis.

Non-Invasive Tests
Lung Function Parameters

Expiratory muscle weakness is often associated with a decrease in the expiratory reserve volume and in the peak expiratory flow or peak cough flow. In addition, when the expiratory muscle weakness affects mainly the muscles of the anterolateral wall, a paradoxical VC increase is usually observed in the supine position relative to the erect position [48].

Expiratory Mouth Pressure

The only test of expiratory muscle strength generally available is maximal expiratory pressure (Pemax), which has the same limitations as the Pimax manoeuvre. Low values are difficult to interpret, as they may result from technical difficulties in performing the test, particularly in patients with facial muscle weakness or bulbar dysfunction [49]. In these situations, the measurement of Pgas during both maximal cough and maximal whistles, which are natural manoeuvres, may represent a useful complementary test (fig. 4). The absence of standardized lung volume is not a major limitation for this test, because it has been shown that lung volume has a very small effect on expiratory muscle strength assessed with non-volitional manoeuvres [50].

Invasive Tests
Cough Gastric Pressure

Coughing is a natural manoeuvre like sniffing. It has recently been proposed that cough Pgas might be a useful additional test of expiratory muscle strength, considering that 6% of patients with normal Pemax were deemed weak by a low cough Pgas (fig. 4) [49].

Twitch Pgas (Non-Volitional Manoeuvres)

It has been demonstrated that twitch Pgas, elicited by magnetic stimulation of the thoracic nerve roots over the tenth thoracic intervertebral space, allowed the generation of a reproducible twitch Pgas in normal subjects [51]. This test is also able to detect expiratory muscle dysfunction in patients unable to perform voluntary tests [52, 53].

EMG of the Expiratory Muscles
The abdominal muscle EMG recording can be used to evaluate the presence of abdominal muscle recruitment in different conditions such as spontaneous breathing [54] and mechanical ventilation [55, 56]. As an example, with this

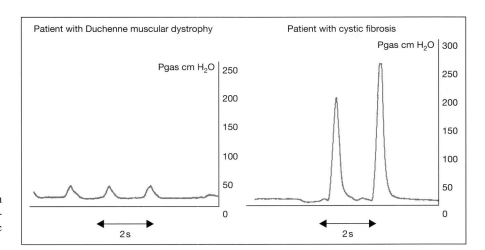

Fig. 4. Gastric pressure (Pgas) during cough in a patient with Duchenne muscular dystrophy (17 cm H_2O) and a patient with cystic fibrosis (233 cm H_2O).

kind of recording it has been demonstrated that the arousal response to an obstructive event during sleep in children was always associated with the presence of abdominal muscle contraction [57].

Indications for the Measurement of Respiratory Muscle Function in Children

Patients with Neuromuscular Disorders

Respiratory failure is one of the main causes of death in patients with neurological and neuromuscular disorders. As such, VC and its rate of decline are strong predictors of mortality in patients with Duchenne muscular dystrophy, with a VC <1 litre being associated with a subsequent 5-year survival of only 8% [58]. Alveolar hypoventilation, especially during sleep, represents one of the most important consequences of respiratory muscle weakness [59, 60]. Systematic evaluation of the level of oxygenation during sleep is recommended when respiratory muscle performance falls below one third of its normal value, and earlier when there is a co-existing respiratory disease. Indeed, clinical symptoms are often absent or minor, mainly because of the progressive course of the majority of neuromuscular diseases. Additionally, children rarely complain of sleep-disordered breathing. Chronic alveolar ventilation is thus frequently diagnosed during acute respiratory failure, underlining the importance of systematic and regular evaluation of lung function parameters in these children. In 49 children and adolescents with progressive neuromuscular disorders, inspiratory VC and peak inspiratory pressure, but not symptom score, correlated with sleep-disordered breathing and severity of nocturnal hypoventilation [61].

The onset of sleep-disordered breathing was predicted by inspiratory VC <60% predicted. Sleep-disordered breathing with nocturnal hypercapnic hypoventilation was predicted by an inspiratory VC <40% predicted and a $PaCO_2$ >40 mm Hg. Thus, the assessment of respiratory muscle force is mandatory to identify those subjects at risk of impending respiratory failure.

Patients with Unexplained Respiratory Failure

An evaluation of the respiratory muscles should also be proposed in children with unexplained or disproportionate breathlessness or those having an adverse outcome defined as, for example, a prolonged requirement of ventilatory support. Indeed, diaphragmatic dysfunction was shown to be associated with prolonged ventilatory support and a protracted stay in intensive care in children who had undergone orthotopic liver transplantation [62]. Magnetic stimulation of the phrenic nerves was also able to document diaphragmatic paralysis in neonates requiring prolonged ventilatory support [29, 36].

Respiratory Muscle Testing in Patients with Lung Disease

The respiratory muscles are the subject of intense research in chronic airway diseases in adults. Indeed, the impairment of respiratory and peripheral muscle function has a major impact on the clinical course in patients with COPD and cystic fibrosis. These patients commonly die of hypercapnic respiratory failure, a terminal consequence of an imbalance between the respiratory muscle load/capacity ratio. The better understanding of the adaptation of the respiratory muscles in these patients can improve their therapeutic management. The analysis of the TwPdi in young patients with cystic fibrosis showed that diaphragm strength was well preserved, and correlated with hyperinflation and nutritional status, assessed by body mass index z-score and fat-free mass [3]. Measuring TwPdi appears to be a valuable non-volitional test that could aid in the evaluation of the effect of nutritional and respiratory interventions on diaphragmatic strength in young patients with CF.

In conclusion, respiratory muscle testing should be performed more routinely in patients with and without neuromuscular disorders. SNIP and magnetic stimulation should be helpful tools in these young patients. Improvements in the evaluation of respiratory muscle endurance need to be continued, which is more difficult but complementary to the assessment of respiratory muscle strength.

References

1 Fauroux B, Cordingley J, Hart N, Clément A, Moxham J, Lofaso F, Polkey MI: Depression of diaphragm contractility by nitrous oxide in humans. Anesth Analg 2002;94:340–345.

2 Polkey MI, Kyroussis D, Hamnegard CH, Mills GH, Green M, Moxham J: Diaphragm strength in chronic obstructive pulmonary disease. Am J Respir Crit Care Med 1996;154:1310–1317.

3 Hart N, Tounian P, Clément A, Boulé M, Moxham J, Girardet JP, Polkey MI, Lofaso F, Fauroux B: Nutritional status is an important predictor of diaphragm strength in young patients with cystic fibrosis. Am J Clin Nutr, in press.

4 Polkey MI, Green M, Moxham J: Measurement of respiratory muscle strength. Thorax 1995; 50:1131–1135.

5 Gaultier C: Tests of respiratory muscle function in children. Am J Respir Crit Care Med 2002; 166:601–609.

6 Seddon PC, Khan Y: Respiratory problems in children with neurological impairment. Arch Dis Child 2003;88:75–78.

7 Gerscovich EO, Cronan M, McGahan JP, Jain K, Jones CD, McDonald C: Ultrasonographic evaluation of diaphragmatic motion. J Ultrasound Med 2001;20:597–604.

8 McCool FD, Benditt JO, Conomos P, Anderson L, Sherman CB, Hoppin FGJ: Variability of diaphragm structure among healthy humans. Am J Respir Crit Care Med 1997;155: 1323–1328.

9 De Bruin PF, Ueki J, Bush A, Khan Y, Watson A, Pride NB: Diaphragm thickness and inspiratory strength in patients with Duchenne muscular dystrophy. Thorax 1997;52:472–475.

10 Pettiaux N, Cassart M, Paiva M, Estenne M: Three-dimensional reconstruction of human diaphragm using spiral computed tomography. J Appl Physiol 1997;82:998–1002.

11 Cassart M, Pettiaux N, Genevois PA, Paiva M, Estenne M: Effect of chronic hyperinflation on diaphragm length and surface area. Am J Respir Crit Care Med 1997;156:504–508.

12 Tobin MJ: Respiratory muscles in disease. Clin Chest Med 1988;9:263–286.

13 Fromageot C, Lofaso F, Annane D, Falaize L, Lejaille M, Clair B, Gajdos P, Raphael JC: Supine fall in lung volumes in the assessment of diaphragmatic weakness in neuromuscular disorders. Arch Phys Med Rehabil 2001;82: 123–128.

14 Wilson SH, Cooke NT, Edwards RHT, Spiro SG: Predicted normal values for maximal respiratory pressures in Caucasian adults and children. Thorax 1984;39:535–538.

15 Gaultier C, Zinman R: Maximal static pressures in healthy children. Respir Physiol 1983;51:45–61.

16 Tomalak W, Pogorzelski A, Prusak J: Normal values for maximal static inspiratory and expiratory pressures in healthy children. Pediatr Pulmonol 2002;34:42–46.

17 Choudhuri D, Aithal M, Kulkarni VA: Maximal expiratory pressure in residential and non-residential school children. Indian J Pediatr 2002;69:229–232.

18 Cook CD, Mead J, Orzalesi MM: Static volume-pressure characteristics of the respiratory system during maximal efforts. J Appl Physiol 1964;19:1016–1022.

19 Shardonofsky F, Perez-Chada D, Carmuega E, Milic-Emili J: Airway pressure during crying in healthy infants. Pediatr Pulmonol 1989;6: 14–18.

20 Shardonofsky F, Perez-Chada D, Milic-Emili J: Airway pressures during crying: An index of respiratory muscle strength in infants with neuromuscular disease. Pediatr Pulmonol 1991;10:172–177.

21 Miller JM, Moxham J, Green M: The maximal sniff in the assessment of diaphragm function in man. Clin Sci 1985;69:91–96.

22 Heritier F, Rahm F, Pasche P, Fitting J-W: Sniff nasal pressure. A noninvasive assessment of inspiratory muscle strength. Am J Respir Crit Care Med 1994;150:1678–1683.

23 Stefanutti D, Fitting J-W: Sniff nasal inspiratory pressure. Reference values in children. Am J Respir Crit Care Med 1999;159:107–111.

24 Rafferty GF, Leech S, Knight L, Moxham J, Greenough A: Sniff nasal inspiratory pressure in children. Pediatr Pulmonol 2000;25: 468–475.

25 Uldry C, Fitting J-W: Maximal values of sniff nasal inspiratory pressure in healthy subjects. Thorax 1995;50:371–375.

26 Iandelli I, Gorini M, Misuri G, Gigliotti F, Rosi E, Duranti R, Scano G: Assessing inspiratory muscle strength in patients with neurologic and neuromuscular diseases (comparative evaluation of two noninvasive techniques). Chest 2001;119:1108–1113.

27 Uldry C, Janssens JP, de Muralt B, Fitting JW: Sniff nasal inspiratory pressure in patients with chronic obstructive pulmonary disease. Eur Respir J 1997;10:1292–1296.

28 Hart N, Polkey MI, Sharshar T, Falaize L, Fauroux B, Raphael JC, Lofaso F: Limitations of sniff nasal pressure in patients with severe neuromuscular disease. J Neurol Neurosurg Psychiatry 2003;74:1685–1687.

29 Rafferty GF, Greenough A, Dimitriou G, Kavadia V, Laubscher B, Polkey MI, Harris ML, Moxham J: Assessment of neonatal diaphragm function using magnetic stimulation of the phrenic nerves. Am J Respir Crit Care Med 2000;162:2337–2340.

30 Stell IM, Tompkins S, Lovell AT, Goldstone JC, Moxham J: An in vivo comparison of a catheter mounted pressure transducer system with conventional balloon catheters. Eur Respir J 1999; 13:1158–1163.

31 Fauroux B, Pigeot J, Polkey MI, Roger G, Boulé M, Clément A, Lofaso F: Chronic stridor caused by laryngomalacia in children. Work of breathing and effects of noninvasive ventilatory assistance. Am J Respir Crit Care Med 2001;64: 1874–1878.

32 Scott C, Nickerson B, Sargen TC, Platzker A, Warburton D, Keens T: Developmental pattern of maximal transdiaphragmatic pressure in infants during crying. Pediatr Res 1983;17: 707–709.

33 Mills GH, Kyroussis D, Hamnegard CH, Polkey MI, Green M, Moxham J: Bilateral magnetic stimulation of the phrenic nerves from an anterolateral approach. Am J Respir Crit Care Med 1996;154:1099–1105.

34 Mills GH, Kyroussis D, Hamnegard C-H, Wragg S, Moxham J, Green M: Unilateral magnetic stimulation of the phrenic nerve. Thorax 1995;50:1162–1172.

35 Rafferty GF, Greenough A, Manczur T, Polkey MI, Harris ML, Heaton ND, Rela M, Moxham J: Magnetic phrenic nerve stimulation to assess diaphragm function in children following liver transplant. Pediatr Crit Care Med 2001;2:122–126.

36 Rafferty GF, Greenough A, Dimitriou G, Polkey MI, Long A, Davenport M, Moxham J: Assessment of neonatal diaphragmatic paralysis using magnetic phrenic nerve stimulation. Pediatr Pulmonol 1999;27:224–226.

37 Polkey MI, Kyroussis D, Keilty SEJ, Hamnegard CH, Mills GH, Green M, Moxham J: Exhaustive treadmill exercise does not reduce twitch transdiaphragmatic pressure in patients with COPD. Am J Respir Crit Care Med 1995;152:959–964.

38 Polkey MI, Kyroussis D, Hamnegard C-H, Hughes PD, Rafferty GF, Moxham J, Green M: Paired phrenic nerve stimuli for the detection of diaphragm fatigue. Eur Respir J 1997; 10:1859–1864.

39 Similowski T, Gauthier AP, Yan S, Macklem PT, Bellemare F: Assessment of diaphragm function using mouth pressure twitches in chronic obstructive pulmonary disease patients. Am Rev Respir Dis 1993;147:850–856.

40 Hamnegard CH, Wragg S, Kyroussis D, Mills G, Bake B, Green M, Moxham J: Mouth pressure in response to magnetic stimulation of the phrenic nerves. Thorax 1995;50:620–624.

41 Sprikkelman AB, van Eykern LA, Lourens MS, Heymans HS, van Aalderen WM: Respiratory muscle activity in the assessment of bronchial responsiveness in asthmatic children. J Appl Physiol 1998;84:897–901.

42 Maarsingh EJW, van Eykern LA, Sprikkelman AB, Hoekstra MO, van Aalderen WM: Respiratory muscle activity measured with a noninvasive EMG technique: Technical aspects and reproducibility. J Appl Physiol 2000;88:1955–1961.

43 Imai T, Shizukawa H, Imaizumi H, Shichinohe Y, Sato M, Kikuchi S, Hachiro Y, Ito M, Kashiwagi M, Chiba S, Matsumoto H: Phrenic nerve conduction in infancy and early childhood. Muscle Nerve 2000;23:915–918.

44 Raimbault J: Technique et résultats de l'exploration électromyographique du diaphragme chez le nourrisson et le jeune enfant. Neurophysiol Clin 1983;13:306–311.

45 Clanton TL, Celli BR, Calverly P: ATS/ERS Statement on respiratory muscle testing: Tests of respiratory muscle endurance. Am J Respir Crit Care Med 2002;166:559–569.

46 Matecki S, Topin N, Hayot M, Rivier F, Echenne B, Prefaut C, Ramonatxo M: A standardised method for the evaluation of respiratory muscle endurance in patients with Duchenne muscular dystrophy. Neuromuscul Disord 2001;11:171–177.

47 Hart N, Hawkins P, Hamnegard C-H, Green M, Moxham J, Polkey MI: A novel clinical test of respiratory muscle endurance. Eur Respir J 2002;19:232–239.

48 Baydur A, Adkins R, Milic-Emili J: Lung mechanics in individuals with spinal cord injury: Effects of injury level and posture. J Appl Physiol 2001;90:405–411.

49 Man WDC, Kyroussis D, Fleming TA, Chetta A, Harraf F, Mustfa N, Rafferty GF, Polkey MI, Moxham J: Cough gastric pressure and maximal expiratory mouth pressure in humans. Am J Respir Crit Care Med 2003;168:714–717.

50 Polkey MI, Luo Y, Guleria R, Hamnegard CH, Green M, Moxham J: Functional magnetic stimulation of the abdominal muscles in humans. Am J Respir Crit Care Med 1999;160:513–522.

51 Kyroussis D, Mills GH, Polkey MI, Hamnegard C-H, Koulouris N, Green M, Moxham J: Abdominal muscle fatigue after maximal ventilation in humans. J Appl Physiol 1996;81:1477–1483.

52 Polkey MI, Lyall RA, Green M, Leigh PN, Moxham J: Expiratory muscle function in amyotrophic lateral sclerosis. Am J Respir Crit Care Med 1998;158:734–741.

53 Polkey MI, Guleria R, Luo YM, Hamnegard C-H, Moxham J, Green M: Functional magnetic stimulation for cough. Am J Respir Crit Care Med 1998;157:A663.

54 Estenne M, Pinet C, De Troyer A: Abdominal muscle strength in patients with tetraplegia. Am J Respir Crit Care Med 2000;161:707–712.

55 Lessard MR, Lofaso F, Brochard L: Expiratory muscle activity increases intrinsic positive end-expiratory pressure independently of dynamic hyperinflation in mechanically ventilated patients. Am J Respir Crit Care Med 1995;143:459–475.

56 Lofaso F, Brochard L, Hang T, Lorino H, Harf A, Isabey D: Home versus intensive care pressure support devices. Experimental and clinical comparison. Am J Respir Crit Care Med 1996;153:1591–1599.

57 Praud JP, D'Allest A, Nedelcoux H, Curzi-Dascalova L, Guilleminault C, Gaultier C: Sleep-related abdominal muscle behavior during partial or complete obstructed breathing in prepubertal children. Pediatr Res 1989;26:347–350.

58 Phillips M, Quinlivan RC, Edwards RH, Calverly PM: Changes in spirometry over time as a prognostic marker in patients with Duchenne muscular dystrophy. Am J Respir Crit Care Med 2001;164:2191–2194.

59 Hukins CA, Hillman DR: Daytime predictors of sleep hypoventilation in Duchenne muscular dystrophy. Am J Respir Crit Care Med 2000;161:166–170.

60 Raguette R, Mellies U, Schwake C, Voit T, Teschler H: Patterns and predictors of sleep disordered breathing in primary myopathies. Thorax 2002;57:724–728.

61 Mellies U, Ragette R, Schwake C, Bochm H, Voit T, Teschler H: Datime predictors of sleep disordered breathing in children and adolescents with neuromuscular disorders. Neuromuscul Disord 2003;13:123–128.

62 Manczur TI, Greenough A, Rafferty GF, Dimitriou G, Baker AJ, Mieli-Vergani G, Rela SM, Heaton N: Diaphragmatic dysfunction after pediatric orthotopic liver transplantation. Transplantation 2002;73:228–232.

Brigitte Fauroux
Pediatric Pulmonology and INSERM E 213
Hôpital Armand Trousseau
Assistance Publique – Hôpitaux de Paris
28 avenue du Docteur Arnold Netter
FR–75012 Paris (France)
Tel. +33 1 44 73 61 74
Fax +33 1 74 67 18
E-Mail brigitte.fauroux@trs.ap-hop-paris.fr

Hammer J, Eber E (eds): Paediatric Pulmonary Function Testing.
Prog Respir Res. Basel, Karger, 2005, vol 33, pp 148–156

Measurements of Thoraco-Abdominal Asynchrony and Work of Breathing in Children

Christopher J.L. Newth[a]   Jürg Hammer[b]

[a]Division of Critical Care Medicine, Children's Hospital Los Angeles, University of Southern California School of Medicine, Los Angeles, Calif., USA;
[b]Division of Intensive Care and Pulmonology, University Children's Hospital Basel, Basel, Switzerland

Abstract

Respiratory muscle fatigue is considered a common cause of respiratory failure, but its detection is hampered by the lack of satisfactory diagnostic tests. Thoraco-abdominal asynchrony, the non-coincident movement of the rib cage and abdomen during breathing, is expressed as a phase angle by applying electrical sine wave theory and analysis. It has been proposed as a clinical index of fatigue, but its sensitivity and specificity as a predictor of outcome are unknown. At this time, it remains a useful, non-invasive indicator of respiratory muscle load, and can be used to determine response to therapy in the individual patient. Energy turnover during muscle activity cannot as yet be measured, so approximate indicators such as work performance and tension-time index are used for this purpose. Work of breathing, pressure-time product, and pressure-rate product are variables that describe the activity of respiratory muscles. While these do not exactly reflect the energy expenditure required for breathing, they are relatively easily measured, if slightly more invasive (oesophageal catheter) than phase angle measurements. They have gained acceptance as useful tools for evaluation of the breathing efforts of critically ill patients.

Thoraco-Abdominal Asynchrony

Thoraco-abdominal asynchrony (TAA), the non-coincident motion of the rib cage (RC) and abdomen (ABD) during breathing, is often used as an indication of respiratory distress. If the RC is sucked in or retracted as abdominal excursions occur (e.g., acute laryngotracheobronchitis), or the ABD is retracted as the RC expands (e.g., diaphragmatic paralysis), or respiratory muscles are activated at different times in the breathing cycle, then asynchrony results. TAA and paradoxical breathing are often observed in infants and children with various forms of respiratory diseases including upper airway obstruction, parenchymal processes (such as hyaline membrane disease, pneumonia, and pulmonary oedema), obstructive lower airways disease [asthma, bronchiolitis, bronchopulmonary dysplasia (BPD)], and neuromuscular diseases. However, this phenomenon has generally been descriptive and referred to as chest wall retractions in clinical scoring systems. It has been previously shown that TAA can be easily detected, quantified and monitored objectively by phase angle analysis of the Lissajous figure [1, 2]. In this technique, RC and ABD movements are recorded by use of an uncalibrated respiratory inductance plethysmograph, the bands of which are placed at the levels of the nipples and upper ABD [see also 3]. The analogue output of the RC and ABD movements is obtained by a computerized data acquisition system that is programmed to calculate continuously phase angles utilizing the method of Agostoni and Mognoni [4]. The phase angle (θ) is thus calculated according to the equation:

$$\sin \theta = m/s$$

where m is the length of the midpoint of the RC excursion and s is the length depicting the ABD excursion (fig. 1). In

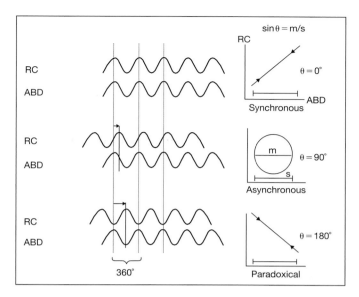

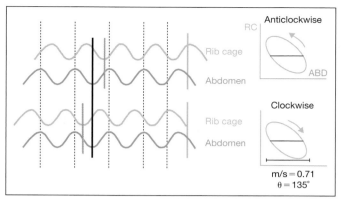

Fig. 1. Lissajous loops and phase angle analysis. The signals from the bands around the RC and the ABD are treated mathematically as sine waves. The phase angle (θ) is thus calculated according to the equation sin θ = m/s, where m is the length of the midpoint of the RC excursion and s is the length depicting the ABD excursion. When the two respiratory compartments are in synchrony (upper panel) the phase angle is zero. As asynchrony appears and worsens the phase angle increases (middle panel) until the two compartments are 180° out of phase (lower panel) where the RC is contracting at the same time the abdominal compartment expands.

Fig. 2. The direction of loop rotation is determined by whether the abdominal muscles contract before or after the intercostal (RC) muscles. Upper panel traces: The diaphragm is the major muscle of respiration and its activity (plotted on the x-axis) usually precedes that of the RC (plotted on the y-axis), where the intercostal muscles react to its contraction. This results in an anticlockwise or counterclockwise loop. Lower panel traces: Here, the intercostal activity precedes the diaphragm motion, as seen on the traces (left) and the plot moves up the y-axis first followed by abdominal movement plotted on the x-axis. A clockwise loop results.

addition, RC and ABD movements can be continuously displayed as an X-Y plot giving optical information about changes in loop shape and loop direction [5].

Except during REM sleep, the RC and ABD expand and decrease in synchrony in normal full-term infants and children, producing a closed or very narrow loop with a positive slope on the X-Y plot. However, during TAA the loop opens and becomes progressively wider as TAA increases. Paradoxical breathing also creates a closed or very narrow loop, but with a negative slope. Important information can further be obtained from the direction of loop rotation. Direction of loop rotation indicates which compartment (RC or ABD) precedes the other. Anticlockwise loops indicate that the ABD compartment (diaphragm) leads the RC as usually observed in normal quiet breathing and most forms of respiratory distress in children. Clockwise loops signify the opposite which is typically associated with bilateral diaphragmatic paralysis (fig. 2). Actual clinical examples are shown in figure 3. In the special case of unilateral paralysis figure-of-eight loops are produced (fig. 4, see below).

A problem often encountered with this technique is that at various times phase angle loops are not based on clear sinusoidal RC and ABD movements, thereby producing numerous types of non-sinusoidal patterns. While the original Lissajous figure (loop) analysis is remarkably strong, Prisk et al. [6] have recently suggested that a sine wave-independent mathematical approach in loop analysis improves the accuracy of phase shift calculations under such circumstances. They concluded that phase angles are best measured using cross-correlation or maximum linear correlation, techniques that are independent of waveform shape, and robust in the presence of noise.

Work of Breathing

Inspiratory work of breathing (WOB) is calculated from the curve of oesophageal pressure (P_{oes}) versus tidal volume (VT). The WOB per breath can be computed from a Campbell diagram by calculating the area enclosed between the recorded P_{oes}-VT curve during inspiration on the one hand, and the static chest wall compliance curve on the other. The WOB can be expressed as joules per litre of ventilation (J/l) and as power normalized by body weight

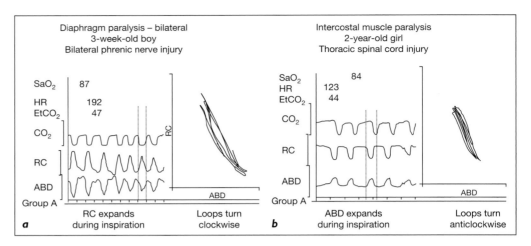

Fig. 3. Clinical examples of paradoxical breathing movements. **a** The patient has bilateral diaphragm paralysis. The RC movement precedes the ABD, and RC and ABD traces move paradoxically with the ABD compartment becoming smaller (more negative) and the RC compartment becoming larger (more positive). The resulting Lissajous loops are 170–180° and clockwise. **b** The patient has a high thoracic spinal cord injury. Again, the RC and ABD traces are paradoxical, but this time the ABD movement precedes the RC with the resulting Lissajous loops being again 170–180° but anticlockwise.

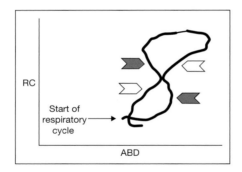

Fig. 4. Representative Lissajous plot of a patient with unilateral diaphragmatic paralysis. Note the initial abdominal excursion and anticlockwise loop of the normal hemidiaphragm (hatched arrows), followed by incursion of the ABD and a clockwise finish as the intercostal muscles contract and pull the other hemidiaphragm up (open arrows).

(J/min/kg or g·cm/kg). The inspiratory muscle load can also be measured using the pressure-time product (PTP) since this is regarded as an index of the oxygen cost of breathing of the respiratory muscles [7] as well as WOB [8]. Under these conditions, the PTP is calculated as the area subtended by the oesophageal pressure tracing and the chest wall static recoil pressure for inspiratory time (fig. 5). Since these measurements require accurate knowledge of inspiratory flow, they are not suitable for application to

infants and children without an artificial airway. Takeuchi et al. [9] extended this technique to non-intubated infants by showing that a modified PTP (PTPmod) using the maximum negative deflection of oesophageal pressure and inspiratory time recorded from a respiratory inductance plethysmography device faithfully followed the original PTP in all situations. The PTP and PTPmod are expressed as $cm H_2O \cdot s \cdot min^{-1}$.

A further modification allowed the 'work' of breathing in both intubated and unintubated infants and children to be measured relatively simply and non-invasively by use of an oesophageal balloon alone to record pleural pressure changes and respiratory rate with subsequent calculation of the pressure-time integral if the pleural pressure signal is integrated (also expressed as $cm H_2O \cdot s \cdot min^{-1}$) or the pressure-time index (PTI) if it is not and the raw signal alone used (recorded as $cm H_2O \cdot min^{-1}$). The latter is now more commonly and accurately referred to as the pressure-rate product (PRP). This index is an estimate of the energy cost of the 'work' of breathing because oxygen consumption by muscle is proportional to the integral of muscle tension (or pressure) with respect to time [10]. Klein and Reynolds [11] demonstrated that when the unintegrated pleural pressure signal was used in the index, they could show a response to therapy with continuous inflating pressure in sleep-related upper airway obstruction. Since breathing slows and inspiratory pressure is greater with upper airway obstruction, the

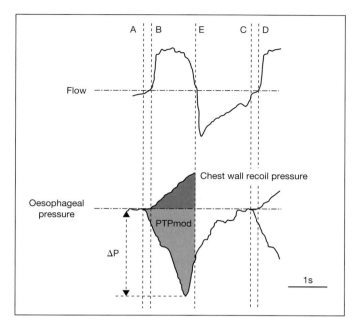

Fig. 5. The upper panel represents flow obtained with inspiration being upwards or positive. The lower panel represents oesophageal pressure with negative deflection during inspiration, and chest wall recoil pressure being positive. Both are plotted over time. During initial inspiratory effort (line A), there is a short time when there is negative oesophageal pressure with no inspiratory flow recorded on the pneumotachograph. This represents the effort required to overcome intrinsic PEEP and initiate inspiration. Thereafter, flow starts (line B) from which point the PTP is measured – the area subtended by the chest wall recoil pressure and the oesophageal pressure. After the patient is extubated there is no direct measurement of airflow. This requires that the inspiratory time be estimated from an independent recording (in this case a respiratory inductance plethysmography device). The area subtended by the negative deflection of the oesophageal trace during the time of inspiration (line A–E) is the PTPmod. The PRP uses the unintegrated or 'raw' oesophageal (pleural) pressure trace. The peak-to-trough negative deflection is ΔP and the respiratory rate is determined from the time of the respiratory cycle (line A–C) [modified from 9].

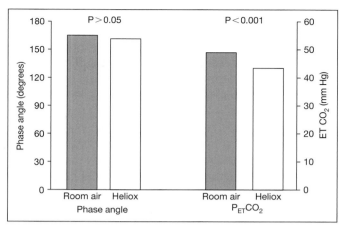

Fig. 6. Ten anaesthetized rhesus monkeys were subjected to graded inspiratory resistances of $1,000 \, \text{cm} \, H_2O \cdot l^{-1} \cdot s^{-1}$. The phase angles increased up to $165°$ as the end-tidal CO_2 ($P_{ET}CO_2$) values went from 39 to 49 mm Hg while breathing room air, indicating respiratory failure. After recording for 10 min at $1,000 \, \text{cm} \, H_2O \cdot l^{-1} \cdot s^{-1}$, heliox was given (79% He/21% O_2) and the respiratory failure resolved with the CO_2 tension returning to normal ($\Delta P_{ET}CO_2$; $p < 0.001$). However, the phase angle remained unchanged ($\Delta PA > 0.05$) confirming that load, not respiratory failure was being measured [modified from 13].

'raw' PTI (or PRP) underestimates the true integrated PTI. Nonetheless, this seems a simple and effective objective measurement for upper airway obstruction.

Clinical Applications and Indications for Measurements of Breathing Pattern and WOB in Children

Thoraco-Abdominal Asynchrony

Continuous phase angle measurement is a promising non-invasive technique for the objective assessment of TAA in a variety of respiratory diseases. However, the technique requires further research to find a better understanding of its predictive value for respiratory fatigue. Earlier work by Tobin et al. [12] in normal adult subjects suggested that TAA reflected respiratory load but not respiratory muscle fatigue. More recently, Hammer et al. [13] have validated phase angle measurements in rhesus monkeys, by showing that they correlated with the level of the imposed respiratory load but did not detect respiratory muscle fatigue, in the setting of acute inspiratory upper airway obstruction. In this study, 10 anaesthetized rhesus monkeys were subjected to graded inspiratory resistances from 5 to $1,000 \, \text{cm} \, H_2O/l/s$. The phase angles increased from normal values of $22°$ up to $165°$ as the end-tidal CO_2 values went from 39 to 49 mm Hg while breathing room air, indicating respiratory failure. There was poor correlation between increasing phase angle and end-tidal CO_2 confirming that the phase angle determined from thoracic and abdominal interaction detected respiratory load well but not respiratory failure. After recording for 10 min at the highest resistance, heliox was given (79% He/21% O_2), and the respiratory failure resolved with the CO_2 tension returning to normal. However, the phase angle remained unchanged confirming that load, not respiratory failure, was being measured (fig. 6).

Phase angles are elevated in cases of acute upper airway obstruction such as infectious croup [14] and postextubation subglottic oedema, and decrease after α-agonist therapy [1]. These responses are consistent with changes in the degree of stridor and are accompanied by improvements in inspiratory flows and tidal volumes. Measurement of TAA has also given valuable insights into mechanisms of chronic upper airway obstruction in infants and young children with adenotonsillar hypertrophy. Reber et al. [15], in a series of studies on anaesthetized children with adenotonsillar hypertrophy, showed that airway opening manoeuvres such as jaw thrust, continuous positive airway pressure (CPAP) and chin lift have distinct effects on TAA. Delivery of CPAP and jaw thrust can be the first airway opening manoeuvres to improve breathing patterns. Most importantly, the authors demonstrated that chin lift without additional CPAP should be used with caution in these patients because it may convert partial into almost complete airway obstruction. This reinforces the use of an oropharyngeal airway when controlling the airway of unconscious children with manual ventilation through a face mask.

In a group of 110 children (ages 1–50 months), Sivan et al. [16] assessed TAA while the children underwent diagnostic daytime polygraphic sleep studies, and correlated the results. TAA was calculated by the phase angle technique and compared to normal values derived from a separate group of 45 control children, matched for age and weight. They concluded that TAA measurement by the phase angle technique may be an important adjunct to the evaluation of breathing disorders during sleep in small children and it may be a good screening test for small children as to their need for more extensive polysomnographic testing.

Phase angle analysis has also been applied in children with obstructive airway diseases such as BPD [17], and in asthmatics and other patients who have shown improvement clinically and by decreasing phase angles after bronchodilator therapy [2].

Bilateral diaphragmatic paralysis (e.g. from phrenic nerve injury following cardiothoracic surgery or liver transplant surgery) can be easily detected at the bedside by the characteristic generation of clockwise loops and highly abnormal phase angles near 180°, even when this may not be very obvious clinically [18]. Infants and young children are predominantly dependent on their diaphragms for respiration and tolerate any diaphragm dysfunction poorly, be it from phrenic nerve injury or from ascites or pneumoperitoneum affecting diaphragm excursion. This phenomenon is age-related, and older children and adults can tolerate weak or absent diaphragm function much better. In the acute situation in the infant or younger child, when the

patient cannot be weaned from the ventilator, mechanical efficiency can be improved by 'medical' plication of the diaphragms and impeding distortion of the RC by elevated positive end-expiratory pressure (PEEP). Less ventilator support is needed using this strategy but the technique does not improve the phase angle [18].

In the case of unilateral paralysis the repeated Lissajous loops with the characteristic figure-of-eight appearance are virtually diagnostic, particularly after cardiothoracic surgery (fig. 4). However, the figure-of-eight Lissajous loop is also observed intermittently in severe BPD [19], and diagnostic caution must be used if such a patient has had recent thoracic or hepatic surgery. It is also noted in cases of unilateral diaphragm dysfunction from other causes (e.g. congenital) and the change in the slope of the Lissajous figures (of eight) with age is shown in figure 7. After surgical plication of the affected diaphragm, there is marked improvement in the figure-of-eight appearance with lessening TAA, but there is not a return to normal.

The use of phase angle analysis to monitor TAA in infants and children with other forms of neuromuscular disease (e.g. infantile botulism, Guillain-Barré syndrome, myopathies, neuropathies, spinal cord injuries) needs to be further clarified. In a group consisting of 31 patients with spinal muscular atrophy and 19 patients with undefined myopathies, Perez et al. [20] noted marked abnormalities of the phase angle and other parameters measured by respiratory inductance plethysmography, which improved nearly back to normal with intermittent positive pressure breathing of 25–30 cm H_2O. In cases of infantile botulism and Guillain-Barré syndrome being observed for the advent of respiratory failure, we have anecdotal experience suggesting that Lissajous loop analysis gives an earlier indication of diaphragm involvement than clinical observation, especially when breathing efforts are stressed such as in crying [21].

WOB, PRP, PTI, PTP, Pressure-Time Integral

In 1986, Klein and Reynolds [11] used the PTI to evaluate the effect on respiratory distress of continuous insufflation of the pharynx (CIP) with warmed, humidified air. They treated 20 children with chronic oropharyngeal airway obstruction in this manner and showed convincingly that breathing frequency and peak-to-trough pleural pressure decreased with CIP, as did their product, the PTI. The latter two variables had highly convincing decreases statistically (fig. 8). Chronic upper airway obstruction caused by laryngomalacia was also reviewed in 2001 when Fauroux et al. [22] recorded the WOB in 5 awake infants and children. They used the PTP (pressure-time integral as defined above) and found it decreased from 541 ± 197 cm

Fig. 7. a Phase angles of acute right diaphragm paralysis of 5 different children at increasing ages from 6 weeks to 5 years are shown. At 6 weeks of age there is a figure-of-eight Lissajous loop with a very abnormal phase angle of close to 180°. This represents almost no intercostal muscle activity to compensate for the poor diaphragm function. As the patients become older, the Lissajous loops still have the figure-of-eight appearance, but the phase angle improves back towards normal, demonstrating the greater ability with age of the intercostal muscles to compensate for the weak hemidiaphragm. **b** The same effect of age is shown in 4 different children (from 2 weeks to 7 years) when the left hemidiaphragm is acutely affected.

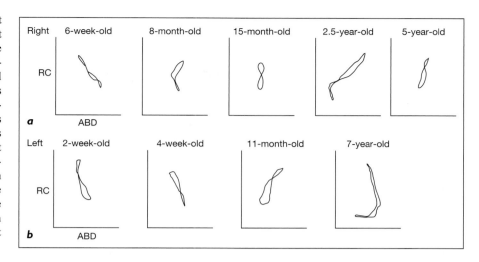

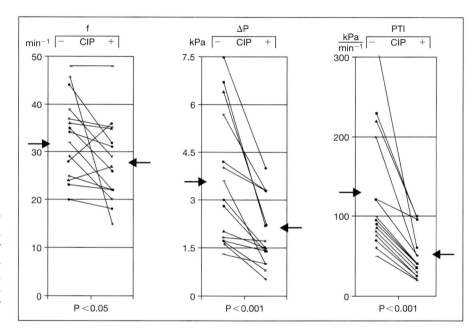

Fig. 8. Effects of CIP on breathing frequency (f), oesophageal pressure change per breath (ΔP) and the PTI or PRP (PTI or PRP = f × ΔP) in 20 sleeping children with obstructive sleep apnoea. Values for each child are the mean of 2–4 brief interruptions of the CIP. Arrows indicate mean values for the group [redrawn from 11].

$H_2O \cdot s \cdot min^{-1}$ while spontaneously breathing to 215 ± 116 cm $H_2O \cdot s \cdot min^{-1}$ when on non-invasive mechanical ventilation support. They also noted an improvement in end-tidal CO_2, and that the PTP decreased with age when spontaneously breathing.

Acute upper airway obstruction in the form of acute laryngotracheobronchitis (croup) was investigated in 20 children by Argent and Klein [23], and compared with 5 normal children. They reported values for WOB of 2,202 (639–7,586) versus 605 (470–1,104) g · cm/kg in croup versus controls. Similarly, the PRP were 2,120 versus 312 cm

$H_2O \cdot min^{-1}$, and the pressure-time integral 1,618 versus 299 cm $H_2O \cdot s \cdot min^{-1}$, respectively.

WOB, PTP and PTPmod were measured in 7 infants while weaning from mechanical ventilation after cardiac surgery [9]. As could be predicted from the previous study [22], the WOB, PTP and PTPmod increased as pressure support ventilation was decreased, and PTPmod declined again after extubation to the level recorded at 4 cm H_2O of pressure support. This work was extended by the same group [24] to the effect of synchronized intermittent mandatory ventilation (SIMV) on respiratory workload in

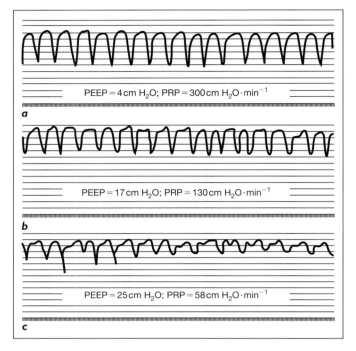

PEEP = 4 cm H$_2$O; PRP = 300 cm H$_2$O·min^{-1}

a

PEEP = 17 cm H$_2$O; PRP = 130 cm H$_2$O·min^{-1}

b

PEEP = 25 cm H$_2$O; PRP = 58 cm H$_2$O·min^{-1}

c

Fig. 9. The decline in the WOB is demonstrated as reflected by the PRP, when a spontaneously breathing but intubated child with severe asthma has external PEEP applied to counterbalance her intrinsic PEEP. *a–c* Oesophageal pressure traces (P$_{oes}$) over time are represented, on the same scales. The PRP is the average peak to trough change in pressure multiplied by the respiratory rate (RR), calculated from the same trace. *a* PRP is calculated at 300 cm H$_2$O·min^{-1} (RR = 60, ΔP$_{oes}$ = 5) when external PEEP is 4 cm H$_2$O. b PRP is calculated at 130 cm H$_2$O · min^{-1} (RR = 35, ΔP$_{oes}$ = 3.7) when external PEEP is 17 cm H$_2$O. *c* PRP is calculated at 58 cm H$_2$O · min^{-1} (RR = 36, ΔP$_{oes}$ = 1.6) when external PEEP is 25 cm H$_2$O. In other words, the effort needed by the patient to initiate a breath is decreased as the applied PEEP is increased.

11 infants aged 2–11 months after cardiac surgery. Five levels of SIMV between 0 and 20 breaths/min were applied randomly. At the lower rates (that is, decreased SIMV support) the WOB and PTP increased.

The role of the PTP in predicting extubation failure was investigated by Manczur et al. [25], who sampled 42 patients (median age 13 months) judged clinically ready to be extubated. The PTP was measured from spontaneous tidal breaths during ventilatory support and was found to be poorly predictive of extubation success under these circumstances (32.0 vs. 32.9 cm H$_2$O · s · min^{-1}, success vs. failure, respectively).

The PRP was used to evaluate the effect on the WOB of applying various levels of PEEP and pressure support breaths to 10 intubated but spontaneously breathing

children with severely obstructed airways [26]. Increasing levels of both pressure support and PEEP, randomly applied, significantly decreased the WOB as reflected by the PRP, but there was a more marked beneficial effect with increasing PEEP (fig. 9). This is consistent with the notion of applying PEEP to negate the effect of intrinsic PEEP in this particular clinical situation and make it easier for the patient to initiate each breath.

Comparative Data: Phase Angles versus PTP and PRP

Takeuchi et al. [9] measured WOB by classical methods, along with PTP in intubated infants, while decreasing the amount of support given for each patient-triggered breath on the ventilator, and again after extubation using a PTPmod. They showed all three measurements increased as support lessened, and decreased again following extubation. They also measured several variables using respiratory inductance plethysmography, reporting a ratio of maximum compartment amplitude to tidal volume where the RC and ABD movements are out of phase when the ratio exceeds 1.0. Unfortunately, they did not report any phase angle measurements. The maximum compartment amplitude to tidal volume ratio was above 1.0 in each case and also increased (worsened) with lessening ventilator support. However, like the WOB measurement it was a poor discriminator statistically between each level of support. Conversely, the PRP and PRPmod were excellent discriminators.

Newth et al. [27] compared the PRP and phase angle measurements in ten anaesthetized rhesus monkeys under conditions of graded increases in inspiratory resistance from 0 to 1,000 cm H$_2$O/l/s. They concluded that while both measurements became more abnormal with increasing respiratory load, PRP was a better discriminator especially when the load exceeded 200 cm H$_2$O/l/s (fig. 10).

There have been no published series of comparisons of PRP and phase angles in humans. However, in a case report by Willis et al. [18], both measurements were taken in a 23-month-old child with bilateral diaphragmatic paralysis after cardiac surgery. The observations were later confirmed in another child with the same condition after a liver transplant. Both children were in respiratory failure requiring mechanically assisted ventilation, and in both cases the phase angles of spontaneous breaths were between 170° and 180° with clockwise loops confirming non-functioning diaphragms. The PRP were high in both while taking unassisted breaths on zero end-expiratory pressure and their breathing was very laboured. The PRP decreased

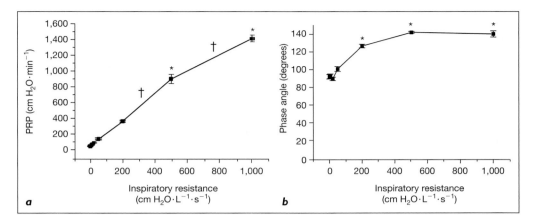

Fig. 10. The PRP and phase angles were measured at the same time in 10 anaesthetized rhesus monkeys under conditions of graded increases in inspiratory resistance from 0 to 1,000 cm $H_2O \cdot l^{-1} \cdot s^{-1}$. *a* PRP plotted against inspiratory resistance. There was a gradual, almost linear, increase in PRP with resistance, with good discrimination between workloads. * $p < 0.05$ from baseline; † $p < 0.05$ from adjacent value. *b* Phase angles plotted against inspiratory resistance. There is a gradual but non-linear increase in phase angles with inspiratory load. * $p < 0.05$ from baseline. The discrimination between loads is not as good as with PRP.

dramatically with increasing PEEP up to 24 cm H_2O, and breathing became comfortable with no mechanical assistance required. However, the phase angles remained unchanged. One reasonable explanation is that in each case while the diaphragms could not be made to function because of the phrenic nerve lesions, their dysfunction was lessened by 'medical plication' from the PEEP. That is, the diaphragms could not move paradoxically with inspiration thus interfering with RC muscle function. The increased pressure also made it easier for the RC muscle activity to initiate inspiration by preventing distortion of the RC itself. In this situation, phase angles are useful in identifying the extent of the problem but cannot reflect the respiratory load – that can be done only by the PRP measurement. It is tempting to speculate that a successful 'medical' plication continued over some days might be predictive of success following surgical plication.

In summary, the PRP has the advantage of directly measuring the work imposed and has the relative disadvantage of being slightly invasive, requiring the insertion of an oesophageal balloon. The phase angle measurement does not directly reflect the work imposed but increasing TAA mirrors the physiological effect on the infant the increased load is causing.

Normal Data: Phase Angles and PRP

There have been several studies which have included measurements of phase angles in normal children. Allen et al. [17] observed 6 infants to have mean phase angles of 8° (range 0–15°). Sivan et al. [1] noted phase angles of 11.5° (range 3–25°) in 30 normal children aged from 1 to 50 months and with a weight from 3.1 to 20 kg irrespective of clinical sleep stage in their first study, and phase angles of 11.8° (range 0–24°) in 45 normal children aged from 1 to 50 months and with a weight from 2 to 22 kg irrespective of polysomnographic sleep stage in their second study [16].

There were slight methodological differences in the measurements of phase angles between the two groups of investigators. However, it appears safe to conclude that in the 1-month-old infant to the 4-year-old child, a normal phase angle is less than 25° regardless of sleep stage.

There is a dearth of published normal values for WOB, PRP, and pressure-time integral, with Argent and Klein [23] reporting 5 children aged 5–31 months who were studied while sedated with chloral hydrate for electroencephalography for the investigation of previous seizures. The mean WOB was 605 g · cm/kg (range 470–1,104), the mean PRP was 312 cm $H_2O \cdot min^{-1}$ (range 196–430), and the mean pressure-time integral was 299 cm $H_2O \cdot s \cdot min^{-1}$ (range 197–537).

The two variables used in PRP and pressure-time integral are respiratory rate and oesophageal pressure, both of which vary with age, the former decreasing and the latter increasing. Hence, normal values need also to be age-related to be useful. In most studies, each patient is used as his own control to show the effect of an intervention.

Measurements of Thoraco-Abdominal Asynchrony and Work of Breathing in Children

References

1 Sivan Y, Deakers TW, Newth CJL: Thoracoabdominal asynchrony in acute upper airway obstruction in small children. Am Rev Respir Dis 1990;142:540–544.

2 Allen JL, Wolfson MR, McDowell K, Shaffer TH: Thoracoabdominal asynchrony in infants with airflow obstruction. Am Rev Respir Dis 1990;141:337–342.

3 Lødrup Carlsen KC, Carlsen K.-H: Tidal breathing measurements; Hammer J, Eber E (eds): Paediatric Pulmonary Function Testing. Prog Respir Res. Basel, Karger, 2005, vol 33, pp 10–19.

4 Agostoni E, Mognoni E: Deformation of chest wall during breathing efforts. J Appl Physiol 1966;21:1827–1832.

5 Henny K, Richardson GA: Principles of Radio, ed 6. New York, Wiley, 1952, pp 576–579.

6 Prisk GK, Hammer J, Newth CJL: Techniques for measurement of thoracoabdominal asynchrony. Pediatr Pulmonol 2002;34:462–472.

7 McGregor M, Becklake MR: The relationship of oxygen cost of breathing to respiratory mechanical work and respiratory force. J Clin Invest 1967;40:971–980.

8 Sassoon CSH, Mahutte CK: Work of breathing during mechanical ventilation; in Marini JJ, Slutsky AS (eds): Physiological Basis of Ventilatory Support. New York, Dekker, 1998, pp 261–310.

9 Takeuchi M, Imanaka H, Miyano H, Kumon K, Nishimura M: Effect of patient-triggered ventilation on respiratory workload in infants after cardiac surgery. Anesthesiology 2000;93:1238–1244.

10 Collett PW, Perry C, Engel LA: Pressure-time product, flow and oxygen cost of resistive breathing in humans. J Appl Physiol 1985;58:1263–1272.

11 Klein M, Reynolds LG: Relief of sleep-related oropharyngeal airway obstruction by continuous insufflation of the pharynx. Lancet 1986;i:935–939.

12 Tobin MJ, Perez W, Guenther SM, Lodato RF, Dantzker DR: Does rib cage-abdominal paradox signify respiratory muscle fatigue? J Appl Physiol 1987;63:851–860.

13 Hammer J, Newth CJ, Deakers TW: Validation of the phase angle technique as an objective measure of upper airway obstruction. Pediatr Pulmonol 1995;19:167–173.

14 Davis GM, Cooper DM, Mitchell I: The measurement of thoraco-abdominal asynchrony in infants with severe laryngotracheobronchitis. Chest 1993;103:1842–1848.

15 Reber A, Bobbia SA, Hammer J, Frei FJ: Effect of airway opening manoeuvres on thoracoabdominal asynchrony in anaesthetized children. Eur Respir J 2001;17:1239–1243.

16 Sivan Y, Ward SD, Deakers T, Keens TG, Newth CJ: Rib cage to abdominal asynchrony in children undergoing polygraphic sleep studies. Pediatr Pulmonol 1991;11:141–146.

17 Allen JL, Greenspan JS, Deoras KS, Keklikian E, Wolfson MR, Shaffer TH: Interaction between chest wall motion and lung mechanics in normal infants and infants with bronchopulmonary dysplasia. Pediatr Pulmonol 1991;11:37–43.

18 Willis BC, Graham AS, Wetzel R, Newth CJL: Respiratory inductance plethysmography used to diagnose bilateral diaphragmatic paralysis: A case report. Pediatr Crit Care Med 2004;5:399–402.

19 Goldman MD, Pagani M, Trang HT, Praud JP, Sartene R, Gaultier C: Asynchronous chest wall movements during non-rapid eye movement and rapid eye movement sleep in children with bronchopulmonary dysplasia. Am Rev Respir Dis 1993;147:1175–1184.

20 Perez A, Mulot R, Vardon G, Barois A, Gallego J: Thoracoabdominal pattern of breathing in neuromuscular disorders. Chest 1996;110:454–461.

21 Hammer J, Frei F, Rutishauser M, Newth CJL: Thoracoabdominal breathing patterns in infants with neuromuscular diseases. Eur Respir J 1997;10(suppl 25):32S.

22 Fauroux B, Pigeot J, Polkey MI, Roger G, Boulé M, Clément A, Lofaso F: Chronic stridor caused by laryngomalacia in children: Work of breathing and effects of noninvasive ventilatory assistance. Am J Respir Crit Care Med 2001;164:1874–1878.

23 Argent AC, Klein M: Pressure time index (PTI): A simple objective measure of airway obstruction in croup. Am Rev Respir Dis 1995;151:A742.

24 Imanaka H, Nishimura M, Miyano H, Uemura H, Yagihara T: Effect of synchronized intermittent mandatory ventilation on respiratory workload in infants after cardiac surgery. Anesthesiology 2001;95:881–888.

25 Manczur TI, Greenough A, Pryor D, Rafferty GF: Assessment of respiratory drive and muscle function in the pediatric intensive care unit and prediction of extubation failure. Pediatr Crit Care Med 2000;1:124–126.

26 Graham AS, Chandrashekharajah G, Citak A, Wetzel R, Newth CJL: Influence of positive end expiratory pressure and pressure support on work of breathing in children with obstructive airways disease. Am J Respir Crit Care Med 2003;167:A515.

27 Newth CJL, Adams JA, Sackner MA, Klein M, Hammer J: Upper airway obstruction in rhesus monkeys: Comparison of pressure-rate product and phase angle measurements. Am J Respir Crit Care Med 1998;157:A471.

Christopher J.L. Newth, MB, FRCPC
Professor of Pediatrics, Mail Stop #12
PICU Administration
Children's Hospital Los Angeles
4650 Sunset Boulevard
Los Angeles, CA 90027 (USA)
Tel. +1 323 669 2557
Fax +1 323 664 0728
E-Mail cnewth@chla.usc.edu

Hammer J, Eber E (eds): Paediatric Pulmonary Function Testing.
Prog Respir Res. Basel, Karger, 2005, vol 33, pp 157–165

Lung Diffusing Capacity

J.C. de Jongste[a]   P.J.F.M. Merkus[a]   H. Stam[b]

[a]Department of Pediatrics, Division of Pediatric Respiratory Medicine and [b]Department of
Pulmonology, Erasmus MC University Medical Center, Sophia Children's Hospital, Rotterdam,
The Netherlands

Abstract

Transfer of oxygen and carbon dioxide over the alveolocapillary membrane is the main function of the lungs and can be
measured by the diffusing capacity for carbon monoxide (CO).
CO has a high affinity for hemoglobin and is absent in
pulmonary capillary blood. After inspiration CO diffuses by the
pressure gradient from the alveoli into the capillary blood and
disappears from the alveolar gas. The reduction of CO in alveolar gas in a fixed time interval quantifies the diffusing capacity
of the lungs and is expressed per unit lung volume. Lung volume
is measured simultaneously with CO diffusion by means of
helium dilution. For children who cannot perform the single-
breath maneuver or who have a lung volume below 1.5 liters
this technique is not feasible. In this case a rebreathing method
can be used where the decay of CO is monitored continuously
in a closed system while the child breathes quietly.

Diffusion measurements have several pitfalls. The measurements are inaccurate in case of severe airway obstruction due
to inadequate time for equilibration of the gases in the airways. At reduced lung volume, diffusion per unit lung volume
increases and this may lead to erroneous interpretation of
data in children with restrictive lung disease. In this case the
use of appropriate reference values, obtained at the relevant
lung volumes, is mandatory. Falsely high diffusing capacity may
be found due to the presence of blood in the airways and
alveoli, or in the case of relative hyperperfusion. Indications
for assessment of diffusing capacity in children include monitoring during and after chemotherapy or irradiation, diagnosis
and monitoring of interstitial lung disease, and monitoring for
pulmonary bleeding disorders. Other possible applications
are assessment of residual lung disease in children with
congenital lung disease or after neonatal lung damage, and
monitoring of lung function in children with chest deformities
and/or neuromuscular disease.

Background

The main function of the lungs is to establish oxygen
(O_2) and carbon dioxide (CO_2) exchange between body tissues and the ambient air. The passage of gases across the
blood-gas barrier can be described by the diffusing capacity
[1]. Several factors affect gas transport across the alveolocapillary membrane:

- the partial pressure gradient of a gas across the membrane,
- the properties (i.e. thickness and surface area) of the
membrane,
- the properties of the gas (i.e. its molecular size and solubility in fluids),
- the matching of ventilation and perfusion of the lung units,
- and the chemical reaction rate with hemoglobin.

Gas diffusion is proportional to the surface area of the
membrane, and to the reciprocal of the membrane thickness.
Furthermore, it depends on the intracapillary resistance that
gas molecules encounter on their way towards hemoglobin.
The diffusing capacity of the lung is expressed as the amount
of a gas that is exchanged in a certain time between alveolar
air and capillary blood per unit partial pressure difference.
As not only diffusion but also chemical reactions affect the
transfer of gases, the term 'transfer' (T) of gas rather than
diffusion is used. Traditionally, gas transfer across the

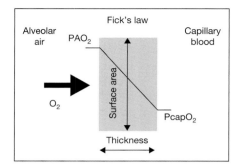

Fig. 1. Schematic illustration of the O_2 transfer across the gas-blood barrier.

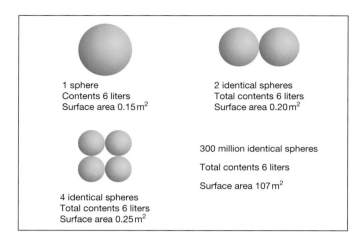

Fig. 2. Schematic representation showing the increase in surface area with the number of alveoli.

alveolocapillary membrane is described in the US by the diffusing capacity for carbon monoxide (DLCO) and in Europe it is called the transfer factor T_{LCO}. However, DLCO and T_{LCO} describe the same variable and are interchangeable.

In figure 1 the O_2 transfer across the gas-blood barrier ($\dot{V}O_2$) is illustrated schematically. $\dot{V}O_2$ is proportional to the surface area of the membrane, that is to say that a doubled surface area doubles $\dot{V}O_2$. On the other hand, $\dot{V}O_2$ is proportional to the reciprocal of the barrier thickness, which means a halving of $\dot{V}O_2$ when membrane thickness doubles. Furthermore, $\dot{V}O_2$ is proportional to the partial O_2 pressure gradient, defined as alveolar PO_2 (PAO_2) minus mean capillary PO_2 ($PcapO_2$). Finally $\dot{V}O_2$ is dependent on the diffusivity (DO_2), which is proportional to the solubility of O_2 in water and inversely proportional to the square root of the molecular weight of O_2.

In formula:

$$\dot{V}O_2 \propto (\text{surface area/barrier thickness}) \cdot DO_2 \cdot (PAO_2 - \text{mean } PcapO_2)$$

The term (surface area/barrier thickness) DO_2 is called the diffusing capacity or transfer factor for O_2, and referred to as DLO_2 or TLO_2, respectively.

In formula:

$$\dot{V}O_2 = TLO_2 \cdot (PAO_2 - \text{mean } PcapO_2)$$

TLO_2 is equal to $\dot{V}O_2$ divided by the pressure gradient, which means that TLO_2 is the conductance of the membrane.

Because the $PcapO_2$ increase is not linear when passing the capillary, mean $PcapO_2$ is difficult to estimate. For that reason the gas carbon monoxide (CO) is used to estimate lung diffusing capacity. CO has the advantage that nearly all CO molecules combine with hemoglobin to form carboxyhemoglobin (HbCO) and the partial CO pressure in the capillary blood (PcapCO) is negligible from the beginning to the end of the capillary. The driving pressure difference across the membrane, the alveolar partial CO pressure minus the partial CO pressure in the capillary blood (PACO – PcapCO), is approximately equal to PACO.

The transfer of CO involves two processes in series: the membrane conductance and a part inside the capillary, which concerns the chemical reaction between hemoglobin and CO. The latter depends on capillary blood volume and hemoglobin concentration.

The membrane conductance (T_{LCO}) measures the surface area of the lung available for gas exchange. As illustrated in figure 2 the surface area is increasing with the number of alveoli. With a radius R the contents of a sphere are $4/3\pi R^3$ and the surface area of the sphere is equal to $4\pi R^2$.

Because surface area is related to alveolar volume, diffusing capacity is normalized per liter alveolar volume. Alveolar volume is routinely assessed simultaneously, using the helium dilution method.

After inspiration of a CO-containing gas mixture, CO disappearance is proportional to the concentration gradient across the alveolar membrane. CO will bind firmly to hemoglobin in erythrocytes. As CO is not normally present in nonsmokers' blood, the driving pressure is entirely determined by the fraction of CO in the alveolar gas. The diffusing capacity can be derived from the amount of CO that disappears from the inhaled gas mixture after a standardized breath hold at total lung capacity (TLC). Recommendations for standardized measurements have been published [2].

Several 'nonpulmonary' factors may affect the diffusing capacity for CO. These include the hemoglobin level and the presence of HbCO.

In general a decreased T_{LCO} can be an expression of loss of surface area, an increased barrier thickness, loss of effective capillary blood volume or a combination of these

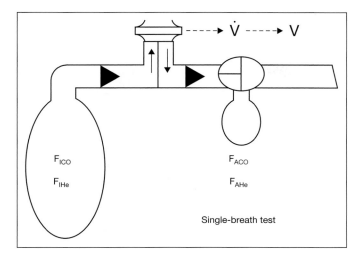

Fig. 3. Schematic representation of equipment for measuring CO diffusing capacity with the single-breath method.

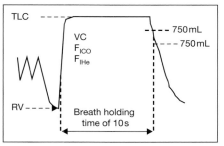

Fig. 4. Spirometric representation of the single-breath maneuver for assessing diffusing capacity. RV = Residual volume.

causes. Because the blood component depends on the hemoglobin concentration correction of T_{LCO} to a normal hemoglobin concentration is necessary, to exclude the possibility that anemia causes a decrease in T_{LCO}.

Commercial equipment may use the normal adult hemoglobin concentration as default standard, and this is clearly inappropriate for young children who have lower normal values; the software should, therefore, be adapted for use in children.

The presence of CO immediately results in the formation of HbCO in the pulmonary capillary blood. The resulting partial CO pressure ('backpressure') impairs CO diffusion. Backpressure results from previous exposition to CO; in practice, significant backpressure is mainly caused by inhalation of cigarette smoke or after inhalation of CO during repeated measurements of CO diffusion.

Techniques of Measuring Lung Diffusing Capacity

Single-Breath Method

To determine the diffusing capacity, the single-breath method is usually applied. The patient is breathing via a two-way valve system (fig. 3). After a maximal expiration (until residual volume) the patient is asked to inspire as deeply as possible (vital capacity, VC) a gas mixture of about 0.3% CO and 5–9% helium (He) from a bag or gas container, until TLC. Flows are measured with a flow transducer (Lilly or Fleisch type) and the inspired and expired volumes are obtained by integration of the flow signal in time. After 10 s of breath-holding time of 10 s the patient exhales and an

alveolar gas sample is collected. Alveolar fractions of CO and He are commonly obtained from a gas sample of 750 ml after discarding the first 750 ml for washout of airways and apparatus dead space (fig. 4). Because the single-breath test is considered as the 'gold standard' in adults the use of this test is preferable in children and adolescents, too. The required measurements are breath-holding time, the initial and final CO and He concentrations and the lung volume at which breath was held. The inert gas He is added to calculate TLC from the dilution of He and VC, according to:

$$TLC = F_{IHe}/F_{AHe} \cdot (VC - V_{DAn} - V_{DApp}) + V_{DAn}$$

where F_{IHe} = helium fraction in inspired gas, F_{AHe} = helium fraction in alveolar gas; V_{Dan} = anatomical dead space; V_{Dapp} = apparatus dead space.

$$\text{maximum alveolar volume } V_{Amax} = TLC - V_{Dan}$$

The initial alveolar CO concentration is calculated from this He dilution and the inspired CO concentration according to:

$$F_{ACO0} = F_{ICO} \cdot F_{AHe}/F_{IHe}$$

where F_{ACO0} = alveolar CO fraction at starting time 0 and F_{ICO} = inspired CO fraction.

During breath-holding, the alveolar fraction of CO decreases exponentially with time (t):

$$FACOt = F_{ACO0} \cdot e^{-kCOt}$$

where kCO = the rate constant for CO uptake per second or minute.

$$lnFACOt = lnF_{ACO0} - kCO \cdot t$$
$$ln(F_{ACO0}/F_{ACOt}) = kCO \cdot t$$

In this equation kCO represents $[T_{LCO} \cdot (P_B - P_{H_2Osat})]/(K_{STPD} \cdot V_{Amax})$ where Pb = barometric pressure, P_{H_2Osat} = saturated water vapor pressure and K_{STPD} = a conversion factor from body temperature, barometric pressure and aturated water vapor pressure conditions (BTPS) to standard temperature (0°C) and pressure (760 mm Hg) and dry conditions (STPD).

Rearrangement gives:

$$TLCO = V_{Amax} \cdot 1/t \cdot K_{STPD}/(P_B - P_{H_2Osat}) \cdot \ln(F_{ACO0}/F_{ACOt})$$

TLCO is expressed in units of conductance: $\mu mol \cdot s^{-1} \cdot kPa^{-1}$ or $mmol \cdot min^{-1} \cdot kPa^{-1}$.

The use of the single-breath test is limited to adults and cooperative children older than 6–8 years who can perform the maneuver and have a VC well exceeding 1.5 liters.

Multiple-Breath Methods

Many children have difficulties in holding their breath for 10 s at TLC or have a VC lower than 1.5 liters. For those, the single-breath method is problematic. An alternative method is the rebreathing technique, for which patients are asked to hyperventilate a gas mixture containing CO and He. However, such a procedure may still be too difficult to perform for small children. Preschool children can be studied using an alternative rebreathing method at normal, spontaneous ventilation, where the patient is connected for several minutes to a closed system filled with a gas mixture containing 0.3% CO and 5% He, while breathing quietly [3]. For small children, the dimensions of the apparatus should be adapted to the smaller gas volumes involved (fig. 5). The rebreathing system essentially consists of a bellows. During the rebreathing procedure CO_2 is absorbed and O_2 kept between 20 and 22%. The ventilation of the patient is measured with a displacement transducer connected to the bellows. He, CO and O_2 concentrations are analyzed continuously. The patient is connected to the bellows at functional residual capacity (FRC) level. FRC is determined by He dilution, and diffusing capacity calculated from the exponential decay in CO. The results are dependent on alveolar ventilation $\dot{V}_A$ and a stable breathing pattern is necessary for reliable measurements [3].

Comparison of Single-Breath and Rebreathing Diffusing Capacity

Theoretically the absolute values of single-breath and rebreathing diffusing capacity should be different, because with the single-breath test measurements are performed at TLC and with the rebreathing method at FRC + ½ tidal volume VT. The diffusing capacity is proportional to the surface area, and a larger volume level means a larger surface area and, thus, a larger diffusing capacity.

When comparing single-breath and rebreathing diffusing capacity, a practical approach is to calculate the results in SDS (or Z) scores of the corresponding predicted values.

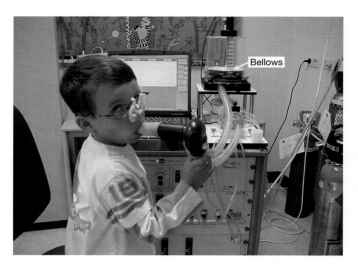

Fig. 5. Measurement of diffusing capacity using the rebreathing method adapted for preschool children. The patient breathes quietly into a closed bellows system filled with a gas mixture containing CO and He. The disappearance of CO from the system and the fall in He due to dilution are continuously monitored (published with permission of the parents and the child).

Interpretation of Measurements

Normative Data for Single-Breath Diffusing Capacity in Children

Reference values have been published [3–7]. In our laboratory lung function parameters are reported as percentage of predicted and the deviation in residual standard deviations (RSD) from predicted. Stam et al. [8] estimated predicted values for single-breath T_{LCO} and transfer coefficient (T_{LCO}/V_A; V_A = alveolar volume) for children and adolescents from 6 to 18 years of age. T_{LCO} increases exponentially with height, whereas T_{LCO}/V_A decreases exponentially with height. The reference equations for single-breath T_{LCO} and T_{LCO}/V_A are:

Boys:
$$T_{LCO} = 39.9\,H^{2.45} \quad \text{RSD of } \ln(T_{LCO}) = 0.10$$
$$T_{LCO}/V_A = 40.1\,H^{-0.60} \quad \text{RSD of } \ln(T_{LCO}/V_A) = 0.11$$

Girls:
$$T_{LCO} = 41.3\,H^{2.23} \quad \text{RSD of } \ln(T_{LCO}) = 0.11$$
$$T_{LCO}/V_A = 43.9\,H^{-0.84} \quad \text{RSD of } \ln(T_{LCO}/V_A) = 0.11$$

where T_{LCO} is in $\mu mol \cdot s^{-1} \cdot kPa^{-1}$, T_{LCO}/V_A in $\mu mol \cdot s^{-1} \cdot kPa^{-1} \cdot l^{-1}$ and height (H) in meters.

These predicted values are comparable with those according to Baran and Englert [4], Bucci et al. [5], Cotes et al. [6] and Nasr et al. [7].

Because TLC increases exponentially with height, T_{LCO} and T_{LCO}/V_A predictions are linearly related with TLC as follows (TLC in liters) [8]:

Boys:
$$T_{LCO} = 29.5 + 22.9\,TLC \quad RSD = 11$$
$$T_{LCO}/V_A = 37.4 - 1.56\,TLC \quad RSD = 3.4$$

Girls:
$$T_{LCO} = 35.8 + 20.2\,TLC \quad RSD = 11$$
$$T_{LCO}/V_A = 41.1 - 2.78\,TLC \quad RSD = 3.0$$

However, there is an important pitfall when assessing gas transfer at lower lung volumes that may be due to restrictive lung disease or impaired chest wall function. The predicted values for T_{LCO} and T_{LCO}/V_A are determined in healthy volunteers, and hence pertain to the predicted normal TLC level. In patients with restrictive lung disease actual TLC is smaller and a comparison with predicted values for T_{LCO} and T_{LCO}/V_A at the larger predicted TLC may be inappropriate. For such cases alveolar volume-dependent T_{LCO}/V_A predicted values for children are available [8].

Boys:
$$T_{LCO}/V_A = 58.9 - (23.1 - 9.98H)V_A$$
$$\left[RSD = \sqrt{2.01V_A^2 - 16.4V_A + 46.6} \right]$$

Girls:
$$T_{LCO}/V_A = 57.6 - (22.5 - 9.52H)V_A$$
$$\left[RSD = \sqrt{1.81V_A^2 - 13.8V_A + 36.7} \right]$$

where V_A is in liters and height (H) in meters.

Normative Values for Rebreathing Diffusing Capacity
Stam et al. [3] described predicted values for the rebreathing T_{LCO} and T_{LCO}/V_A in children from 6 to 18 years of age. These predicted values were not only dependent on $\dot{V}_A$, but also depended on V_A and height, just like the single-breath values described above:

Boys:
$$T_{LCO} = 7.8\,V_A + 2.8\,\dot{V}_A + 23.1\,H - 28.4 \quad RSD = 5.2$$
$$T_{LCO}/V_A = 27.9 - (19.2 - 7.5\,H)V_A + 1.3\,\dot{V}_A \quad RSD = 2.8$$

Girls:
$$T_{LCO} = 6.4\,V_A + 2.7\,\dot{V}_A + 28.0\,H - 32.7 \quad RSD = 4.5$$
$$T_{LCO}/V_A = 31.7 - (29.8 - 12.4\,H)V_A + 1.5\,\dot{V}_A \quad RSD = 2.7$$

where $\dot{V}_A$ is in $l \cdot min^{-1}$, V_A in liters and height (H) in meters.

Interpretation in Obstructive Lung Disease
During a single-breath assessment of gas transfer, the helium dilution technique is used to determine TLC.

However, in spirometry He is washed in and diluted in several minutes, while in the single-breath procedure only 10 s are available to obtain equilibration of helium concentrations within the airspaces. In case of unequal ventilation this may be too short, leading to inaccurate TLC measurement. As the well-ventilated lung areas are mainly measured, the diffusing capacity of these lung areas is estimated. An indication of the degree of unequal ventilation distribution is, therefore, important. One indication for ventilation inhomogeneity is the ratio between TLC determined with the single-breath test (TLCsb) and TLC determined with the multiple-breath helium dilution method (TLCmb). A TLCsb/TLCmb ratio >0.85 has been proposed as indicative for normal and ≤0.85 for unequal distribution of ventilation. To examine if a small TLCsb/TLCmb ratio is caused by unequal ventilation or related to a submaximal inspiration, VC determined with the single-breath test (VCsb) and VC during spirometry (VCmb) should be compared, too. Only when VCsb and VCmb are similar a small TLCsb/TLCmb ratio reflects unequal ventilation. In such cases the single-breath technique estimates the diffusion characteristics of the well-ventilated lung areas. Surprisingly, children with severe obstructive lung disease due to cystic fibrosis show a (nearly) normal diffusing capacity [9]. The reason for this is unclear but may be partly due to binding of CO by free hemoglobin in the airways (see below) or hypervascularity of the bronchial mucosa. An increased transfer of CO to the lung has also been observed in patients with airflow obstruction of different origins [10, 11], including cystic fibrosis patients aged 9–25 years [12]. There are many ways in which diffusing capacity of the lung may be affected by alterations of lung parenchyma, airway patency, pulmonary blood flow and posture [13–15]. It has been speculated that whole lung CO transfer in symptomatic cystic fibrosis patients becomes elevated because (1) more blood is sucked into the lung following increased pressure swings due to dyspnea [12, 16], (2) pulmonary circulation is increased in the best-ventilated regions due to hypoxia-induced vasoconstriction [16, 17], and (3) bronchiectasis causes an increased bronchial circulation [16].

Interpretation in Restrictive Lung Disease
Commonly, diffusing capacity is normalized for alveolar volume [13]. However, this assumes that the volume and the surface of the alveolocapillary membrane are proportional. This may not be the case especially in children with thoracic cage deformity or neuromuscular disease, who have essentially normal lungs that are restricted by their deformed chest and/or respiratory muscle weakness. The presence of a normal-sized lung in a small chest will lead to a relatively large surface for diffusion per unit of

lung volume and an apparently normal or even supranormal T_{LCO}/V_A. Preferably, measured values in such patients should be normalized for diffusing capacity at the same reduced lung volumes as in healthy controls [8].

Interpretation in Pulmonary Bleeding Disorders

As the measurement of CO diffusing capacity is based on the high affinity binding of CO to hemoglobin, the test results will be unreliable in any condition where there is blood present in the alveoli or airways. A falsely high diffusing capacity will result when CO binds to hemoglobin in the airways before crossing the alveolocapillary membrane [18]. This does not mean that measurement of diffusing capacity is useless in pulmonary bleeding disorders. Monitoring T_{LCO} and T_{LCO}/V_A can help to detect bleeding in patients with primary pulmonary hemosiderosis, Wegener's disease and other bleeding disorders and may be helpful when deciding about a change in treatment.

Pediatric Indications for Measurement of T_{LCO} and T_{LCO}/V_A

In adults, diffusing capacity measurement is important to quantify and monitor functional impairment due to interstitial lung disease, COPD and emphysema. These are rare diagnoses in children. The main clinical indications to assess diffusing capacity in childhood are limited and include the following.

Monitoring during and after Treatments That Are Toxic to the Lungs

- Chemotherapy, especially when it includes bleomycin, commonly used for treatment of Hodgkin's lymphoma or bone tumors. A dramatic reduction in T_{LCO} may occur during a course of chemotherapy and may go unnoticed when not properly monitored. Very little is known about reversibility of such toxic effects in children. Adjustment of the treatment protocol may be necessary. An important pitfall is that children who undergo chemotherapy will have varying hemoglobin levels, which may affect the diffusing capacity. Appropriate corrections should be made. Many other drugs may affect diffusing capacity, including methotrexate, nitrofurantoin, sulfa-containing products, azathioprine, penicillamine and cyclophosphamide.
- Chest radiation. At present this is a rare treatment option, but radiation-induced lung damage may lead to progressive and irreversible diffusion impairment.
- Systemic treatment for autoimmune and rheumatic diseases, including systemic lupus erythematosus, vasculitis, Sturge-Weber syndrome, Goodpasture syndrome, juvenile

chronic arthritis, mixed connective tissue disease, dermatomyositis.
- Immunosuppressive regimens used after organ transplant have been associated with severe obstructive and restrictive lung disease.

Diagnosis, Monitoring and Follow-Up of Patients with Chronic Interstitial Lung Disease

Here, the diffusing capacity is one of the early signs of disease, and an important indicator of progression and treatment effects.
- Interstitial fibrosis syndromes
- Extrinsic allergic alveolitis
- Systemic lupus erythematosus
- Pulmonary vasculitis syndromes

Monitoring of Children with Pulmonary Bleeding Disorders

An increase in diffusing capacity may predict a relapse or indicate ongoing disease sometimes at an otherwise subclinical level. On the other hand, in the long term, therapy-resistant hemosiderosis may lead to fibrosis and restrictive lung disease, with impaired diffusing capacity at times when there is no active bleeding.
- Primary pulmonary hemosiderosis
- Goodpasture syndrome
- Wegener's disease

Assessment of Functional Impairment in Children with Progressive Thoracic Cage Deformities and/or Neuromuscular Disease

In such children, diffusing capacity may be wrongly interpreted as preserved despite a low lung volume (see above). In long-standing restriction, the lung tissue may adapt and diffusing capacity per unit lung volume may decrease.

Long-Term Follow-Up Evaluation of Lung Function in Children after Prematurity, Lung Damage due to Intensive Care and Artificial Ventilation, Severe Pneumonia, or Congenital Malformations of the Lungs
- Bronchopulmonary dysplasia
- Meconium aspiration
- Congenital diaphragmatic hernia
- Lung cysts

Case Presentations

To illustrate the use of T_{LCO} and T_{LCO}/V_A measurements in pediatric practice, we present a few cases where diffusion measurement was important in monitoring and diagnosis.

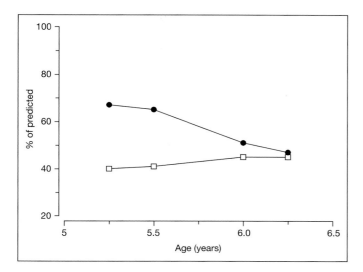

Fig. 6. Diffusing capacity and VC in a boy with systemic vasculitis of unknown origin. T_{LCO} is corrected to normal hemoglobin concentration. ● = Rebreathing T_{LCO}; □ = VC.

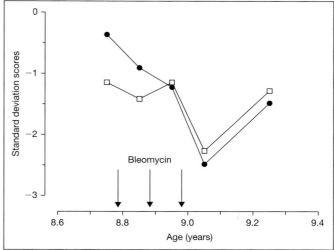

Fig. 7. Diffusing capacity and TLC in a girl with Hodgkin's disease treated with bleomycin. y-axis depicts diffusion and volumes as standard deviation scores. ● = Single-breath T_{LCO}; □ = TLCHe.

Case 1

A 4-year-old boy with atopic asthma and eczema developed severe systemic vasculitis of unknown origin, unresponsive to high-dose anti-inflammatory treatment. His older sisters died aged 9 and 11 because of the same disorder, both having interstitial lung disease. This boy had no specific respiratory symptoms, apart from his mild asthma. Chest X-ray was within normal limits; a CT scan of the lungs was suggestive of minor interstitial lung disease. However, measurement of rebreathing diffusing capacity showed severe and progressive impairment of diffusion. Lung volumes were reduced too, but without clear progression (fig. 6). In view of the bad prognosis, the fatal course of the disease in his sisters, and the steady decline of diffusing capacity without effect of immunosuppressives, a bone marrow transplant was successfully carried out.

Case 2

An 8-year-old girl was diagnosed to have Hodgkin's lymphoma and received a chemotherapy regimen which included bleomycin. Diffusing capacity was routinely measured at baseline and before each bleomycin application. The longitudinal course of total lung capacity assessed with helium dilution (TLCHe) and of single-breath diffusing capacity, corrected for alveolar volume and hemoglobin, showed that diffusing capacity started to decrease well before TLC, declining almost 2 SD scores (fig. 7). TLC shows rapid recovery to baseline values after cessation of bleomycin treatment, whereas recovery of diffusing capacity is markedly slower and still incomplete.

Case 3

A 16-year-old boy was treated for Hodgkin's disease. His lung function was monitored before and after treatment and showed a significant drop in diffusing capacity from baseline without concomitant changes in TLC. As the baseline value of diffusing capacity

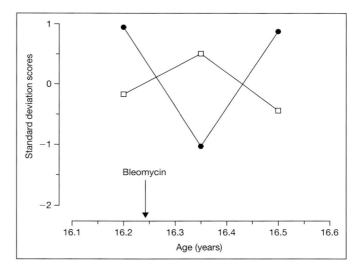

Fig. 8. Diffusing capacity, corrected for alveolar volume and hemoglobin, and TLC in a boy with Hodgkin's disease treated with bleomycin. ● = Single-breath T_{LCO}/V_A; □ = TLCHe.

was relatively high, the diffusing capacity remained within normal limits despite the significant drop (fig. 8). This illustrates the importance of obtaining baseline values before the start of the treatment.

Case 4

An 11-year-old boy with a height of 1.57 m had a restriction of lung volume due to neuromuscular disease. His actual TLC was 2.86

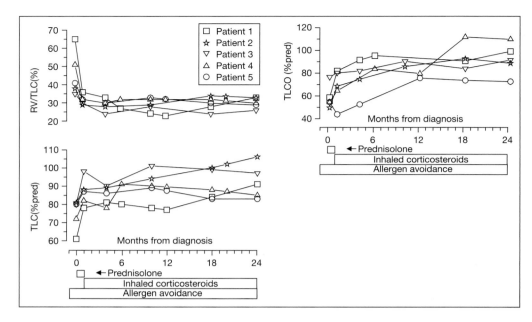

Fig. 9. Diffusing capacity, TLC, and residual volume (RV)/TLC ratio in five children from a family, in which all developed severe extrinsic allergic alveolitis due to exposure to pigeon excreta. The initial response to corticosteroids was dramatic, followed by various degrees of recovery after allergen avoidance [19].

liters, which was 65% of predicted normal. His T_{LCO}/V_A at the actual, restricted TLC was 150% of predicted T_{LCO}/V_A at predicted normal TLC. However, if we calculated his predicted value corrected for the reduced lung volume of 2.86 liters his T_{LCO}/V_A was 96% of predicted. In other words, the correction for a reduced V_A resulted in a lower diffusing capacity.

At the age of 14 the boy was measured again. At that time his height was 1.75 m and his TLC was 4.50 liters, which was 78% of predicted. T_{LCO}/V_A at the actual small TLC was 131% of the predicted normal T_{LCO}/V_A at normal TLC. More realistically, T_{LCO}/V_A was 96% of the predicted T_{LCO}/V_A at the actual TLC of 4.50 liters.

When using T_{LCO}/V_A predictions at predicted normal TLC, the conclusion might be that the T_{LCO}/V_A had decreased from 150 to 131%. However, when using T_{LCO}/V_A predictions at the actual reduced TLC, T_{LCO}/V_A had remained unchanged at 96%.

Case 5

Five children from one family were diagnosed with extrinsic allergic alveolitis due to excessive exposure to city pigeon excreta [19]. A short time before, their mother had died from respiratory insufficiency, in retrospect most likely due to the same disease. All five children showed varying degrees of respiratory distress and hypoxemia, one child requiring intensive care. Lung function including diffusing capacity was measured in all children, and was found markedly reduced, consistent with the diagnosis of extrinsic allergic alveolitis (fig. 9). The children were treated with systemic corticosteroids for 1 month and inhaled steroids for 24 months, while antigen exposure was reduced as much as possible. All five children showed a quick clinical recovery and a slow normalization of pulmonary function indices, especially of the diffusing capacity, during a follow-up of 24 months. In the course of the next years, lung volumes and diffusing capacity showed further gradual improvement towards normalization in all five children.

References

1 Krogh M: The diffusion of gases through the lungs of man. J Physiol 1915;49:271–300.

2 American Thoracic Society: Single-breath carbon monoxide diffusing capacity (transfer factor). Recommendations for a standard technique – 1995 update. Am J Respir Crit Care Med 1995;152:2185–2198.

3 Stam H, Van der Beek A, Grünberg K, De Ridder MAJ, De Jongste JC, Versprille A: A rebreathing method to determine carbon monoxide diffusing capacity in children: Reference values for 6–18 year olds and validation in adult volunteers. Pediatr Pulmonol 1998;25:205–212.

4 Baran D, Englert M: Les valeurs normales du facteur de transfert pulmonaire d'oxyde de carbone et de la 'perméabilité' alvéolo-capillaire chez l'enfant. Bull Eur Physiopathol Respir 1968;4:659–672.

References

1 Kharitonov SA, Barnes PJ: Exhaled markers of pulmonary disease. Am J Respir Crit Care Med 2001;163:1693–1722.

2 Nightingale JA, Rogers DF, Barnes PJ: Effect of repeated sputum induction on cell counts in normal volunteers. Thorax 1998;53:87–90.

3 Kharitonov SA, Barnes PJ: Clinical aspects of exhaled nitric oxide. Eur Respir J 2000;16:781–792.

4 Kharitonov SA: Exhaled markers of inflammatory lung diseases: Ready for routine monitoring? Swiss Med Wkly 2004;134:175–192.

5 Kharitonov SA: Exhaled nitric oxide and carbon monoxide in asthma. Eur Respir J 1999;9:212–218.

6 Kharitonov SA, Alving K, Barnes PJ: Exhaled and nasal nitric oxide measurements: Recommendations. Eur Respir J 1997;10:1683–1693.

7 Recommendations for standardized procedures for the online and offline measurement of exhaled lower respiratory nitric oxide and nasal nitric oxide in adults and children. Am J Respir Crit Care Med 1999;160:2104–2117.

8 Jones SL, Kittelson J, Cowan JO, Flannery EM, Hancox RJ, McLachlan CR, et al: The predictive value of exhaled nitric oxide measurements in assessing changes in asthma control. Am J Respir Crit Care Med 2001;164:738–743.

9 Kharitonov SA, Yates DH, Chung KF, Barnes PJ: Changes in the dose of inhaled steroid affect exhaled nitric oxide levels in asthmatic patients. Eur Respir J 1996;9:196–201.

10 Jatakanon A, Lim S, Barnes PJ: Changes in sputum eosinophils predict loss of asthma control. Am J Respir Crit Care Med 2000;161:64–72.

11 http://www.fda.gov/bbs/topics/ANSWERS/2003/ANS01219.html. FDA report, 2003.

12 Wildhaber JH, Hall GL, Stick SM: Measurements of exhaled nitric oxide with the single-breath technique and positive expiratory pressure in infants. Am J Respir Crit Care Med 1999;159:74–78.

13 Franklin PJ, Turner SW, Mutch RC, Stick SM: Comparison of single-breath and tidal breathing exhaled nitric oxide levels in infants. Eur Respir J 2004;23:369–372.

14 Silkoff PE, Bates CA, Meiser JB, Bratton DL: Single-breath exhaled nitric oxide in preschool children facilitated by a servo-controlled device maintaining constant flow. Pediatr Pulmonol 2004;37:554–558.

15 Uasuf CG, Jatakanon A, James A, Kharitonov SA, Wilson NM, Barnes PJ: Exhaled carbon monoxide in childhood asthma. J Pediatr 1999;135:569–574.

16 Jobsis Q, Raatgeep HC, Hop WC, de Jongste JC: Controlled low flow off line sampling of exhaled nitric oxide in children. Thorax 2001;56:285–289.

17 Buchvald F, Bisgaard H: FeNO measured at fixed exhalation flow rate during controlled tidal breathing in children from the age of 2 yr. Am J Respir Crit Care Med 2001;163:699–704.

18 Steerenberg PA, Janssen NA, de Meer G, Fischer PH, Nierkens S, van Loveren H, et al: Relationship between exhaled NO, respiratory symptoms, lung function, bronchial hyperresponsiveness, and blood eosinophilia in school children. Thorax 2003;58:242–245.

19 Paredi P, Loukides S, Ward S, Cramer D, Spicer M, Kharitonov SA, et al: Exhalation flow and pressure-controlled reservoir collection of exhaled nitric oxide for remote and delayed analysis. Thorax 1998;53:775–779.

20 Jobsis Q, Schellekens SL, Kroesbergen A, Hop WC, de Jongste JC: Off-line sampling of exhaled air for nitric oxide measurement in children: Methodological aspects. Eur Respir J 2001;17:898–903.

21 Kissoon N, Duckworth LJ, Blake KV, Murphy SP, Taylor CL, Silkoff PE: FE(NO): Relationship to exhalation rates and online versus bag collection in healthy adolescents. Am J Respir Crit Care Med 2000;162:539–545.

22 Koenig JQ, Jansen K, Mar TF, Lumley T, Kaufman J, Trenga CA, et al: Measurement of offline exhaled nitric oxide in a study of community exposure to air pollution. Environ Health Perspect 2003;111:1625–1629.

23 Gungor A, Vural C: A method for off-line nasal nitric oxide measurement. Ear Nose Throat J 2002;81:449–453.

24 Franklin PJ, Turner SW, Mutch RC, Stick SM: Measuring exhaled nitric oxide in infants during tidal breathing: Methodological issues. Pediatr Pulmonol 2004;37:24–30.

25 Baraldi E, Dario C, Ongaro R, Scollo M, Azzolin NM, Panza N, et al: Exhaled nitric oxide concentrations during treatment of wheezing exacerbation in infants and young children. Am J Respir Crit Care Med 1999;159:1284–1288.

26 Kharitonov SA, Chung FK, Evans DJ, O'Connor BJ, Barnes PJ: The elevated level of exhaled nitric oxide in asthmatic patients is mainly derived from the lower respiratory tract. Am J Respir Crit Care Med 1996;153:1773–1780.

27 Silkoff PE, McClean PA, Slutsky AS, Furlott HG, Hoffstein E, Wakita S, et al: Marked flow-dependence of exhaled nitric oxide using a new technique to exclude nasal nitric oxide. Am J Respir Crit Care Med 1997;155:260–267.

28 Pijnenburg MW, Lissenberg ET, Hofhuis W, Ghiro L, Ho WC, Holland WP, et al: Exhaled nitric oxide measurements with dynamic flow restriction in children aged 4–8 yrs. Eur Respir J 2002;20:919–924.

29 Kharitonov SA, Barnes PJ: Nasal contribution to exhaled nitric oxide during exhalation against resistance or during breath holding. Thorax 1997;52:540–544.

30 Kharitonov SA, Yates DH, Robbins RA, Logan-Sinclair R, Shinebourne EA, Barnes PJ: Increased nitric oxide in exhaled air of asthmatic patients. Lancet 1994;343:133–135.

31 Baraldi E, de Jongste JC: Measurement of exhaled nitric oxide in children, 2001. Eur Respir J 2002;20:223–237.

32 Kharitonov SA, Gonio F, Kelly C, Meah S, Barnes PJ: Reproducibility of exhaled nitric oxide measurements in healthy and asthmatic adults and children. Eur Respir J 2003;21:433–438.

33 Dupont LJ, Demedts MG, Verleden GM: Prospective evaluation of the validity of exhaled nitric oxide for the diagnosis of asthma. Chest 2003;123:751–756.

34 Baraldi E, Carraro S, Alinovi R, Pesci A, Ghiro L, Bodini A, et al: Cysteinyl leukotrienes and 8-isoprostane in exhaled breath condensate of children with asthma exacerbations. Thorax 2003;58:505–509.

35 Hall GL, Reinmann B, Wildhaber JH, Frey U: Tidal exhaled nitric oxide in healthy, unsedated newborn infants with prenatal tobacco exposure. J Appl Physiol 2002;92:59–66.

36 Malmberg LP, Pelkonen AS, Haahtela T, Turpeinen M: Exhaled nitric oxide rather than lung function distinguishes preschool children with probable asthma. Thorax 2003;58:494–499.

37 Wilson NM, Bridge P, Spanevello A, Silverman M: Induced sputum in children: Feasibility, repeatability, and relation of findings to asthma severity. Thorax 2000;55:768–774.

38 Belda J, Parameswaran K, Keith PK, Hargreave FE: Repeatability and validity of cell and fluid-phase measurements in nasal fluid: A comparison of two methods of nasal lavage. Clin Exp Allergy 2001;31:1111–1115.

39 Hamid Q, Springall DR, Riveros-Moreno V, Chanez P, Howarth PH, Redington A, et al: Induction of nitric oxide synthase in asthma. Lancet 1993;342:1510–1513.

40 Saleh D, Ernst P, Lim S, Barnes PJ, Giaid A: Increased formation of the potent oxidant peroxynitrite in the airways of asthmatic patients is associated with induction of nitric oxide synthase: Effect of inhaled glucocorticoid. FASEB J 1998;12:929–937.

41 Wechsler ME, Grasemann H, Deykin A, Silverman EK, Yandava CN, Israel E, et al: Exhaled nitric oxide in patients with asthma. Association with NOS1 genotype. Am J Respir Crit Care Med 2000;162:2043–2047.

42 Chatkin JM, Ansarin K, Silkoff PE, McClean P, Gutierrez C, Zamel N, et al: Exhaled nitric oxide as a noninvasive assessment of chronic cough. Am J Respir Crit Care Med 1999;159:1810–1813.

43 Dupont LJ, Demedts MG, Verleden GM: Prospective evaluation of the accuracy of exhaled nitric oxide for the diagnosis of asthma. Am J Respir Crit Care Med 1999;159:A861.

44 Ekroos H, Tuominen J, Sovijarvi AR: Exhaled nitric oxide and its long-term variation in healthy non-smoking subjects. Clin Physiol 2000;20:434–439.

45 Smith AD, Cowan JO, Filsell S, McLachlan C, Monti-Sheehan G, Jackson P, et al: Diagnosing asthma: Comparisons between exhaled nitric oxide measurements and conventional tests. Am J Respir Crit Care Med 2004;169:473–478.

46 Artlich A, Busch T, Lewandowski K, Jonas S, Gortner L, Falke KJ: Childhood asthma: Exhaled nitric oxide in relation to clinical symptoms. Eur Respir J 1999;13:1396–1401.

47 Baraldi E, Azzolin NM, Zanconato S, Dario C, Zacchello F: Corticosteroids decrease exhaled nitric oxide in children with acute asthma. J Pediatr 1997;131:381–385.

48 Lanz MJ, Leung DY, White CW: Comparison of exhaled nitric oxide to spirometry during emergency treatment of asthma exacerbations with glucocorticosteroids in children. Ann Allergy Asthma Immunol 1999;82:161–164.

49 Lanz MJ, Leung DY, McCormick DR, Harbeck R, Szefler SJ, White CW: Comparison of exhaled nitric oxide, serum eosinophilic cationic protein, and soluble interleukin-2 receptor in exacerbations of pediatric asthma. Pediatr Pulmonol 1997;24:305–311.

50 van Den Toorn LM, Prins JB, Overbeek SE, Hoogsteden HC, de Jongste JC: Adolescents in clinical remission of atopic asthma have elevated exhaled nitric oxide levels and bronchial hyperresponsiveness. Am J Respir Crit Care Med 2000;162:953–957.

51 van Den Toorn LM, Overbeek SE, de Jongste JC, Leman K, Hoogsteden HC, Prins JB: Airway inflammation is present during clinical remission of atopic asthma. Am J Respir Crit Care Med 2001;164:2107–2113.

52 Sovijärvi ARA, Saarinen A, Helin T, Malmberg P, Haahtela T, Linholm H, et al: Increased nitric oxide in exhaled air in patients with asthmatic symptoms not fulfilling the functional criteria of asthma. Eur Respir J 1998;12:431S.

53 Withers NJ, Bale KL, Laszlo G: Levels of exhaled nitric oxide as a screening tool for undiagnosed asthma: Results of a pilot study. Eur Respir J 1998;12:393S.

54 Adisesh LA, Kharitonov SA, Yates DH, Snashal DC, Newman-Taylor AJ, Barnes PJ: Exhaled and nasal nitric oxide is increased in laboratory animal allergy. Clin Exp Allergy 1998;28:876–880.

55 Stirling RG, Kharitonov SA, Campbell D, Robinson D, Durham SR, Chung KF, et al: Exhaled NO is elevated in difficult asthma and correlates with symptoms and disease severity despite treatment with oral and inhaled corticosteroids. Thorax 1998;53:1030–1034.

56 van Amsterdam JG, Verlaan AP, van Loveren H, Vos SG, Opperhuizen A, Steerenberg PA: The balloon technique: A convenient method to measure exhaled NO in epidemiological studies. Int Arch Occup Environ Health 1999;72:404–407.

57 Henriksen AH, Lingaas-Holmen T, Sue-Chu M, Bjermer L: Combine use of exhaled nitric oxide and airway hyperresponsiveness in characterizing asthma in a large population survey. Eur Respir J 2000;15:849–855.

58 Kharitonov SA, Barnes PJ: Does exhaled nitric oxide reflect asthma control? Yes, it does! Am J Respir Crit Care Med 2001;164:727–728.

59 Meyts I, Proesmans M, De Boeck K: Exhaled nitric oxide corresponds with office evaluation of asthma control. Pediatr Pulmonol 2003;36:283–289.

60 Leuppi JD, Salome CM, Jenkins CR, Anderson SD, Xuan W, Marks GB, et al: Predictive markers of asthma exacerbation during stepwise dose reduction of inhaled corticosteroids. Am J Respir Crit Care Med 2001;163:406–412.

61 Kharitonov SA, Barnes PJ, O'Connor BJ: Reduction in exhaled nitric oxide after a single dose of nebulised budesonide in patients with asthma. Am J Respir Crit Care Med 1996;153:A799.

62 Kharitonov SA, Donnelly LE, Montuschi P, Corradi M, Collins JV, Barnes PJ: Dose-dependent onset and cessation of action of inhaled budesonide on exhaled nitric oxide and symptoms in mild asthma. Thorax 2002;57:889–896.

63 Kharitonov SA, Yates DH, Barnes PJ: Inhaled glucocorticoids decrease nitric oxide in exhaled air of asthmatic patients. Am J Respir Crit Care Med 1996;153:454–457.

64 Yates DH, Kharitonov SA, Barnes PJ: Effect of short- and long-acting inhaled beta2-agonists on exhaled nitric oxide in asthmatic patients. Eur Respir J 1997;10:1483–1488.

65 Bisgaard H, Loland L, Oj JA: NO in exhaled air of asthmatic children is reduced by the leukotriene receptor antagonist montelukast. Am J Respir Crit Care Med 1999;160:1227–1231.

66 Lipworth BJ, Dempsey OJ, Aziz I, Wilson AM: Effects of adding a leukotriene antagonist or a long-acting beta(2)-agonist in asthmatic patients with the glycine-16 beta(2)-adrenoceptor genotype. Am J Med 2000;109:114–121.

67 Buchvald F, Bisgaard H: Comparisons of the complementary effect on exhaled nitric oxide of salmeterol vs montelukast in asthmatic children taking regular inhaled budesonide. Ann Allergy Asthma Immunol 2003;91:309–313.

68 Duiverman EJ, Jobsis Q, Essen-Zandvliet EE, van Aalderen WM, de Jongste JC: Guideline 'Treating asthma in children' for pediatric pulmonologists (2nd revised edition). I. Diagnosis and prevention. Ned Tijdschr Geneeskd 2003;147:1905–1908.

69 Leung DY, Nelson HS, Szefler SJ, Busse WW: Exhaled nitric oxide: Does it add anything to asthma management? J Allergy Clin Immunol 2003;112:817.

70 Ludviksdottir D, Janson C, Hogman M, Hedenstrom H, Bjornsson E, Boman G: Exhaled nitric oxide and its relationship to airway responsiveness and atopy in asthma. BHR-Study Group. Respir Med 1999;93:552–556.

71 Moody A, Fergusson W, Wells A, Bartley J, Kolbe J: Increased nitric oxide production in the respiratory tract in asymptomatic Pacific Islanders: An association with skin prick reactivity to house dust mite. J Allergy Clin Immunol 2000;105:895–899.

72 Langley SJ, Goldthorpe S, Custovic A, Woodcock A: Relationship among pulmonary function, bronchial reactivity, and exhaled nitric oxide in a large group of asthmatic patients. Ann Allergy Asthma Immunol 2003;91:398–404.

73 Frey U, Kuehni C, Roiha H, Cernelc M, Reinmann B, Wildhaber JH, et al: Maternal atopic disease modifies effects of prenatal risk factors on exhaled nitric oxide in infants. Am J Respir Crit Care Med, 2004.

74 Lehtimaki L, Turjanmaa V, Kankaanranta H, Saarelainen S, Hahtola P, Moilanen E: Increased bronchial nitric oxide production in patients with asthma measured with a novel method of different exhalation flow rates. Ann Med 2000;32:417–423.

75 Tsoukias NM, George SC: A two-compartment model of pulmonary nitric oxide exchange dynamics. J Appl Physiol 1998;85:653–666.

76 Brindicci C, Cosio B, Gajdocsi R, Collins JV, Bush A, Abdallah S, et al: Extended exhaled NO measurements at different exhalation flows may differentiate between bronchial and alveolar inflammation in patients with asthma and COPD. Eur Respir J 2002;20:174s.

77 Paska C, Maestrelli P, Formichi B, Monti S, Baldi S, Miniati M, et al: Increased expression of inducible NOS in peripheral lung of severe COPD patients. Eur Respir J 2002;20:95s.

78 Williams O, Rafferty GF, Hannam S, Milner AD, Greenough A: Nasal and lower airway levels of nitric oxide in prematurely born infants. Early Hum Dev 2003;72:67–73.

79 Corbelli R, Hammer J: Measurement of nasal nitric oxide; Hammer J, Eber E (eds): Paediatric Pulmonary Function Testing. Prog Respir Res. Basel, Karger, 2005, vol 33, pp 179–187.

80 Gannon PF, Belcher J, Pantin CF, Burge PS: The effect of patient technique and training on the accuracy of self-recorded peak expiratory flow. Eur Respir J 1999;14:28–31.

Dr. Sergei A. Kharitonov
Department of Thoracic Medicine
National Heart and Lung Institute
Imperial College
Dovehouse Street
London SW3 6LY (UK)
Tel. +44 207 351 8006
Fax +44 207 351 8126
E-Mail s.kharitonov@imperial.ac.uk

Hammer J, Eber E (eds): Paediatric Pulmonary Function Testing.
Prog Respir Res. Basel, Karger, 2005, vol 33, pp 181–189

· ·

Measurement of Exhaled Markers

Measurement of Nasal Nitric Oxide

Regula Corbelli   Jürg Hammer

Division of Intensive Care and Pulmonology, University Children's Hospital Basel,
Basel, Switzerland

Abstract

The major part of nitric oxide (NO) in exhaled air originates from the nasal airways, with only minor contribution from the lower airways and the oral cavity. The physiological role of the very high local NO concentration in the paranasal sinuses is still unclear. The most widely used and best-standardized method to sample nasal NO in isolation from the lower respiratory tract is aspiration at a fixed flow through the nasal passages in series. Important technical considerations include the choice of the correct transnasal flow and the ability of children to perform a breath-holding manoeuvre. The effects of age and height on nasal NO values have yet to be defined in a larger population of healthy children using the recommended aspiration technique. Presently, there is no validated technique available to measure nasal NO in infants and small children. The measurement of nasal NO concentrations has evoked interest in its potential to serve as a non-invasive and simple diagnostic tool for upper and lower respiratory tract disorders. Measurements of nasal NO concentrations are helpful to screen children with clinical symptoms suggestive of primary ciliary dyskinesia and to exclude this disease in those with high nasal NO concentrations with high certainty. Nasal NO measurements are, however, of no diagnostic utility in distinguishing between other conditions such as asthma, cystic fibrosis, bronchiectasis, sinusitis or rhinitis, or in monitoring therapeutic interventions in any such disorder.

Origin of Nasal Nitric Oxide

Nitric oxide (NO) is produced endogenously within the respiratory tract and was first documented in exhaled air in humans and mammals in 1991 [1]. It was then shown that the major part of NO in exhaled air originates from the nasal airways, with only a minor contribution from the lower airways and the oral cavity [2]. NO is present in the nasal airways and paranasal sinuses in very high concentrations, close to the acute exposure levels set by occupational health guidelines for short-term exposure at the workplace [3, 4].

Biochemical Pathway and Cellular Origin

NO is generated from the semi-essential amino acid *L*-arginine by the enzyme NO synthase (NOS), which can be divided into two major categories: constitutive NOS (cNOS) and inducible NOS (iNOS). The constitutive enzyme, which according to its location may be named endothelial NOS (eNOS) or neuronal NOS (nNOS), is activated by calcium and calmodulin. It produces small amounts of NO to modulate physiological processes, and can be stimulated by bradykinin, acetylcholine, histamine, leukotrienes, and several other mediators. Calmodulin is an enzyme cofactor regulating electron transport. It is also identified in close juxtaposition to the cilia of the upper airway epithelium, and is thought to be involved in ciliary motility. The iNOS, which was first isolated in macrophages, is calcium- and calmodulin-independent and activated by a variety of pro-inflammatory cytokines and endotoxins. The induction of iNOS requires gene transcription. Hence, an increase in NO production takes hours, but it may continue for days. When activated, iNOS produces up to 1,000 times more NO than cNOS. Corticosteroids only inhibit iNOS [5]. The different NOS are coded by genes on chromosomes 7 (eNOS), 12 (nNOS), and 17 (iNOS). NOS requires oxygen and nicotinamide adenine dinucleotide phosphate as cosubstrates to oxidize L-arginine to L-citrulline and NO.

Many cells in the upper and lower respiratory system produce cNOS including parasympathetic vasodilator nerves, endothelial cells, and ciliated mucosa cells. iNOS has been reported to be present not only in epithelium but also in macrophages, fibroblasts, neutrophils, endothelium and vascular smooth muscle. The NOS found in abundance in the apical regions of the maxillary sinus epithelium most closely resembles the inducible isoform. It is, however, constantly expressed and not inhibited by steroids which are characteristics commonly associated with cNOS rather than iNOS [3]. It is localized mainly within cilia and microvilli and held responsible for the high NO concentrations within the sinus lumen of healthy humans [3, 6].

Anatomic Origin

The epithelial cells of the paranasal sinuses were identified as a major source of NO production in the respiratory tract. NO concentrations inside the paranasal sinus are several hundred times higher than in exhaled air from lower airways [3,000–25,000 parts per billion (ppb)]. The sinuses communicate with the nasal cavity through their ostia and the rate of gas exchange between these cavities is dependent on several factors such as the size of the ostia, the volume of the sinuses, the nasal airflow, and intranasal pressure. There is still some controversy whether the majority of NO measured in nasal air originates from the paranasal sinuses or from the mucosa of the nasal cavity. The low concentrations of NO found intranasally during an acute sinusitis as well as its increase after antibiotic therapy have preferentially been explained by obstruction and opening of the sinus ostia, respectively [7]. Recent data, however, suggest that iNOS expression is markedly reduced in the sinus epithelium of patients with maxillary sinusitis [6]. Hence, patency of sinus ostia is not the only factor affecting nasal NO concentration during sinusitis. High concentrations of NO are found in the nose of neonates shortly after birth, even before the sinuses have developed [8]. In a unique study, the osteomeatal complex and sphenoethmoidal recess were occluded in one volunteer to isolate the nose from the sinuses. It was shown that, when all the sinus ostia are blocked, nasal NO output is decreased by only 12%. Interestingly, after ostial occlusion paranasal sinus NO concentration reached a plateau at about 30,000 ppb. This suggests a negative feedback mechanism limiting NO output above a certain local concentration. Further measurements also suggested that, although the NO output per square unit of mucosa was smaller in the nose than in the sinuses, the majority of nasal NO is still derived from the nose itself, because of its larger surface area [9].

Physiological Role of Nasal NO

NO production is commonly enhanced at sites of inflammation. The physiological role of the very high local NO concentration in the paranasal sinuses is still unclear. NO is bacteriostatic at such high concentrations and may contribute to the local host defence of these cavities [3]. It may also play an important role in the regulation of ciliary function [10, 11]. Pulmonary vascular resistance is decreased in humans during nasal breathing compared to that during mouth breathing, intubation or after tracheotomy [12, 13]. This implies that nasally derived NO acts by autoinhalation as an aerocrine messenger to modulate the pulmonary vascular tone and to improve ventilation/perfusion matching.

Methodology of Measuring Nasal NO [14]

Many brilliant experimental techniques have been used to measure NO production at the various sites of the upper airways to arrive at the current understanding of nasal NO physiology. The measured NO concentrations differed widely, because they depend highly on the technology and measurement techniques used. Therefore, international task forces have tried to set standards for NO measurements to enable the comparison of results from different laboratories. This chapter will review the currently recommended technique to measure nasal NO concentrations for diagnostic purposes in clinical practice [15, 16].

Terminology and Units

The nasal airway is a complex system of communicating cavities composed of the nasal cavities, paranasal sinuses, the middle ear, and the nasopharynx. Measurements of nasal NO provide no information with respect to the anatomical source of the gas or the physiological processes that generate the NO. The fractional concentration of nasal NO is termed nasal FE_{NO} and expressed in ppb, which is equivalent to nanolitres per litre. Nasal NO output represents the amount of nasal NO exhaled per time unit, and is denoted nasal $\dot{V}_{NO}$. It is calculated from the product of NO

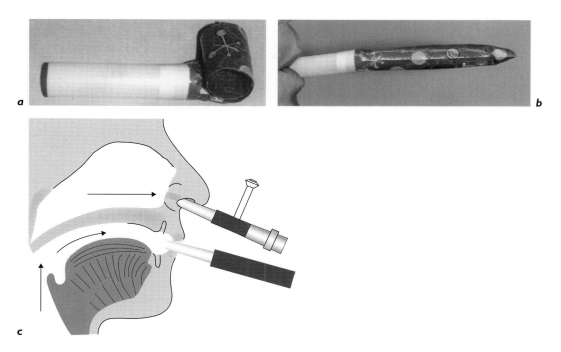

Fig. 1. *a* Party toy. *b* Party toy inflated. *c* Velopharyngeal closure achieved with inflation of party toy [reproduced with permission from 21].

concentration in nanolitres per litre and expiratory flow rate in litres per minute, corrected to BTPS.

NO Analyzer

NO is measured in exhaled air by chemiluminescence which is based on the emission of light from the reaction of NO with ozone (O_3) to NO_2. The quantity of light emitted is proportional to the concentration of NO [17]. The extremely high sensitivity and fast response time of modern NO analyzers permit continuous on-line measurements of NO in exhaled air. Minimum standards for suitable chemiluminescence NO analyzers have been described in detail with respect to linearity and accuracy ($\pm 1\%$ full range), lower detectable limit (≤ 1 ppb), response time (fast lag time and rise time), and measurement range (0.1–10,000 ppb) [15].

Description of Standard Technique

Measurement of nasal NO output requires generation of air flow through the nasal cavity (transnasal air flow). While the velum is closed, transnasal flow can be achieved by various aspiration or insufflation methods which generate flow through the nasal cavities in series (air circulates from one naris to the other) or in parallel. Aspiration at a fixed flow through the nasal passages in series is currently the most widely used and best-validated method to sample nasal NO in isolation from the lower respiratory tract.

Velum Closure

Measurements have to be performed during velum closure to exclude air entry from the lower respiratory tract and to prevent a loss of nasal air via the posterior velopharyngeal aperture. Recommended methods to achieve velum closure are: (1) inhalation to total lung capacity and exhalation against an expiratory resistance while targeting a mouth pressure of 10 cm H_2O [18], (2) breath holding [19], (3) pursed lip breathing [20], and (4) sustained inflation of a party toy [21].

Slow oral exhalation against a resistance of at least 10 cm H_2O has been chosen as the preferred method in adults, but any method that can reliably close the velum is acceptable. It is our experience and the experience of others that in older children velum closure can be reliably achieved by breath holding or exhalation into a balloon or 'party toys' which can act as expiratory resistors (fig. 1) [21, 22]. The children are asked to keep the party toy inflated until a maximum plateau NO concentration is reached. The sustained inflation of the party toy indicates that palatal closure is reliably achieved. Simultaneous measurement of nasal CO_2 is used

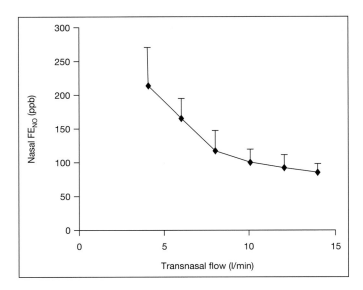

Fig. 2. Inverse correlation of nasal NO concentration (FE_{NO}) with transnasal flow rate [reproduced with permission from 16].

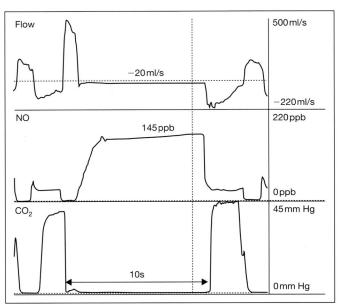

Fig. 3. Simultaneous measurements of flow, NO concentration and CO_2 level against time. The NO trace shows a washout phase and steady plateau at a fixed transnasal flow of 20 ml/s. The CO_2 signal confirms the absence of contamination with alveolar air.

to verify velum closure and to demonstrate the absence of contamination with exhaled air from the lower airways. There is, however, no validated technique to measure nasal NO concentrations in infants and young children who are unable to perform velum closure manoeuvres.

Aspiration or Sampling Flow

It is essential to measure the NO concentration at a known and fixed aspiration flow, because nasal NO concentration is inversely related to transnasal flow rate (fig. 2) [23]. The transnasal or aspiration flow should be measured and recorded against time together with the NO concentration and CO_2 level. The constant transnasal flow produces a washout phase of NO followed by the establishment of a steady plateau documented in the profile of NO (fig. 3). It has been demonstrated that nasal NO output varies with the magnitude of aspiration flow, despite the achievement of a steady-state plateau of NO concentration in the aspired air. NO output is higher when measured at transnasal flows in the magnitude of 2.7–3.7 l/min compared with lower flows of 0.2–0.7 l/min. The higher flows produce a turbulent instead of a laminar flow pattern and facilitate ventilation of the narrow peripheral parts of the nasal airway. It is also argued that the efficacy of NO removal from the nasal mucosa is higher with turbulent flow, as is water and heat transfer. These turbulent flows also most closely resemble physiological flows during quiet nasal breathing.

Hence, NO measurements obtained at low laminar flows may underestimate NO output compared to measurements at higher and more physiological transnasal flow rates. By reporting the NO output instead of the NO concentration, measurements at different flows become comparable, provided the aspiration flow is within the flow range that provides maximal and stable NO concentrations (0.9–6.0 l/min) [24]. An ATS task force defined 3.0 l/min as the optimal flow to measure nasal NO concentration in adults [16]. However, no specific recommendations were made for optimal transnasal flows in children, which are likely to be lower. The optimal range of flows was later reported to be 3.2–5.2 l/min in adults and 2.2–3.2 l/min in children [25]. We obtained steady plateau NO concentrations in children with transnasal flows at 1.2 l/min [22]. It is recommended to increase aspiration flow rates up to 6 l/min, if a steady NO plateau is not achieved. The precise flow used should be documented for each subject.

Technique

Nasal NO is measured in the child sitting with an olive introduced approximately 1 cm inside one nostril ensuring a tight seal while the contralateral nostril is left open

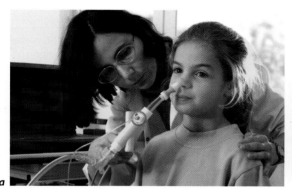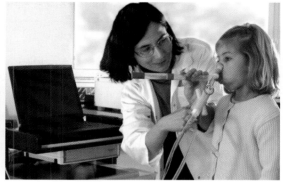

Fig. 4. Measurements of nasal NO output during breath hold (**a**) and during constant insufflation into an expiratory resistor (**b**). Aspiration flow is measured by an ultrasonic spirometer connected to a vacuum source and CO_2 by capnography, respectively.

(eventually with the help of another nozzle). This olive should be composed of a soft, non-traumatizing material, and be of sufficient diameter and appropriate shape to occlude the naris. Air is aspirated at a constant flow rate by a suction pump while the velum is closed by an appropriate technique for at least 10 s. A side port just distal to the olive samples gas for NO analysis (fig. 4). A tight-fitting mask covering the nose may also be used for nasal NO measurements.

Humming and Assessment of Sinus Ventilation
Nasal NO concentrations increase largely (15-fold) during humming compared to silent exhalation [26]. This is explained by an increased washout of air, and hence NO, from the paranasal sinuses into the nasal cavity by the oscillating sound waves. The increase in nasal NO during humming is absent if the sinus ostia are completely obstructed. Hence, combined nasal NO measurements with and without humming could be of use to estimate sinus ventilation and to assess the relative contribution of the nasal cavity and the sinuses to nasal NO output [27]. Nasal NO is markedly decreased following repeated consecutive humming manoeuvres and recovers to baseline concentrations after a 3-min period of silence. This pattern fits well with the notion that humming empties the sinuses and that a period of silence will allow for NO to accumulate again. It is of interest that posthumming nasal NO measurements are characterized by less intrasubject variability in comparison with measurements performed after a short period of speaking or silence [28]. Posthumming measurements may serve as a measure of NO output from the nasal cavity mucosa.

Factors Influencing Nasal NO Values

There is only limited knowledge on whether and how physiological, pharmacological, and external factors affect nasal NO output. It is evident that breath holding or nose occlusion increase nasal NO measurements.

Ambient Air
Ambient NO concentrations are highly variable and can reach concentrations that may cause considerable errors if ambient air is used as the gas source for transnasal flow. This is of utmost concern if ambient NO concentrations are higher than nasal NO concentrations, e.g. in conditions with very low nasal NO output such as primary ciliary dyskinesia (PCD). The use of NO-free air as gas source for transnasal flow is recommended to eliminate this problem. In any case, the ambient NO concentration should be recorded and taken into consideration for correct interpretation of nasal NO measurements.

Smoking
The effect of prenatal or postnatal tobacco smoke exposure on nasal NO concentration has not been investigated in children. Nasal NO concentrations are slightly lower in smokers [29].

Age
It has been hypothesized that nasal NO concentrations rise from birth until the age of 10 years with pneumatization of the sinuses, although when related to body weight NO output in preterm infants was shown to be similar to

Table 1. Published studies measuring nasal NO in healthy children

Study	n	Age years	Technique	Aspiration flow, l/min	No output, nl/min	NO concentration, ppb
Corbelli et al. [22]	24	12.4 (4.5–24)	Breath hold	1.2		223.7 (90–950)
Daya et al. [21]	30	10.7 (3.3–17.5)	Breath hold	3	458 (131–1,424)	
Narang et al. [48]	53	10.7 (5.5–19)	Breath hold	0.25		716 (398–1,437)
Karadag et al. [36]	20	~10.8	Breath hold	0.25		553 (116–1,437)
Baraldi et al. [38]	133	6–15	Tidal breathing	0.7		216 (95% CI 204–228)
Balfour-Lynn et al. [37]	54	12.2 (6–17)	Breath hold	0.25		1,024 (158–2,502)
Lundberg et al. [40]	19	5–15	Tidal breathing	0.7		239 (SD 20)
Dötsch et al. [46]	37	4–18	Tidal breathing	0.7		101 (SD 49)

Data represent mean or median with the range in parentheses except where stated otherwise. CI = Confidence interval; SD = standard deviation.

adults [30]. More work is needed to clarify age-related changes in nasal NO output from infancy to adulthood using comparable methods. Nasal NO concentrations in adults are not affected by aging.

Physical Exercise

Nasal NO concentrations decrease by about 50% during physical exercise and reach normal baseline concentrations in about 15–20 min [31, 32]. The reason for the decrease in nasal NO output during exercise has not yet been elucidated.

Drugs

Data on the effect of pharmacological substances on nasal NO output is limited. Nasal decongestants, such as oxymetazoline and xylometazoline, decrease nasal NO concentrations by about 15% and have a dose-dependent inhibitory effect on total iNOS activity in vitro [33, 34]. Histamine, topical and systemic steroids, and antibiotics have no effect on nasal NO concentrations in healthy persons [35].

Normal Data of Nasal NO Measurements in Children

Data obtained from healthy children demonstrate considerable intersubject variation resulting in a broad range of normal nasal NO output [21]. Normal values have yet to be established in a larger population of healthy children of different ages using the recommended aspiration technique

Table 2. Effect of diseases on nasal NO concentrations in children

Disease	Nasal NO concentration
Common cold, upper respiratory tract infection	Unchanged
Allergic rhinitis	Increased (decreased with topical steroids)
Asthma	Unchanged
Acute sinusitis	Decreased
Cystic fibrosis	Decreased
Non-cystic fibrosis or non-PCD bronchiectasis	Decreased
PCD	Extremely low

during breath holding. Previous studies reporting nasal NO concentrations in healthy children are summarized in table 1. Intrasubject coefficients of variation of repeated measurements by the aspiration technique are between 4 and 8% in healthy children [36–38].

Diagnostic Use in Paediatric Respiratory Diseases

Nasal NO concentrations are increased in asthma, allergic rhinitis, and viral respiratory infections, but are reduced in sinusitis, cystic fibrosis, PCD, bronchiectasis, chronic cough, diffuse panbronchiolitis, and after exposure to tobacco and alcohol (table 2) [37, 39–46]. The most

Table 3. Published studies reporting sensitivity and specificity of nasal NO concentrations in discriminating between patients with PCD and non-PCD bronchiectasis

Study	Aspiration flow, l/min	Cutoff level, ppb	Sensitivity, %	Specificity, %	Positive predictive value, %	Negative predictive value, %
Horvath et al. [51]	0.25	187	93	95	87	97
Narang et al. [48]	0.25	250	97	90	83	97
Corbelli et al. [22]	1.2	105	94	88	89	94

comprehensive and significant changes in nasal NO concentrations in relation to normal values can be documented in patients with PCD. Current knowledge suggests that the measurement of nasal NO concentrations may be of clinical value in clarifying diagnostic problems in patients with clinical suspicion of PCD. Nasal NO measurements are, however, of no diagnostic utility in distinguishing between conditions such as asthma, cystic fibrosis, bronchiectasis, sinusitis or rhinitis, or in monitoring therapeutic interventions in any such disorder.

Primary Ciliary Dyskinesia

PCD constitutes a recessively inherited group of disorders of ciliary structure and/or function resulting in impaired mucociliary clearance. Typical structural ciliary abnormalities include absent inner or outer dynein arms, and radial spoke and tubular defects. The clinical manifestations are recurrent or chronic respiratory tract infections with mucus retention as there are rhinitis, sinusitis, serous otitis media, and bronchitis. Mirror image arrangement occurs in 50% of the patients (Kartagener syndrome) [47].

Measurements of nasal NO concentrations in patients with PCD are extremely low compared to healthy children or children with other respiratory disorders [22, 36, 48–52]. There is no relationship between the different structural defects in PCD and the levels of nasal NO concentration [52]. The reason for the low nasal NO concentrations in patients with PCD has not yet been clarified. Several observations suggest that NO plays an important role in signal transduction associated with ciliary motility. The epithelial NOS is localized at the basal body of the microtubules of the cilia, and NO has been found to stimulate ciliary beat frequency [6, 53]. It seems, however, unlikely that the lower levels of nasal and also exhaled NO concentrations in PCD are the results of reduced NOS activity, because levels of NO metabolites are not different between patients with PCD and healthy subjects [54].

Measurements of nasal NO concentrations are helpful to screen children with clinical symptoms suggestive of PCD and to decide on the need for further, more invasive testing. This is strengthened by the high sensitivity and specificity of nasal NO concentrations to discriminate between PCD and other disorders with chronic airway inflammation, such as cystic fibrosis and non-PCD bronchiectasis (table 3). If nasal NO concentration is unexpectedly low in a patient with recurrent respiratory infections, the diagnosis of PCD should be actively excluded. This is done by assessing the ciliary beat frequency by light microscopy, and searching for the typical ultrastructural defects of the cilia by electron microscopy in mucosal biopsy specimens.

References

1 Gustafsson LE, Leone AM, Persson MG, Wiklund NP, Moncada S: Endogenous nitric oxide is present in the exhaled air of rabbits, guinea pigs and humans. Biochem Biophys Res Commun 1991;181:852–857.

2 Alving K, Weitzberg E, Lundberg JM: Increased amount of nitric oxide in exhaled air of asthmatics. Eur Respir J 1993;6:1368–1370.

3 Lundberg JO, Farkas-Szallasi T, Weitzberg E, Rinder J, Lidholm J, Anggaard A, Hokfelt T, Lundberg JM, Alving K: High nitric oxide in human paranasal sinuses. Nat Med 1995;1:370–373.

4 Occupational Health Guideline for Nitric Oxide. National Institute for Occupational Safety and Health. Occupational Health Guidelines for Chemical Hazards. DHHS (NIOSH) Publication 1981; http://www.cdc.gov/niosh/pdfs/0448.pdf

5 Asano K, Chee CB, Gaston B, Lilly CM, Gerard C, Drazen JM, Stamler JS: Constitutive and inducible nitric oxide synthase gene expression, regulation and activity in human lung epithelial cells. Proc Natl Acad Sci USA 1994;91:10089–10093.

6 Deja M, Busch T, Bachmann S, Riskowski K, Campean V, Wiedmann B, Schwabe M, Hell B, Pfeilschifter J, Falke KJ, Lewandowski K: Reduced nitric oxide in sinus epithelium of patients with radiologic maxillary sinusitis and sepsis. Am J Respir Crit Care Med 2003;168:281–286.

7 Baraldi E, Azzolin NM, Biban P, Zacchello F: Effect of antibiotic therapy on nasal nitric oxide concentration in children with acute sinusitis. Am J Respir Crit Care Med 1997;155:1680–1683.

8 Williams O, Rafferty GF, Hannam S, Milner AD, Greenough A: Nasal and lower airway levels of nitric oxide in prematurely born infants. Early Hum Dev 2003;72:67–73.

9 Haight JS, Djupesland PG, Qjan W, Chatkin JM, Furlott H, Irish J, Witterick I, McClean P, Fenton RS, Hoffstein V, Zamel N: Does nasal nitric oxide come from the sinuses? J Otolaryngol 1999;28:197–204.

10 Kim JW, Min YG, Rhee CS, Lee CH, Koh YY, Rhyoo C, Kwon TY, Park SW: Regulation of mucociliary motility by nitric oxide and expression of nitric oxide synthase in the human sinus epithelial cells. Laryngoscope 2001;111:246–250.

11 Lindberg S, Cervin A, Runer T: Low levels of nasal nitric oxide (NO) correlate to impaired mucociliary function in the upper airways. Acta Otolaryngol 1997;117:728–734.

12 Settergren G, Angdin M, Astudillo R, Gelinder S, Liska J, Lundberg JO, Weitzberg E: Decreased pulmonary vascular resistance during nasal breathing: Modulation by endogenous nitric oxide from the paranasal sinuses. Acta Physiol Scand 1998;163:235–239.

13 Lundberg JO, Settergren G, Gelinder S, Lundberg JM, Alving K, Weitzberg E: Inhalation of nasally derived nitric oxide modulates pulmonary function in humans. Acta Physiol Scand 1996;158:343–347.

14 Kissoon N, Duckworth L, Blake K, Murphy S, Silkoff PE: Exhaled nitric oxide measurements in childhood asthma: Techniques and interpretation. Pediatr Pulmonol 1999;28:282–296.

15 Kharitonov S, Alving K, Barnes PJ: Exhaled and nasal nitric oxide measurements: Recommendations. The European Respiratory Society Task Force. Eur Respir J 1997;10:1683–1693.

16 American Thoracic Society: Recommendations for standardized procedures for the online and offline measurement of exhaled lower respiratory nitric oxide and nasal nitric oxide in adults and children. Am J Respir Crit Care Med 1999;160:2104–2117.

17 Archer S: Measurement of nitric oxide in biological models. FASEB J 1993;7:349–360.

18 Silkoff PE, McClean PA, Slutsky AS, Furlott HG, Hoffstein E, Wakita S, Chapman KR, Szalai JP, Zamel N: Marked flow-dependence of exhaled nitric oxide using a new technique to exclude nasal nitric oxide. Am J Respir Crit Care Med 1997;155:260–267.

19 Kimberly B, Nejadnik B, Giraud GD, Holden WE: Nasal contribution to exhaled nitric oxide at rest and during breathholding in humans. Am J Respir Crit Care Med 1996;153:829–836.

20 Rodenstein DO, Stanescu DC: Absence of nasal air flow during pursed lips breathing. The soft palate mechanisms. Am Rev Respir Dis 1983;128:716–718.

21 Daya H, Qian W, McClean P, Haight J, Zamel N, Papsin BC, Forte V: Nasal nitric oxide in children: A novel measurement technique and normal values. Laryngoscope 2002;112:1831–1835.

22 Corbelli R, Bringolf-Isler B, Amacher A, Sasse B, Spycher M, Hammer J: Nasal nitric oxide measurements to screen children for primary ciliary dyskinesia? Chest 2004;126:1054–1059.

23 Silkoff PE, Chatkin J, Qian W, Chakravorty S, Gutierrez C, Furlott H, McClean P, Rai S, Zamel N, Haight J: Nasal nitric oxide: A comparison of measurement techniques. Am J Rhinol 1999;13:169–178.

24 Imada M, Iwamoto J, Nonaka S, Kobayashi Y, Unno T: Measurement of nitric oxide in human nasal airway. Eur Respir J 1996;9:556–559.

25 Qian W, Djupesland PG, Chatkin JM, McClean P, Furlott H, Chapnik JS, Zamel N, Haight JS: Aspiration flow optimized for nasal nitric oxide measurement. Rhinology 1999; 37:61–65.

26 Weitzberg E, Lundberg JO: Humming greatly increases nasal nitric oxide. Am J Respir Crit Care Med 2002;166:144–145.

27 Maniscalco M, Weitzberg E, Sundberg J, Sofia M, Lundberg JO: Assessment of nasal and sinus nitric oxide output using single-breath humming exhalations. Eur Respir J 2003;22:323–329.

28 Maniscalco M, Sofia M, Weitzberg E, Carratu L, Lundberg JO: Nasal nitric oxide measurements before and after repeated humming maneuvers. Eur J Clin Invest 2003;33:1090–1094.

29 Olin AC, Hellgren J, Karlsson G, Ljungkvist G, Nolkrantz K, Toren K: Nasal nitric oxide and its relationship to nasal symptoms, smoking and nasal nitrate. Rhinology 1998;36:117–121.

30 Artlich A, Bush T, Lewandowsky K: Exhaled nitric oxide in preterm infants. Respir Physiol 1998;114:195–200.

31 Phillips CR, Giraud GD, Holden WE: Exhaled nitric oxide during exercise: Site of release and modulation by ventilation and blood flow. J Appl Physiol 1996;80:1865–1871.

32 Lundberg JON, Rinder J, Weitzberg E, Alving K: Heavy physical exercise decreases nitric oxide levels in the nasal airways in humans. Acta Physiol Scand 1997;159:51–57.

33 Ferguson EA, Eccles R: Changes in nasal nitric oxide concentration associated with symptoms of common cold and treatment with a topical nasal decongestant. Acta Otolaryngol 1997;117:614–617.

34 Westerveld GJ, Voss HP, van der Hee RM, de Haan-Koelewijn GJ, den Hartog GJ, Scheeren RA, Bast A: Inhibition of nitric oxide synthase by nasal decongestants. Eur Respir J 2000;16:437–444.

35 Lundberg JON, Weitzberg E, Lundberg JM, Alving K: Nitric oxide in exhaled air. Eur Respir J 1996;9:2671–2680.

36 Karadag B, James AJ, Gultekin E, Wilson NM, Bush A: Nasal and lower airway level of nitric oxide in children with primary ciliary dyskinesia. Eur Respir J 1999;13:1402–1405.

37 Balfour-Lynn IM, Laverty A, Dinwiddie R: Reduced upper airway nitric oxide in cystic fibrosis. Arch Dis Child 1996;75:319–322.

38 Baraldi E, Azzolin NM, Cracco A, Zacchello F: Reference values of exhaled nitric oxide for healthy children 6–15 years old. Pediatr Pulmonol 1999;27:54–58.

39 Baraldi E, Azzolin NM, Carra S, Dario C, Marchesini L, Zacchello F: Effect of topical steroids on nasal nitric oxide production in children with perennial allergic rhinitis: A pilot study. Respir Med 1998;92:558–561.

40 Lundberg JON, Nordvall SL, Weitzberg E, Kollberg H, Alving K: Exhaled nitric oxide in paediatric asthma and cystic fibrosis. Arch Dis Child 1996;75:323–326.

41 Arnal JF, Didier A, Rami J, M'Rini C, Charlet JP, Serrano E, Besombes JP: Nasal nitric oxide is increased in allergic rhinitis. Clin Exp Allergy 1997;27:358–362.

42 Kharitonov SA, Rajakulasingam K, O'Connor B, Durham SR, Barnes PJ: Nasal nitric oxide is increased in patients with asthma and allergic rhinitis and may be modulated by nasal glucocorticoids. J Allergy Clin Immunol 1997;99:58–64.

43 Thomas SR, Kharitonov SA, Scott SF, Hodson ME, Barnes PJ: Nasal and exhaled nitric oxide is reduced in adult patients with cystic fibrosis and does not correlate with cystic fibrosis genotype. Chest 2000;117:1085–1089.

44 Nakano H, Ide H, Imada M, Osanai S, Takahashi T, Kikuchi K, Iwamoto J: Reduced nasal nitric oxide in diffuse panbronchiolitis. Am J Respir Crit Care Med 2000;162:2218–2220.

45 Lindberg S, Cervin A, Runer T: Low levels of nasal nitric oxide (NO) correlate to impaired mucociliary function in the upper airways. Acta Otolaryngol 1997;117:728–734.

46 Dötsch J, Demirakca S, Terbrack HG, Huls G, Rascher W, Kuhl PG: Airway nitric oxide in asthmatic children and patients with cystic fibrosis. Eur Respir J 1996;9:2537–2540.

47 Bush A, Cole P, Hariri M, Mackay I, Phillips G, O'Callaghan C, Wilson R, Warner JO: Primary ciliary dyskinesia: Diagnosis and standards of care. Eur Respir J 1998;12:982–988.

48 Narang I, Ersu R, Wilson NM, Bush A: Nitric oxide in chronic airway inflammation in children: Diagnostic use and pathophysiological significance. Thorax 2002;57:586–589.

49 Lundberg JO, Weitzberg E, Nordvall SL, Kuylenstierna R, Lundberg JM, Alving K: Primarily nasal origin of exhaled nitric oxide and absence in Kartagener's syndrome. Eur Respir J 1994;7:1501–1504.

50 Wodehouse T, Kharitonov SA, Mackay IS, Barnes PJ, Wilson R, Cole PJ: Nasal nitric oxide measurements for the screening of primary ciliary dyskinesia. Eur Respir J 2003; 21:43–47.

51 Horvath I, Loukides S, Wodehouse T, Csiszer E, Cole PJ, Kharitonov SA, Barnes PJ: Comparison of exhaled and nasal nitric oxide and exhaled carbon monoxide levels in bronchiectatic patients with and without primary ciliary dyskinesia. Thorax 2003;58:68–72.

52 Noone PG, Leigh MW, Sannuti A, Minnix SL, Carson JL, Hazucha M, Zariwala MA, Knowles MR: Primary ciliary dyskinesia. Diagnostic and phenotypic features. Am J Respir Crit Care Med 2004;169:459–467.

53 Doran SA, Tran CH, Eskicioglu C, Stachniak T, Ahn KC, Goldberg JI: Constitutive and permissive roles of nitric oxide activity in embryonic ciliary cells. Am J Physiol Regul Integr Comp Physiol 2003;285:R348–R355.

54 Csoma Z, Bush A, Wilson NM, Donnelly L, Balint B, Barnes PJ, Kharitonov SA: Nitric oxide metabolites are not reduced in exhaled breath condensate of patients with primary ciliary dyskinesia. Chest 2003;124:633–638.

Prof. Dr. med. Jürg Hammer
Head, Division of Intensive Care
and Pulmonology
University Children's Hospital Basel
Römergasse 8, CH–4005 Basel (Switzerland)
Tel. +41 61 685 65 65
Fax +41 61 685 50 59
E-Mail juerg.hammer@unibas.ch

Hammer J, Eber E (eds): Paediatric Pulmonary Function Testing.
Prog Respir Res. Basel, Karger, 2005, vol 33, pp 190–202

Measurement of Exhaled Markers

Exhaled Breath Condensate and Other Markers in Exhaled Air

Alexander Moeller[a]   Bogumila Kielbasa[a, b]

[a]Division of Respiratory Medicine, University Children's Hospital Zürich, Zürich, Switzerland;
[b]Department of Medicine, Jagiellonian University School of Medicine Krakow, Krakow, Poland

Abstract

Airway inflammation and oxidative stress are hallmarks of chronic lung diseases, such as asthma, cystic fibrosis, and primary ciliary dyskinesia. Especially in young children and infants, where there is a lack of objective measures a reliable non-invasive technique is necessary. The analyses of exhaled gases and exhaled breath condensate (EBC) in children represent challenging new techniques, and have the potential as non-invasive measures to assess and to monitor airway inflammation, oxidative stress, and metabolic processes. The techniques are simple to perform, may be repeated frequently, and are ideally suited for young or disabled patients. Several volatile chemicals (nitric oxide, carbon monoxide, ethane), and many non-volatile molecules (mediators, oxidation and nitration products, proteins) have been measured in exhaled air. These mediators have been reported to be altered in a range of conditions. However, the technique has yet to be standardized and numerous methodological questions have to be answered before the analysis of EBC for the assessment of childhood respiratory disease can become a clinical tool. In this chapter we provide a detailed update on the techniques currently used to obtain EBC in children, and the methods used for the measurement of markers within the EBC. We summarize the current knowledge of EBC contents and discuss the available paediatric data.

Introduction

Based on the hypothesis that aerosol particles exhaled in human breath reflect the composition of bronchoalveolar extracellular lining fluid, there is increased interest in different techniques to assess inflammation and oxidative stress in the lungs indirectly by the analysis of various non-volatile and volatile breath components [1, 2].

Exhaled breath is saturated with water vapour. As exhaled air cools below the dew point on a chilled condenser surface, condensation occurs on available aerosolized particles. The enlarged droplets of exhaled breath condensate (EBC) impact and collect on the condenser wall. For the most part the condensate consists of water, but it also contains aerosol particles, which allow non-volatile and soluble substances to be transported from the lower respiratory tract [3]. The number of particles detected in exhaled air during tidal breathing varies over a range from less than 0.1 to about 4 particles/cm^3, with a mean diameter of particles less than 0.3 μm [4, 5]. It is assumed that aerosols are disrupted from the extracellular surface fluid layer by turbulent flow and airflow deviation in branching points of the bronchi and alveoli, and that the amount may depend on the current velocity of the passing air and the surface tension [6]. Therefore, condensate components reflect different markers and molecules derived from oropharynx, airways, and alveoli.

The first studies identifying surface-active properties of EBC were published in Russia in the 1980s [7]. Since then a wide range of inflammatory markers has been reported to be present in the EBC. Nitric oxide (NO) metabolites, markers of oxidative stress, eicosanoids, cytokines, and pH have all been measured in the EBC. Mediators have been reported to be altered in a range of conditions including asthma, chronic obstructive pulmonary disease as well as cystic fibrosis (CF) [8–16]. Most of the studies have been carried out in adults but there is also a raising number of studies in children with various respiratory conditions. The collection of EBC requires only minimal patient cooperation and may therefore be ideally suited for young or disabled patients. The EBC offers a potentially important step forward in the development of the non-invasive clinical diagnosis and monitoring of respiratory disease. Especially in young children and infants, where there is a lack of objective measures, there is a strong need for a reliable non-invasive technique.

Methods

Different systems to obtain EBC have been used by different research groups; however, the principle to cool or freeze the exhaled air is the same for all condenser systems used. The collection involves rapid cooling of the exhaled air with consecutive condensation of water vapour as well as sedimentation and impaction of aerosol particles to cold surfaces.

Generally, the child is breathing tidally via a mouthpiece trough a two-way non-rebreathing valve by inhaling normal room air and exhaling into a condenser. The most simple and originally widely used design included Teflon-lined tubing immersed in an ice-filled bucket [17]. Formanek et al. [11] used an adaptation of this system. Briefly, a mouthpiece including a saliva trap and a two-way valve is attached to a polyvinyl chloride tube (length 55 cm, internal diameter 1 cm), which is passed through a section of pipe packed with ice. The EBC is collected into a small container attached to the free end of the tube. This technique allowed EBC to be collected in children as young as 3 years of age. Several investigators used a condensing device formed by two glass chambers. The inner glass chamber is cooled by ice and is suspended in a larger glass chamber. The EBC is collected between the two glass surfaces. The exhaled air enters the chamber by a two-way non-rebreathing valve and leaves the cooling chamber by a one-way valve at the outlet, keeping the chamber closed [9, 18].

Two commercially available systems have been used so far. In the ECOScreen system (Erich Jaeger, Hoechberg, Germany) the exhaled air is conducted through a lamellar condenser to which a sample collection vial is connected. The condenser is inserted into a cuff containing circulating cooling liquid (electric refrigerator). The condenser maintains a temperature of $-10°C$ throughout a 10- to 15-min collection period, which may be an important point in the attempt to standardize the collection of EBC. The

disadvantage of this system is the size of the equipment which may limit its use in field studies. The Rtube breath condensate collector (Respiratory Research, Charlottesville, Va., USA) is a portable device and consists of a disposable polypropylene tube acting as condenser and collector, which is placed into a precooled aluminum sleeve. The device uses an exhalation valve that also serves as a syringe-style plunger to pool fluid from the condenser walls, which allows to reduce collection time.

All presented condenser systems have been used in children with minimal or no adaptation. Specific issues have to be considered when EBC is collected from infants and newborns. Small children are not able to cooperate, and they are preferential nose breathers. In addition, the tidal volume and hence the minute ventilation are small; therefore, the amount of condensate which is collected is small, and additional volume loss can occur in the sampling system. Breath condensates have been obtained from nasally exhaled air in children as young as 4 weeks and older using nasal prongs serially connected via two 50-ml polypropylene tubes submerged into frozen 10% salt water to an electric air suction pump. With this technique minimal cooperation is needed but there are some important limitations. Only parameters which are not produced in significant amounts within the nasal airways can be assessed in EBC collected from nasal breathing. The method allows the collection of a fraction of only 20–30% of the exhaled water vapour; therefore, the obtained volumes are very small in infants, and collection time may become an important issue [19]. A recently developed method to collect EBC during both oral and nasal breathing in infants allows the collection of 75–500 µl within 10 min. Briefly, the cooling device consists of a mouthpiece attached to two connected 60-ml syringes (Plastipack, Becton Dickinson) fixed in series in an insulation box. Two ice packs ($-10°C$) are wrapped around the syringes. The infant is assessed during induced sleep and is breathing tidally into the collector system. Using this device we found no significant difference in NO metabolites between EBC collected during oral or nasal breathing but there was a high degree of variability in the short-term repeatability of measurements [20].

The collection of EBC has been shown to be safe. There are no adverse effects in children, even during asthma exacerbation [18, 21], and infants [20]. The most important issue in the collection of EBC in childhood is the cooperation to breath quietly trough a mouthpiece for 10–15 min. The cooperation can be obtained by adequate instruction of the child and the parents, and by a certain distraction, for example by showing video cartoons. Many of the inflammatory markers, such as eicosanoids [thromboxane B_2, leukotriene B_4 (LTB_4), prostaglandin F_2 (PGF_2)], and nitrate and nitrite, are found in significant concentrations in the saliva [22, 23]. It is, therefore, important to prevent salivary contamination of the EBC. In many studies salivary contamination has been monitored by measuring amylase, and it has been shown that a saliva trap, introduced between mouthpiece and sampling system, prevents efficiently salivary contamination [3, 24, 25]. Nevertheless, coughing into the sampling system or forced exhalation manoeuvres can lead to salivary contamination of the condensate and should therefore be avoided. The child should rinse his mouth prior to collection and try to keep the mouth dry by periodically swallowing the saliva. The effect of wearing nose clips to ease the collection remains controversial and has not been standardized yet. The use of a nose clip may prevent the velum to close and thereby lead to contamination of the exhaled air with nasal air [26, 27].

Current Knowledge

The biochemical and pathophysiological features of the different markers that have been measured in EBC of children will be discussed, and the methodologies for the measurement of the mentioned markers are described below.

Markers of Oxidative Stress

Hydrogen peroxide (H_2O_2) is thought to be an important reactive oxygen species which may cause cellular injury by the conversion to hydroxyl radical and lipid peroxidation products [28]. Eosinophils, activated phagocytes, and neutrophils are important sources of H_2O_2 [29], which is soluble and therefore diffuses into the extracellular airway lining fluid and is partially exhaled. Lipid peroxidation is a central feature of oxidative stress, and can be assessed by a number of methods. 8-Isoprostane is a prostaglandin-like compound formed by peroxidation of arachidonic acid on membrane phospholipids [30], and has been assessed as a marker of oxidative stress in asthma [9, 31], CF [32], severe respiratory failure in infants [33], and other respiratory diseases. Secondary carbonyl compounds, such as aldehydes, are formed together with unstable lipid hydroperoxides by a chain reaction caused by oxidation of cell membrane phospholipids [34, 35]. Malondialdehyde is generated mainly by arachidonic acid and docosahexaenoic acid and can be measured in exhaled air [36]. Glutathione is a protective antioxidant and is therefore important in the balance with oxidative and nitrosative stress, and has a key role in inflammation control, immune modulation, and tissue protection [36].

Methods for the Measurement of Markers of Oxidative Stress

H_2O_2 can be measured using a colorimetric assay. The condensate is mixed with 100 ml of 420 mM 3'3'5'5-tetramethylbenzidine in 0.42 M citrate buffer pH 3.8 and 10 ml of horseradish peroxidase (52.5 U/ml). The samples are incubated at room temperature for 20 min and the reaction has to be stopped by the addition of 10 ml of 2 N sulfuric acid. The product is then measured spectrophotometrically at 450 nm by a microplate reader. Detection limits vary between 0.1 µmol/l and 0.1 mmol/l [37]. Two different methods to measure 8-isoprostane in EBC have been reported: the use of specific enzyme immunoassays (EIA) or specific radioimmunoassays (RIA). There is a significant difference in the sensitivity of these methods with median 8-isoprostane levels in healthy children varying from 2.6–3.8 pg/ml with the former [38, 39] to 33.6–34.2 pg/ml with the latter method [31]. Malondialdehyde and reduced glutathione can be measured by high-performance liquid chromatography separation and fluorescence detection, or by liquid chromatography-tandem mass spectrometry after derivatization [36, 40].

NO Metabolites, Nitrogen-Reactive Species

NO is generated by three isoforms of NO synthases (types I–III). This enzyme catalyzes the oxidation of *L*-arginine to NO and *L*-citrulline [41]. As an unstable molecule, NO has a short half-life that is often attributed to a rapid oxidation to end products including nitrite (NO_2^-), nitrate (NO_3^-) and S-nitrosothiols (RSNO) [42]. The primary decomposition product of NO in aerobic aqueous solution is NO_2^-, and further oxidation to NO_3^- requires the presence of additional oxidizing species such as oxyhaemoproteins [43, 44]. RSNO are formed by an interaction between NO and cysteine and glutathione. 3-Nitrotyrosine is a metabolite from the reaction of peroxynitrite with tyrosine residues in proteins. Peroxynitrite is a highly reactive species which is formed by the reaction of NO with superoxide anions, and may be regarded as a marker of nitrosative-oxidative stress in airways [45].

Methods for the Measurement of Nitrogen-Reactive Species

The determination of NO_2^- using a colorimetric assay based on the Griess reaction [46] is very simple. The EBC sample is (1:1) reacted with Griess reagent (0.1% naphthylethylenediamine dihydrochloride, 1% sulphanilamide,

3% H_3PO_4) and measured at an absorbance wavelength of 550–570 nm with a microplate reader. Levels are quantified on standard curves. The incubation of samples with NO_3^- reductase allows the NO_3^- present in the sample to be measured by various assays after being converted to NO_2^-. Total NO_2^- and NO_3^- can be measured using an adaptation of a rapid response NO analyzer. Briefly, using microsyringe aliquots of 20 µl of the condensate are instilled into a heated reaction cylinder which contains a saturated solution of vanadium (lll) chloride (VCl_3) in 1 M HCl. The NO_3^- is reduced by the VCl_3 to NO_2^-, which is further reduced to gaseous NO. Levels are then calculated from standard curves generated prior to analysis.

RSNO can be measured following the release of NO_2^- from RSNO by 2 mM Hg_2Cl using the above-mentioned procedures [47], or after treatment with cuprous chloride and cysteine as gaseous NO by chemiluminescence [48].

3-Nitrotyrosine is usually measured with a specific EIA; however, the condensate samples may have to be concentrated using freeze-dry processes [10].

Eicosanoids

Cysteinyl leukotrienes (cys-LT; LTE_4, LTC_4, LTD_4) are strong pro-inflammatory mediators generated from arachidonic acid metabolism by the 5-lipoxygenase pathway, and are released primarily by eosinophils and mast cells [49]. Cys-LT are found in high levels in asthmatic patients and their production is further upregulated during asthma exacerbation and as a response to allergen challenge [49]. Particularly high levels can be found in patients with aspirin-induced asthma [50]. Cys-LT are important in the pathophysiology of asthma as they potently induce bronchoconstriction, increase vascular permeability and mucous secretion, and lead to impaired mucociliary clearance [51–53]. Furthermore, there is some evidence for their role in airway remodeling processes in chronic asthma [49]. PGE_2 has bronchoprotective and inhibitory effects on inflammatory cells, and there is some evidence that impaired production of PGE_2 may contribute to the pathogenesis of asthma [54]. LTB_4 is another lipid mediator derived from arachidonic acid metabolism, and is an important chemoattractant and activator for neutrophils. LTB_4 increases neutrophil-endothelial interactions and further stimulates neutrophil activation [55], and may play an important part in severe asthma, which is associated with increased neutrophilic airway inflammation [56]. High levels of LTB_4 are found in EBC of patients suffering from CF, where it is well known that high numbers of neutrophils can be found even in the absence of bacterial colonization or clinical signs of infection [57–60].

Methods for the Measurement of Eicosanoids

Eicosanoids can be readily measured by EIA using commercially available kits. The detection limits may vary between 4 and 15 pg/ml (e.g. for LTB_4 and cys-LT kits, Cayman Chemical, Ann Arbor, Mich., USA). Recently, the measurement of LTB_4 in EBC has been validated using reverse-phase high-performance liquid chromatography [61]. Prostaglandins are measured using EIA or specific RIA. A new method is the measurement with mass spectrometry-gas chromatography [62].

Cytokines

Cytokines reported in EBC collected from children include interleukin-4 (IL-4), IL-8, and tumour necrosis factor-α. Cytokines are peptides with a relatively low molecular mass (<80 kD). However, the measurement of proteins is difficult due to very low concentrations of these molecules in the EBC [62]. To date there is no sufficient data published regarding cytokines in EBC to be a useful clinical tool in the assessment of pathological processes within the lung and airways, though this is an area of active investigation.

Methods for the Measurement of Cytokines

The analysis of cytokines within EBC is performed usually by EIA, using commercially available detection kits. Recent developments include flow-cytometric bead array systems which make it possible to assess various cytokines in very small volumes.

Airway Acidity

The airway surface fluid is slightly alkaline in healthy subjects with a pH in the range of 7–8 [64]. Bronchoscopy studies revealed reduced pH in human airway inflammation [65]. It is well known that altering the pH of the airway environment affects airway function, e.g. application of nebulized citric acid can induce bronchoconstriction [66]. In addition, low pH conditions in the airways may favour protonation of NO_2^- liberating NO, indicating a critical pH dependency of the bioactivity of the nitrogen-reactive species [67]. Low pH levels may have additional consequences such as a reduction of the ciliary beating frequency [68], and an increase of airway mucus viscosity, hence leading to impaired mucociliary clearance [69]. The pH of EBC has been found to be low in asthmatic [14, 70] and CF patients [71]. Recently, Vaughan et al. [72] investigated different methodological aspects, such as the effects of ventilatory pattern during EBC collection, its duration, temperature, and induced bronchoconstriction on the pH of the condensate, and found the EBC pH to be a robust and reproducible assay to investigate airway acidity.

Methods for the Measurement of pH

The pH of condensate samples has to be measured within a short time of collection since pH may change due to other components of the EBC such as NO_2^- or ammonia. The measurement itself is very simple using a pH micro-electrode. The system has to be recalibrated before each analysis. To prevent changes of pH, stabilization can be achieved by deaeration of the condensate with argon (350 ml/min) for 10 min [14].

EBC: Expected Changes in Respiratory Diseases and Normal Values

Asthma

A variety of markers within the EBC have been investigated as possible measures of disease activity of asthma in children.

H_2O_2 in EBC has been found to be 4-fold elevated in children with stable asthma compared to healthy controls [8, 17], whereas a subgroup of steroid naïve asthmatics showed a 5-fold increase of median H_2O_2 levels [8]. There was a further increase in a subgroup of asthmatic patients who were sick at the moment of EBC collection [17]. A correlation between expired breath H_2O_2 levels and clinical status was shown, but not between H_2O_2 levels and lung function parameters [17]. To date no controlled intervention study using H_2O_2 in EBC has been carried out in children. There are some methodological issues to be resolved, such as the question of flow dependency and intraindividual variability [73]; however, there is some evidence that H_2O_2 may be useful as a biochemical marker of oxidative stress and airway inflammation in childhood asthma.

Products of lipid peroxidation in EBC such as 8-isoprostanes have been investigated only in few studies in children. Levels of 8-isoprostane have been found to be significantly elevated in mild asthmatic children when compared to healthy controls; however, no difference was found between steroid-treated and steroid-naïve asthmatic children [31]. Furthermore, no difference could be found in children suffering from unstable asthma compared to steroid-treated or steroid-naïve mild asthmatic children [38]. In children with acute asthma exacerbation 8-isoprostane levels decreased significantly after a 5-day course of oral steroids but did not reach levels of healthy controls [39]. No correlation was found to clinical status, lung function parameters, and fractional exhaled nitric oxide (FeNO), and there was a certain overlap in 8-isoprostane concentrations between healthy children and children with asthma [31, 38, 39].

To establish the clinical utility of exhaled 8-isoprostane measurement in the diagnosis and management of children with asthma larger and longitudinal studies are required. The changes of aldehyde levels in childhood asthma have been evaluated only in one study. Corradi et al. [36] found levels of malondialdehyde significantly higher in children with asthma exacerbation than in control subjects, and oral steroids reduced these levels to normal. Conversely glutathione, a protective antioxidant, was halved in asthma exacerbation and increased after steroid treatment. Whereas malondialdehyde and glutathione were negatively correlated to each other, no correlation was found to clinical measures such as pulmonary function tests [36]. Even though this study showed pathophysiologically interesting results, there is not enough evidence that these markers of oxidative stress may be useful in the assessment and management of childhood asthma.

Levels of nitrite, a stable end product of NO, were found to be 5-fold higher in asthmatic children compared to healthy controls in a study by Formanek et al. [11]. In this study nitrite levels were not correlated with age, asthma severity, or steroid treatment. Another study found levels being more than doubled in asthmatic children, and after treatment with inhaled corticosteroids there was a significant reduction in nitrite in patients with clinical improvement [74]. Our group showed that high-altitude climate therapy significantly reduced nitrite levels in asthmatic children [74]. In this study, significant correlations could be shown for nitrite and maximal expiratory flow at 50% of forced vital capacity (MEF_{50}), airway responsiveness to methacholine, and symptoms [74]. In infants with recurrent wheeze we found total nitrite/nitrate levels not different from concentrations in healthy controls, whereas there were significantly higher levels in infants with subacute respiratory syncytial virus infection. This may be due to the relatively small patient groups and the heterogeneity of recurrent wheeze in infancy [20].

3-Nitrotyrosine levels have been found to be elevated in condensates from asthmatic compared to normal children; however, in the same study no correlation was observed between FeNO and 3-nitrotyrosine [76]. Measurements of cys-LT in EBC collected from asthmatic children demonstrated heterogeneous variances but were found to be repeatable [77]. In children with mild persistent and moderate to severe persistent asthma cys-LT were found to be higher than in children with mild intermittent asthma and healthy controls [75]. Interestingly, the authors found an inverse correlation to levels of LTB_4 in EBC, which acts as a potent neutrophil attractant. This correlation has been discussed as a potential contrary effect of steroids on eosinophil and neutrophil survival [75]. On the other hand, no correlation was found with pulmonary function (forced expiratory volume in 1 s, FEV_1) and FeNO [39, 75]. In children with asthma exacerbation, cys-LT levels in EBC were 3 times higher than in healthy children, and after 5 days of treatment with oral corticosteroids levels decreased significantly to levels found in the healthy control group [39]. Cys-LT levels were up to 10-fold increased in children with unstable asthma compared to stable asthmatics on or without inhaled steroids. In the same study the authors found a correlation between cys-LT levels and FeNO in the subgroup of steroid-naïve children [38]. Avoiding house dust mites for 3 months in asthmatic children led to reduced cys-LT levels in EBC, which were parallel to a significant reduction of 8-isoprostane levels and eosinophil percentage in induced sputum. As neutrophil count in sputum did not change, no change was found in EBC LTB_4 levels in the same study [76]. Exhaled PGE_2 concentrations were found to be not different in EBC obtained from healthy, steroid-naïve, or steroid-treated asthmatic children [39]. The role of LTB_4 in asthmatic airway inflammation is not yet completely clear. LTB_4 was reported to be significantly increased in EBC collected from children with mild persistent and moderate to severe persistent asthma compared with children with mild intermittent asthma and healthy controls [75]. These findings suggest that LTB_4 may play a role in the pathogenesis of more severe asthma. Interestingly, isocapnic hyperventilation of cold air in children with stable asthma led to a significant increase in LTB_4 levels, whereas there was no increase in healthy children [80].

In asthma there is an imbalance between T helper 2 (Th2) cells, secreting IL-4, and Th1 cells, secreting interferon-γ (IFN-γ). IL-4 levels were found to be similar in steroid-treated asthmatics and healthy controls, whereas they were significantly higher in steroid-naïve asthmatic children [15]. On the other hand, IFN-γ was significantly lower in steroid-naïve asthmatic children. There was no correlation between these two markers for Th2 and Th1 activity and pulmonary function, FeNO, or atopy status [15]. No other studies investigating cytokines in EBC have been published so far; therefore, the value of these findings cannot be regarded as established. Low pH values were observed in EBC of children with asthma compared to controls; furthermore, a relationship between EBC pH and severity of asthma was found [78]. Another study revealed no significant correlation between EBC pH, lung function, exhaled carbon monoxide and FeNO [82]. These investigators suggested that airway acidification may explain increased levels of exhaled NO, and proposed that serial measurements of pH might be helpful in titrating anti-inflammatory therapy in children with asthma.

Despite the lack of long-term prospective studies and the existence of only few intervention studies the prospective to use biomarkers from EBC in childhood asthma appears to be promising. Overall the assessment of markers in EBC may prove a valuable diagnostic tool by providing an objective measure to define the severity of asthma and to guide anti-inflammatory treatment. If changes in biomarkers precede those of physiological parameters, there would be a further utility of these measurements in the management of asthma. Paediatric data on markers in EBC in asthma are summarized in table 1.

Cystic Fibrosis

Lung disease is the predominant cause of morbidity and mortality in CF and is initiated early in childhood [60]. Therefore, early recognition of airway inflammation and infection may lead to a better therapeutic management and hence allow a better clinical outcome. Activated neutrophils and macrophages are major sources of oxygen-free radicals including H_2O_2 [79]. Serial H_2O_2 measurements in children with CF suffering from pulmonary exacerbation showed a significant decrease of H_2O_2 during intravenous antibiotic treatment [80]. Most of the children showed a concomitant increase of FEV_1 values, while in some of the children H_2O_2 levels decreased but no change in lung function could be obtained. Changes in FEV_1 and levels of H_2O_2 were weakly correlated [80]. The limitation of this study is the lack of a control group. Other markers of oxidative stress in EBC of CF children such as 8-isoprostane or malondialdehyde have not been reported to date. In CF children our group found 5-fold higher median levels of NO_2^- compared to healthy controls or children suffering from a non-specific cough. Cunningham et al. [13] found similar levels of NO_2^- in EBC of children with stable CF. In none of these studies a correlation could be found between NO_2^- levels and lung function or clinical scores. In contrast to FeNO, NO_2^- may represent a more sensitive marker of NO production in the lower respiratory tract due to its greater stability relative to NO. In a longitudinal study in children with CF, where EBC was collected during 1 year, no correlation could be found to clinical changes, whereas intravenous antibiotic treatment reduced total NO_2^-/NO_3^- levels in children with exacerbation of lung disease [own unpublished data, 2004]. We found a tendency towards higher concentrations of total NO_2^-/NO_3^- in infants with CF compared to healthy controls; however, the difference did not reach statistical significance [own unpublished data, 2004]. Horak et al. [85]

Table 1. Markers in EBC in asthma

Marker	Asthma, stable	Asthma, unstable	Asthma, acute/severe	Asthma, OCS	Asthma, no ICS	Asthma, ICS	Reference no.
H_2O_2, μmol/l	0.54–0.81		1.50		0.80	0.45	8, 17
8-Isoprostane (EIA), pg/ml			12.0–29.7	8.40	16.20	18.60	30, 37
8-Isoprostane (RIA), pg/ml					56.40	47.20	38
Malondialdehyde, nmol			30.20	18.5			35
Glutathione, nmol			5.96	8.44			35
Nitrite (NO_2^-), μmol/l	2.10					1.27	11, 72
Total NO_2^-/NO_3^-, μmol/l[a]					12.10		20
3-Nitrotyrosine, ng/ml						13.5	76
Cys-LT, pg/ml	27.90	106.00	12.7–1.50	5.2	10.8	12.7–14.2	37, 38, 73, 74
LTB_4, pg/ml	52.7		131.9			2.36	73, 74
IL-4, pg/ml					53.7	37.5	15
Interferon-γ, pg/ml					4.1	3.7	15

OCS = Oral corticosteroids; ICS = inhaled corticosteroids.
[a] Infants with current wheeze.

found no significant differences between NO_2^- levels in EBC obtained from infants with CF compared to normals using a copper condensate sampler. 3-Nitrotyrosine levels did not differentiate between children with CF and healthy subjects, and there was no correlation with lung function [86]. Only few studies have been reported assessing cytokines or eicosanoids in children with CF. Cunningham et al. [13] detected IL-8, the most important neutrophil chemoattractant in only a third of clinically stable CF patients included in the study. Although the levels showed a tendency to be higher in CF children, there was no statistically significant difference compared to healthy controls. This was mostly due to the small group of patients where IL-8 was detectable [13]. We found LTB_4 detectable in most EBC collected from stable CF patients, and levels were reduced after 3 weeks of intravenous antibiotic treatment [own unpublished data, 2004]. The pH of EBC was decreased in CF patients during pulmonary exacerbations, but there was no significant difference between stable CF patients and healthy controls [81]. The reduced pH was associated with a lower level of EBC ammonium [88].

In summary, data from the studies presented suggest a potential role for the determination of biomarkers of oxidative stress and airway inflammation in EBC in the management of CF patients. Paediatric data on markers in EBC in CF are summarized in table 2.

Other Respiratory Conditions

Only few studies have been reported regarding the collection of EBC in children with conditions other than

Table 2. Markers in EBC in CF

Marker	CF, stable	CF, exacerbation	CF, intravenous antibiotics	Reference no.
H_2O_2, μmol/l		0.28	0.16	77
Nitrite (NO_2^-), μmol/l	2.02–3.00			11, 13
Total NO_2^-/NO_3^-[a], μmol/l	18.4 (11–29.1)[b]			20
3-Nitrotyrosine, ng/ml	1.69			86
LTB_4, pg/ml	6.8 (5.3–10.6)[b]			own unpublished data, 2004
IL-8, pg/ml	47 (8–90)[b]			13

[a] Infants.
[b] Quartile range.

CF or asthma. In children with primary ciliary dyskinesia (PCD) Csoma et al. [82] found no differences in levels of NO metabolites in EBC compared to healthy controls with similar concentrations of NO_2^-, total NO_2^-/NO_3^- and S-nitrosothiols in both groups. Levels of FeNO were not correlated to its metabolites, and there were no correlations to lung function. The same group did not find differences in LTB_4 and cys-LT levels comparing children with PCD and healthy controls, whereas PGE_2 was decreased in the

Table 3. Normal values of markers in EBC

Marker	Level	Patient number	Reference no.
H_2O_2, µmol/l	0.15–0.25	31	8, 17
H_2O_2, µmol/l	0.13 (0.01–0.48)[b]	93	20
H_2O_2[a], µmol/l	0.49 (0.47–0.61)[b]	141	19
8-Isoprostane (EIA), pg/ml	3.5–4.3	32	37, 38
8-Isoprostane (RIA), pg/ml	34.2 (24.3–44.0)[b]	12	30
Malondialdehyde, nmol	19.40 (±1.9)	12	35
Glutathione, nmol	14.1 (±0.8)	12	35
Nitrite (NO_2^-), µmol/l	0.41 (0.13–1.83)	13	11, 13
Nitrite (NO_2^-), µmol/l	0.4 (0.0–1.9)[c]	73	100
Cys-LT, pg/ml	3.5–18.5	40	37, 38, 73
LTB_4, pg/ml	47.9 (±4.1)	11	73
IL-4, pg/ml	35.70 (±6.2)	11	15
IL-8, pg/ml	10 (5–49)[d]	10	13
Interferon-γ, pg/ml	5.10 (±0.4)	11	15

Data are presented as range or mean (±SD).
[a] Nasally collected in infants and older children.
[b] 95% confidence interval.
[c] 10th to 90th centiles.
[d] Quartile range.

PCD group [82]. Reported reference data on markers in EBC from healthy children are summarized in table 3.

Measurement of Exhaled Gases (other than NO) in Children

Carbon Monoxide

There are three major sources of CO in exhaled air: enzymatic oxidation of haem, which is the largest portion, non-haem-related production (e.g. lipid peroxidation), and exogenous CO. The enzyme haemoxygenase (HO) exists in three isoforms. The HO-1, thought to be involved in airway inflammation, can be induced in various cells by oxidant agents, pro-inflammatory cytokines, and other forms of cellular stress [26, 84]. HO-1 converts haem and haemin to biliverdin with the formation of CO. Bilirubin, the end product of the biliverdin metabolism, acts as a potent antioxidant. The predominant site of CO production in the lung are the alveoli although the airways contribute to the exhaled CO concentration [85].

The first use of exhaled CO as a marker of different diseases was described in 1972 by Russian investigators [87]. High concentrations of exhaled CO have been suggested to reflect airway inflammation or indicate oxidative stress in the lung [1, 84, 88].

Methods for the Measurement of CO in Exhaled Air

CO can be measured by a number of different techniques. In most of the studies electrochemical CO sensors have been used. CO can also be measured by laser spectrophotometer and conventional multigas emission analyzers [89]. The sensitivity of CO analyzers varies from 0 to 1,000 parts per million (ppm) with resolutions between 0.1 and 1 ppm. End-tidal exhaled CO measurements can be made during single exhalations, and can be performed easily by children as young as 5 years of age [92]. The technique is usually a deep inhalation with consecutive breath holding for 15–20 s followed by exhalation. The exhalation is either uncontrolled and rapid [92], controlled for flow (5–6 litres/min) [88, 93], or into a bag collector system [94]. Bronchodilatation and hence airway calibre does not influence CO levels measured in exhaled air [94]. Levels of exhaled CO were found unaffected by different flows during collection but increased with breath hold, suggesting an origin in the alveoli rather than the conducting airways [89].

Expected Changes of Exhaled CO in Childhood Respiratory Disease

Uasuf et al. [92] showed significantly increased values of CO in exhaled air of children with persistent asthma compared to those with infrequent episodic asthma, and twice as high levels compared to healthy controls. On the other hand, there was no such difference in CO levels when children with infrequent episodes were compared to healthy children. Asthmatic subjects with acute upper airway infection showed raised levels of CO similar to those found in persistent asthma. The authors found no correlation to lung function (FEV_1) or bronchial responsiveness assessed by a methacholine challenge [92]. Ece et al. [96] also found higher CO concentrations in asthmatic compared to healthy children. Parental smoking habits significantly influenced CO levels in both asthmatic and healthy children, with higher levels in those exposed to passive smoking. Asthmatic children receiving inhaled corticosteroids had lower levels than steroid-naïve children [96]. Zanconato et al. [94] found significantly increased exhaled CO concentrations in children with an acute asthma exacerbation compared to healthy children. Interestingly, CO levels were higher in asthmatic children who were on long-term inhaled steroids prior to the exacerbation than in

Table 4. Exhaled carbon monoxide in children with disease and healthy controls

Disease	Patient group, ppm		Healthy controls, ppm		Reference no.
	median/mean value	number of subjects	median/mean value	number of subjects	
Asthma, persistent	2.17 ± 0.21[a]	16	1.01 ± 0.12[a]	40	85
Asthma, episodic	1.39 ± 0.18[a]	13			85
Asthma, exacerbation	3.2 ± 0.2[a]	30	2.0 ± 0.2[a]	21	87
Asthma, stable	1.32 ± 1.50[b]	54	0.86 ± 1.35[b]	235	88
Cystic fibrosis[c]	1.2 ± 0.4[b]	21	1.3 ± 0.4[b]	30	89
Healthy with URTI	2.16 ± 0.33[a]	12	1.01 ± 0.12[a]		85

URTI = Upper respiratory tract infection.
[a] Standard error of the mean (SEM).
[b] Standard deviation (SD).
[c] End tidal CO.

steroid-naïve asthmatic children. Despite a significant improvement in lung function after 5 days' treatment with oral corticosteroids, no significant change in exhaled CO could be documented. No correlation could be found between exhaled CO concentrations and FeNO or lung function parameters. Because of the relatively small changes in CO concentrations due to treatment there is not a great chance that the changes might have become significant with a bigger patient group [94]. Only one study is available in which exhaled CO was assessed in children with CF. These patients showed no difference in tidal exhaled CO (ETCO) levels compared with control subjects. In this study, the authors found a strong relation between ETCO and total lung capacity as assessed by the multiple-breath helium wash-in method (TLC-He) in healthy control subjects, and that TLC-He was significantly lower in patients with CF. When corrected for TLC-He, ETCO concentrations were significantly higher in CF patients compared with control subjects [97].

The number of studies using CO in the assessment of childhood respiratory disease is still limited, and the findings are not consistent. In addition, the overlap between asthmatics and healthy subjects is considerable. This limits the potential application of this method in individual patients. Furthermore, the role of exhaled CO as a measure of airway inflammation and oxidative stress in the lung is not yet clear. Therefore, more research is needed before exhaled CO measurements can be used in a clinical setting.

Volatile Hydrocarbons
Ethane and pentane are hydrocarbons released in biological tissues during lipid peroxidation. Although

ethane in exhaled air has been analyzed since the 1960s, the research in this area has only progressed slowly due to technical and practical problems. Usually ethane has been measured by gas chromatography. Drury et al. [98] assessed the feasibility and reproducibility of pentane measurements in preterm infants ventilated for the respiratory distress syndrome. Despite a relatively high intra-individual variability the authors concluded that the measurement of exhaled pentane allows an accurate quantification of endogenous breath pentane in ventilated infants, making it possible to follow longitudinal changes. To date no other studies have been reported assessing the concentration of exhaled hydrocarbons in children. Paediatric data on exhaled gases are summarized in table 4.

Potential Value of EBC in Paediatric Respiratory Medicine and Future Considerations

The analysis of EBC in children is a challenging new technique and has the potential as a non-invasive measure to assess and to monitor airway inflammation, oxidative stress and metabolic processes. There is a wide array of biologically relevant compounds in the EBC, and alterations of these mediators during pathological processes may be predictable. Therefore, the measurement of inflammatory mediators in EBC may provide insights into the pathophysiology of inflammatory lung diseases. The technique is simple and does not need cooperation, and may therefore also be applied in small children, infants and disabled patients. In addition, the collection of EBC is completely non-invasive, and hence allows repeated measurements. Nevertheless, the apparent potential of EBC in children must not be overstated as there are several problems still to be resolved. The direct relationship between markers measured in the condensate and local inflammatory processes in the airways is still an open question. The correlation of products measured in the EBC and measures of lung function and airway responsiveness as indirect assessment of airway inflammation is discussed controversially in the literature. While several authors found an inverse correlation between markers of inflammation in the condensates and lung function parameters [25, 80] or airway responsiveness [24], others showed no correlation [12, 16, 17]. There is a confusing lack of correlation among methods, and inconsistency between studies. Differences may be partially explained by the heterogeneity of respiratory disease in childhood. On the other hand, only little information is available about levels of inflammatory products in EBC in a wide range of healthy subjects.

The collection and analysis of EBC are a rapidly expanding area of research. There is now a need for moving away from the evaluation of single markers to patterns of changes in different diseases. Patterns of markers may reflect more accurately the complex pathophysiological processes in respiratory disease, and could meet the fact that markers of airway inflammation are differently affected in different diseases. This may in the future lead to disease-characteristic profiles and a diagnostic fingerprint for respiratory diseases, and may enlarge our understanding of the disease processes, and hence may provide the potential for more appropriate customized therapy. For EBC to become a clinical tool for daily practice (easy to perform, cheap, and reliable), the technique has to be standardized for (1) flow and time dependence, (2) nasal contamination, (3) saliva and sputum contamination, and (4) the influence of temperature and humidity. Further efforts have to be directed towards optimizing the condenser and collector systems, standardizing the analysis, and improving the sensitivity of assays for the measurement of markers. The intra-individual variability in concentrations of most EBC contents leads to a considerable overlap between disease and health, and makes the evaluation of therapeutic interventions difficult. Much of the variation found in concentrations of non-volatile soluble substances in EBC is probably related to differences in the dilution of respiratory droplets by water vapour. A more quantitative assessment of the concentrations of markers within the condensate can be estimated from the concentrations of non-volatile constituents in the condensate [99]. However, to date there is no reliable reference indicator. This does not necessarily limit the utility of EBC. The same difficulties have limited the utility of bronchoalveolar lavage, induced sputum, or FeNO measurements. Ratios of solutes that do not depend on dilution factors will provide important information.

Further research is needed (1) to identify reference values of the different inflammatory markers in healthy subjects, (2) to evaluate the reproducibility of measurements, (3) to assess changes in disease longitudinally, and (4) to investigate correlations between EBC markers and symptoms, and parameters derived from pulmonary function testing (including assessment of bronchial responsiveness) and standard methods for the quantification of airway inflammation (e.g. bronchoalveolar lavage, biopsy). In the end many of the open questions regarding dilution and variability may be addressed by investigating the mechanism of EBC formation and its relationship with airway lining fluid. The assessment of the airway lining fluid by direct microcapillary sampling techniques may provide a gold standard to compare true changes in concentrations of mediators within the airway lining fluid to findings in EBC.

Longitudinal and interventional studies are required to investigate the usefulness of these measurements in a clinical setting; furthermore, less sophisticated and cheaper devices are required to allow day to day use of these techniques in the clinical management of inflammatory lung disease. However, whether and, if so, when analysis of EBC for the clinical assessment of childhood respiratory disease will be introduced is difficult to predict.

References

1 Kharitonov SA, Barnes PJ: Biomarkers of some pulmonary diseases in exhaled breath. Biomarkers 2002;7/1:1–32.
2 Barnes PJ, Belvisi MG: Nitric oxide and lung disease. Thorax 1993;48:1034–1043.
3 Scheideler L, Manke HG, Schwulera U, Inacker O, Hammerle H: Detection of non-volatile macromolecules in breath. A possible diagnostic tool? Am Rev Respir Dis 1993; 148:778–784.
4 Fairchild CI, Stampfer JF: Particle concentration in exhaled breath. Am Ind Hyg Assoc J 1987;48:948–949.
5 Papineni RS, Rosenthal FS: The size distribution of droplets in the exhaled breath of healthy human subjects. J Aerosol Med 1997;10/2: 105–116.
6 Mutlu GM, Garey KW, Robbins RA, Danziger LH, Rubinstein I: Collection and analysis of exhaled breath condensate in humans. Am J Respir Crit Care Med 2001; 164:731–737.
7 Sidorenko GI, Zborovskii EI, Levina DI: Surface-active properties of the exhaled air condensate (a new method of studying lung function). Ter Arkh 1980;52/3:65–68.
8 Jobsis Q, Raatgeep HC, Hermans PW, de Jongste JC: Hydrogen peroxide in exhaled air is increased in stable asthmatic children. Eur Respir J 1997;10:519–521.

9 Montuschi P, Corradi M, Ciabattoni G, Nightingale J, Kharitonov SA, Barnes PJ: Increased 8-isoprostane, a marker of oxidative stress, in exhaled condensate of asthma patients. Am J Respir Crit Care Med 1999;160/1: 216–220.

10 Hanazawa T, Kharitonov SA, Barnes PJ: Increased nitrotyrosine in exhaled breath condensate of patients with asthma. Am J Respir Crit Care Med 2000;162:1273–1276.

11 Formanek W, Inci D, Lauener RP, Wildhaber JH, Frey U, Hall GL: Elevated nitrite in breath condensates of children with respiratory disease. Eur Respir J 2002;19:487–491.

12 Ho LP, Innes JA, Greening AP: Nitrite levels in breath condensate of patients with cystic fibrosis is elevated in contrast to exhaled nitric oxide. Thorax 1998;53:680–684.

13 Cunningham S, McColm JR, Ho LP, Greening AP, Marshall TG: Measurement of inflammatory markers in the breath condensate of children with cystic fibrosis. Eur Respir J 2000;15:955–957.

14 Hunt JF, Fang K, Malik R, Snyder A, Malhotra N, Platts-Mills TA, Gaston B: Endogenous airway acidification. Implications for asthma pathophysiology. Am J Respir Crit Care Med 2000;161:694–699.

15 Shahid SK, Kharitonov SA, Wilson NM, Bush A, Barnes PJ: Increased interleukin-4 and decreased interferon-gamma in exhaled breath condensate of children with asthma. Am J Respir Crit Care Med 2002;165: 1290–1293.

16 Ganas K, Loukides S, Papatheodorou G, Panagou P, Kalogeropoulos N: Total nitrite/nitrate in expired breath condensate of patients with asthma. Respir Med 2001;95:649–654.

17 Dohlman AW, Black HR, Royall JA: Expired breath hydrogen peroxide is a marker of acute airway inflammation in pediatric patients with asthma. Am Rev Respir Dis 1993;148: 955–960.

18 Baraldi E, Ghiro L, Piovan V, Carraro S, Zacchello F, Zanconato S: Safety and success of exhaled breath condensate collection in asthma. Arch Dis Child 2003;88:358–360.

19 Griese M, Latzin P, Beck J: A noninvasive method to collect nasally exhaled air condensate in humans of all ages. Eur J Clin Invest 2001;31:915–920.

20 Moeller A, Franklin PJ, Hall GL, Stick SM: Limitations of breath condensates in infants. Am J Respir Crit Care Med 2003;167:A978.

21 Jobsis Q, Raatgeep HC, Schellekens SL, Hop WC, Hermans PW, de Jongste JC: Hydrogen peroxide in exhaled air of healthy children: Reference values. Eur Respir J 1998;12: 483–485.

22 Mozalevskii AF, Travianko TD, Iakovlev AA, Smirnova EA, Novikova NP, Sapa I: Content of arachidonic acid metabolites in blood and saliva of children with bronchial asthma. Ukr Biokhim Zh 1997;69/5–6:162–168.

23 Zetterquist W, Pedroletti C, Lundberg JO, Alving K: Salivary contribution to exhaled nitric oxide. Eur Respir J 1999;13:327–333.

24 Horvath I, Donnelly LE, Kiss A, Kharitonov SA, Lim S, Fan Chung K, Barnes PJ: Combined use of exhaled hydrogen peroxide and nitric oxide in monitoring asthma. Am J Respir Crit Care Med 1998;158:1042–1046.

25 Loukides S, Horvath I, Wodehouse T, Cole PJ, Barnes PJ: Elevated levels of expired breath hydrogen peroxide in bronchiectasis. Am J Respir Crit Care Med 1998;158: 991–994.

26 Kharitonov SA, Barnes PJ: Exhaled markers of pulmonary disease. Am J Respir Crit Care Med 2001;163:1693–1722.

27 Montuschi P, Barnes PJ: Analysis of exhaled breath condensate for monitoring airway inflammation. Trends Pharmacol Sci 2002; 23/5:232–237.

28 Tonnel AB, Wallaert B: Oxidants and bronchial inflammatory processes. Eur Respir J 1990;3:987–988.

29 Joseph BZ, Routes JM, Borish L: Activities of superoxide dismutases and NADPH oxidase in neutrophils obtained from asthmatic and normal donors. Inflammation 1993;17: 361–370.

30 Morrow JD, Roberts LJ: The isoprostanes: Their role as an index of oxidant stress status in human pulmonary disease. Am J Respir Crit Care Med 2002;166/12:S25–30.

31 Baraldi E, Ghiro L, Piovan V, Carraro S, Ciabattoni G, Barnes PJ, Montuschi P: Increased exhaled 8-isoprostane in childhood asthma. Chest 2003;124/1:25–31.

32 Montuschi P, Kharitonov SA, Ciabattoni G, Corradi M, van Rensen L, Geddes DM, Hodson ME, Barnes PJ: Exhaled 8-isoprostane as a new non-invasive biomarker of oxidative stress in cystic fibrosis. Thorax 2000;55/3:205–209.

33 Goil S, Truog WE, Barnes C, Norberg M, Rezaiekhaligh M, Thibeault D: Eight-epi-PGF2alpha: A possible marker of lipid peroxidation in term infants with severe pulmonary disease. J Pediatr 1998;132:349–351.

34 Rahman I, MacNee W: Oxidative stress and regulation of glutathione in lung inflammation. Eur Respir J 2000;16:534–554.

35 Liebler DC, Reed DJ: Free-radical defence and repair mechanisms; in Wallance KB (ed): Free Radical Toxicology. New York, Taylor & Francis, 1999, pp 141–171.

36 Corradi M, Folesani G, Andreoli R, Manini P, Bodini A, Piacentini G, Carraro S, Zanconato S, Baraldi E: Aldehydes and glutathione in exhaled breath condensate of children with asthma exacerbation. Am J Respir Crit Care Med 2003;167:395–399.

37 Gallati H, Pracht I: Horseradish peroxidase: Kinetic studies and optimization of peroxidase activity determination using the substrates H_2O_2 and 3,3′,5,5′-tetramethylbenzidine. J Clin Chem Clin Biochem 1985;23:453–660.

38 Zanconato S, Carraro S, Corradi M, Alinovi R, Pasquale MF, Piacentini G, Zacchello F, Baraldi E: Leukotrienes and 8-isoprostane in exhaled breath condensate of children with stable and unstable asthma. J Allergy Clin Immunol 2004;113:257–263.

39 Baraldi E, Carraro S, Alinovi R, Pesci A, Ghiro L, Bodini A, Piacentini G, Zacchello F, Zanconato S: Cysteinyl leukotrienes and 8-isoprostane in exhaled breath condensate of children with asthma exacerbations. Thorax 2003;58:505–509.

40 Larstad M, Ljungkvist G, Olin AC, Toren K: Determination of malondialdehyde in breath condensate by high-performance liquid chromatography with fluorescence detection. J Chromatogr B Analyt Technol Biomed Life Sci 2002;766/1:107–114.

41 Gaston B, Drazen JM, Loscalzo J, Stamler JS: The biology of nitrogen oxides in the airways. Am J Respir Crit Care Med 1994;149:538–551.

42 Marletta MA, Yoon PS, Iyengar R, Leaf CD, Wishnok JS: Macrophage oxidation of L-arginine to nitrite and nitrate: Nitric oxide is an intermediate. Biochemistry 1988;27:8706–8711.

43 Moncada S, Higgs A: The L-arginine-nitric oxide pathway. N Engl J Med 1993;329: 2002–2012.

44 Nathan C: Nitric oxide as a secretory product of mammalian cells. FASEB J 1992;6:3051–3064.

45 Ischiropoulos H, Zhu L, Chen J, Tsai M, Martin JC, Smith CD, Beckman JS: Peroxynitrite-mediated tyrosine nitration catalyzed by superoxide dismutase. Arch Biochem Biophys 1992;298:431–437.

46 Schulz K, Kerber S, Kelm M: Reevaluation of the Griess method for determining NO/NO_2^- in aqueous and protein-containing samples. Nitric Oxide 1999;3:225–234.

47 Balint B, Donnelly LE, Hanazawa T, Kharitonov SA, Barnes PJ: Increased nitric oxide metabolites in exhaled breath condensate after exposure to tobacco smoke. Thorax 2001;56:456–461.

48 Gaston B, Sears S, Woods J, Hunt J, Ponaman M, McMahon T, Stamler JS: Bronchodilator S-nitrosothiol deficiency in asthmatic respiratory failure. Lancet 1998;351:1317–1319.

49 Bisgaard H: Leukotriene modifiers in pediatric asthma management. Pediatrics 2001;107: 381–390.

50 Antczak A, Montuschi P, Kharitonov S, Gorski P, Barnes PJ: Increased exhaled cysteinyl-leukotrienes and 8-isoprostane in aspirin-induced asthma. Am J Respir Crit Care Med 2002;166:301–306.

51 Barnes NC, Piper PJ, Costello JF: Comparative effects of inhaled leukotriene C4, leukotriene D4, and histamine in normal human subjects. Thorax 1984;39:500–504.

52 Drazen JM, Austen KF, Lewis RA, Clark DA, Goto G, Marfat A, Corey EJ: Comparative airway and vascular activities of leukotrienes C-1 and D in vivo and in vitro. Proc Natl Acad Sci USA 1980;77:4354–4358.

53 Marom Z, Shelhamer JH, Bach MK, Morton DR, Kaliner M: Slow-reacting substances, leukotrienes C4 and D4, increase the release of mucus from human airways in vitro. Am Rev Respir Dis 1982;126:449–451.

54 Pavord ID, Tattersfield AE: Bronchoprotective role for endogenous prostaglandin E2. Lancet 1995;345:436–438.

55 Busse WW: Leukotrienes and inflammation. Am J Respir Crit Care Med 1998; 157/6: S210–213, S247–248.

56 Jatakanon A, Uasuf C, Maziak W, Lim S, Chung KF, Barnes PJ: Neutrophilic inflammation in severe persistent asthma. Am J Respir Crit Care Med 1999;160/5:1532–1539.

57 Carpagnano GE, Barnes PJ, Geddes DM, Hodson ME, Kharitonov SA: Increased leukotriene B4 and interleukin-6 in exhaled breath condensate in cystic fibrosis. Am J Respir Crit Care Med 2003;167:1109–1112.

58 Rosenfeld M, Gibson RL, McNamara S, Emerson J, Burns JL, Castile R, Hiatt P, McCoy K, Wilson CB, Inglis A, Smith A, Martin TR, Ramsey BW: Early pulmonary infection, inflammation, and clinical outcomes in infants with cystic fibrosis. Pediatr Pulmonol 2001;32:356–366.

59 Konstan MW, Berger M: Current understanding of the inflammatory process in cystic fibrosis: Onset and etiology. Pediatr Pulmonol 1997;24/2:137–142, 159–161.

60 Khan TZ, Wagener JS, Bost T, Martinez J, Accurso FJ, Riches DW: Early pulmonary inflammation in infants with cystic fibrosis. Am J Respir Crit Care Med 1995;151:1075–1082.

61 Montuschi P, Ragazzoni E, Valente S, Corbo G, Mondino C, Ciappi G, Barnes PJ, Ciabattoni G: Validation of leukotriene B4 measurements in exhaled breath condensate. Inflamm Res 2003;52/2:69–73.

62 Griese M, Noss J, von Bredow C: Protein pattern of exhaled breath condensate and saliva. Proteomics 2002;2:690–696.

63 Sanak M, Kielbasa B, Bochenek G, Szczeklik A: Exhaled eicosanoids following oral aspirin challenge in asthmatic patients. Clinical and Experimental Allergy 2004, in press.

64 Jack CI, Calverley PM, Donnelly RJ, Tran J, Russell G, Hind CR, Evans CC: Simultaneous tracheal and oesophageal pH measurements in asthmatic patients with gastro-oesophageal reflux. Thorax 1995;50/2:201–204.

65 Guerrin F, Voisin C, Macquet V, Robin RA, Lequien P: Apport de la pH métrie bronchique in situ. Prog Respir Res 1971;6:372–383.

66 Ricciardolo FL, Rado V, Fabbri LM, Sterk PJ, Di Maria GU, Geppetti P: Bronchoconstriction induced by citric acid inhalation in guinea pigs: Role of tachykinins, bradykinin, and nitric oxide. Am J Respir Crit Care Med 1999;159:557–562.

67 Govindaraju K, Cowley EA, Eidelman DH, Lloyd DK: Microanalysis of lung airway surface fluid by capillary electrophoresis with conductivity detection. Anal Chem 1997;69:2793–2797.

68 Luk CK, Dulfano MJ: Effect of pH, viscosity and ionic-strength changes on ciliary beating frequency of human bronchial explants. Clin Sci 1983;64:449–451.

69 Holma B, Hegg PO: pH- and protein-dependent buffer capacity and viscosity of respiratory mucus. Their interrelationships and influence on health. Sci Total Environ 1989;84:71–82.

70 Kostikas K, Papatheodorou G, Ganas K, Psathakis K, Panagou P, Loukides S: pH in expired breath condensate of patients with inflammatory airway diseases. Am J Respir Crit Care Med 2002;165:1364–1370.

71 Tate S, MacGregor G, Davis M, Innes JA, Greening AP: Airways in cystic fibrosis are acidified: Detection by exhaled breath condensate. Thorax 2002;57:926–929.

72 Vaughan J, Ngamtrakulpanit L, Pajewski TN, Turner R, Nguyen TA, Smith A, Urban P, Hom S, Gaston B, Hunt J: Exhaled breath condensate pH is a robust and reproducible assay of airway acidity. Eur Respir J 2003;22:889–894.

73 Schleiss MB, Holz O, Behnke M, Richter K, Magnussen H, Jorres RA: The concentration of hydrogen peroxide in exhaled air depends on expiratory flow rate. Eur Respir J 2000;16:1115–1118.

74 Straub DA, Ehmann R, Hall GL, Moeller A, Hamacher J, Frey U, Sennhauser FH, Wildhaber JH: Correlation of nitrites in breath condensates and lung function in asthmatic children. Pediatr Allergy Immunol 2004;15/1:20–25.

75 Csoma Z, Kharitonov SA, Balint B, Bush A, Wilson NM, Barnes PJ: Increased leukotrienes in exhaled breath condensate in childhood asthma. Am J Respir Crit Care Med 2002;166:1345–1349.

76 Petrovski FI, Salnikov AV, Petrovskaia IA, Ogorodova LM, Serebrov VY: Nitrite levels in breath condensate of children with bronchial asthma. Eur Respir J 2001;18:269s.

77 Bodini A, Peroni D, Vicentini L, Loiacono A, Baraldi E, Ghiro L, Corradi M, Alinovi R, Boner A, Piacentini G: Exhaled breath condensate eicosanoids and sputum eosinophils in asthmatic children: A pilot study. Pediatr Allergy Immunol 2004;15/1:6–31.

78 Carpagnano GE, Barnes PJ, Francis N, Wilson M, Bush A, Kharitonov SA: Breath condensate pH in children with cystic fibrosis and asthma: A new noninvasive marker of airway inflammation? Chest 2004;125:2005–2010.

79 McGrath LT, Mallon P, Dowey L, Silke B, McClean E, McDonnell M, Devine A, Copeland S, Elborn S: Oxidative stress during acute respiratory exacerbations in cystic fibrosis. Thorax 1999;54:518–523.

80 Jobsis Q, Raatgeep HC, Schellekens SL, Kroesbergen A, Hop WC, de Jongste JC: Hydrogen peroxide and nitric oxide in exhaled air of children with cystic fibrosis during antibiotic treatment. Eur Respir J 2000;16/1:95–100.

81 Cain D, MacGregor G, Ho LP, Innes JA, Greening A, Cunningham S: Breath condensate is acidified during infective exacerbations in children with cystic fibrosis. Eur Respir J 2002;20:527s.

82 Csoma Z, Bush A, Wilson NM, Donnelly L, Balint B, Barnes PJ, Kharitonov SA: Nitric oxide metabolites are not reduced in exhaled breath condensate of patients with primary ciliary dyskinesia. Chest 2003;124:633–638.

83 Vogelberg C, Hirsch T, Rosen-Wol A, Leupold W: Effect of isocapnic hyperventilation with cold air on breath condensate volume and LTB4-concentration in breath condensate. Eur Respir J 2002;20:411s.

84 Horvath I, Donnelly LE, Kiss A, Paredi P, Kharitonov SA, Barnes PJ: Raised levels of exhaled carbon monoxide are associated with an increased expression of heme oxygenase-1 in airway macrophages in asthma: A new marker of oxidative stress. Thorax 1998;53:668–672.

85 Kharitonov SA, Barnes PJ: Exhaled ammonia in ammoniain asthma, cystic fibrosis and upper airway tract infection. Am J Respir Crit Care Med 2000;161:A307.

86 Van Iersel M, Rosias PPR, Joebsis Q, Pennings HJ, Hendriks JJE, Dompeling E: The relationship between control of childhood asthma, NO and CO in exhaled air, acidity of and cytokines in exhaled breath condensate. Am J Respir Crit Care Med 2002;165:A486.

87 Nikberg II, Murashko VA, Leonenko IN: Carbon monoxide concentration in the air exhaled by the healthy and the ill. Vrach Delo 1972;12:112–114.

88 Paredi P, Leckie MJ, Horvath I, Allegra L, Kharitonov SA, Barnes PJ: Changes in exhaled carbon monoxide and nitric oxide levels following allergen challenge in patients with asthma. Eur Respir J 1999;13/1:48–52.

89 Zetterquist W, Marteus H, Johannesson M, Nordval SL, Ihre E, Lundberg JO, Alving K: Exhaled carbon monoxide is not elevated in patients with asthma or cystic fibrosis. Eur Respir J 2002;20/1:92–99.

90 Horak FJ, Stoer H, Hoeller B, Putschoegl B, Eichler I, Frischer T, Urbanek R: Measurement of nitrite in the breathing condensate of healthy infants and infants with cystic fibrosis. Am J Respir Crit Care Med 2002;165:A485.

91 MacGregor G, Tate S, Davis M, Leadbetter K, Ho LP, Cunningham S, Innes JA, Greening AP: Nitrotyrosine levels of exhaled breath condensate in cystic fibrosis adults and children. Am J Respir Crit Care Med 2002;165:A278.

92 Uasuf CG, Jatakanon A, James A, Kharitonov SA, Wilson NM, Barnes PJ: Exhaled carbon monoxide in childhood asthma. J Pediatr 1999;135:569–574.

93 Paredi P, Kharitonov SA, Barnes PJ: Analysis of expired air for oxidation products. Am J Respir Crit Care Med 2002;166/12:S31–S37.

94 Zanconato S, Scollo M, Zaramella C, Landi L, Zacchello F, Baraldi E: Exhaled carbon monoxide levels after a course of oral prednisone in children with asthma exacerbation. J Allergy Clin Immunol 2002;109:440–445.

95 MacGregor G, Cain D, Ellis S, Davis M, Cunningham S, Innes JA, Greening AP: Low ammonium levels in exhaled breath condensate in cystic fibrosis adults and children. Am J Respir Crit Care Med 2003;167:A916.

96 Ece A, Gurkan F, Haspolat K, Derman O, Kirbas G: Passive smoking and expired carbon monoxide concentrations in healthy and asthmatic children. Allergol Immunopathol 2000;28/5:255–260.

97 Terheggen-Lagro SW, Bink MW, Vreman HJ, van der Ent CK: End-tidal carbon monoxide corrected for lung volume is elevated in patients with cystic fibrosis. Am J Respir Crit Care Med 2003;168:1227–1231.

98 Drury JA, Nycyk JA, Cooke RW: Pentane measurement in ventilated infants using a commercially available system. Free Radic Biol Med 1997;22:895–900.

99 Effros RM, Hoagland KW, Bosbous M, Castillo D, Foss B, Dunning M, Gare M, Lin W, Sun F: Dilution of respiratory solutes in exhaled condensates. Am J Respir Crit Care Med 2002;165:663–669.

100 Moeller A, Straub DA, Waser M, Babians A, Wildhaber JH, Braun-Fahrländer C, Lauener RP, Frey U, Hall GL: Airway reactivity, offline exhaled nitric oxide and nitrite are correlated in school aged children. Am J Respir Crit Care Med 2002;165:A485.

Dr. Alexander Moeller
Division of Respiratory Medicine
University Children's Hospital Zürich
Steinwiesstrasse 75
CH–8032 Zürich (Switzerland)
Tel. +41 1 266 71 11
Fax +41 1 266 71 71
E-Mail alexander.moeller@kispi.unizh.ch

Clinical Application of Pulmonary Function Testing in Common Paediatric Respiratory Diseases

Hammer J, Eber E (eds): Paediatric Pulmonary Function Testing.
Prog Respir Res. Basel, Karger, 2005, vol 33, pp 204–214

....

Childhood Asthma and Wheezing Disorders

Pavel Basek[a]   Daniel Straub[b]   Johannes H. Wildhaber[b]

[a]Department of Paediatrics, University Hospital, Hradec Kralove, Czech Republic, and
[b]Swiss Paediatric Respiratory Research Group, Division of Respiratory Medicine,
University Children's Hospital Zürich, Zürich, Switzerland

Abstract

Pulmonary function tests, mainly spirometry (FEV_1), are generally considered the standard tools for objective evaluation and re-evaluation in childhood asthma. However, since most asthmatic children have FEV_1 values in the normal range, independent of disease severity, the value of commonly used pulmonary function tests in short- and long-term evaluations of childhood asthma remains controversial. Other parameters may be more valuable for this purpose. Wheezing disorders in infancy are common and their prevalence has increased in the last decade. Clinically, it is often difficult to distinguish whether an obstructive episode is a transient 'viral wheeze' or the beginning of allergic asthma, which tends to persist in adulthood. There is an increased availability of techniques and commercial equipment for pulmonary function tests for this age group. Infant pulmonary function tests have been helpful in distinguishing between wheezy and healthy children and may have some predictive value, however for the time being, they are mainly research tools.

The pathophysiology of asthma as it is currently understood consists of variable airway obstruction, as first described by Salter more than hundred years ago, bronchial hyperresponsiveness, as described in 1960, chronic airway inflammation, recognized over the last few decades to be the key mechanism of asthma, and airway remodelling, a number of structural changes considered over the last few years to be a primary key factor.

Based on our understanding of the pathophysiology, combined assessment of the degree of airway obstruction, bronchial responsiveness, airway inflammation and airway remodelling would appear to be the best approach to diagnose and monitor asthma. In spite of this, diagnosis and monitoring of asthma in clinical praxis are still mainly based on symptom evaluation.

The impact of airway remodelling on the natural course of the disease is still little understood. Assessment of airway inflammation has so far mostly been proven to be too invasive, too expensive, not sensitive or specific enough, and not insufficiently validated and standardized to be used in clinical practice and hence, at the moment, still mainly remains a research tool. In addition, despite there being some indications that the assessment of bronchial responsiveness is helpful not only in diagnosing but also in monitoring the disease, these techniques are rarely used in clinical practice.

Therefore, although asthma is now recognized as a chronic inflammatory disease of the airways, reversible airway obstruction is still the main objective outcome measure recommended by most guidelines for the diagnosis and monitoring of asthma in childhood. However, some of the lung function parameters used, such as peak expiratory flow (PEF) and forced expiratory volume in 1 s (FEV_1), have been lately shown not to be as helpful in the care of children with asthma.

Whereas asthma is a well-defined disorder in children over 5 years of age, the diagnosis of asthma in younger children remains a challenge. Children presenting with wheeze at an early age belong to a heterogeneous group, and little is understood about the pathophysiology of wheeze in young children; hence, the diagnosis and monitoring of wheezy disorders in young children are difficult. The tools available for the assessment of airway inflammation and/or reversible airway constriction and bronchial responsiveness in this young age group are not yet available for clinical practice, but remain mainly available for research purposes.

This chapter will cover the use of lung function tests in the initial evaluation and follow-up of both asthma in children older than 5 years and wheezy disorders in children younger than 5 years.

Children Older Than 5 Years

Pathophysiology

Asthma should be regarded as a syndrome and not as a single disease entity. Like other syndromes, asthma has its characteristic features, which are expressed to a variable extent in affected individuals. The main pathophysiological characteristics are [1–4]:

- Reversible airway obstruction
- Bronchial hyperresponsiveness
- Airway inflammation
- Structural airway changes (airway remodelling)

Surprisingly, current strategies for the management of asthma as outlined in guidelines do generally not focus on the assessment of all of the above characteristics for diagnosing asthma and for monitoring the effectiveness of treatment.

Reversible Airway Obstruction and Bronchial Hyperresponsiveness

Increased resistance to airflow is the most important functional abnormality in asthma. It is the basis of the clinical manifestations of asthma, including dyspnoea and wheeze. Increased airway resistance in asthma may be partly due to poor function of pulmonary surfactant [5, 6]. However, the main mechanisms leading to increased airway resistance are decreased airway diameter as a consequence of bronchial constriction, luminal narrowing due to airway wall oedema and luminal obstruction resulting from hypersecretion of mucus. Normally, airflow limitation is reversible; however, there may be fixed airway obstruction, which is mainly seen in later disease stages or may also be

an expression of a specific asthma phenotype [7–10]. Methods to assess airflow obstruction include, among others, body plethysmography, spirometry, forced oscillation technique and the interrupter technique.

The Childhood Asthma Management Program (CAMP) study looking at the effect of an inhaled steroid compared to nedocromil and placebo on the improvement of lung function using postbronchodilator percent predicted FEV_1 as the primary outcome has shown an initial improvement [11]. However, postbronchodilator percent predicted FEV_1 gradually diminished by the end of the treatment period over 4–6 years and did not differ from those in the nedocromil and placebo groups. This finding may be indicative for pathophysiological processes (airway remodelling) other than airway inflammation which are not influenced by an anti-inflammatory treatment with inhaled steroids.

While functional abnormalities of airflow in asthmatics have mainly been attributed to changes in resistance of large and medium-sized airways, studies have shown that small airways and terminal airways also contribute to airway resistance [5, 6, 12]. Bronchial obstruction leads to air trapping and hence, to an increased volume of gas remaining in the respiratory system at the end of tidal expiration (functional residual capacity; FRC), and at the end of complete expiration (residual volume; RV). Using capnometry and a multiple-breath nitrogen wash-out technique, it has been shown that the obstruction of peripheral airways diminishes the distribution of air during inspiration and causes a ventilation/perfusion mismatch [13].

Another functional abnormality is airway hyperresponsiveness to stimuli provoking airway narrowing. Children with asthma often have normal lung function and only develop severe bronchial obstruction during an exacerbation. This finding may be explained by an underlying bronchial hyperresponsiveness. Weiss et al. [14] have shown a relationship between the severity of asthma and the degree of bronchial hyperresponsiveness in children with a normal FEV_1. Thus, the measurement of bronchial responsiveness may be helpful in the initial assessment of asthma severity as well as in the follow-up assessments of asthma control. The measurement of bronchial responsiveness is discussed in detail in the chapter by Barben and Riedler [15].

Airway Inflammation

Airway inflammation is the dominant feature of asthma and is present even at the earliest stage of mild disease [3]. The inflammatory response is associated with the accumulation of chronic inflammatory cells, including lymphocytes, macrophages, and plasma cells that are abundant in the lamina propria in larger airways and in the adventitial connective tissue in smaller airways [16, 17]. So far, assessment of airway inflammation has been too invasive or not feasible for use in children. However, there are some new promising tools for the non-invasive assessment of airway inflammation such as the measurement of exhaled nitric oxide or other markers in exhaled air or breath condensate.

Airway Remodelling

Airway remodelling refers to a variety of structural changes in the airway wall [3, 4]. Most prominent is the accumulation of collagens and other matrix components in the subepithelial region of the airway wall. In addition, there is smooth muscle hypertrophy and/or hyperplasia, epithelial proliferation, and mucous cell hyperplasia/metaplasia, as well as increased vascularity of the mucosa. The alterations in airway wall thickness could have two opposite effects on airway mechanics [18]. Firstly, when the increase in thickness predominantly affects the inner layers of the airway wall, pronounced narrowing of the airway with concomitant flow limitation will be the result. Secondly, when the outer layer of the airway enlarges, there will be increased stiffness without a remarkable effect on airway resistance. Currently, bronchoscopy with bronchial biopsy is the most commonly used technique for determining the extent of airway remodelling [19, 20]. However, apart from invasivity and unavoidable risks of this procedure, bronchoscopically obtained specimens do not permit an evaluation of the peripheral airways and their surrounding parenchyma. The high-speed interrupter technique allows studying the changes in airway wall mechanical properties, as anti-resonance phenomena occurring in the airway at high frequencies contain information on airway wall mechanics [21]. High-resolution computed tomography (CT), magnetic resonance imaging (MRI), and single-photon emission computed tomography (SPECT) may also be helpful in the assessment of airway abnormalities in asthmatic patients [22–25].

Pulmonary Function Testing in Asthmatic Children

National and international guidelines recommend an initial evaluation followed by regular re-evaluations for the assessment of the severity and the control of asthma [26, 27]. The initial evaluation guides therapy based on the level of severity, whereas the regular re-evaluations assess the response to therapy based on the level of control. Guidelines recommend a number of outcome measures for the initial evaluation and the regular re-evaluations. Pulmonary function tests, mainly spirometry, are generally considered the standard tools for objective evaluation and re-evaluation.

Outcome Measures in the Assessment of Asthma

The various outcome measures listed by guidelines are symptoms, nocturnal awakenings, rescue β_2-agonist use, and lung function parameters. Despite all of these measures being predictive for either short (exacerbations)- and/or long-term outcomes, they do not necessarily correlate with each other. There is new evidence that the measurement of bronchial responsiveness and inflammatory markers in exhaled air may be helpful for initial evaluation as well as for follow-up evaluations [28, 29].

Rationale to Measure Lung Function

Despite the advantage of objective assessment of variable, reversible airway obstruction by pulmonary function testing and the recommendation of most guidelines to perform lung function tests in the initial assessment as well as in the follow-up of asthma, lung function tests are not widely available in private practice. A medical diagnosis of asthma based on symptoms and clinical signs followed by a therapy trial, is still common standard in the assessment of asthma in general practice. It was shown in the AIRE (Asthma Insights and Reality Europe) study, that only 29% of asthmatic children reported that their doctor had given them a lung function test in the past year, and over 50% of children with asthma had never undergone any lung function test [30]. This is in agreement with epidemiological asthma studies, where the inclusion of patients was entirely based on a general practitioner's diagnosis [31]. On the other hand, particularly FEV_1, is often used as the primary outcome variable for efficacy studies in asthma [11].

Initial Assessment
The initial assessment of asthma as stated by guidelines, with FEV_1 being the only objective measure, serves to evaluate the severity of the disease. Children with mild persistent asthma have FEV_1 values of more than 80% of predicted, children with moderate persistent asthma have values of 60–80% of predicted, and children with severe persistent asthma have values of less than 60% of predicted [26, 27]. However, since most asthmatic children have FEV_1 values in the normal range independent of disease severity, as discussed latter, it may be necessary to redefine asthma severity in future guidelines [32].

Follow-Up
Regular monitoring of lung function may have some benefits for the patient as well as the doctor. The clinical

assessment of asthma by the general practitioner can be verified by an objective measure. Many asthmatics, especially children are poor symptom perceivers. In addition, another rationale to regularly monitor lung function is that reduced lung function is a poor prognostic factor for the outcome of asthma later in life [33, 34].

Poor Perception of Asthma Symptoms

According to guidelines, children's and parents' reports on asthma symptoms are important in assessing asthma severity and control [26, 27]. Dyspnoea, cough and wheeze, as well as exercise-induced symptoms are helpful to guide treatment decisions. However, it is well known that many children and their parents do not adequately perceive or report asthma symptoms [35]. There is evidence to support the hypothesis that poor perception of airway obstruction is a clinically relevant problem in children with asthma. Considerable airway obstruction may be present in asymptomatic patients with asthma [36]. Children with long-standing airway obstruction are less likely to report dyspnoea than children with acute onset of airway obstruction [37]. Such poor perceivers are more likely to present with hypoxia during an acute exacerbation, predisposing to severe or life-threatening attacks [38]. Reported symptoms do not reliably correlate with lung function parameters in asthmatic children, and correlation is dependent on the instrument used [39].

Reduced Lung Function as a Poor Prognostic Factor of Asthma Outcome

A recent retrospective study in a large number of asthmatic children showed that children with significant airway obstruction were twice as likely to develop an asthmatic attack in subsequent years as children with more or less normal lung function [40]. However, many children with life-threatening asthma episodes have FEV_1 values on hospital admission >80% predicted [41]. This implies that the number and severity of exacerbations should also be taken into account when assessing asthma severity. A large body of evidence shows that airway obstruction in children with asthma is associated with ongoing respiratory morbidity and reduced lung function in adulthood, both in cohorts of children with mild disease from the general population and in hospital-based cohorts of patients with more severe asthma [42–47]. These studies have demonstrated a small annual decline in lung function among patients with asthma, with a decline of approximately 1% FEV_1 of predicted per year. Thus, the degree of airway obstruction in children with asthma has both short-term and long-term

prognostic significance. Ideally, lung function should be measured serially over time as a change in lung function over time may provide valuable information regarding the natural course of the disease [48, 49]. However, when and how often lung function should be tested in asthmatic children remains controversial. Besides the initial assessment of asthma severity, lung function testing is doubtless indicated if symptoms deteriorate, are unexplained and/or do not respond to usual anti-asthma therapy.

Evidence for the Usefulness of Lung Function Measurements

Two recent reviews on the usefulness of monitoring lung function in asthma have clearly stated that despite there being a rationale for the recommendation to monitor lung function there is apparently no firm evidence [32, 50]. There has so far not been a single randomized trial to test the usefulness of monitoring lung function for short- and long-term outcomes in asthmatic children.

Peak Flow Measurements

Portable peak flow meters have been advocated as tools to assess asthma control, and were included in guidelines for a more effective asthma management in order to reduce morbidity and mortality based on the above rationales, mainly the poor perception of symptoms by children [51]. However, no or only weak correlations were reported between PEF and individual symptom scores and/or bronchial responsiveness in asthmatic children [52–56]. It has also been shown that changes in PEF do not correlate with changes in lung function measured by spirometry. Clinically relevant falls in PEF were found to occur in the absence of changes in other lung function parameters, and significant falls in other lung function measures occurred that were not reflected by a fall in PEF [57]. In addition, it has been shown that the information provided in a PEF diary by apparently well-motivated children with asthma and their families is unreliable [58]. Not only do some patients cheat by inventing PEF values, but they also may misreport the readings they have made. Asthmatic children and their parents are more likely to use PEF meters to get an objective measure during symptomatic episodes; however, daily use is likely to be an unrealistic expectation [59]. In summary, there is no evidence to support the general use of PEF measurements for home monitoring in asthma management in childhood. Home monitoring may be beneficial in asthmatic children facing extra challenges as a result of disease severity, sociodemographic, or health care system characteristics [60]. New portable electronic devices measuring PEF and FEV_1 may allow a more accurate and controllable objective measure for home monitoring in asthmatic children [61–64].

Spirometry

Fuhlbrigge et al. [40] performed an analysis of spirometry in more than 3,000 children with asthma who were observed for up to 15 years and found >90% of all FEV_1 values to be >80% of predicted. Over 50% of asthmatic children from the CAMP study with moderate persistent asthma based on frequency of symptoms had mean pre- and postbronchodilator FEV_1 values between 94 and 103% of predicted [11]. Bacharier et al. [65] found that the mean FEV_1 was 95.1% of predicted in children with mild persistent asthma, 90.2% of predicted in those with moderate persistent asthma, and 83.8% of predicted in those with severe persistent asthma. This general finding that most asthmatic children have FEV_1 values in the normal range has major implications for its usefulness in the initial assessment of asthma severity as well as in the follow-up of asthma control. If the diagnosis and/or the management of asthma greatly rely on FEV_1 measurements, there is a risk of underdiagnosing and/or undertreating asthmatic children. On the other hand, a low FEV_1 seen at follow-up visits may likely be explained by gross undertreatment or unexplained disease progression. There is also a lack of correlation between FEV_1 and individual symptom scores in asthmatic children [52, 53]. Thus, asthma status may be better characterized by parent-reported symptoms, health care utilization, and functional health status measures than by FEV_1 [66]. In contrast to baseline FEV_1, a β_2-agonist response in FEV_1 assessed by pre- and postbronchodilator spirometry correlates with airway inflammation [67, 68]. As discussed earlier, small airways and terminal airways contribute to airway resistance in asthma. This may explain why pulmonary function parameters (PEF, FEV_1) thought to represent larger airways, do not correlate well with other asthma outcome parameters (symptoms, inflammatory parameters), whereas some recent studies found a better correlation between pulmonary function parameters (maximal expiratory flow at 50 and 25% of forced vital capacity (FVC), MEF_{50} and MEF_{25}, respectively) thought to represent smaller airways and other asthma outcome parameters [52, 69, 70, 71, 72]. In summary, bronchodilator response in FEV_1 should be obtained and analysed together with other parameters derived from the flow-volume curve (MEF_{50}, MEF_{25}) for the critical assessment of asthma severity and control [71]. Brand et al. [50] call the process of looking at the entire expiratory flow-volume

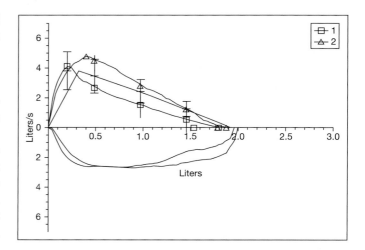

Fig. 1. Flow-volume curve in a 9-year-old boy with asthma, showing normal PEF and FEV_1 values, but a concave shape of the expiratory loop before bronchodilator (□) and a significant improvement following administration of a bronchodilator (Δ).

curve 'eyeballing', where a concave pattern in the curve may be seen despite a normal FEV_1 (fig. 1). The limitation of FEV_1 as an inclusion/exclusion criterion for efficacy studies has to be stressed [32].

Other Pulmonary Function Parameters

The most useful tool in the assessment of severe acute asthma exacerbation is pulse oxymetry. The measurement of oxyhaemoglobin saturation reflects ventilation-perfusion mismatch rather than lung function. However, it is clinically relevant and readily available. The importance of non-invasive assessment of gas exchange arises from the observation that pulmonary gas exchange abnormalities resulting from alveolar hypoventilation and ventilation-perfusion mismatch are present even in the clinically mildest form of asthma; furthermore, the correlation with FEV_1 is only weak. This fact implies the importance of peripheral airway involvement [72–74].

It is known, that in mild or moderate asthma, at times when FVC and FEV_1 values are entirely normal, the measurement of lung volume may identify the presence of air trapping [74]. The RV is the most sensitive parameter of airway obstruction in children, and a decrease in RV after bronchodilator administration appears to be more specific for asthma diagnosis than an increase in FEV_1 [75]. Currently, however, there are no data supporting the clinical utility of static lung volume measurements in the management of childhood asthma.

Children Less Than Five Years of Age

Pulmonary Function Testing in Wheezy Disorders

Due to the age-dependent lack or limitation of cooperation, lung function measurements in young children are difficult to perform [76]. Newborns and infants are not cooperative at all and therefore pulmonary function can only be assessed passively. Some techniques, like tidal breathing measurements, interrupter techniques, and gas-dilution measurements may be performed in non-sedated sleeping infants, whereas measurements of forced expiratory flows as well as body plethysmographic measurements require sedation. In preschool children, tidal breathing measurements and measurements using interrupter or oscillation techniques can provide reasonable results while only minimal cooperation is required.

Pathophysiology

The interaction between airway and/or lung disease and growth and development influences the function and structure of the respiratory system in early childhood (fig. 2 [77]).

Rationale to Measure Lung Function

Wheezy disorders consist of a heterogeneous group. Hence, it would be important to distinguish between early transient, late-onset, and persistent wheeze according to Martinez et al. [78]. The majority of infants with wheeze do not have an increased risk of asthma later in life. Because wheezy disorders are difficult to distinguish clinically, it would be helpful to have some objective measures for diagnosis. Asthma starts early in life, and hence, objective measures applicable to all age groups would be helpful to guide treatment from early childhood into adulthood. In addition, there are data showing that in a minority of infants, reduced lung function and increased airway responsiveness are probably related to persistent asthma [79]. The disagreement between the mother's perception of her infant's health and objective lung function parameters and the general practitioner's health assessment has also been demonstrated, stressing the importance of objective measurements [80].

Outcome Measures in the Assessment of Wheezing Disorders

Clinical symptoms are widely used as outcome measures [81–84]. There is growing evidence that measurements of lung function and inflammatory markers may support the evaluation of wheezy disorders in early childhood [80, 85].

Summary of Commonly Used Methods

Tidal forced expiration (rapid thoraco-abdominal compression technique; RTC) and the raised volume rapid thoraco-abdominal compression technique (RVRTC) have been widely used to measure airflow at flow limitation. Using tidal breathing analysis, a range of physiological parameters related to respiratory control and pulmonary function can be obtained. As in older children lung volume measurements can be performed using gas dilution techniques or whole-body plethysmography. The mechanic properties of airway and lung tissue can be evaluated by the forced oscillation technique or interrupter technique, and several approaches have been used in infants to assess airway response to inhaled bronchoconstrictive or bronchodilator agents.

Evidence for the Usefulness of Lung Function Measurements

Evidence for the usefulness of infant lung function testing is limited by the lack of standardized equipment and relatively large inter- and intra-subject variations with some techniques.

Tidal Volume Measurements

The ratio time to peak tidal expiratory flow/total expiratory time (t_{PTEF}/t_E) calculated from tidal breathing flow curves, in epidemiological studies has been shown to predict the development of recurrent wheezing over the subsequent 3 years of life [86, 87]. This approach allows to distinguish between asthmatic and healthy preschool children [88–90], and to evaluate the response to methacholine, histamine [91, 92], or bronchodilators [93–95].

Forced Expiratory Maneuvers

The RTC technique, suitable for measurements of maximal expiratory flow at FRC ($V'_{max,FRC}$), has been widely used to investigate aspects of lung development and lung disease. Regarding the long-term course, a reduced $V'_{max,FRC}$ in the first month of life, correlating independently with airway hyperresponsiveness at the age of 11 years, could be demonstrated in wheezy infants [33]. As the RVRTC technique has been introduced relatively recently, the number of studies published is still small. Expiratory flows obtained by the RVRTC technique distinguish better between healthy infants and infants with recurrent wheeze than $V'_{max,FRC}$ as measured by the RTC technique [96]. Forced expiratory maneuvers have been used to show that asymptomatic infants with recurrent

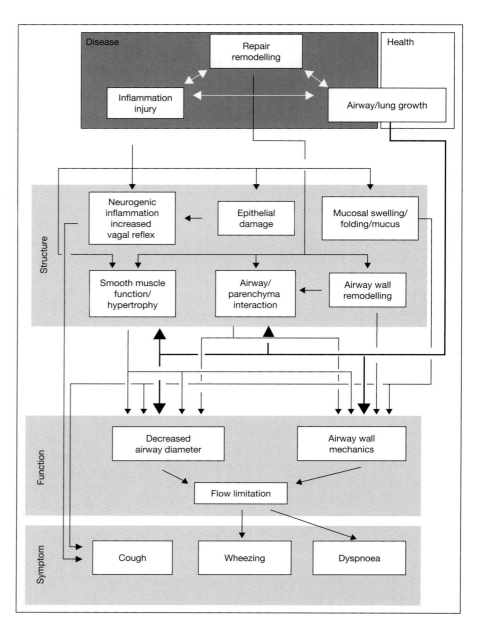

Fig. 2. Complex interactions between injury, natural healing processes, including remodelling, and lung growth/development represent a dynamic equilibrium in health and may be disturbed in disease. The classical concept of wheezing is based on flow limitation due to airway narrowing. However, there is growing evidence that not only airway diameter but also airway wall function and lung volume may be altered in wheezing disorders in infants. Any given increase in airway resistance may reflect differing combinations of altered airway wall compliance, airway smooth muscle shortening and relative thickness of airway wall due to mucosal swelling. Infants are particularly prone to wheeze due to developmental differences in airway mechanics compared to adults. Furthermore, while in adults inflammation and remodelling alone may explain structural and functional changes in wheezing disorders, in infants inflammation, remodelling and airway development have to be considered as a continuously interacting system. Whether or not wheezing will persist may be understood as a function of this dynamic system. The dynamic interaction between airway/lung disease and growth and development of respiratory system in early childhood influence the function of the respiratory system in later life. The airways are not the same in adults and small children, and what may appear to be irreversible in an adult may not be so in a growing child. From Frey [77] with permission).

wheeze have a lower forced expiratory volume in 0.5 s ($FEV_{0.5}$) than healthy infants [97], to investigate the airway tone and the airway response to a β_2-agonist in healthy young children, and to demonstrate that in asymptomatic recurrently wheezing infants β_2-agonists as well as anti-inflammatory treatment cause no significant improvement in lung function [98–100]. Furthermore, forced expiratory manoeuvers have been used to assess airway responsiveness in challenge tests [101, 102].

Measurement of Functional Residual Capacity by Gas Dilution Techniques

There are only few studies in this age group. Using the multiple breath nitrogen and the sulphur hexafluoride washout technique in infants, the involvement of peripheral airways has been documented in asthma [103–105]. Recently, a new method has been published which aimed at solving the problem of measuring trapped gas [106].

Measurement of lung mechanics

Forced Oscillation Technique (FOT). With the low-frequency forced oscillation technique (LFOT) it has been shown that asymptomatic wheezy infants have altered respiratory tissue mechanics, and that infants with a family history of asthma have elevated respiratory system resistance and reduced elastance [97, 107]. The LFOT was found to be a suitable method to study bronchodilator responsiveness in infants [108]. Investigating airway responsiveness to methacholine has shown conflicting results: in preschool children FOT was found to be unreliable when determining respiratory system resistance using frequencies of 6 and 8 Hz [109–111]. However, using a frequency spectrum of 0.5–20 Hz in infants, respiratory tissue mechanics were significantly altered after methacholine challenge, correlating with a decline in $FEV_{0.5}$ [102]. Furthermore, using a spectrum of high frequencies a dramatic change in airway wall mechanics after methacholine challenge could be demonstrated [112].

The Interrupter Technique. In preschool children with asthma, interrupter resistance (R_{int}) may be helpful in monitoring lung function. It has been shown to correlate with FEV_1 but to underestimate airway resistance compared with body plethysmography [113]. Furthermore, it has good short-term repeatability and can therefore be used to examine bronchodilator response in children with asthma [114–116]. With the interrupter technique, higher resistance values were measured in children with persistent wheeze as compared with healthy children [117].

On the other hand, some investigators mention a number of theoretical and technical problems requiring further exploration, and call for studies standardizing the equipment and identifying the most appropriate analysis technique for application in infants [118, 119].

The high-speed interrupter technique has been used for investigations in infants mainly by one study group who demonstrated altered airway wall mechanics in asymptomatic infants with a history of wheeze [120].

Airway Responsiveness in Infancy

Bronchial challenge tests have been found to be a safe and tolerable tool even in infants, when using appropriate monitoring [121]. By assessing airway responsiveness, it could be demonstrated, that bronchial responsiveness in the neonatal period and male sex are risk factors for wheezing in infancy. Increased airway responsiveness at the age of 1 month is associated with physician-diagnosed asthma and decreased lung function at the age of 6 years [122, 123].

Clinical Usefulness

Some pulmonary function tests distinguish well between healthy children and children with wheezy disorders. Therefore, pulmonary function tests could be valuable tools to evaluate and monitor disease state in wheezy disorders and may even have prognostic value when used in combination with other tests. However, there are some disadvantages and unsolved problems, which have so far limited their application in clinical practice.

For example, RVRTC is a promising method to assess airway function in infancy; however the number of published studies using RVRTC is still small, the reference values are limited and there is no definite consensus regarding standardization. After resolving these problems, this method may provide data comparable to those obtained from spirometric measurements in cooperative children and adults and may allow true longitudinal assessment of airway function in health and disease. FOT is an attractive approach as well, as the measurement is non-invasive, does not require cooperation and may be quickly repeated. The commercial FOT equipment that has become available may lead to expansion of clinical studies in preschool children in the next years. These studies should verify the validity and usefulness of FOT in clinical practice and augment the reference data.

Lung function testing in infants and preschool children is a feasible but complicated procedure. Using light sedation, a variety of measurements (airway resistance, lung volumes and forced expiratory) can be performed even in infants and young children. However, while the measurement of lung mechanics in early childhood provides valuable information regarding type and severity of functional abnormality; the unsatisfactory sensitivity and specificity of most pulmonary function tests limit their use in diagnosis.

In summary, there is currently lack of lung function test for infants and young children that would be at once sufficiently reproducible, easy, cheap and quickly, and able to reflect the clinical situation. Hence the indication and purpose of any test session should be clearly defined and, pending the demonstration of the superiority of objective parameters over clinical assessment in wheezy disorders, pulmonary function tests should be restricted to research in this age group.

References

1 Salter HH: The pathology of asthma – Its absolute nature; in Brewis RAL (ed): Classic Papers in Asthma. London, Science Press, 1990, pp 106–142.

2 Hilman B: NHLBI guidelines for diagnosis and management of asthma. Bethesda, National Heart, Lung, and Blood Institute; 1997. NIH publication No 97–4051.

3 Bousquet J, Jeffery PK, Busse WW, Johnson M, Vignola AM: From bronchoconstriction to airways inflammation and remodelling. Am J Respir Crit Care Med 2000;161:720–1745.

4 Davies DE, Wicks J, Powell RM, Puddicombe SM, Holgate ST: Airway remodelling in asthma: New insights. J Allergy Clin Immunol 2003;111:215–225.

5 Hohlfeld JM, Ahlf K, Enhorning G, Balke K, Erpenbeck VJ, Petschalles J, Hoymann HG, Fabel H, Krug N: Dysfunction of pulmonary surfactant in asthmatics after segmental allergen challenge. Am J Respir Crit Care Med 1999;159:1803–1809.

6 Jarjour NN, Enhorning G: Antigen-induced airway inflammation in atopic subjects generates dysfunction of pulmonary surfactant. Am J Respir Crit Care Med 1999;160:336–341.

7 Finucane KE, Greville HW, Brown PJE: Irreversible airflow obstruction: Evolution in asthma. Med J Aust 1985;142:602–604.

8 Strachan DP, Griffiths JM, Johnston IDA, Anderson HR: Ventilatory function in British adults after asthma or wheezing illness at ages 0–35. Am J Respir Crit Care Med 1996;154:1629–1635.

9 Lange P, Parner J, Vestbo J, Schnohr P, Jensen G: A 15-year follow-up study of ventilatory function in adults with asthma. N Engl J Med 1998;339:1194–1200.

10 Bush A: Phenotype specific treatment of asthma in childhood. Paediatr Respir Rev 2004;5 (suppl A):S93-S101.

11 The Childhood Asthma Management Program Research Group: Long-term effects of budesonide or nedocromil in children with asthma. N Engl J Med 2000;343:1054–1063.

12 Wagner EM, Liu MC, Weinmann GG: Peripheral lung resistance in normal and asthmatic subjects. Am Rev Respir Dis 1990;141:584–588.

13 Stromberg NO, Gustafsson PM: Ventilation inhomogeneity assessed by nitrogen washout and ventilation-perfusion mismatch by capnography in stable and induced airway obstruction. Pediatr Pulmonol 2000;29:94–102.

14 Weiss ST, Van Natta ML, Zeiger RS: Relationship between increased airway responsiveness and asthma severity in the Childhood Asthma Management Program. J Allergy Clin Immunol 1999;103:376–387.

15 Barben J, Riedler J: Measurements of bronchial responsiveness in children; Hammer J, Eber E (eds): Paediatric Pulmonary Function Testing. Prog Respir Res. Basel, Karger, 2005, vol 33, pp 125–136.

16 Laitinen LA, Laitinen A, Haahtela T: Airway mucosal inflammation even in patients with newly diagnosed asthma. Am Rev Respir Dis 1993;147:697–704.

17 Haley KJ, Sunday ME, Wiggs BR, Kozakewich HP, Reilly JJ, Mentzer SJ, Dugarbaker DJ, Doerschuk CM, Drazen JM: Inflammatory cell distribution within and along asthmatic airways. Am J Respir Crit Care Med 1998;158:565–572.

18 McParland BE, Macklem PT, Pare PD: Airway wall remodeling: Friend or foe? J Appl Physiol 2003;95:426–434.

19 Jeffery PK, Wardlaw AJ, Nelson FC, Collins JV, Kay AB: Bronchial biopsies in asthma: An ultrastructural, quantitative study and correlation with hyperreactivity. Am Rev Respir Dis 1989;140:1745–1753.

20 Roche WR, Beasley R, Williams JH, Holgate ST: Subepithelial fibrosis in the bronchi of asthmatics. Lancet 1989;i:520–524.

21 Frey U, Makkonen K, Wellman T, Beardsmore C, Silverman M: Alterations in airway wall properties in infants with a history of wheezing disorders. Am J Respir Crit Care Med 2000;161:1825–1829.

22 Muller NL, Miller RR: Diseases of the bronchioles: CT and histopathologic findings. Radiology 1995;196:3–12.

23 Awadh N, Muller NL, Park CS, Abboud RT, Fitzgerald JM: Airway wall thickness in patients with near fatal asthma and control groups: Assessment with high resolution computed tomographic scanning. Thorax 1998;53:248–253.

24 King GG, Muller NL, Pare PD: Evaluation of airways in obstructive pulmonary disease using high-resolution computed tomography. Am J Respir Crit Care Med 1999;159:992–1004.

25 King GG, Eberl S, Salome CM, Young IH, Woolcock AJ: Differences in airway closure between normal and asthmatic subjects measured with single-photon emission computed tomography and technegas. Am J Respir Crit Care Med. 1998;158:1900–1906.

26 National Heart Lung and Blood Institute, World Health Organisation Global Initiative for Asthma: Global strategy for asthma management and prevention: NHLBI & sol; WHO workshop report. Bethesda, National Institutes of Health, 1995, pp 1–176.

27 Scottish Intercollegiate Guidelines Network and the British Thoracic Society in association with the British Association of Accident and Emergency Medicine, the General Practice Airways Group, the National Asthma Campaign, the Royal College of Paediatrics and Child Health, the Royal Paediatric Respiratory Society and Royal College of Physicians of London: The British guidelines on the management of asthma. Thorax 2003;58 (suppl 1):i1-i94.

28 Sont JK, Willems LN, Bel EH, van Krieken JH, Vandenbroucke JP, Sterk PJ: Clinical control and histopathologic outcome of asthma when using airway hyperresponsiveness as an additional guide to long-term treatment. The AMPUL Study Group. Am J Respir Crit Care Med 1999;159:1043–1051.

29 Strunk RC, Szefler SJ, Phillips BR, Zeiger RS, Chinchilli VM, Larsen G, Hodgdon K, Morgan W, Sorkness CA, Lemanske RF: Relationship of exhaled nitric oxide to clinical and inflammatory markers of persistent asthma in children. J Allergy Clin Immunol 2003;112:883–892.

30 Rabe KF, Vermeire PA, Soriano JB, Maier WC: Clinical management of asthma in 1999: The Asthma Insights and Reality Europe (AIRE) study. Eur Respir J 2000;16:802–807.

31 International Study of Asthma and Allergies in Childhood (ISAAC) Steering Committee: Worldwide variation in prevalence of symptoms of asthma, allergic rhinoconjunctivitis, and atopic eczema: ISAAC. Lancet 1998;351:1225–1232.

32 Spahn JD, Cherniack R, Paull K, Gelfand EW: Is forced expiratory volume in one second the best measure of severity in childhood asthma? Am J Respir Crit Care Med 2004;784–786.

33 Turner SW, Palmer LJ, Rye PJ, Gibson NA, Judge PK, Cox M, Young S, Goldblatt J, Landau LI, Le Souëf PN: The relationship between infant airway function, childhood airway responsiveness, and asthma. Am J Respir Crit Care Med 2004;169:921–927.

34 Sears MR, Greene JM, Willan AR, Wiecek EM, Taylor DR, Flannery EM, Cowan JO, Herbison GP, Silva PA, Poulton R: A longitudinal, population-based, cohort study of childhood asthma followed to adulthood. N Engl J Med 2003;349:1414–1422.

35 Yoos HL, Kitzman H, McMullen A, Sidora K: Symptom perception in childhood asthma: How accurate are children and their parents? J Asthma 2003;40:27–39.

36 Clough JB, Holgate ST: Episodes of respiratory morbidity in children with cough and wheeze. Am J Respir Crit Care Med 1994;150:48–53.

37 Rietveld S, Everaerd W: Perceptions of asthma by adolescents at home. Chest 2000;117:434–439.

38 Male I, Richter H, Seddon P: Children's perception of breathlessness in acute asthma. Arch Dis Child 2000;83:325–329.

39 Horak E, Grässl G, Skladal D, Ulmer H: Lung function and symptom perception in children with asthma and their parents. Pediatr Pulmonol 2003;35:23–28.

40 Fuhlbrigge AL, Kitch BT, Paltiel AD, Kuntz KM, Neumann PJ, Dockery DW: FEV_1 is associated with risk of asthma attacks in a pediatric population. J Allergy Clin Immunol 2001;107:61–67.

41 Jenkins HA, Cherniack R, Szefler SJ, Covar R, Gelfand EW, Spahn JD: A comparison of the clinical characteristics of children and adults with severe asthma. Chest 2003;124:1318–1324.

42 Rasmussen F, Taylor DR, flannery EM, Cowan JO, Herbison GP: Risk factors for hospital admission for asthma from childhood to young adulthood: A longitudinal population study. J Allergy Clin Immunol 2002;110:220–227.

43 Jenkins MA, Hopper JL, Bowes G, Carlin JB, Flander LB, Giles GG: Factors in childhood as predictors of asthma in adult life. BMJ 1994;309:90–93.

44 Grol MH, Gerritsen J, Postma DS: Asthma: From childhood to adulthood. Allergy 1996; 51:855–869.

45 Roorda RJ, Gerritsen J, van Aaalderen WMC, Schouten JP, Veltman JC, Weiss ST: Follow-up of asthma from childhood to adulthood: Influence of potential childhood risk factors on the outcome of pulmonary function and bronchial hyperresponsiveness in adulthood. J Allergy Clin Immunol 1994;93:575–584.

46 Brown PJ, Greville HW, Finucane KE: Asthma and irreversible airflow obstruction. Thorax 1984;39:131–136.

47 Peat JK, Woolkock AJ, Cullen K: Rate of decline of lung function in subjects with asthma. Eur J Respir Dis 1987;70:171–179.

48 Eid N, Yandell B, Howell L, Eddy M, Sheikh S: Can peak flow predict airflow obstruction in children with asthma? Pediatrics 2000;105: 354–358.

49 Rasmussen F, Taylor DR, Flannery EM, Cowan JO, Greene JM, Herbison GF, Sears MR: Risk factors for airway remodelling in asthma manifested by a low postbronchodilator FEV_1/vital capacity ratio: A longitudinal population study from childhood to adulthood. Am J Respir Crit Care Med 2002;165:1480–1488.

50 Brand PLP, Roorda RJ: Usefulness of monitoring lung function in asthma. Arch Dis Child 2003;88:1021–1025.

51 Sly PD, Landau LI, Weymouth R: Home recording of peak expiratory flow rates and perception of asthma. Am J Dis Child 1985; 139:479–482.

52 Verini M, Rossi N, Dalfino T, Verrotti A, Di Gioacchino M, Chiarelli M: Lack of correlation between clinical patterns of asthma and airway obstruction. Allergy Asthma Proc 2001;22:293–294.

53 Mitra AD, Ogston S, Crighton A, Mukhopadhyay S: Lung function and asthma symptoms in children: Relationship and response to treatment. Acta Paediatr 2002;91: 789–792.

54 Sly PD: Relationship between change in PEF and symptoms: Questions to ask in paediatric clinics. Eur Respir J Suppl 1997;24:S80–S83.

55 Brand PL, Duiverman EJ, Postma DS, Waalkens HJ, Kerrebijn KF, van Essen-Zandvliet EE: Peak flow variation in childhood asthma: Relationship to symptoms, atopy, airways obstruction and hyperresponsiveness. Dutch CNSLD study Group. Eur Respir J 1997;10:1242–1247.

56 Gern JE, Eggleston PA, Schuberth KC, Eney ND, Goldstein EO, Weiss ME, Adkinson NF Jr: Peak flow variation in childhood asthma: A three-year analysis. J Allergy Clin Immunol 1994;93:706–716.

57 Sly PD, Cahill P, Willet K, Burton P: Accuracy of mini peak flow meters in indicating changes in lung function in children with asthma. BMJ 1994;308:572–574.

58 Kamps AWA, Roorda RJ, Brand PLP: Peak flow diaries in childhood asthma are unreliable. Thorax 2001;56:180–182.

59 McMullen AH, Yoos HL, Kitzman H: Peak flow meters in childhood asthma: Parent report of use and perceived usefulness. J Pediatr Health Care 2002;16:67–72.

60 Yoos HL, Kitzman H, McMullen A, Henderson C, Sidora K: Symptom monitoring in childhood asthma: A randomized clinical trial comparing peak expiratory flow rate with symptom monitoring. Ann Allergy Asthma Immunol 2002;88:283–291.

61 Pelkonen AS, Nikander K, Turpeinen M: Reproducibility of home spirometry in children with newly diagnosed asthma. Pediatr Pulmonol 2000;29:34–38.

62 Mortimer KM, Fallot A, Balmes JR, Tager IB: Evaluating the use of a portable spirometer in a study of pediatric asthma. Chest 2003;123: 1899–1907.

63 Wensley DC, Silverman M: The quality of home spirometry in school children with asthma. Thorax 2001;56:183–185.

64 Bastian-Lee Y, Chavasse R, Richter H, Seddon P: Assessment of a low-cost home monitoring spirometer for children. Pediatr Pulmonol 2002;33:388–394.

65 Bacharier LB, Mauger DT, Lemanske RF, Schend V, Sorkness C, Strunk RC: Classifying asthma severity in children: Is measuring lung function helpful? J Allergy Clin Immunol 2002;109:S266.

66 Sharek PJ, Mayer ML, Loewy L, Robinson TN, Shames RS, Umetsu DT, Bergman DA: Agreement among measures of asthma status: A prospective study of low-income children with moderate to severe asthma. Pediatrics 2002;110:797–804.

67 Covar RA, Szefler SJ, Martin R, Sundstrom D, Silkoff P, Murphy J, Young DA, Spahn JD: Relations between exhaled nitric oxide levels and measures of disease activity among children with mild to moderate asthma. J Pediatr 2003;142:469–475.

68 Szefler SJ, Martin RJ, Sharp King T, Boushey HA, Cherniack RM, Chinchilli VM, Craig TJ, Dolivich M, Drazen JM, Fagan JK, Fahy JV, Fish JE, Ford JG, Israel E, Kiley J, Kraft M, Lazarus SC, Lemanske RF Jr, Mauger E, Peters SP, Sorkness CA: Significant variability in response to inhaled corticosteroids for persistent asthma. J Allergy Clin Immunol 2002;109:410–418.

69 Straub DA, Ehmann R, Hall GL, Moeller A, Hamacher J, Frey U, Sennhauser FH, Wildhaber JH: Correlation of nitrites in breath condensates and lung function in asthmatic children. Pediatr Allergy Immunol 2004;15: 20–25.

70 Bahceciler NN, Barlan IB, Nuhoglu Y, Basaran MM: Risk factors for the persistence of respiratory symptoms in childhood asthma. Ann Allergy Asthma Immunol 2001;86:449–455.

71 Brand PLP: Practical interpretation of lung function tests in asthma; in David TJ, (ed): Recent Advances in Paediatrics. Edinburgh, Churchill Livingstone, 2000, vol 18, pp 77–109.

72 Wagner PD, Hedenstierna G, Rodriguez-Roisin R: Gas exchange, expiratory flow obstruction and the clinical spectrum of asthma. Eur Respir J 1996;9:1278–1282.

73 Ferrer A, Roca J, Wagner PD, Lopez FA, Rodriguez-Roisin R: Airway obstruction and ventilation-perfusion relationships in acute severe asthma. Am Rev Respir Dis. 1993;147:579–584.

74 Belessis Y, Dixon S, Thomsen A, Duffy B, Rawlinson W, Henry R, Morton J: Risk factors for an intensive care unit admission in children with asthma. Pediatr Pulmonol 2004;37:201–209.

75 Walamies MA: Diagnostic role of residual volume in paediatric patients with chronic symptoms of the lower airways. Clin Physiol 1998;18:49–54.

76 Kanengiser S, Dozor AJ: Forced expiratory maneuvers in children aged 3 to 5 years. Pediatr Pulmonol 1994;18:144–149.

77 Frey U: Why are infants prone to wheeze? Physiological aspects of wheezing disorders in infants. Swiss Med Wkly 2001;131:400–406.

78 Martinez FD, Helms PJ: Types of asthma and wheezing. Eur Respir J 1998;12(suppl 27): 3S–8S.

79 Turner SW, Palmer LJ, Rye PJ, Gibson NA, Judge PK, Young S, Landau LI, Le Souef PN: Infants with flow limitation at 4 weeks: Outcome at 6 and 11 years. Am J Respir Crit Care Med 2002;165:1294–1298.

80 Wildhaber JH, Dore ND, Devadason SG, Hall GL, Hamacher J, Arheden L, Le Souef PN: Comparison of subjective and objective measures in recurrently wheezy infants. Respiration 2002;69:397–405.

81 Csonka P, Kaila M, Laippala P, Iso-Mustajarvi M, Vesikari T, Ashorn P: Oral prednisolone in the acute management of children age 6 to 35 months with viral respiratory infection-induced lower airway disease: A randomized, placebo-controlled trial. J Pediatr 2003;143: 725–730.

82 Oommen A, Lambert PC, Grigg J: Efficacy of a short course of parent-initiated oral prednisolone for viral wheeze in children aged 1–5 years: Randomised controlled trial. Lancet 2003;362:1433–1438.

83 Delacourt C, Dutau G, Lefrancois G, Clerson P: Comparison of the efficacy and safety of nebulized beclometasone dipropionate and budesonide in severe persistent childhood asthma. Respir Med 2003;97(suppl B): S27–S33.

84 Scott MB, Ellis MH, Cruz-Rivera M, Fitzpatrick S, Smith JA: Once-daily budesonide inhalation suspension in infants and children < 4 and > or = 4 years of age with persistent asthma. Ann Allergy Asthma Immunol 2001;87:488–495.

85 Spahn J: Clinical trial efficacy: What does it really tell you? J Allergy Clin Immunol 2003;112(suppl):S102–S106.

86 Martinez FD, Morgan WJ, Wright AL, Holberg C, Taussig LM: Initial airway function is a risk factor for recurrent wheezing respiratory illnesses during the first three years of life. Am Rev Respir Dis 1991;143:312–316.

87 Martinez FD, Morgan WJ, Wright AL, Holberg CJ, Taussig LM: Diminished lung function as a predisposing factor for wheezing respiratory illness in infants. N Engl J Med 1988;319:1112–1117.

88 van der Ent CK, Brackel HJ, van der Laag J, Bogaard JM: Tidal breathing analysis as a measure of airway obstruction in children three years of age and older. Am J Respir Crit Care Med 1996;153:1253–1258.

89 Carlsen KH, Lodrup Carlsen KC: Tidal breathing analysis and response to salbutamol in awake young children with and without asthma. Eur Respir J 1994;7:2154–2159.

90 Lodrup Carlsen KC, Stenzler A, Carlsen KH: Determinants of tidal flow volume loop indices in neonates and children with and without asthma. Pediatr Pulmonol 1997;24:391–396.

91 Benoist MR, Brouard JJ, Rufin P, Delacourt C, Waernessyckle S, Scheinmann P: Ability of new lung function tests to assess methacholine-induced airway obstruction in infants. Pediatr Pulmonol 1994;18:308–316.

92 Young S, Le Souef PN, Geelhoed GC, Stick SM, Turner KJ, Landau LI: The influence of a family history of asthma and parental smoking on airway responsiveness in early infancy. N Engl J Med 1991;324:1168–1173.

93 Lodrup Carlsen KC, Carlsen KH: Inhaled nebulized adrenaline improves lung function in infants with acute bronchiolitis. Respir Med 2000;94:709–714.

94 Lodrup Carlsen KC, Halvorsen R, Ahlstedt S, Carlsen KH: Eosinophil cationic protein and tidal flow volume loops in children 0–2 years of age. Eur Respir J 1995;8:1148–1154.

95 Prendiville A, Green S, Silverman M: Paradoxical response to nebulised salbutamol in wheezy infants, assessed by partial expiratory flow-volume curves. Thorax 1987;42:86–91.

96 Turner DJ, STick SM, Le Souef KL, Sly PD, Le Souef PN: A new technique to generate and assess forced expiration from raised lung volume in infants. Am J Respir Crit Care Med 1995;151:1441–1450.

97 Hall GL, Hantos Z, Sly PD: Altered respiratory tissue mechanics in asymptomatic wheezy infants. Am J Respir Crit Care Med 2001;164:1387–1391.

98 Goldstein AB, Castille RG, Davis SD, Filbrun DA, Flucke RL, McCoy KS, Tepper RS: Bronchodilator responsiveness in normal infants and young children. Am J Respir Crit Care Med 2001;164:447–454.

99 Hayden MJ, Wildhaber JH, Le Souef PN: Bronchodilator responsiveness testing using raised volume forced expiration in recurrently wheezing infants. Pediatr Pulmonol 1998;26:35–41.

100 Moeller A, Franklin P, Hall GL, Turner S, Straub DA, Wildhaber JH, Stick SM: Inhaled fluticasone dipropionate decreases levels of nitric oxide in recurrently wheezy infants. Pediatr Pulmonol, in press.

101 Hayden MJ, Devadason SG, Sly PD, Wildhaben JH, Le Souef PN: Methacholine responsiveness using the raised volume forced expiration technique in infants. Am J Respir Crit Care Med 1997;155:1670–1675.

102 Hall GL, Hantos Z, Wildhaber JH, Petak F, Sly PD: Methacholine responsiveness in infants assessed with low frequency forced oscillation and forced expiration techniques. Thorax 2001;56:42–47.

103 Verbanck S, Schuermans D, Noppen M, Van Muylem A, Paiva M Vincken W: Evidence of acinar airway involvement in asthma. Am J Respir Crit Care Med 1999;159:1545–1550.

104 Verbanck S, Schuermans D, Paiva M, Vincken W: Nonreversible conductive airway ventilation heterogeneity in mild asthma. J Appl Physiol 2003;94:1380–1386.

105 Gustafsson PM, Ljungberg HK, Kjellman B: Peripheral airwa involvement in asthma assessed by single-breath SF6 and He washout. Eur Respir J 2003;21:1033–1039.

106 Gustafsson PM, Kallman S, Ljungberg H, Lindblad A: Method for assessment of volume of trapped gas in infants during multiple-breath inert gas washout. Pediatr Pulmonol 2003;35:42–49.

107 Hall GL, Hantos Z, Petak F, Wildhaber JH, Tiller K, Burton PR, Sly PD: Airway and respiratory tissue mechanics in normal infants. Am J Respir Crit Care Med 2000;162:1397–1402.

108 Delacourt C, Lorino H, Herve-Guillot M, Reinert P, Harf A, Housset B: Use of the forced oscillation technique to assess airway obstruction and reversibility in children. Am J Respir Crit Care Med 2000;161:730–736.

109 Hayden MJ, Petak F, Hantos Z, Hall G, Sly PD: Using low-frequency oscillation to detect bronchodilator responsiveness in infants. Am J Respir Crit Care Med 1998;157:574–579.

110 Duiverman EJ, Neijens HJ, Van der Snee-van Smaalen M, Kerrebijn KF: Comparison of forced oscillometry and forced expirations for measuring dose-related responses to inhaled methacholine in asthmatic children. Bull Eur Physiopathol Respir 1986;22:433–436.

111 Wilson NM, Bridge P, Phagoo SB, Silverman M: The measurement of methacholine responsiveness in 5 year old children: Three methods compared. Eur Respir J 1995;8:364–370.

112 Frey U, Jackson AC, Silverman M: Differences in airway wall compliance as a possible mechanisme for wheezing disorders in infants. Eur Respir J 1998;12:136–142.

113 Bisgaard H, Klug B: Lung function measurement in awake young children. Eur Respir J 1995;8:2067–2075.

114 Oswald-Mammosser M, Llerena C, Speich JP, Donata L, Lonsdorfer: Measurements of respiratory system resistance by the interrupter technique in healthy and asthmatic children. Pediatr Pulmonol 1997;24:78–85.

115 Chan EY, Bridge PD, Dundas I, Pao CS, Healy MJ, McKenzie SA: Repeatability of airway resistance measurements made using the interrupter technique. Thorax 2003;58:344–347.

116 Beydon N, Amsallem F, Bellet M, Boule M, Chaussain M, Denjean A, Matran R, Wuyam B, Alberti C, Gaultier C: Pre/postbronchodilator interrupter resistance values in healthy young children. Am J Respir Crit Care Med 2002;165:1388–1394.

117 Brussee JE, Smit HA, Koopman LP, Wijga AH, Kerkhof M, Corver K, Vos AP, Gerritsen J, Grobbee DE, Brunekreef B, Merkus PJ, de Jongste JC: Interrupter resistance and wheezing phenotypes at 4 years of age. Am J Respir Crit Care Med 2004;169:209–213.

118 Hall GL, Wildhaber JH, Cernelc M, Frey U: Evaluation of the interrupter technique in healthy, unsedated infants. Eur Respir J 2001;18:982–988.

119 Chavasse RJ, Bastian-Lee Y, Seddon P: Comparison of resistance measured by the interrupter technique and by passive mechanics in sedated infants. Eur Respir J 2001;18:330–334.

120 Frey U, Makkonen K, Wellman T, Beardsmore C, Silverman M: Alterations in airway wall properties in infants with a history of wheezing disorders. Am J Respir Crit Care Med 2000;161:1825–1829.

121 Bez C, Sach G, Jarisch A, Rosewich M, Reichenbach J, Zielen S: Safety and tolerability of methacholine challenge in infants with recurrent wheeze. J Asthma 2003;40:795–802.

122 Clarke JR, Salmon B, Silverman M: Bronchial responsiveness in the neonatal period as a risk factor for wheezing in infancy. Am J Respir Crit Care Med 1995;15:1434–1440.

123 Palmer LJ, Rye PJ, Gibson NA, Burton PR, Landau LI, Le Souëf PN: Airway responsiveness in early infancy predicts asthma, lung function, and respiratory symptoms by school age. Am J Respir Crit Care Med 2001;163:37–42.

Johannes Wildhaber, MD, PhD
Head of Respiratory Medicine
University Children's Hospital
Steinwiesstrasse 75
CH–8032 Zürich (Switzerland)
Tel. +41 1 266 7690
Fax +41 1 266 7171
E-Mail johannes.wildhaber@kispi.unizh.ch

Hammer J, Eber E (eds): Paediatric Pulmonary Function Testing.
Prog Respir Res. Basel, Karger, 2005, vol 33, pp 215–223

Cystic Fibrosis

Felix Ratjen   Hartmut Grasemann

Children's Hospital, University of Essen, Essen, Germany

Abstract

Cystic fibrosis (CF) lung disease is caused by isotonic fluid depletion of airway surface liquid that results in obstructive lung disease primarily involving the small airways. Lung function measurements are an important tool to diagnose the extent of pulmonary involvement, follow its progression, assess the response to treatment, demonstrate the presence of airway hyperreactivity and define candidates for lung transplantation. To date, no better criterion than a forced expiratory volume in 1 s (FEV_1) of less than 30% predicted in conjunction with other clinical indicators has been identified for the referral to lung transplantation in CF. Despite all the efforts to develop other lung function techniques that were hoped to be more sensitive to small airways disease, forced expiratory maneuvers have been found to be the most useful lung function tests in CF. FEV_1 is the single best lung function parameter in older patients. Flows at lower lung volumes often show abnormalities in patients with limited disease in whom other lung function tests including FEV_1 are in the normal range. Modifications of forced expiratory maneuvers such as the rapid thoracoabdominal compression technique have been developed for noncooperative children and infants. This technique has been thoroughly evaluated and is now considered feasible for the use in clinical studies assessing pulmonary interventions in CF.

Cystic Fibrosis Pathophysiology and Its Effect on Lung Function

The underlying pathophysiology of cystic fibrosis (CF) lung disease is characterized by isotonic fluid depletion, which results in decreased periciliary liquid as a consequence of abnormal sodium absorption from the airway lumen coupled with a failure of the cystic fibrosis transmembrane regulator (CFTR) protein to secrete chloride [1]. Water loss increases mucus viscosity and impairs mucociliary clearance and cough clearance. Bacteria invading the CF lung are trapped in this viscous mucus layer on top of respiratory epithelial cells. Bacterial infections lead to an exaggerated, sustained and prolonged inflammatory response dominated by neutrophils. The combination of mucus retention, bacterial infection and inflammation results in obstructive lung disease. Histological data from patients with limited respiratory disease as well as lung function studies suggest that the disease process starts in the small airways rather than the lung parenchyma [2, 3]. The expression of the CFTR protein follows the same regional distribution as it is primarily expressed in bronchial tissue and not in alveoli [4, 5]. As the disease process is not uniformly distributed throughout the lower respiratory tract, it is also characterized by inhomogeneity of ventilation. Restrictive alterations develop secondary to the damage of lung parenchyma by inflammatory changes and by neutrophil degradation products.

The evolution of CF lung disease from a primarily small airways disease to the involvement of larger airways, development of bronchiectasis and destruction of lung tissue has implications for the lung function abnormalities observed in CF patients. Early lung function studies in CF that included patients with a wide range of disease severity have shown lung hyperinflation with increased residual volume (RV), decreased vital capacity

(VC), decreased compliance and increased resistance [6]. Studies using body plethysmography have also provided evidence for trapped gas in the majority of patients [7]. Esophageal pressure measurements have shown that there is a marked frequency dependence of compliance indicative of airway obstruction, whereas alterations in lung elastic recoil were found only in a subgroup of patients [6, 8]. This has not been confirmed in a subsequent study where reduction in static elastic recoil was observed in more than half of the patients [9]. However, the reduction in lung elastic recoil in any of these studies was not pronounced and did not account for a major loss in the pressure driving expiratory flow, a finding which would imply that the major reason for reduced expiratory flows in CF patients is airway obstruction and not loss of elastic recoil. This is unlike classical emphysema as seen in adult patients with α_1-antitrypsin deficiency.

As the disease process progresses, bronchial obstruction leads to tissue destruction with bronchiectasis and eventually the development of areas of pulmonary emphysema and fibrosis. In more advanced disease, the destruction of lung tissue leads to decreased compliance that parallels the decline in forced expiratory volume in 1 s (FEV_1) [10]. This increases respiratory load and favors a rapid and shallow breathing pattern that further impairs gas exchange in CF patients.

Due to the large surface area of small airways, their contribution to airway resistance is relatively small. This explains why airway resistance (or conductance) is not a sensitive test to detect early alterations in patients with CF. Airway resistance measurements are normal in many patients with CF until they develop more advanced disease involving the larger airways [8]. This is in contrast to measurements of lung volumes with body plethysmography, since the ratio of RV to total lung capacity (TLC) that indicates hyperinflation, a key feature of CF lung disease, has been found to correlate with disease severity in numerous studies [7, 8, 11].

Since airway obstruction primarily affects the small airways, at least in patients with limited lung disease, lung function abnormalities are first observed with tests that can detect alterations in this area of the respiratory tract. Tests that have been used to assess small airway function include frequency dependence of compliance, RV as a fraction of TLC, closing volume, flows of the lower portion of the maximal expiratory flow volume (MEFV) curve, MEFV curves with gases of different density (heliox curves), and arterial blood gases [3, 8, 11–16]. Frequency dependence of compliance has been observed in the majority of patients that have been studied, but the

invasive nature of this technique makes it unsuitable for routine clinical use [8]. Closing volume measured by the nitrogen washout method has been studied in a large population of CF patients and was found to be less sensitive than the RV/TLC ratio, MEFV curves, and arterial blood gases [12]. The comparison of MEFV curves breathing room air and a mixture of 80% helium and 20% oxygen was introduced, since helium has a lower density under conditions of laminar flow, and it has been postulated that the point where flow is similar for both gas mixtures (point of isoflow) is reached earlier in patients with small airways disease [3].

Among the tests for small airway function, flow between 75 and 25% of VC or maximal flow at 50% VC have been found to be the most useful tests of lung function [14–16]. These tests often show abnormalities in patients in whom other lung function tests including FEV_1 are in the normal range. However, the large interindividual variability makes these tests problematic for cross-sectional analysis of lung function [17]. It is also important to note that flows at lower lung volumes are only useful in patients with mild disease in the absence of marked hyperinflation, because shifts of the MEFV curve to higher lung volumes result in spuriously increased expiratory flows.

Arterial oxygen tension has been reported to be decreased before lung function abnormalities occur [13], and has been considered by some authors to show the best correlation with the severity of CF lung disease [7]. This may reflect the fact that uneven ventilation is seen early in the disease [18, 19].

Despite all the efforts to develop other lung function techniques that were hoped to be more sensitive to small airways disease, forced expiratory maneuvers have been found to be the most useful lung function tests in CF [14, 15, 20]. Among these tests, FEV_1 is the most reliable test to determine disease progression and is currently considered the 'gold standard' for lung function testing in CF. Longitudinal studies using large data bases have shown that the natural course of the disease is reflected by a mean annual rate of decline in FEV_1 of 2–4% [21]. However, the rate of decline depends upon the level of baseline function and patients with less severe disease have been found to show a more rapid decline in lung function [22] (see below). FEV_1 is also the single best predictor of survival and is used for selecting suitable candidates for lung transplantation (see below). The loss of lung volume that develops in patients due to tissue destruction as well as the hyperinflation decrease forced vital capacity (FVC), which explains why the FEV_1/FVC ratio is not a useful test in CF patients and may be normal even in patients with severe disease [8]. A subgroup of CF patients also develops a primarily restrictive lung disease for reasons that are at present poorly understood [23].

Lung Function Tests in Infants and Small Children with CF

Newborns with CF are born with essentially normal lungs, but the majority of infants develop pulmonary disease manifestations in the first years of life. A number of lung function tests have been developed to detect these abnormalities. So far none of these tests has been shown to be clinically useful, and no single test can be used throughout different age groups for longitudinal lung function assessments [21]. Problems with lung function tests in infants involve the necessity to sedate infants beyond 6 weeks of age, and that tests are time consuming and require experienced personnel. In addition, intra- and interindividual variability of all tests have been found to be relatively larger in infants compared to older, cooperative subjects. However, infant pulmonary function tests have yielded important information on early abnormalities and some of the newer techniques, at least partially, resolved some of the problems of previously utilized techniques [24].

Lung volume measurements in infants with CF have been performed with body plethysmography and gas dilution techniques, but comparative data are not available. Elevated thoracic gas volume has been found in CF infants although some of the studies were subjected to methodological problems that lead to an overestimation of thoracic gas volume [25, 26]. Airway resistance was reported to be elevated in a proportion of infants with CF despite the fact that most cooperative children have normal airway resistance at the age of 6 years [27]. Airway resistance measurements in infants are complicated by the fact that measurements are performed with a face mask and that the upper airway, which contributes about 50% to total airflow resistance, cannot be excluded. Total respiratory system resistance and compliance have been tested in CF infants with the occlusion techniques that utilize the Hering-Breuer reflex. These techniques rely on the assumption that time constants are uniformly distributed among the respiratory tract and that the respiratory system can be modeled as a one-compartment system. This is unlikely to be the case in a heterogeneously distributed disease such as CF. Regional differences in the pressure volume relationship also limit the usefulness of respiratory system compliance measurements, which have been found to be

decreased in a fraction of CF infants [28]. However, some interesting data have been generated with compliance measurements, such as in the study by Dakin et al. [29], where specific compliance was found to be correlated to the degree of airway infection and inflammation in CF patients.

Among the tests that have been developed for this age group, quite similar to older patients with CF, measurements of forced expiratory flows have been found to be the most useful method to determine lung function abnormalities. These can be obtained in sedated subjects with the rapid thoracoabdominal compression technique by squeezing the chest wall with an inflatable jacket [see 30]. Initial studies have used the rapid thoracoabdominal compression technique from end-inspiration [31, 32]. While flow limitation has been shown to be achievable with this technique, it yields only a partial expiratory flow volume curve [33, 34]. A modification of this technique that enables inflation of the sedated infants to a predetermined pressure (e.g. 20 cm H_2O) has been introduced in recent years and was found to be more sensitive in detecting abnormalities in both wheezy infants and infants with CF [35–37]. These tests have been thoroughly evaluated and larger cohorts of normal infants have been tested, so that this technique is now considered feasible for the use in clinical studies assessing pulmonary interventions in CF [38]. Interestingly, lung function abnormalities have already been found with this technique in infants that were considered to be asymptomatic by their physician [39, 40]. In addition, lung function tests have been shown to remain abnormal even after initiation of specialized care [41] (fig. 1, 2).

As ventilation inhomogeneity is considered to be one of the earliest abnormalities in CF, more recent studies have focused on assessing the time for washout of an inert gas. This can then be quantified using the lung clearance index, which is remarkably stable throughout life and can be studied both in awake and sedated subjects with a similar technique [19, see 42]. Future studies will show whether this test will turn out to be a useful lung function test for infants with CF.

The Use of Pulmonary Function Tests in Monitoring CF Patients

Pulmonary function testing with spirometry or body plethysmography is the principal measure of pulmonary status in CF patients older than 5–6 years of age. FEV_1 is the most widely used lung function parameter in CF

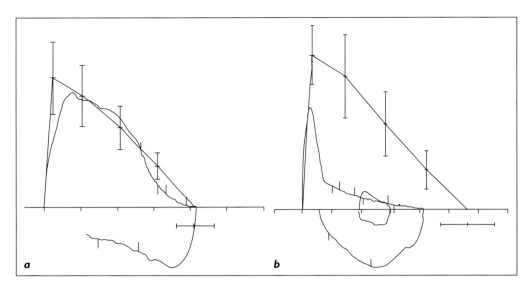

Fig. 1. Representative examples of flow-volume curves during forced expiration in a CF patient with early lung disease (**a**) and a CF patient with more advanced lung disease (**b**). Note that flows are normal during most of the expiration except for flows at lower lung volumes (**a**) and decreased throughout expiration (**b**).

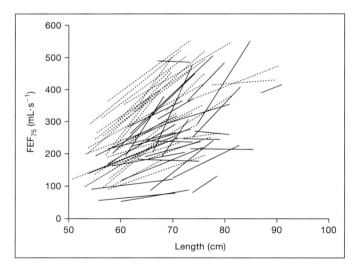

Fig. 2. Association of forced expiratory flow when 75% of FVC had been expired (FEF_{75}) with length. The dashed and solid lines indicate airway function of healthy infants and infants with CF, respectively [41].

patients with obstructive lung disease [43–45]. Pulmonary function testing, at least spirometry with FEV_1, should be assessed at every visit to the clinic. FEV_1 is not only used in day-to-day clinical practice as the primary marker for airway disease to predict decline in health status and survival [45–50], but also as a primary outcome parameter in clinical studies of new therapeutics in CF [44, 51, 52].

Severity of lung disease in CF is usually classified by the degree of impairment in FEV_1 and FVC. Patients with an FEV_1 below 30% or an FVC below 40% of predicted values are considered to have severe disease. Mild lung disease is present when FVC and FEV_1 are still within the normal range. However, in some studies, an FEV_1 below 75% has been used to separate moderate from mild lung disease [52]. The average annual decline in FEV_1 in the US CF population is 2% [53]. However, patients may be stable for many years and then show periods of more rapid progression. Most important, the slope of decline, among other factors that are listed below, depends upon baseline pulmonary function, as patients with better function have a steeper initial decline [53]. The individual decline in FEV_1 is not strongly related to the CFTR genotype, although so-called mild CFTR mutations and pancreatic sufficiency are associated with slower rates of decline [46, 54]. Poor nutritional status [55], airway colonization with *Pseudomonas aeruginosa* [46, 56], and *Burkholderia cepacia* [57, 58], frequent pulmonary exacerbations [46], and comorbidity from diabetes mellitus [59, 60] have

Table 1. Definition of pulmonary exacerbation [61]

Symptoms
  Increased frequency, duration, and intensity of cough
  Increased or new onset of sputum production
  Change in sputum appearance
  New onset or increased hemoptysis
  Increased shortness of breath and decreased exercise tolerance
  Decrease in overall well-being, increased fatigue, weakness,
    fever, poor appetite
Physical signs
  Increased work of breathing, intercostal retractions and use of
    accessory muscles
  Increased respiratory rate
  New onset or increased crackles on chest examination
  Increased air trapping
  Fever
  Weight loss
Laboratory findings
  Decrease in FEV_1 $\geq$10% compared with best value in previous
    6 months
  Increased air trapping and/or new infiltrate on chest radiograph
  Leukocytosis
  Decreased SaO_2

Table 2. Improvement in FEV_1 after intravenous antibiotics

	n	Improvement in FEV_1, %	Range, %
Bosworth and Nielson [66]	32	23	n.r.
Smith et al. [67]	54	18	−40 to +140
Ordonez et al. [68]	55	10	−6 to +32
Cunningham et al. [69]	14	27	n.r.

n.r. = Not reported.

been shown to accelerate the deterioration in pulmonary function.

Response to Therapy for Pulmonary Exacerbation

Pulmonary function tests are used to monitor stability of lung disease and any significant change in lung function should prompt a thorough investigation into the possible causes of this finding. Due to the intrinsic variability of the test, a change in FEV_1 $\geq$12% is generally considered a significant change from baseline. A decrease in FEV_1 $\geq$12% is used as one criterion in defining a pulmonary exacerbation (table 1) [61], and is also utilized to monitor response to treatment. Controlled trials on the optimal duration of treatment are lacking, but most centers use the return of FEV_1 to its baseline value with improvement in respiratory symptoms as criteria to document a successful treatment (table 2) [62–64].

There is significant overlap in the clinical features of CF pulmonary exacerbation and allergic bronchopulmonary aspergillosis (ABPA). However, the decline of pulmonary function is usually greater in ABPA, and is unresponsive to both antibiotics and bronchodilators. Therapy of ABPA includes oral corticosteroids and, in case of poor clinical or serologic response, itraconazole. The goal of treatment is to restore and preserve baseline pulmonary function [65].

Airway Responsiveness in CF

Bronchial hyperresponsiveness (BHR) occurs in about 20–50% of patients with CF, depending on the age and methods used to determine pulmonary function [70, 71]. The etiology of BHR in CF is multifactorial and differs from that in asthma. Bronchial responsiveness has also been shown to be inconsistent over time in patients with CF [72]. Bronchial responsiveness has been assessed in CF patients both by bronchial provocation tests and the response to β-adrenergic agents. Methacholine, cold air, histamine and exercise challenge tests have all been performed in cohorts of CF patients with the highest rate of BHR being reported for methacholine challenge [73]. In most normal populations the variability of this test (defined as the mean response + 2 SD) is below 12%; therefore, a test is considered positive, if it exceeds this level [73]. Most studies have demonstrated that, while the absolute threshold of these responses does not correlate with disease severity, the absolute frequency of positive responses does [73–76]. These data are consistent with the hypothesis that airway hyperreactivity in patients with CF is associated with more rapid pulmonary deterioration, and is an unfavorable prognostic finding. BHR should, therefore, be routinely assessed in CF patients.

In clinical practice, bronchial provocation tests are rarely used in CF patients and bronchial responsiveness is usually assessed as bronchodilator response to β-adrenergic agents [77, 78]. While FEV_1 improves in 50–60% of patients, approximately 20–30% show no change, and 10–20% patients show reduced lung function in response to short-acting inhaled bronchodilators [79]. The results of short-term studies on the effect of bronchodilators on pulmonary function in CF are inconclusive; however, longitudinal studies of short-acting β-agonists over 1–2 years show that almost all patients improved in FEV_1 on at least one evaluation. On average, subjects had a bronchodilator response on approximately 25% of the days tested [80, 81].

Reduction in lung function induced by β-adrenergic agents has been proposed to reflect airway instability that is worsened by decreasing bronchomotor tone. This has been assessed by superimposing MEFV and partial expiratory flow volume curves with subsequent extrapolation of flow transients to calculate the 'volume of airway contribution' [82]. This theory has subsequently been challenged, as flows in a given forced expiratory curve are affected by the relative hysteresis of lung and airway parenchyma [83]. In CF patients, similar to asthma, a predominance of parenchyma hysteresis is observed that worsens after administration of bronchodilators. Negative responses to bronchodilator may, therefore, have multiple reasons that are not easily detected in routine pulmonary function testing.

The development of long-acting β-agonist drugs has provided an additional rationale for considering bronchodilator therapy in CF. However, in spite of the widespread use of long-acting bronchodilators, there are very few long-term studies of their effects in CF patients available. Further research into the most appropriate utilization of these medications in patients with CF is needed [84].

Lung Transplantation

Median age of survival in patients with CF in the US has increased from 14 years in 1969 to 32 years in 1999. Approximately 80% of patients with CF still die due to end-stage lung disease [85]. A final treatment option for some patients with CF is lung transplantation. With 114–136 transplants having been performed annually in patients with CF between 1996 and 1999 [85], CF is currently the second leading indication for bilateral lung transplantation in the US [86]. The criteria with which to guide the selection of appropriate candidates and the timing of referral to lung transplantation remain controversial. On one hand, shortage of donor organs results in waiting times between listing for transplantation and receiving lungs of up to 2 years [86], so that delayed referral may result in death before transplant. On the other hand, lung transplantation carries a risk of 40% 3-year mortality rate [87], so that premature referral for transplantation could shorten life expectancy.

Current US and European guidelines for CF transplantation recommend an FEV_1 of less than 30% predicted in conjunction with other clinical indicators, such as rapidly progressive respiratory deterioration, hypercarbia, hypoxia, and female gender, as criteria with which to identify patients with CF potentially within the transplant window [87–90]. These guidelines are based on several models of short-term mortality among patients with CF [91–96].

In a recent analysis of data obtained from 14,572 patients of the CF Foundation National Patient Registry a model was developed to identify the best clinical predictors of 2-year mortality [97]. In this study FEV_1, as well as age, height, respiratory microbiology, number of hospitalizations for pulmonary exacerbations, and number of home intravenous antibiotic courses were all significant predictors of 2-year mortality. A comparison of the model developed in this study when used to guide referral for lung transplantation with that of the widely used criterion of an FEV_1 of less than 30% predicted showed, however, no better diagnostic accuracy of this well-fitting model than of the simpler FEV_1 criterion. Both had high negative predictive values (98 and 97%, respectively) but only modest positive predictive values (33 and 28%, respectively). Therefore, to date, no better criterion than an FEV_1 of less than 30% (in conjunction with other clinical indicators) has been identified for the referral to lung transplantation in CF.

Monitoring Pulmonary Function after Lung Transplantation [see also 90]

Lung transplant recipients are at risk of opportunistic infections, as well as acute or chronic rejection. Early intervention, which is essential to improve long-term survival, is dependent on the earliest possible detection of an infection or rejection event. FEV_1 is the most reliable and consistent pulmonary function test parameter providing an indication of graft dysfunction [98]. Several studies have shown that home spirometry detects lung function decline associated with acute events earlier than pulmonary function tests performed at routine clinical visits [99–101]. Regular home spirometry was also shown to help detecting the progression of the bronchiolitis obliterans syndrome [102], a condition defined as chronic allograft dysfunction in the absence of confirming histology [98]. The goal of therapeutic interventions initiated for events of infection or rejection in allograft recipients is to restore baseline posttransplant pulmonary function.

References

1 Ratjen F, Döring G: Seminar: Cystic fibrosis. Lancet 2003;361:681–689.

2 Bedrossian CW, Greenberg SD, Singer DB, Hansen JJ, Rosenberg HS: The lung in cystic fibrosis. A quantitative study including prevalence of pathologic findings among different age groups. Hum Pathol 1976;7:195–204.

3 Fox WW, Bureau MA, Taussig LA, Martin RR, Beaudry PH: Helium flow-volume curves in the detection of early small airway disease. Pediatrics 1974;54:293–299.

4 Tizzano EF, O'Brodovich H, Chitayat D, Benichou JC, Buchwald M: Regional expression of CFTR in developing human respiratory tissues. Am J Respir Cell Mol Biol 1994;10: 355–362.

5 Engelhardt JF, Zepeda M, Cohn JA, Yankaskas JR, Wilson JM: Expression of the cystic fibrosis gene in adult human lung. J Clin Invest 1994;93:737–749.

6 Cook CD, Helliesen PJ, Kulczycki L, Barrie H, Friedlander L, Agathan A, Harris GBC, Shwachman H: Studies of respiratory physiology in children. II. Lung volumes and mechanics of respiration in 64 patients with cystic fibrosis of the pancreas. Pediatrics 1959;24: 181–193.

7 Beier FR, Renzetti AD Jr, Mitchell M, Watanabe S: Pulmonary pathophysiology in cystic fibrosis. Am Rev Respir Dis 1966;94: 430–440.

8 Landau LI, Phelan PD: The spectrum of cystic fibrosis. Am Rev Respir Dis 1973;108: 593–602.

9 Mansell A, Dubrawsky C, Levison H, Bryan AC, Crozier DN: Lung elastic recoil in cystic fibrosis. Am Rev Respir Dis 1974;109: 190–197.

10 Hart N, Polkey MI, Clement A, Boule M, Moxham J, Lofaso F, Fauroux B: Changes in pulmonary mechanics with increasing disease severity in children and young adults with cystic fibrosis. Am J Respir Crit Care Med 2002;166:61–66.

11 Landau LI, Mellis C, Phelan P, Bristowe B, McLennan L: Small airway disease in children: No test is the best. Thorax 1979;34:217–223.

12 Cooper DM, Doron I, Mansell AL, Bryan AC, Levison H: The relative sensitivity of closing volume in children with cystic fibrosis. Am Rev Respir Dis 1974;109:519–524.

13 Lamarre A, Reilly BJ, Bryan AC, Levison H: Early detection of pulmonary function abnormalities in cystic fibrosis. Pediatrics 1972;50: 291–297.

14 Featherby EA, Tzong-Ruey W, Crozier DN, Duic A, Reilly BJ, Levison H: Dynamic and static lung volumes, blood gas tensions, and diffusion capacity in patients with cystic fibrosis. Am Rev Respir Dis 1970;102: 737–749.

15 Zapletal A, Motoyama EK, Gibson LE, Bouhuys A: Pulmonary mechanics in asthma and cystic fibrosis. Pediatrics 1971;48:64–72.

16 Corey M, Levison H, Crozier D: Five to seven year course of pulmonary function in cystic fibrosis. Am Rev Respir Dis 1976;114: 1085–1092.

17 Hoffstein V, Brown I, Taylor R, McLean P, Zamel N: Maximum flow ratios at mid-vital capacity in young healthy adults. Chest 1986; 90:857–860.

18 Tam CH, Mansell A, Levison H, Reilly BJ, Aspin N: Dynamic regional lung function studies patients with asthma and cystic fibrosis. Am Rev Respir Dis 1973;108:283–293.

19 Gustafsson PM, Aurora P, Lindblad A: Evaluation of ventilation maldistribution as an early indicator of lung disease in children with cystic fibrosis. Eur Respir J 2003;22:972–979.

20 Landau LI, Taussig LM, Macklem PT, Beaudry PH: Contribution of inhomogeneity of lung units to the maximal expiratory flow volume curve in children with asthma and cystic fibrosis. Am Rev Respir Dis 1975;111: 725–731.

21 Ramsey BW, Boat TF: Outcome measures for clinical trials in cystic fibrosis. Summary of a Cystic Fibrosis Foundation consensus conference. J Pediatr 1994;124:177–192.

22 Davis PB, Byard PJ, Konstan MW: Identifying treatments that halt progression of pulmonary disease in cystic fibrosis. Pediatr Res 1997;41: 161–165.

23 Ries AL, Sosa G, Prewitt L, Friedman PJ, Harwood IR: Restricted pulmonary function in cystic fibrosis. Chest 1988;94:575–579.

24 Gappa M, Ranganathan SC, Stocks J: Lung function testing in infants with cystic fibrosis: Lessons from the past and future directions. Pediatr Pulmonol 2001;32:228–245.

25 Beardsmore CS, Bar-Yishaw E, Maayan C, Yahav Y, Katznelson D, Godfrey S: Lung function in infants with cystic fibrosis. Thorax 1988;43:545–551.

26 Kraemer R: Early detection of lung function abnormalities in infants with cystic fibrosis. J R Soc Med (Suppl) 1989;82:21–25.

27 Beardsmore CS, Stocks J, Silverman M: Problems in measuring thoracic gas volume in infancy. J Appl Physiol 1982;52:995–999.

28 Tepper RS, Hiatt PW, Eigen H, Smith J: Total respiratory system compliance in asymptomatic infants with cystic fibrosis. Am Rev Respir Dis 1987;135:1075–1079.

29 Dakin CJ, Numa AH, Wang H, Morton JR, Vertzyas CC, Henry RL: Inflammation, infection, and pulmonary function in infants and young children with cystic fibrosis. Am J Respir Crit Care Med 2002;165:904–910.

30 Modl M, Eber E: Forced expiratory flow-volume measurements; Hammer J, Eber E (eds): Paediatric Pulmonary Function Testing. Prog Respir Res. Basel, Karger, 2005, vol 33, pp 34–43.

31 Adler SM, Wohl MEB: Flow-volume relationship at low lung volumes in healthy term newborn infants. Pediatrics 1978;61:636–640

32 Taussig L, Landau L, Godfrey S, Arad I: Determinants of forced expiratory flows in newborn infants. J Appl Physiol 1982;53: 1220–1227.

33 Ratjen F, Zinman R, Wohl MEB: A new technique to demonstrate flow limitation in partial expiratory flow-volume curves in infancy. J Appl Physiol 1989;67:1662–1669.

34 Ratjen F, Grasemann H, Wolstein R, Wiesemann HG: Isovolume pressure/flow curves of rapid thoracoabdominal compressions in healthy infants. Pediatr Pulmonol 1998;26: 197–203.

35 Turner DJ, Lanteri CJ, LeSouef PN, Sly PD: Improved detection of abnormal respiratory function using forced expiratory flow from raised lung volume in infants with cystic fibrosis. Eur Respir J 1994;7:1995–1999.

36 Henschen M, Stocks J: Assessment of airway function using partial expiratory flow-volume curves: How reliable are measurements of maximal expiratory flow at FRC during early infancy? Am J Respir Crit Care Med 1999; 159:480–486.

37 Ranganathan SC, Bush A, Dezateux C, Carr SB, Hoo AF, Lum S, Madge S, Price J, Stroobant J, Wade A, Wallis C, Wyatt H, Stocks J; London Collaborative Cystic Fibrosis Study: Relative ability of full and partial forced expiratory maneuvers to identify diminished airway function in infants with cystic fibrosis. Am J Respir Crit Care Med 2002;166: 1350–1357.

38 Jones M, Castile R, Davis S, Kisling J, Filbrun D, Flucke R, Goldstein A, Emsley C, Ambrosius W, Tepper RS: Forced expiratory flows and volumes in infants. Normative data and lung growth. Am J Respir Crit Care Med 2000;161: 353–359.

39 Ranganathan SC, Dezateux C, Bush A, Carr SB, Castle R, Madge S, Price J, Stroobant J, Wade A, Wallis C, Stocks J; London Collaborative Cystic Fibrosis Study: Airway function in infants newly diagnosed with cystic fibrosis. Lancet 2001;358:1964–1965.

40 Ranganathan SC, Goetz I, Hoo AF, Lum S, Stocks J: Assessment of tidal breathing parameters in infants with cystic fibrosis. Eur Respir J 2003;22:761–766.

41 Ranganathan SC, Stocks J, Dezateux C, Bush A, Wade A, Carr S, Castle R, Dinwiddie R, Hoo AF, Lum S, Price J, Stroobant J, Wallis C: The evolution of airway function in early childhood following clinical diagnosis of cystic fibrosis. Am J Respir Crit Care Med 2004; 169:928–933.

42 Gustafsson PM, Ljungberg H: Measurement of functional residual capacity and ventilation inhomogeneity by gas dilution techniques; Hammer J, Eber E (eds): Paediatric Pulmonary Function Testing. Prog Respir Res. Basel, Karger, 2005, vol 33, pp 54–65.

43 Davis PB, Byard PJ, Konstan MW: Identifying treatments that halt progression of pulmonary disease in cystic fibrosis. Pediatr Res 1997;41: 161–165.

44 Ramsey BW, Boat TF: Outcome measures for clinical trials in cystic fibrosis: Summary of a Cystic Fibrosis Foundation Consensus Conference. J Pediatr 1994;124:177–192.

45 Corey M, Edwards L, Levison H, Knowles M: Longitudinal analysis of pulmonary function decline in patients with cystic fibrosis. J Pediatr 1997;131:809–814.

46 Emerson J, Rosenfeld M, McNamara S, Ramsey B, Gibson RL: *Pseudomonas aeruginosa* and other predictors of mortality and morbidity in young children with cystic fibrosis. Pediatr Pulmonol 2002;34: 91–100.

47 Kerem E, Reisman J, Corey M, Canny GJ, Levison H: Prediction of mortality in patients with cystic fibrosis. N Engl J Med 1992;326: 1187–1191.

48 Corey M, Levison H, Crozier D: Five- to seven-year course of pulmonary function in cystic fibrosis. Am Rev Respir Dis 1976;114: 1085–1092.

49 Liou TG, Adler FR, Fitzsimmons SC, Cahill BC, Hibbs JR, Marshall BC: Predictive 5-year survivorship model of cystic fibrosis. Am J Epidemiol 2001;153:345–352.

50 Hamblett N, Rosenfeld M, Emerson J, Goss CH, Aitken ML: Developing cystic fibrosis lung transplant referral criteria using predictors of 2-year mortality. Am J Respir Crit Care Med 2002;166:1550–1555.

51 Fuchs HJ, Borowitz DS, Christiansen DH, Morris EM, Nash ML, Ramsey BW, Rosenstein BJ, Smith AL, Wohl ME: Effect of aerosolized recombinant human DNase on exacerbations of respiratory symptoms and on pulmonary function in patients with cystic fibrosis. The Pulmozyme Study Group. N Engl J Med 1994;331:637–642.

52 Ramsey B, Pepe M, Quan JM, Otto KL, Montgomery AB, Williams-Warren J: Efficacy and safety of chronic intermittent administration of inhaled tobramycin in patients with cystic fibrosis. N Engl J Med 1999;340: 23–30.

53 Davis PB, Byard PJ, Konstan MW: Identifying treatments that halt progression of pulmonary disease in cystic fibrosis. Pediatr Res 1997;41: 161–165.

54 Schaedel C, de Monestrol I, Hjelte L, Johannesson M, Kornfalt R, Lindblad A, Strandvik B, Wahlgren L, Holmberg L: Predictors of deterioration of lung function in cystic fibrosis. Pediatr Pulmonol 2002;33:483–491.

55 Steinkamp G, Wiedemann B: Relationship between nutritional status and lung function in cystic fibrosis: Cross-sectional and longitudinal analyses from the German CF quality assurance (CFQA) project. Thorax 2002;57: 596–601.

56 Demko CA, Byard PJ, Davis PB: Gender differences in cystic fibrosis: *Pseudomonas aeruginosa* infection. J Clin Epidemiol 1995; 48:1041–1049.

57 Thomassen MJ, Demko CA, Klinger JD, Stern RC: *Pseudomonas cepacia* colonization among patients with cystic fibrosis: A new opportunist. Am Rev Respir Dis 1985;131: 791–796.

58 Isles A, Maclusky I, Corey M, Gold R, Prober C, Fleming P, Levison H: *Pseudomonas cepacia* infection in cystic fibrosis: An emerging problem. J Pediatr 1984;104:206–210.

59 Lanng S, Thorsteinsson B, Nerup J, Koch C: Diabetes mellitus in cystic fibrosis: Effect of insulin therapy on lung function and infections. Acta Paediatr 1994;83:849–853.

60 Milla CE, Warwick WJ, Moran A: Trends in pulmonary function in patients with cystic fibrosis correlate with the degree of glucose intolerance at baseline. Am J Respir Crit Care Med 2000;162:891–895.

61 Gibson RL, Burns JL, Ramsey BW: Pathophysiology and management of pulmonary infections in cystic fibrosis. Am J Respir Crit Care Med 2003;168:918–951.

62 Regelmann WE, Elliott GR, Warwick WJ, Clawson CC: Reduction of sputum *Pseudomonas aeruginosa* density by antibiotics improves lung function in cystic fibrosis more than do bronchodilators and chest physiotherapy alone. Am Rev Respir Dis 1990;141:914–921.

63 Redding GJ, Restuccia R, Cotton EK, Brooks JG: Serial changes in pulmonary functions in children hospitalized with cystic fibrosis. Am Rev Respir Dis 1982;126:31–36.

64 Michel BC: Antibacterial therapy in cystic fibrosis: A review of the literature published between 1980 and February 1987. Chest 1988; 94:129S–140S.

65 Stevens DA, Moss RB, Kurup VP, Knutsen AP, Greenberger P, Judson MA, Denning DW, Crameri R, Brody AS, Light M, Skov M, Maish W, Mastella G; Participants in the Cystic Fibrosis Foundation Consensus Conference: Allergic bronchopulmonary aspergillosis in cystic fibrosis – State of the art: Cystic Fibrosis Foundation Consensus Conference. Clin Infect Dis 2003;37(suppl 3):S225–S264.

66 Bosworth DG, Nielson DW: Effectiveness of home versus hospital care in the routine treatment of cystic fibrosis. Pediatr Pulmonol 1997;24:42–47.

67 Smith AL, Fiel SB, Mayer-Hamblett N, Ramsey B, Burns JL: Susceptibility testing of *Pseudomonas aeruginosa* isolates and clinical response to parenteral antibiotic administration: Lack of association in cystic fibrosis. Chest 2003;123:1495–1502.

68 Ordonez CL, Henig NR, Mayer-Hamblett N, Accurso FJ, Burns JL, Chmiel JF, Daines CL, Gibson RL, McNamara S, Retsch-Bogart GZ, Zeitlin PL, Aitken ML: Inflammatory and microbiologic markers in induced sputum after intravenous antibiotics in cystic fibrosis. Am J Respir Crit Care Med 2003;168: 1471–1475.

69 Cunningham S, McColm JR, Mallinson A, Boyd I, Marshall TG: Duration of effect of intravenous antibiotics on spirometry and sputum cytokines in children with cystic fibrosis. Pediatr Pulmonol 2003;36:43–48.

70 Mitchell I, Corey M, Woenne R, Krastins IR, Levison H: Bronchial hyperreactivity in cystic fibrosis and asthma. J Pediatr 1978;93: 744–748.

71 Nielsen KG, Pressler T, Klug B, Koch C, Bisgaard H: Serial lung function and responsiveness in cystic fibrosis during early childhood. Am J Respir Crit Care Med 2004;169: 1209–1216.

72 Weinberger M: Airways reactivity in patients with CF. Clin Rev Allergy Immunol 2002;23: 77–85.

73 Mellis CM, Levison H: Bronchial reactivity in cystic fibrosis. Pediatrics 1978;61:446–450.

74 Holzer FJ, Olinsky A, Phelan PD: Variability of airways hyper-reactivity and allergy in cystic fibrosis. Arch Dis Child 1981;56: 455–459.

75 Darga LL, Eason LA, Zach DM, Polgar G: Cold air provocation of airway hyperreactivity in patients with cystic fibrosis. Pediatr Pulmonol 1986;2:82–88.

76 Eggleston PA, Rosenstein BJ, Stackhouse CM, Alexander MF: Airway hyperreactivity in cystic fibrosis: Clinical correlates and possible effects on the course of the disease. Chest 1988;94:360–365.

77 Landau LI, Phelan P: The variable effect of a bronchodilating agent on pulmonary function in cystic fibrosis. J Pediatr 1973;82: 863–868.

78 Shapiro GG, Bamman J, Kanarek P, Bierman CW: The paradoxical effect of adrenergic and methylxanthine drugs in cystic fibrosis. Pediatrics 1976;58:740–743.

79 Brand PL: Bronchodilators in cystic fibrosis. J R Soc Med 2000;93:37–39.

80 Konig P, Gayer D, Barbero GJ, Shaffer J: Short-term and long-term effects of albuterol aerosol therapy in cystic fibrosis: A preliminary report. Pediatr Pulmonol 1995;20:205–214.

81 Hordvik NL, Konig P, Morris D, Kreutz C, Barbero GJ: A longitudinal study of bronchodilator responsiveness in cystic fibrosis. Am Rev Respir Dis 1985;131:889–893.

82 Zach M, Oberwaldner B, Forche G, Polgar G: Bronchodilators increase airway instability in cystic fibrosis. Am Rev Respir Dis 1985; 131:537–543.

83 Zinman R, Wohl ME, Ingram RH Jr: Non-homogeneous lung emptying in cystic fibrosis patients. Volume history and bronchodilator effects. Am Rev Respir Dis 1991;143: 1257–1261.

84 Colombo JL: Long-acting bronchodilators in cystic fibrosis. Curr Opin Pulm Med 2003; 9:504–508.

85 Cystic Fibrosis Foundation: Patient Registry 1999 Annual Data Report. Bethesda, Cystic Fibrosis Foundation, 2000.

86 United Network for Organ Sharing: 1999 Annual Report of the US Scientific Registry for Transplant Recipients and the Organ Procurement and Transplantation Network: Transplant Data: 1989–1998. Rockville, US Department of Health and Human Services, Health Resources and Services Administration, Office of Special Programs, Division of Transplantation, 1999.

87 Yankaskas JR, Mallory GB: Lung transplantation in cystic fibrosis: Consensus conference statement. Chest 1998;113:217–226.

88 American Society for Transplant Physicians: American Thoracic Society, European Respiratory Society, and International Society for Heart and Lung Transplantation: International guidelines for the selection of lung transplant candidates. Am J Respir Crit Care Med 1998; 158:335–339.

89 Kotloff RM, Zuckerman JB: Lung transplantation for cystic fibrosis: Special considerations. Chest 1996;109:787–798.

90 Tablizo MA, Woo MS: Lung transplantation in pediatric patients; Hammer J, Eber E (eds): Paediatric Pulmonary Function Testing. Prog Respir Res. Basel, Karger, 2005, vol 33, pp 224–232.

91 Kerem E, Reisman J, Corey M, Canny GJ, Levison H: Prediction of mortality in patients with cystic fibrosis. N Engl J Med 1992; 326:1187–1191.

92 Milla CE, Warwick WJ: Risk of death in cystic fibrosis patients with severely compromised lung function. Chest 1998;113:1230–1234.

93 Knoke JD, Stern RC, Doershuk CF, Boat TF, Matthews LW: Cystic fibrosis: The prognosis for five-year survival. Pediatr Res 1978;12: 676–679.

94 Hayllar KM, Williams SG, Wise AE, Pouria S, Lombard M, Hodson ME, Westaby D: A prognostic model for the prediction of survival in cystic fibrosis. Thorax 1997;52:313–317.

95 Aurora P, Wade A, Whitmore P, Whitehead B: A model for predicting life expectancy of children with cystic fibrosis. Eur Respir J 2000;16:1056–1060.

96 Grasemann H, Wiesemann HG, Ratjen F: The importance of lung function as a predictor of 2-year mortality in mucoviscidosis. Pneumologie 1995;49:466–469.

97 Mayer-Hamblett N, Rosenfeld M, Emerson J, Goss CH, Aitken ML: Developing cystic fibrosis lung transplant referral criteria using predictors of 2-year mortality. Am J Respir Crit Care Med 2002;166:1550–1555.

98 Cooper JD, Billingham M, Egan T, Hertz MI, Higenbottam T, Lynch J, Mauer J, Paradis I, Patterson GA, Smith C, et al: A working formulation for the standardization of nomenclature and for clinical staging of chronic dysfunction in lung allografts. International Society for Heart and Lung Transplantation. J Heart Lung Transplant 1993;12:713–716.

99 Otulana BA, Higenbottam TW, Scott JP, Clelland C, Hutter JA, Wallwork J: Pulmonary function monitoring allows diagnosis of rejection in heart-lung transplant recipients. Transplant Proc 1989;21:2583–2584.

100 Bjortuft O, Johansen B, Boe J, Foerster A, Holter E, Geiran O: Daily home spirometry facilitates early detection of rejection in single lung transplant recipients with emphysema. Eur Respir J 1993;6:705–708.

101 Finkelstein SM, Hertz MI, Snyder M, et al: Early detection of infection and rejection in lung transplantation. Proc Eng Med Biol Soc 1994;16:862–863.

102 Finkelstein SM, Snyder M, Stibbe CE, Lindgren B, Sabati N, Killoren T, Hertz MI: Staging of bronchiolitis obliterans syndrome using home spirometry. Chest 1999;116: 120–126.

Prof. Dr. med. Felix Ratjen
Children's Hospital, University of Essen
Hufelandstrasse 55, DE–45122 Essen
(Germany)
Tel. +49 201 723 3350
Fax +49 201 723 5721
E-Mail f.ratjen@uni-essen.de

Hammer J, Eber E (eds): Paediatric Pulmonary Function Testing.
Prog Respir Res. Basel, Karger, 2005, vol 33, pp 224–232

Lung Transplantation in Pediatric Patients

Mary Anne Tablizo   Marlyn S. Woo

Children's Hospital Los Angeles, Keck School of Medicine at the University of Southern California,
Los Angeles, Calif., USA

Abstract

Lung transplantation is indicated in selected children with end-stage lung disease, which is unresponsive to conventional medical or surgical therapy. Unlike adult lung transplant candidates, pediatric patients are most frequently referred for cystic fibrosis, congenital heart disease, and primary pulmonary hypertension. Pulmonary function testing is an essential component of most pediatric lung transplant evaluations. Response to treatments and lung disease progression are revealed in serial pulmonary function tests. Evaluation of lung volumes, expiratory flow rates, diffusing capacity, arterial blood gases, and response to bronchodilators is also mandatory in the assessment of prospective lobar donors for living donor lobar lung transplant procedures. Pulmonary function testing, particularly spirometry, is the standard method of monitoring postlung transplant recipients for early evidence of rejection. The type and frequency of monitoring vary from center to center, as well as by patient interval posttransplant. However, new tools for pulmonary function assessment, such as infant pulmonary function testing, home/remote spirometry equipment; high-resolution computed tomography scans, and magnetic resonance imaging, are becoming more widely available to help us better detect early signs of lung graft dysfunction in children.

Introduction

In 1968 Dr. Cooley performed the first pediatric heart-lung transplant in a 2-month-old infant. Since that time, advances in both surgical technique and antirejection regimens have made lung transplantation a therapeutic option in selected pediatric patients with end-stage lung disease. No longer considered an experimental procedure, pediatric lung transplantation is performed in a small number of specialized centers around the world. Outcome of pediatric lung transplant is now equivalent to adult lung transplant survival. Hence, understanding the indications for lung transplant, as well as the evaluation and monitoring of the pediatric patient is important for all medical practitioners involved in the care of children with acute or chronic lung disease. Pulmonary function testing is an important tool used for evaluation of potential lung transplant candidates as well as for screening potential living lobar donors.

Indications

Irreversible pulmonary parenchymal and vascular diseases are generally the indications for lung transplant [1] (table 1). The indications for lung transplant in children vary with age. The 2003 Pediatric Registry of the International Society for Heart and Lung Transplantation (ISHLT) reported that congenital heart disease was the most common indication for lung transplant among infants. For children more than 1 year of age, cystic fibrosis (CF) was the most common lung transplant indication followed by primary pulmonary hypertension. However, CF continues to be the leading indication in adolescents, accounting for 67%

Table 1. Indications for lung transplantation in children [2, 11, 16]

CF
Primary pulmonary hypertension
Pulmonary hypertension associated with congenital heart disease
Bronchopulmonary dysplasia

BO
Retransplant due to BO
Retransplant not due to BO
Bronchiectasis
Chronic obstructive pulmonary disease/emphysema
Idiopathic pulmonary fibrosis
Congenital surfactant protein disorders
Collagen vascular disease
Other pulmonary fibrotic disorders
Pulmonary alveolar proteinosis
Pulmonary alveolar microlithiasis
Pulmonary hypertension associated with parenchymal lung disease
    and congenital abnormalities of lung development
Pulmonary vein stenosis

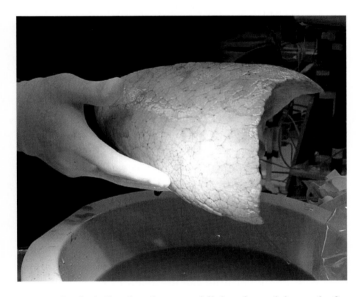

Fig. 1. Newly inflated and prepared living donor lobe ready for transplantation.

of lung transplantations in this age group [2]. Although improvement in long-term outcomes for lung transplant recipients lags behind heart, liver, and renal transplantation, it still offers the child with advanced lung disease the possibility of improved quality of life and longer life expectancy.

Types of Lung Transplantation

The lung for transplantation can come from a cadaver or from a living donor. Because the waiting period for cadaveric organs is lengthening, an alternative in selected patients is the living donor lobar lung procedure (fig. 1). Human living donor lobar lung transplantation was first performed by Dr. Starnes in 1990 as a single lobe transplant [3, 4] and then in 1993 as a bilateral lobe transplant surgery [5]. It is now an alternative for selected patients who are too ill and unable to wait for cadaveric organs [6].

Single lung transplant is common in adults, but it is rarely utilized in children [7]. Bilateral sequential lung transplant surgery is the most common pediatric lung transplant method. The lungs can come as whole lungs from a cadaver, lower lobes from a cadaver or living donors, or are obtained by the split cadaveric lung method [8, 9]. En bloc heart and lung transplant is indicated for patients with severe pulmonary vascular disease due to uncorrectable cardiac lesions, end-stage lung disease with significant left ventricular dysfunction, or pulmonary hypertension with right ventricle failure [10].

Contraindications

All patients considered for transplantation should be evaluated for medical and psychological contraindications. Patients referred for transplantation should have maximized all available medical and surgical methods. Patients who are critically ill/medically unstable or who suffer from other irreversible organ dysfunction should be excluded unless multisolid organ transplantation is under consideration. The creatinine clearance should be near normal and left ventricular function should be normal [11]. Psychosocial problems, such as poor family support or medical nonadherence, are contraindications. Other relative contraindications vary from center to center (table 2). The presence of a pan-resistant organism is not an absolute contraindication, but patients harboring such an organism may have a higher morbidity and mortality risk after transplantation. The presence of symptomatic osteoporosis has to be treated aggressively before and after transplantation. High chronic systemic corticosteroid use is a relative contraindication due to poor postoperative healing. Hence, attempts should be made to wean off or decrease the overall steroid dose before transplant surgery [10]. A history of prior thoracic surgery and/or pleurodesis were previously considered strict contraindications, but these procedures are now relative contraindications in most experienced

Table 2. Relative contraindications for lung transplantation [10, 11]

Severe malnutrition
Diabetes mellitus, poorly controlled
Significant neurologic deficit
Active collagen vascular disease
Musculoskeletal abnormalities with significant impairment in
  pulmonary mechanics
Serious psychiatric disability and inability to comply with
  medication regimen
HIV infection

Severe congenital immunodeficiency
Hepatic dysfunction
Neuromuscular weakness
Active tuberculosis
Hepatitis B antigen positivity
Hepatitis C, active disease
Cigarette smoking
Ventilator-dependent respiratory failure
Recent malignancy

centers [11]. Exclusion criteria vary amongst different transplant centers, depending on each transplant center's experience and resources. A patient who is refused at one center may be accepted at another transplant center.

Lung Transplant Candidate Evaluation

Because of the shortage of suitable donor organs, it is important to select appropriate transplant candidates. The evaluation team should consist of transplant surgeons, pulmonologists, transplant nurse coordinators and social workers. Other specialists (infectious disease, psychiatry, endocrinology, pathology, psychology) should also be consulted about candidate suitability, depending on the patient's primary diagnosis and condition.

The timing of transplant referral is based on the natural history of the underlying disease [12]. There is no perfect measure in assessing the timing and selection of a lung transplant candidate. Similarly, exclusion criteria are also not well established. Patient referrals made too early may result in delay transplanting other more critically ill lung transplant candidates. However, it is more common that potential lung transplant candidates are referred too late. These late-referral patients will often not have the opportunity to undergo lung transplant, let alone to survive any major surgery. A lung transplant candidate needs to be sufficiently ill to benefit from transplantation, yet well enough to survive the stress and potential complications inherent in this surgery [13].

For CF patients, pulmonary function tests are used to measure the progression of respiratory disease. Specifically, the forced expiratory volume in 1 s (FEV_1) is used by most centers as criterion for a CF patient to be considered as a possible candidate for lung transplantation. This criterion is based on a study by Kerem et al. [14], which showed that FEV_1 of less than 30% of the predicted value was associated with a 2-year survival of approximately 50%. Thus, CF patients with FEV_1 of less than 30% predicted are considered for lung transplantation. However, the deterioration in lung function of CF children is unpredictable, making it difficult to determine the appropriate window for both referral and timing of transplantation. Therefore, while the FEV_1 remains an important marker of CF lung disease severity, other factors (patient age, gender, rate of deterioration) must also be considered.

Other survival models have attempted to define optimal referral timing for CF patients for lung transplantation. One of the most commonly cited survival models was proposed by Liou et al. [15]. The paper concluded that CF patients with a predicted 5-year survival of ≤30% should be referred for lung transplant evaluation. The ISHLT, the American Thoracic Society, the American Transplant Physicians, and the European Respiratory Society developed an international guideline for CF lung transplant referral. This guideline includes FEV_1 <30% predicted, rapid respiratory deterioration with FEV_1 >30% predicted, increased frequency of hospitalizations, rapid fall in FEV_1, presence of massive hemoptysis, progressive weight loss despite optimal medical management, PaO_2 <55 mm Hg, $PaCO_2$ >50 mm Hg, female CF patient with rapid deterioration regardless of physiological criteria but meets other criteria, and other quality of life issues [16]. For other lung diseases there are few data available to identify risk factors that will predict optimal timing for referral and transplantation [7].

For young patients under 2 years of age who are unable to perform standard pulmonary function tests, infant pulmonary function testing can be used for pretransplant evaluation. It can determine the presence of restrictive lung disease and airway obstruction by applying a variety of techniques [17].

Donor Evaluation

The selection of appropriate donor organs is an important component of successful lung transplantation. In addition to being blood group compatible, the donor lung and the potential recipient's required lung sizes should be matched as closely as possible. This size matching is critical

Table 3. Criteria for evaluation of potential donors for living donor procedures [18, 20]

Age ≥18 and preferably ≤55 years
No recent viral infections
No significant past medical history
Clear chest x-ray
FEV_1 and FVC >85% predicted
No previous thoracic surgery on donor side
Normal electrocardiogram
Normal echocardiogram
Oxygen tension >80 mm Hg on room air
No significant pulmonary pathology on CT (completely normal on donor side)

---

to the success of a transplant [11]. Various size-matching criteria have been used, which include measurements of donor and recipient height, width, parameters from chest x-ray, chest circumference and pulmonary function tests. Most centers now use height and/or predicted total lung capacity (TLC) to match the size of the donor and recipient. Using TLC, which is a function of height, weight and gender, predicted values for both donor and recipient can be compared using well-established reference values [18]. Bronchial size matching is based on height with a range of 3–4 inches above and below the height of the recipient. Potential donors also undergo bronchoscopy to look for anatomic abnormality, evidence of aspiration of blood or gastrointestinal contents and presence of purulent secretions, which are contraindications for lung donation [12].

There are several accepted parameters for the donors of living donor lobar procedures (table 3). The organ from a living lobar donor must meet the same standards as those for cadaveric lung transplantation. The potential living lobar donor should be able to tolerate removal of either the left or right lower lobe without resulting obvious functional limitations. The living lobar donors undergo detailed physical examination, extensive cardiopulmonary testing and psychological evaluation by a 'donor advocate team' at another institution. The cardiopulmonary function of the donor should be normal. This includes FEV_1 >85% of predicted value, PaO_2 >80 mm Hg, and normal cardiac function [19]. A comprehensive workup, such as ABO blood group compatibility with the recipient, arterial blood gas analysis, echocardiography, serology titers for hepatitis (A, B, and C), HIV, varicella, EBV, HSV, CMV, and pulmonary function tests (including lung volume, spirometry, and diffusion capacity), is done [20]. Computed tomography (CT) and/or magnetic resonance imaging (MRI) of the chest may also be used for volumetric assessment of the lobes.

Post transplantation

Complications

Despite the improvement in surgical techniques, diagnostic tools and immunosuppressive therapies, complications continue to occur. Both infant and standard pulmonary function tests are important tools to evaluate and follow patients for these potential complications. Other noninvasive tools are radiological studies, such as chest radiographs, CT, MRI, nuclear perfusion scan and others. Tissue biopsy, either by transbronchial or open lung method, remains the gold standard in diagnosing and differentiating between these conditions [21].

Surgical and Airway Complications

The airway and vascular anastomoses are potential sources of major surgical complications. Partial or complete dehiscence of the airway anastomosis is a rare, but dangerous complication that can occur in the immediate postoperative period. Evaluation of this problem includes nuclear perfusion scan, intraoperative esophageal echocardiography, and bronchoscopy to evaluate the anastomosis site. Transesophageal echocardiography should be used to assess patency of vascular anastomoses at the time of surgery and whenever the suspicion of postoperative graft ischemia arises.

Tracheal or bronchial stenosis at the anastomotic site is another complication. Symptoms may be absent in mild cases but wheezing and dyspnea may develop with progressive narrowing of the anastomosis [21]. Spirometry will often show an obstructive pattern and a biphasic flow-volume loop. Vocal cord and hemidiaphragm paresis and paralysis are other surgical complications that usually resolve within a few months after transplant [7]. On pulmonary function testing, hemidiaphragm paresis will show a decrease in mean inspiratory pressure while vocal cord paralysis will show flattening of the inspiratory loop. Lung transplant patients with a history of previous thoracic surgery or with 'clam-shell' incisions are at increased risk for diaphragm complications.

Infection

Infection is a major cause of morbidity and mortality after lung transplantation. In the 2003 ISHLT registry report, non-CMV infection was the most common cause of death in the period between 30 days and 1 year in pediatric lung transplant recipients, and the second most common cause of mortality in children between 1 and 3 years post-transplant [2]. Immunosuppression, denervation of the transplanted lung, interruption of bronchial and lymphatic

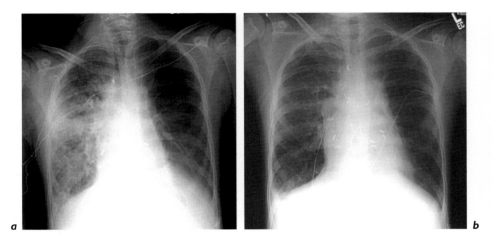

a   b

Fig. 2. Acute rejection: pre- and posttreatment with corticosteroids. Chest x-ray of acute cellular rejection with associated pleural effusion (*a*). Chest x-ray of the same patient 1 week after treatment completed with 3 days of intravenous corticosteroids with resolution of infiltrates (*b*).

circulation, impaired recruitment of antibody-forming cells in the transplanted lung, abnormal cough reflexes (from postoperative pain and phrenic nerve complications), and impairment in mucociliary clearance (from graft dysfunction and mechanical barrier at the anastomoses) make all lung transplant recipients vulnerable to infection. During an infection, there can be a decrease in maximal expiratory flow rates, and it may be difficult to distinguish pulmonary infection from acute cellular rejection. In fact, the lung transplant recipient may have both infection and acute rejection occurring at the same time. Hence, early use of bronchoscopy is often required to identify the causative microbial agent, and to select the most appropriate therapy in these immunocompromised patients.

Rejection

Rejection is classified into three clinical patterns: hyperacute, acute, and chronic. Although now rare, hyperacute rejection usually manifests itself within minutes after initial perfusion of the new lung graft. It results from preformed antibodies directed at blood group, HLA/MHC group, or endothelial antigens, which lead to activation and proliferation of complement and cell-mediated graft injury [22]. Acute cellular rejection can occur in the first few weeks to months after transplant. The donor cells are perceived as foreign, which causes activation, differentiation and proliferation of T lymphocytes. Perivascular mononuclear infiltrate and lymphocytic bronchitis are the characteristic histology. The ISHLT established a classification of acute rejection by histological grading. Acute rejection is graded from 0 to 4: grade 0 has no abnormality and 1 through 4 is mild to severe disease, respectively [23]. The chest x-ray may be clear or there can be infiltrates and pleural effusion (fig. 2). The small airways of the transplanted lung are affected, which is usually reflected as a decrease in expiratory flow rates. A sudden 15–20% decrease in FEV_1 and forced expiratory flow rate at 25–75% of forced vital capacity ($FEF_{25-75\%}$) can be a sign of acute cellular injury. However, it is difficult to determine if the reduced expiratory flow rates are due to infection, rejection or both infection with rejection. The stable posttransplant patient with persistent decrease in maximal expiratory flow rates (after repeated spirometry) should undergo bronchoscopy and possible transbronchial biopsy within 1 week to establish the diagnosis and choose appropriate treatment [21]. Clinical improvement is expected with return of maximal expiratory flow rates to baseline.

Chronic rejection can occur from only a few months to several years after lung transplantation. It is characterized by fibroproliferative obliteration of the bronchioles and vessels that cause scarring and fibrosis of the small airways [22, 24]. Chronic lung rejection leads to bronchiolitis obliterans (BO), which is a significant cause of morbidity and mortality in lung transplant recipients.

Bronchiolitis obliterans

BO is the most common cause of mortality in lung transplant patients who are 1–3 years posttransplant [2]. It remains the single most common cause of death (45%) of patients who survive 3 years after lung transplant. In

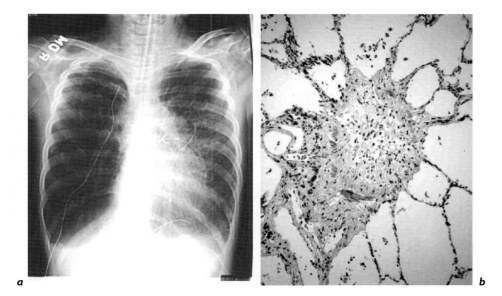

Fig. 3. BO. *a* Chest x-ray of lung transplant patient with respiratory failure secondary to severe BO. Note bilateral cystic lesions. *b* Photomicrograph of post lung transplant BO, showing granulation tissue filling the bronchial lumen.

all lung transplant survivors, it is the third most common cause of morbidity [2]. BO is presumed to be a form of chronic allograft rejection. Diagnosis is based both on histology and clinical presentation. The histopathology is characterized by a fibroproliferative process from lymphohistiocytic-mediated cytotoxicity resulting in a dense fibrous scar tissue affecting the small airways (fig. 3). Clinical presentation is based on persistent airway obstruction with pulmonary function changes such as a decrease in FEV_1 and $FEF_{25-75\%}$ after lung transplantation [25]. The histological diagnosis of BO is by examination of lung tissue. However, the nonuniform distribution of the rejection process makes diagnostic tissue biopsy difficult and not sufficiently sensitive for diagnosis [26, 27]. In 1993, the ISHLT defined a clinical staging of BO based on pulmonary function changes or bronchiolitis obliterans syndrome (BOS). The original BOS was defined by a >20% decrease from baseline in the FEV_1, which was defined as BOS stage 1 [28]. In the highest stage (stage 3) there is a decrease in FEV_1 >50%. The most recent staging criteria added stage 0-p to detect early deterioration in allograft function that might predict stage 1. Potential BOS stages 0-p were defined as 10–19% decrease in FEV_1 or decrease ≥25% in $FEF_{25-75\%}$ from baseline [25]. Other pulmonary function changes associated with BO include a decrease in diffusing capacity and in TLC [29].

For pediatric lung transplant patients who can perform standard pulmonary function testing, the decline in function should be expressed in terms of percent predicted instead of absolute values to account for lung and airway growth [25]. One study revealed that $FEF_{25-75\%}$ was a more sensitive indicator of lung function deterioration in pediatric patients with BOS; decline in FEV_1 and maximal expiratory flow ($\dot{V}$ max) occurred after the decline in $FEF_{25-75\%}$ [30]. Patients suspected of having BO should undergo bronchoscopy to differentiate other etiologies of airway obstruction, such as infection, acute rejection, bronchial stenosis and/or bronchomalacia.

Infants and young children not able to perform standard pulmonary function testing can be assessed by rapid chest compression techniques. These techniques measure maximal forced expiratory flows or timed volumes that will help assess presence or absence of significant airway obstruction. They can also be used to determine treatment response of BOS by serial lung function testing. However, these tests require deep sedation or anesthesia and are available only in specialized centers [for details see 31].

Other diagnostic tools to identify BOS are bronchoscopy with bronchoalveolar lavage showing neutrophilia and elevated cytokine levels, measurement of exhaled nitric oxide, assessment of air trapping on expiratory CT scans, bronchial hyperresponsiveness, and ventilation distribution [25].

BO is usually treated by augmented immunosuppression. However, there is no long-term effective treatment. Response to treatment should be assessed by following the pulmonary function tests [improvement in FEV_1, $FEF_{25-75\%}$, and FEV_1/forced vital capacity (FVC) ratio]. At this time, the only successful 'cure' for BO is retransplantation.

Lung Growth

Most pediatric lung transplant recipients can expect some increase in their linear height. Adequate growth of the transplanted lung proportionate to linear height growth is important in order to prevent restrictive lung disease and development of pulmonary hypertension.

In infants and older children, it has been shown that pulmonary function values can return to the normal range posttransplant. There is proportionate increase in lung volumes versus body length when immature lungs are transplanted into young infants and children [32, 33]. In one study using serial infant pulmonary function testing, the St. Louis group reported the same rate of increase in lung volume in both young stable lung transplant recipients (<3 years) and normal young toddlers [20, 33]. The mechanism for the improvement in lung volume is still unclear – whether it is from an increase in the number of alveoli or from alveolar hyperinflation.

Do mature lobes grow new tissue when transplanted into children? Children who underwent bilateral living donor lobar transplantation have a proportionate increase in TLC with linear growth [34]. This proportionate increase in lung volume was felt to be secondary to alveolar dilatation rather than new lung/alveolar growth. This conclusion was based on finding a decrease in diffusing capacity of the lung for carbon monoxide adjusted for lung volume (DLCO/VA) despite an increase in TLC in the first year following bilateral lobar lung transplantation. While the pediatric cadaveric lung transplant recipients also showed an increase in TLC in the first year posttransplant, their DLCO/VA values did not decrease but remained relatively constant [35].

Pulmonary Function Tests

Posttransplant, patients are closely monitored using serial pulmonary function tests. Maximal expiratory flows, as well as measurement of lung volume, are used to monitor the graft function and lung growth. There is significant improvement in lung volume and expiratory flow rates for both adult and pediatric recipients after lung transplantation. The expiratory flow rates are usually normal by 6 months after cadaveric lung transplantation, and continue to improve until 12 months for living donor lobar recipients [20, 36]. There is significant improvement in FEV_1 and

FVC observed at all time intervals up to 2 years after transplant in CF patients [37].

Infants who undergo lung transplantation can be monitored by infant pulmonary function testing. Serial measurement of functional residual capacity is used to measure lung growth [17]. Deterioration in expiratory flow rates should trigger suspicion of acute or chronic cellular rejection. Appropriate diagnostic tests should follow as soon as possible.

Exercise Testing in Posttransplant Patients

Exercise testing has been used to assess functional outcome after lung transplantation. Posttransplant exercise testing for adult patients without acute surgical, infectious, and immunologic complications shows marked improvement, if not normalization in pulmonary function and hemodynamics. A moderate level of activity compatible with normal lifestyle can be achieved. However, most lung transplant recipients have persistent exercise impairment with decrease in maximum oxygen uptake and work rate. The amount of exercise limitation is the same in different types of transplant procedures (single-lung, bilateral-lung, and heart-lung transplants) and regardless of primary underlying disease. Ventilatory abnormalities were not noted as limiting factors to exercise. Gas exchange abnormalities, although particularly noted to occur in single-lung transplant recipients, were generally not limiting [38]. In one study done in pediatric heart, heart-lung and lung transplant, exercise testing results showed a decrease in exercise tolerance as reflected in reduced peak work capacity and peak oxygen uptake. The reduced exercise tolerance was attributed to several factors, such as reduced cardiovascular and ventilatory responses, subnormal nutritional status, physical deconditioning, preexisting abnormal muscle structure and function, pharmacologic side effects, or a combination of these factors [39].

Protocol: Pulmonary Function in Children after Lung Transplantation

There are no universally accepted guidelines for post-lung-transplant patients. At the Children's Hospital Los Angeles, complete pulmonary function tests are obtained 1 week after the final chest tube has been removed. After hospital discharge, lung transplant recipients are routinely seen in the transplant clinic with pulmonary function tests (both lung volume measurement and spirometry) weekly during the first month, then every 2 weeks for another month, and then monthly thereafter until the patients are 1 year posttransplant. Then they are monitored every 3 months when they are well and seen more frequently in the event of illness.

Conclusion

Advances in the surgical techniques, immunosuppressive therapy, and diagnostic techniques have enabled lung transplantation to become a viable therapy for selected children and adults with end-stage lung disease. Pulmonary function testing plays an integral role in the evaluation of the transplant recipient both pre- and posttransplantation as well as in the evaluation of potential donors for living donor lobar procedures. The role of pulmonary function tests is fundamental in following lung growth posttransplantation in children, and for monitoring of potential complications related to lung transplantation.

References

1 Huddleston CB, Bloch JB, Sweet SC, Dela Morena M, Patterson A, Mendeloff EM: Lung transplantation in children. Ann Surg 2002; 236:270–276.
2 Boucek MM, Edwards LB, Keck BM, Trulock EP, Taylor DO, Mohacsi PJ, Hertz MI: The Registry of the International Society for Heart and Lung Transplantation: Sixth Official Pediatric Report 2003. J Heart Lung Transplant 2003;22:636–652.
3 Goldsmith M: Mother to child: First living donor lung transplant (news). JAMA 1990;264: 2724.
4 Starnes VA, Lewiston NJ, Luikart H, Theodore J, Stinson EB, Shumway NE: Current trends in lung transplantation. Lobar transplantation and expanded use of single lungs. J Thorac Cardiovasc Surg 1992;104:1060–1066.
5 Starnes VA, Barr ML, Cohen RG: Lobar transplantation: Indications, technique, outcome. J Thorac Cardiovasc Surg 1994;108:403–411.
6 Starnes VA, Bowdish ME, Woo MS, Barbers RG, Schenkel FA, Horn MV, Passotto R, Sievers EM, Baker CJ, Cohen RG, Bremner RM, Wells WJ, Barr ML: A decade of living lobar lung transplantation: Recipient outcomes. J Thorac Cardiovasc Surg 2004;127/1:114–122.
7 Sweet SC: Pediatric lung transplantation: Update 2003. Pediatr Clin North Am 2003;50: 1393–1417.
8 Coeutil JA, Tolan MJ, Loulmet DF, Guinvarch A, Chevalier PG, Achkar A, Birmbaum P, Carpentier AF: Pulmonary bipartitioning and lobar transplantation: A new approach to donor organ shortage. J Thorac Cardiovasc Surg 1997;113: 529–537.
9 Artemiou O, Birsan T, Taghavi S, Eichler I, Wisser W, Wolner E, Klepetko W: Bilateral lobar transplantation with the split lung technique. J Thorac Cardiovasc Surg 1999;118: 369–370.
10 MacLaughlin EF: Recipient characteristics, original disease and pre-transplant recipient evaluation; in Tejani AH, Harmon WE, Fine RN (eds): Pediatric Solid Organ Transplantation. Copenhagen, Munksgaard, 2000, pp 463–470.
11 Fullerton DA: Pediatric lung transplantation; Part D. Lung transplantation; in Stuart F, Abecassis D, Kaufman D (eds): Organ Transplantation. Georgetown, Vademecum Landes Bioscience, 2000, pp 305–314.
12 Conte JV Jr, Orens J: Lung transplantation; in Kuo PC, Schroeder RA, Johnson LB (eds): Clinical Management of the Transplant Patient. London, Arnold, 2001, pp 169–200.

13 Maurer JR: Patient selection for lung transplantation. JAMA 2001;286:2720–2721.
14 Kerem E, Reisman J, Corey M, Canny GJ, Levison H: Prediction of mortality in patients with cystic fibrosis. N Engl J Med 1992;326: 1187–1191.
15 Liou TG, Adler FR, Fitzsimmons S, Cahill BC, Hibbs JR, Marshall BC: Predictive 5-year survivorship model of cystic fibrosis. Am J Epidemiol 2001;153:345–352.
16 Maurer JR, Frost AE, Estenne M, Higenbottam T, Glanville AR: International guidelines for the selection of lung transplant candidates. Transplantation 1998;66:951–956.
17 Hamvas A, Nogee LM, Mallory GB Jr, Spray TL, Huddleston CB, August A, Dehner LP, DeMelllo DE, Moxley M, Nelson R, Cole SF, Colten HR: Lung transplantation for treatment of infants with surfactant protein B deficiency. J Pediatr 1997;130/2:231–239.
18 Orens JB, Boehler A, De Perrot M, Estenne MS, Glanville AR, Keshavjee S, Kotloff R, Morton J, Studer SM, Van Raemdonck D, Waddel T, Snell GI: A review of lung transplant donor acceptability criteria. J Heart Lung Transplant 2003;22:1183–1200.
19 Mallory GB Jr, Cohen AH: Donor considerations in living-related donor lung transplantation. Clin Chest Med 1997;18/2:239–244.
20 Woo MS, MacLaughlin EF, Horn MV, Wong PC, Rowland JM, Barr ML, Starnes VA: Living donor lobar lung transplantation: The pediatric experience. Pediatr Transplant 1998;2:185–190.
21 Woo MS: Lung graft dysfunction: Etiologies and management; in Tejani AH, Harmon WE, Fine RN (eds): Pediatric Solid Organ Transplantation. Copenhagen, Munksgaard, 2000, pp 482–490.
22 King-Biggs MB: Acute pulmonary allograft rejection. Mechanism, diagnosis and management. Clin Chest Med 1997;18:301–310.
23 Yousem SA, Berry GJ, Cagle PT, Chamberlain D, Husain AN, Hruban RH, Marchevsky A, Ohori NP, Ritter J, Stewart S, Tazelaar HD: Revision of the 1990 working formulation for the classification of pulmonary allograft rejection. Lung rejection study group. J Heart Lung Transplant 1996;15:1–15.
24 Phadke SM: Post-transplant complications. Pediatr Pulmonol Suppl 2004;26:119–120.
25 Estenne M, Maurer JR, Boehler A, Egan JJ, Frost A, Hertz M, Mallory GB Jr, Snell GI, Yousem S: Bronchiolitis obliterans syndrome 2001: An update of the diagnostic criteria. J Heart Lung Transplant 2002;21:297–310.

26 Kramer MR, Stoehr C, Whang JL, Berry GJ, Sibley R, Marshall SE, Patterson GM, Starnes VA, Theodore J: The diagnosis of obliterative bronchiolitis after heart-lung and lung transplantation: Low yield of transbronchial biopsy. J Heart Lung Transplant 1993;12:675–681.
27 Chamberlain D, Maurer J, Chaparro C, Idolor L: Evaluation of transbronchial lung biopsy specimens in the diagnosis of bronchiolitis obliterans after lung transplantation. J Heart Lung Transplant 1994;13:963–971.
28 Cooper JD, Billingham M, Egan T, Hertz MI, Higenbottam T, Lynch J, Maurer J, Paradis I, Patterson A, Smith C, Trulock EP, Vreim C, Yousem S: A working formulation for the standardization of nomenclature and for clinical staging of chronic dysfunction in lung allografts. J Heart Lung Transplant 1993;12: 713–716.
29 Kelly K, Hertz MI: Obliterative bronchiolitis. Clin Chest Med 1997;18:319–338.
30 Sritippayawan S, Keens TG, Horn MV, Starnes VA, Woo MS: What are the best pulmonary function test parameters for early detection of post-lung transplant bronchiolitis obliterans syndrome in children? Pediatr Transplant 2003;7:200–203.
31 Modl M, Eber E: Forced expiratory flow-volume measurements; Hammer J, Eber E (eds): Paediatric Pulmonary Function Testing. Prog Respir Res. Basel, Karger, 2005, pp 34–43.
32 Huddleston CB, Sweet SC, Mallory GB Jr, Hamvas A, Mendeloff EN: Lung transplantation in very young infants. J Thorac Cardiovasc Surg 1999;118:796–804.
33 Cohen AH, Mallory GB Jr, Ross K, White DK, Mendeloff E, Huddleston CB, Kemp JS: Growth of lungs after transplantation in infants and children younger than 3 years of age. Am J Respir Crit Care Med 1999;159: 1747–1751.
34 Woo MS, MacLaughlin EF, Horn MV, Starnes VA: Pulmonary volume increases with linear growth in pediatric living donor lobar lung transplant recipients. Am J Respir Crit Care Med 1999;159:A540.
35 Sritippawayan S, Keens TG, Horn MV, MacLaughlin EF, Barr ML, Starnes VA, Woo MS: Does lung growth occur when mature lobes are transplanted into children? Pediatr Transplant 2002;6:500–504.

36 Starnes VA, Woo MS, MacLaughlin EF, Horn MV, Wong PC, Rowland JM, Durst CL, Wells WJ, Barr ML: Comparison of outcome between living donor and cadaveric lung transplantation in children. Ann Thorac Surg 1999;68:2279–2283.

37 Mendeloff EN, Huddleston CB, Mallory GB, Trulock EP, Cohen AH, Sweet SC, Lynch J, Sundaresan S, Cooper JD, Patterson GA: Pediatric and adult lung transplantation for cystic fibrosis. J Thorac Cardiovas Surg 1998;115:404–414.

38 Howard DK, Iademarco EJ, Trulock EP: The role of cardiopulmonary exercise testing in lung and heart-lung transplantation. Clin Chest Med 1994;15:405–420.

39 Nixon PA, Fricker FJ, Noyes BE, Webber SA, Orenstein DM, Armitage JM: Exercise testing in pediatric heart, heart-lung, and lung transplant recipients. Chest 1995;107:1328–1335.

Marlyn S. Woo, MD, Medical Director,
Cardiothoracic Transplant Program
Division of Pediatric Pulmonology
Mailstop #83, Children's Hospital
Los Angeles, 4650 Sunset Boulevard
Los Angeles, CA 90027 (USA)
Tel. +1 323 669 2101, Fax +1 323 664 9758
E-Mail mwoo@chla.usc.edu

Hammer J, Eber E (eds): Paediatric Pulmonary Function Testing.
Prog Respir Res. Basel, Karger, 2005, vol 33, pp 233–246

Neuromuscular Disorders

Uwe Mellies   Christian Dohna-Schwake

Department of General Pediatrics and Neuropediatrics, University of Essen,
Children's Hospital, Essen, Germany

Abstract

In children with both inherited and acquired neuromuscular disorders (NMD) deterioration of the respiratory function contributes to relevant morbidity and is often responsible for a high mortality with these diseases. Respiratory manifestation of NMD depends on the pattern of muscle and/or nerve involvement and the rate of progression. Some NMD have little or no respiratory involvement whereas others present with a continuous deterioration of the respiratory system. The latter is the rule in the most common pediatric NMD, Duchenne muscular dystrophy, spinal muscular atrophy and congenital muscular dystrophies. But it is important to be aware that some disorders may present with considerable asynchrony in trunk and limb muscular weakness on the one hand and respiratory muscle weakness on the other hand. Hence, patients who are still ambulatory may present with unsuspected respiratory complications. Normally, chronic respiratory muscle failure develops slowly over a period of several years. Initially, it presents with disordered breathing apparent only during sleep, followed by continuous progression to severe hypoventilation, cor pulmonale and eventually frank respiratory failure in end-stage disease. In patients with preexisting respiratory compromise respiratory failure may also present acutely, in most cases as a result of a chest infection. The use of the respiratory function testing in neuromuscular patients has been investigated extensively and many tests have proven to be helpful. However, most studies have been done in adolescents with Duchenne muscular dystrophies and adults with other neuromuscular conditions. But there has been only very little research on how to assess respiratory function in infants and toddlers with NMD. In fact, assessing and interpreting respiratory function in young children is often difficult. This is above all due to the patients' limited cooperation but also to a lack of standardized-test normative data for respiratory function testing other than the measurement of lung volumes. Other difficulties may occur in connection with underlying disabilities of the children such as facial dysmorphia with an inability of mouth closure, bulbar and swallowing dysfunction or an inability of unassisted sitting in a body chamber. Distribution and severity of respiratory muscle involvement differs in distinct NMD, may change in the individual patient over time and often deteriorates during sleep. Respiratory function testing should make it possible to differentiate between inspiratory and expiratory muscle weakness and/or upper airway muscle involvement. Therefore, wherever feasible, basic evaluation should include assessment of pulmonary function, inspiratory and expiratory muscle strength and peak cough flow. It is important to recall that results of respiratory function testing vary considerably in how they are ultimately affecting breathing and gas exchange. Therefore, in patients with pathological respiratory function testing advanced evaluation should include an examination of the breathing pattern and blood gases during wakefulness and sleep. A sleep study with continuous recording of respiration, oxygen saturation and carbon dioxide tension is the most valuable single test, though expensive. Moreover, it makes possible the assessment of respiratory function in children who are not able to cooperate in classic respiratory function testing. Given that NMD patients are at high risk of respiratory complications frequent and early evaluation is crucial. Where possible patients should be diagnosed and treated in an interdisciplinary approach including pediatric neurologists, pulmonologists, orthopedics and physiotherapists with thorough training in pediatric NMD. The aim of periodic respiratory assessment is to detect respiratory malfunction and to predict complications on time. It is coupled with a consequent therapeutic program aimed to prevent and treat respiratory complications. This chapter will review the respiratory disturbances in different NMD, discuss the indications and clinical value of respiratory function testing and describe the assessment and interpretation of respiratory function testing in children with NMD.

Neuromuscular Disorders

Duchenne Muscular Dystrophy

Duchenne muscular dystrophy (DMD) is an X-linked (gene location Xp21) hereditary muscular dystrophy. The defect leads to an abnormality of dystrophin, a product of the muscle basal membrane. DMD affects 1 of 3,500 live male births and is the most frequent muscular dystrophy. Although the clinical course may vary between patients, DMD is probably the most homogeneous group of neuromuscular disorders (NMD). In the majority of patients psychomotor development after birth is normal although some boys may present with mild mental retardation. Symptoms such as tiptoe gait, pseudohypertrophy of calves, Gower's sign or slightly delayed motor development appear in three quarters of patients before the age of 4 years. The weakness progresses steadily. Almost all patients lose their ability to walk between the ages of 7 and 13 years and develop progressive contractures and scoliosis in the following years. Patients who become wheelchair-dependent beyond 16 years of age are likely to have Becker muscular dystrophy [1].

The lung function parallels the clinical course and can be divided into three phases [2]. (1) In the ambulatory patient the lung volume increases with age and predicted values are mostly normal [3] (ascending phase). (2) When Duchenne boys need assistance to walk until they are completely wheelchair-bound the vital capacity (VC) remains stable but predictive values begin to decline (plateau phase). (3) In the following years VC steadily declines by about 200 ml or 6–8% predicted per year [4, 5] (descending phase).

The decline of lung function in DMD is strongly related to inspiratory muscle weakness causing a restrictive ventilatory defect [6]. Inspiratory muscle weakness seems to occur earlier than lung volume restriction and worsens as the disease progresses [4]. A comparative study showed maximum inspiratory pressures (Pi_{max}) of $37\,cm\,H_2O$ in DMD patients and $80\,cm\,H_2O$ in healthy controls [7]. Koessler et al. [8] showed that Pi_{max} decreased with age from $72\,cm\,H_2O$ in 12-year-old boys to $54\,cm\,H_2O$ in 19-year-old patients. Intrinsic lung disease does not contribute to the decline of lung function. Airway resistance, CO diffusion capacity and respiratory drive have been shown to be normal [9, 10].

Interestingly in DMD a predominant diaphragm involvement apparent by a drop of VC in the supine position is rare. Although an ultrasound study showed less diaphragm thickening during a maximal inspiratory maneuver in 10-year-old Duchenne patients [7], lung volumes and flow rates did not drop significantly after the change from the erect to the supine position [10].

Scoliosis occurs after the loss of ambulation in almost all patients. Its contribution to the decline of lung function remains unclear. Most retrospective analyses of scoliosis correction surgery failed to demonstrate a gain or slower decline of lung function when compared with patients who refused the operation [11, 12].

The rate of respiratory complications increases with the progression of respiratory muscle weakness. Nocturnal hypoventilation becomes likely with inspiratory vital capacity (IVC) <40% and frank respiratory failure with IVC <25% or <1 liter [13–15]. If VC falls below 1 liter 5-year survival is very poor unless patients are treated with mechanical ventilation. Noninvasive ventilation became the treatment of choice in patients with hypercapnic respiratory failure and resulted in a 5-year survival of 73% [16–18].

With increasing life expectancy cardiac involvement becomes more evident and at a certain time almost all patients develop cardiomyopathy. In a recent study 22% of the patients died due to left ventricular dysfunction [19]. Therefore, evaluation of the cardiac function completes the patient's investigation and should be carried out annually [20].

Spinal Muscular Atrophy

Patients with spinal muscular atrophy (SMA) comprise a heterogeneous group with different clinical courses. The autosomal recessively inherited disease is caused by mutations in the SMN gene on chromosome 5. The disease is characterized by degeneration of the anterior horn cell (alpha motor neuron) in the spinal cord. Prevalence rates are about 1:10,000 live births. The clinical picture is characterized by proximal muscle weakness and muscular atrophy.

Although there is an infinitely variable picture of the clinical severity patients can be divided into three main groups: (1) Type I (Werdnig-Hoffmann disease) with onset at birth or within the first few months of life and death before the age of 2. These patients never sit. (2) Type II (intermediate form) with onset between 3 and 15 months of age and survival beyond 4 years. Patients never learn to stand without assistance. (3) Type III (Kugelberg-Welander disease) with onset after 24 months and a more benign course. However, the individual patient may not follow these criteria. A probably more accurate classification differentiates between severe SMA type 1.1–1.9, intermediate SMA type 2.1–2.9 and mild SMA 3.1–3.9. The higher the classification the better the clinical course [1].

Pulmonary function has been mainly investigated in patients with SMA types II and III. Survival probabilities at ages 2, 4, 10 and 20 years were 32, 18, 8 and 0% in SMA I and 100, 100, 98 and 77% in SMA II. These data were reported in a large cohort study of 445 SMA patients [21]. Mortality is almost completely related to respiratory complications, especially in SMA I and II. Treatment of SMA with invasive or noninvasive ventilation and assisted coughing procedures may improve survival [22].

Although SMA patients experience stable phases in their clinical courses, pulmonary function in general decreases with age. In 39 SMA II children followed from the age of 10 to 16 mean VC declined from 54.9 to 37.4% predicted, in another 24 patients with SMA III followed from the age of 12 to 18 the VC dropped from 87 to 73% [23].

Many patients develop severe scoliosis during adolescence. Like in DMD patients the contribution of the spine deformity to the loss of pulmonary function remains unclear. One study reported no correlation between Cobb angle and VC [24]. In contrast another study found a loss of 4.7% VC for each 10° scoliosis angle [25]. In a few studies surgery for scoliosis correction led to a small postoperative improvement or a less marked reduction of VC (7.7 vs. 3.8% annual decrease) [26, 27].

A typical clinical feature of inspiratory muscle weakness is atrophy of intercostal muscles leading to the typical bell-shaped thorax. Since normal alveolar ventilation mainly depends on diaphragmatic strength, which is well preserved in SMA, no differences in VC measured in the sitting and supine postures have been reported [3, 28]. Weakness of intercostal muscles reduces compliance of the rib cage apparent from paradoxical thoracoabdominal movement and impairs alveolar ventilation of the upper lobes of the lungs [29]. Thus atelectasis is a frequent complication.

Due to a relatively well-preserved diaphragmatic function alveolar ventilation is well maintained until advanced disease [30, 31]. For SMA II patients it has been shown that maximum expiratory pressures were significantly lower than maximum inspiratory pressures [32]. In fact recurrent chest infections may occur early and are mainly due to a predominance of expiratory muscle weakness with insufficient cough and retention of airway secretions. Thus, assisted coughing maneuvers are the most important therapeutic techniques to prevent respiratory tract infections and are instituted before noninvasive ventilation.

Spinal Muscular Atrophy with Respiratory Distress Type 1

Autosomal recessive SMA with respiratory distress is another anterior horn cell disorder but clinically and genetically distinct from SMA. Mutations on chromosome 11q13 have recently been identified [33]. Most patients present at age 1–6 months with respiratory distress caused by diaphragmatic paralysis. A large retrospective study showed that all patients (29/29) developed respiratory failure mostly during the 1st year of life. Spinal muscular atrophy with respiratory distress type 1 is also associated with progressive muscle weakness predominantly of distal lower limb muscles.

Myotonic Dystrophy

Myotonic dystrophy is an autosomal dominant inherited NMD. An abnormal chloride conductance of the muscle fiber membrane and a reduced ability to inactivate sodium channels lead to the clinical picture of persistent contracture of skeletal muscle following stimulation. Heart, eyes, ears and bowels may also be involved in this disease. Affected individuals normally have an expansion of greater than 50 CTG repeats in the responsible gene on chromosome 19 [34]. The degree of the amplification of trinucleotide repeats correlates with the severity of disease and age of onset [35].

Congenital myotonic dystrophy is rare and infants often present with severe muscular weakness and respiratory failure at birth [36]. In these patients the need for mechanical ventilation longer than 30 days is associated with poor psychomotor development. Furthermore, it is a strong negative predictor of survival [37, 38]. However, in some patients survival is possible despite prolonged mechanical ventilation in the neonatal period [39, 40].

For adults with myotonic dystrophy it has been shown that VC and respiratory muscle strength as well as myotonia of the diaphragm play a role [41, 42]. Sleep-disordered breathing (SDB) and successful treatment of respiratory failure with noninvasive ventilation have been reported for adults with myotonic dystrophy [43–45].

Congenital Muscular Dystrophies

Congenital muscular dystrophies (CMD) are a heterogeneous group of autosomal recessively inherited muscle disorders. Laminin α2-negative CMD (MDC1A) constitutes approximately 40% of all CMD. The loss of pulmonary function is strongly correlated with general motor function in these patients. Wheelchair-bound patients are very likely to present with a severe restrictive ventilatory defect and either nocturnal or diurnal hypoventilation. On the other hand, ambulatory patients are likely to have a normal gas exchange.

The remaining CMD are caused by strongly reduced or absent proteins of the basal membrane of the muscle cell. The disease courses differ widely between patients. Patients with the rigid spine syndrome (RSMD-1) and Ullrich CMD typically present with diaphragm weakness when they are still ambulatory. The severity of respiratory compromise is likely to be underestimated if spirometry in the supine position has not been performed. In RSMD-1 CMD diaphragm involvement with the consequence of nocturnal hypoventilation usually develops during the 1st decade. Patients with secondary laminin deficiency (MDC1C) may present with a Duchenne-like disease course. Early cases with respiratory failure have been described [46].

Myopathies

Structural congenital myopathies comprise, for example, central core myopathy, minicore myopathy, nemaline myopathy or myotubular myopathies. Furthermore, metabolic myopathies such as acid maltase deficiency also affect respiratory muscles. Congenital myopathies tend to present in a nonspecific way. Patients may present as floppy infants or later in childhood with distinct muscle weakness.

Respiratory failure due to involvement of respiratory muscles has been described in case reports for mini-/multicore myopathy and nemaline myopathy [47, 48]. In X-linked myotubular myopathy death due to respiratory failure normally occurs in infancy or early childhood. One multicenter study of 40 boys reported the need for mechanical ventilation in three quarters of patients aged 1 year or older [49]. In centronuclear myopathy the involvement of the respiratory system is milder [50].

Acid maltase deficiency (Pompe's disease) is a rare glycogen storage disease that results in the loss of functional tissue in heart and skeletal muscle. The clinical course depends on residual acid maltase enzyme activity. In the infantile type death usually occurs in the 1st year of life due to respiratory and cardiac failure. Patients with late-onset disease develop proximal limb muscle weakness between childhood and the 5th decade. However, the majority

remains ambulatory. In late onset disease involvement of the diaphragm is an inevitable complication leading to nocturnal hypoventilation and respiratory failure on average 10 years after the onset of limb muscle weakness [51].

Myasthenia gravis

The etiology of myasthenia gravis (MG) is heterogeneous and can be divided into hereditary congenital myasthenic syndromes and 'pure' MG, which is acquired and autoimmune. The majority of these patients will test positive for serum acetylcholine receptor antibodies. MG is a syndrome of changing skeletal muscle weakness that worsens with use and improves with rest [52].

Autoimmune MG in childhood is rare comprising 10–20% of all myasthenic patients [53]. Studies regarding respiratory function in adults with MG reported only slight decreases of VC and respiratory muscle pressures [54, 55]. Nevertheless, a myasthenic crisis may be associated with severe respiratory muscle weakness and respiratory failure and mechanical ventilation is necessary for a limited period of time [56, 57].

The congenital myasthenic syndromes are characterized by the onset of symptoms within the 1st month of life. Clinical appearance and involvement of respiratory muscles varies largely; some patients present as 'floppy infants' with early respiratory failure and the need for mechanical ventilation [58, 59].

Periodic Assessment of Children with NMD

The first goal of periodic respiratory function testing in children with NMD is the description of the patient's individual respiratory status and disease course. A regular follow-up will make it possible to assess the disease progression and has important clinical implications for the detection and prediction of respiratory complications and for introducing treatment on time.

According to the guidelines recently published jointly by pulmonologists and neurologists in a workshop report of the European Neuromuscular Conference (ENMC) on ventilatory support in pediatric NMD, the basic assessment should include techniques to assess lung function, respiratory muscle pressures, cough and symptoms [60]. Further investigation is indicated in patients with abnormal results in this basic assessment and suspicious features in their history or physical examination; it may include the measurement of VC in the supine position, blood gas monitoring and polysomnography. Complete ENMC recommendations are listed in table 1.

Mellies/Dohna-Schwake

Table 1. Guidelines for respiratory evaluation in children with NMD [adapted from the 117th ENMC workshop report, 60]

Basic evaluation

Lung function

FVC (in % predicted) in sitting position should be performed annually; when FVC is abnormal (<80%) an additional measurement in supine position should be performed to detect potential diaphragm weakness (indicated by >20% drop from baseline)

FVC <60% indicates a risk of SDB

FVC <40% and diaphragm weakness constitute a significant risk of nocturnal hypoventilation

Cough

PCF should be measured annually during a steady state

With PCF <200 liters/min or recurrent episodes of chest infections assisted coughing techniques and chest physiotherapy are indicated

Symptoms

Features of respiratory impairment may include the following, which should be specifically investigated and documented:

Diaphragmatic involvement (suggested by >20% drop in supine FVC, dyspnea in the supine position, paradoxical breathing)

Frequent chest infections

Bulbar dysfunction

Feeding difficulties

Failure to thrive

SDB

Typically present in these patients before frank respiratory failure; symptoms of SDB should be investigated and documented at every appointment; these may include:

Night: frequent nocturnal awakening, nightmares, scary dreams, frequent need for turning, night sweating

Morning: drowsiness, difficulty in getting going, no appetite in the morning, nausea, headache

Day: drop in energy levels, need for a rest after school/frequent naps during the day, concentration levels at school dropping, loss of appetite, bad mood

However, SDB may be present in the absence of symptoms

Further investigations should be initiated at a center with adequate expertise if pulse oximetry is abnormal and/or there are symptoms suggesting SDB

Respiratory muscle pressures

Peak inspiratory and peak expiratory muscle pressures may be used to monitor the severity and course of respiratory muscle weakness

Advanced evaluation

Blood gases

Punctual: from arterial puncture or arterialized ear lobe blood: pH, PaO_2, $PaCO_2$, base excess

Continuous: (pulse) oximetry: SaO_2, transcutaneous carbon dioxide tension ($PtcCO_2$), end-tidal carbon dioxide tension ($PetCO_2$)

In patients

With symptoms suggesting current respiratory failure

Presenting with current or recurrent lower airway infections

With abnormal overnight pulse oximetry and/or capnometry

With FVC <40% predicted

Polysomnography

Including capnometry is also indicated if overnight pulse oximetry is not diagnostic in the presence of symptoms suggestive of SDB such as obstructive and nonobstructive apnea, hypopnea or hypoventilation; polysomnography should be performed according to the guidelines of the American Sleep Disorders Association

---

The frequency of such an assessment will need to be individualized depending on the underlying disorder and rate of respiratory function decay. As a general rule an evaluation should be performed biannually when VC is >60% of predicted values, peak inspiratory pressure is >4 kPa, peak cough flow (PCF) is >200 liters/min and the patient is in a stable condition. The frequency should be increased when measurements are lower or if the patient had already had respiratory complications. In patients less than 5 years old or patients in whom VC cannot be measured for other reasons nocturnal pulse oximetry (and end-tidal or transcutaneous CO_2 if available) is an alternative technique to roughly estimate the respiratory function.

Furthermore, respiratory function tests are valuable tools to assess the preoperative risk, especially prior to spinal stabilization. They give valuable data for the decision regarding the initiation of mechanical ventilation and assisted coughing and are helpful in monitoring the effects of treatment.

History and Physical Examination

Even though laboratory tests are of unequivocal value, the history and physical examination of the child remain the first and most important indicators for further investigation. Particular attention needs to be paid to signs and symptoms indicating SDB or chronic respiratory failure (summarized in table 1). They should be investigated and documented at every visit. Sensitive indicators of a respiratory compromise are paradoxical breathing in the supine position pointing to diaphragm weakness and use of accessory muscles during quiet breathing or during speech. It is important to recall that nonambulatory children with chronic respiratory muscle weakness normally do not develop dyspnea; if they do it is an alarming sign indicating impending respiratory failure.

Respiratory Function Testing

Laboratory tests commonly used to assess, diagnose and follow up patients with NMD are listed in table 2.

Pulmonary Function
In patients with NMD a decrease of VC is an early sign of respiratory impairment. Development of a restrictive ventilatory defect is usually closely linked to a weakness of inspiratory muscles [6, 15, 61] and will occur over time as the disease progresses [10, 62]. For patients with DMD it has been shown that VC is relatively normal until patients

Table 2. Tests used to assess respiratory function in children with NMD

Lung volumes
  Static lung volumes
    Total lung capacity (TLC)
    Functional residual capacity (FRC)
    Residual volume (RV)
    Vital capacity (VC) in upright and supine position
    Maximum insufflation capacity (MIC)
  Spirometry
    Forced vital capacity (FVC)
    Forced expiratory volume in 1 s (FEV_1)
    Flow-volume loop
Respiratory muscle function
  Static mouth pressures
    Peak (maximum) inspiratory pressure (PIP/MIP)
    Peak (maximum) expiratory pressure (PEP/MEP)
  Respiratory drive
    Mouth occlusion pressure at 0.1 s ($P_{0.1}$)
  Others
    Sniff nasal pressure
    Transdiaphragmatic pressure
Cough
  Peak cough flow (PCF)
Respiration
  During wakefulness
    Physical examination
    Maximum minute ventilation (MMV)
  During sleep
    Cardiorespiratory polygraphy (PG)
    Cardiorespiratory polysomnography (PSG)
Gas exchange
  Punctual
    Arterial blood gases: pH, PaO_2, $PaCO_2$, base excess
  Continuous
    (Pulse) oximetry: SaO_2
    Transcutaneous carbon dioxide tension ($PtcCO_2$)
    End-tidal carbon dioxide tension ($PetCO_2$)

lose ambulation followed by a continuous decline of VC of a mean of 200 ml per year [2]. However, this highly predictable course of VC in Duchenne patients has not been described for any other NMD and VC may increase with growth, stay unchanged over a long period, decrease slowly or fall rapidly. Deterioration may occur continuously or stepwise, the latter often after a period of illness.

VC measurement with spirometry is highly reproducible and reliable if performed by a cooperative patient. But spirometry in children with NMD may cause some difficulties. A significant number of children will develop respiratory compromise before an age at which they are able to cooperate in the examination. Some NMD are associated with mental retardation, thus making cooperation a problem. Other difficulties interfering with proper spirometry might occur from facial dysmorphia with the inability to achieve an airtight seal with the mouthpiece, bulbar and swallowing dysfunction or the inability of unassisted sitting.

Experience shows that best results are achieved when spirometry is performed at bedside, when parents or caregivers are present to support the child and when tests are performed by a trained person familiar with the special features of respiratory function testing in these patients.

Because VC measurement depends on full inspiration followed by a maximal expiratory maneuver it reflects the strength of both inspiratory and expiratory muscles. IVC measured after slow exhalation to residual volume (RV) and forced expiratory vital capacity (FVC) can be used equally; in adult patients with NMD a close correlation between IVC and FVC was found (r = 0.98) [15]. Forced expiratory volume in 1 s may be of interest when additional obstruction, mostly during a period of chest infection, is suspected.

Static lung volume measurements in patients with advanced NMD usually demonstrate restriction. Total lung capacity (TLC) is reduced secondary to low IVC and other factors that add to reduced chest wall and lung compliance. Scoliosis seems to be an independent factor contributing significantly to VC decline; it has been shown that severe restriction may also develop in patients with idiopathic scoliosis and no muscle disease [63, 64]. Thus, in children with NMD progression of scoliosis will significantly contribute to VC decline [65]. On the other hand, treatment of scoliosis with spinal stabilization did not prevent further VC decay in patients with SMA and DMD [11, 26, 66]. This suggests that spinal surgery does not preserve lung function and therefore the indication for surgery should be based on other parameters. Chest wall compliance may be further reduced as a result of fibrotic reconstruction of dystrophic chest wall muscles and contractures of costovertebral joints. Whether microatelectasis contributes to a relevant reduction of lung compliance or not remains controversial [67–69].

Despite a reduction in VC and TLC, a relative increase in RV is observed in many patients and the increased RV/TLC ratio is sometimes misinterpreted as hyperinflation. Actually, this phenomenon reflects that the effort- and strength-dependent VC decline is more marked and precedes TLC decline. A relative RV increase has been attributed to the predominant weakness of expiratory muscles [10, 61] and has been shown to be an early indicator of

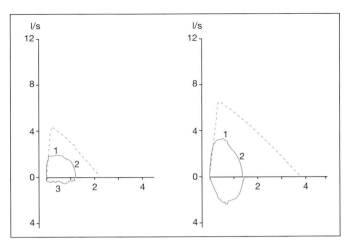

Fig. 1. Flow-volume curves in children with NMD demonstrating: (1) diminished peak expiratory flow, (2) sudden end-expiratory drop of expiratory flow and (3) diminished mid-inspiratory flow.

respiratory muscle weakness in adults with amyotrophic lateral sclerosis [70]. However, measurement of static lung volumes requires examination in a body plethysmograph, which is difficult and unpleasant for severely handicapped children. Furthermore, measurements of TLC and RV rarely add clinically relevant information to simple spirometry.

Children with NMD demonstrate reduced flow rates that parallel a decrease in lung volumes; thus flow volume curves usually appear normal. A detailed studying of flow volume curves, however, often reveals that respiratory muscle weakness results in a characteristic loop providing additional information. This loop though cannot be distinguished from that obtained from an individual who exerts a submaximal effort. For adults with NMD it has been shown that expiratory muscle weakness is characterized by a diminished initial sharp peak expiratory flow and a rapid vertical drop of forced expiratory flow near RV [71]. Decreased inspiratory effort may become apparent as diminished forced mid-inspiratory flow and upper airway obstruction due to bulbar involvement as additional inspiratory flow oscillation [72]. Figure 1 displays flow-volume curves in children with respiratory muscle weakness.

Additional important information is provided by spirometry in the erect and supine positions. A drop of 25% from baseline or more after supine positioning is a highly specific indicator of diaphragm weakness. VC decline in the supine position is attributed to the upward shift of the abdominal contents, which cannot be counteracted due to diaphragm weakness. At least 30 cm H_2O transdiaphragmatic pressure is required to overcome the additional pressure of abdominal contents in the lying position [73]. For children no data are available, but studies in adults suggest that supine VC is a simple, sensitive and specific test for diaphragm weakness and can replace invasive diagnostic procedures [74, 75].

For the interpretation of a child's individual pulmonary function it is essential to follow up and document VC in absolute numbers and percent predicted, the latter always in relation to the child's actual height. Inaccuracies in calculating VC in percent predicted may arise from difficulties to determine patients' standing height either because the patient is nonambulatory or joint contractures and scoliosis impair measurement. As a helpful rule the standing height (SH in centimeters) can be estimated from forearm length (FL) or ulna length (UL) using the equation: $SH = 3.497 \times FL + 9.595$ or $SH = 6.332 \times UL + 1.157$, respectively [76].

Periodic assessment of VC has important clinical implications since thresholds of VC have been identified to predict treatable complications and outcome in patients with NMD. A VC below 60% is a sensitive and specific predictor of the onset of SDB; VC below 40% predicts nocturnal alveolar hypoventilation and VC <25%, or <1 liter in Duchenne patients, is strongly associated with respiratory failure and poor survival [15, 18, 31, 60, 77, 78].

Tests to Evaluate Respiratory Muscle Strength

In the following only common and noninvasive tests to assess respiratory muscle strength in children with NMD are discussed [for further details, please see 79].

Several invasive and noninvasive methods have been reported to be of value in testing respiratory muscle strength in patients with NMD [80]. However, since respiratory muscle strength and muscle strength in general strongly depend on the child's age, reliable assessment in children requires normative data which are only available for maximum inspiratory and expiratory mouth pressures and nasal sniff pressures.

Maximum inspiratory mouth pressure (MIP or Pi_{max}) and maximum expiratory mouth pressure (MEP or Pe_{max}) are common tests used to assess and follow muscle strength in patients with NMD. MIP and MEP are measured as static mouth pressures with the child seated wearing a nose clip. In a child that has been well instructed before the test accurate measurements can be obtained at approximately 6–7 years of age. At least 3–5 consecutive measurements are needed. Since proper tests are strenuous for a child with weak respiratory muscles more frequent investigations may result in increasing muscle fatigue and should therefore be avoided.

Maximum Inspiratory Pressure

Measurements of static inspiratory mouth pressure are obtained against occluded airways using a spirometer with a shutter valve or a simple manometer. Each effort should be maintained for 1 s. Simultaneous measurement of the lung volume at which the pressure is generated is helpful (fig. 2). MIP can be measured either during tidal breathing from functional residual capacity (FRC) or after maximum exhalation from RV. MEP can be measured either at FRC or after maximum inspiration at TLC.

Normal values and predicting equations in large samples including children of all age groups have only been reported in few studies. Gaultier and Zinman [81] studied maximum static pressures at different lung volumes in 119 schoolchildren aged 7–13 years, and found that MIP and MEP at RV and TLC, respectively, were higher than pressures generated at FRC.

Wilson et al. [82] studied MIP at RV and MEP at TLC in 235 children aged 6–17 years. Our group studied MIP at RV in 300 healthy children aged 6–17 years. Normal values and prediction equations of MIP of both studies are given in table 3. A systematic difference of about 10% lower mean values in our patients compared to Wilson et al. may be due to a different age distribution.

Static mouth pressures in healthy children are generally higher during expiration than inspiration, and boys, even before puberty, generate significantly higher pressures than girls. Maximum pressures strongly depend on age and therefore on height, weight, and also on VC [83]. In boys, throughout the period of growth mean MIP increases from about 50 cm H_2O at 6–7 years of age to 90 cm H_2O at 16–17 years of age. In girls it increases from about 45 to 75 cm H_2O. However, marked interindividual variability of respiratory muscle pressures in healthy children makes data interpretation difficult. Values between 40 and 100 cm H_2O are within the normal range in all subjects. Intraindividual variability is at least 10% [80, 81].

To assess respiratory muscle weakness in children it is helpful to know that for both girls and boys between 6 and 16 years of age the 5th percentile of MIP is approximately 30–40 cm H_2O. This means that 95% of healthy children are able to generate higher pressures (unpubl. data). Values repeatedly below this threshold should be considered suggestive of inspiratory muscle weakness and require further investigation.

Despite difficulties in interpreting a patient's single MIP measurement a regular follow-up provides additional information on the course of inspiratory muscle strength. Low MIP is always suggestive of predominant diaphragm weakness and should entail additional VC and MIP

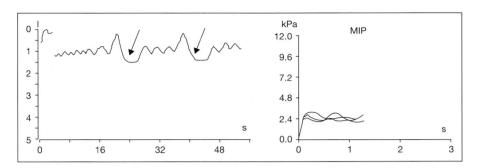

Fig. 2. Measurement of MIP from RV in an 8-year-old patient with SMA II. Left: Spirometry during measurement of MIP. Arrows: Expiration to RV followed by maximum inspiratory effort against the occluded airways. Right: Reproducible measurements with an MIP of 2.7 kPa = 27 cm H_2O.

Table 3. Normal values and prediction equations for MIP measured at RV in children aged 6–17 years

	n	MIP cm H_2O	Equation MIP cm H_2O
Wilson et al. [82]			
Girls	98	63 ± 21	40 + (weight × 0.57)
Boys	137	75 ± 23	45.5 + (weight × 0.75)
Mellies et al. [83]			
Girls	153	58 ± 24	[2.43 + (age × 0.28)] × 10
Boys	147	68 ± 31	[2.58 + (age × 0.39)] × 10

measurements in the supine position. In patients with diaphragm weakness a VC decline of 25% or more following supine positioning is associated with an MIP decline of 10–20% as well [15, 51]. In contrast, VC and MIP in the supine position did not fall more than 5% of baseline in 60 healthy schoolchildren (unpubl. data).

In some patients the measurement of MIP may also help to differentiate between whether a restrictive lung defect is primarily due to scoliosis or to progressive inspiratory muscle weakness.

Where possible MIP should be obtained with every spirometry and values in absolute numbers and the difference to the age-adjusted mean value should be documented. Difficulties in obtaining accurate MIP measurements in handicapped children are similar to those with spirometry. In some children additional inaccuracy may arise from problems with maintaining a maximum and sustained effort against the occluded airways (fig. 2).

Maximum Expiratory Pressures

Since expiration during tidal breathing is entirely passive, activation of expiratory muscles only contributes to respiration in case of increased respiratory drive, e.g. during exertion, fever or hypoxemia. Therefore, in a nonambulatory child in stable condition, expiratory muscles normally do not significantly contribute to alveolar ventilation, though they are essential for effective cough and airway clearance of secretions. In patients with muscular dystrophies MEP >45 cm H_2O has been found to be necessary for an effective cough [51, 84].

Expiratory muscles that contribute to MEP are primarily the abdominal muscles and their strength normally exceeds that of the inspiratory muscles [80]. Therefore MEP < MIP indicates prevailing expiratory muscle weakness, a finding characteristic for children with SMA. The following equations can be used to estimate mean MEP: boys: 35 + (5.5 × age) cm H_2O; girls 24 + (4.8 × age) cm H_2O [82].

However, the relevance of MEP measurements is limited since the consequence of expiratory muscle weakness – impaired cough flow – can be measured directly.

Sniff Nasal Pressure

Sniff nasal pressure (P_{sniff}) is an established test of inspiratory muscle strength in adults but recently this technique has also been applied to children and normal values have been published [85]. Pressures are measured using a catheter occluding one nostril during maximal sniffs performed through the contralateral nostril from FRC.

In patients with NMD noninvasive P_{sniff} measurement has potential advantages. Due to the ease and natural character of the maneuver the test is well tolerated [80, 86].

Weak children who could not perform an MIP maneuver were able to perform reproducible P_{sniff} [85].

P_{sniff} predominately reflects the diaphragmatic component of inspiratory muscle strength and interestingly, dynamic P_{sniff} pressures are higher than static inspiratory mouth pressures. In 180 children of 6–17 years P_{sniff} measured at FRC was 104 ± 26 cm H_2O in boys and 93 ± 23 cm H_2O in girls. Values were similar to those in adults [85].

Peak Cough Flow

Mucus retention, atelectasis and recurrent pneumonia, the results of impaired coughing, are severe complications in patients with NMD [87, 88]. Reduced PCF is primarily due to reduced vital capacity expiratory muscle weakness. PCF can be easily measured by letting the child perform a maximum cough into a simple peak flowmeter. The nostrils should be occluded with a nose clip.

In adults with NMD PCF below 160–200 liters/min are associated with insufficient clearance of airway secretions and clinical experience confirms a similar threshold in children. Since effective methods of assisted coughing are available periodic assessment of PCF has clinical implications and treatment should be initiated when PCF has fallen below 200 liters/min [60].

Gas Exchange

Gas exchange can be measured punctually and continuously, during wakefulness and sleep, using the techniques listed in table 2; details are summarized in table 1.

In patients with respiratory complications calculation of alveolar-arterial O_2 gradient (AaO_2) is particularly helpful to distinguish whether hypoxemia is primarily due to impaired gas exchange or to alveolar hypoventilation. AaO_2 can be calculated using the equation:

$$AaO_2 = (FiO_2\%/100) \times (P_{atm} - 47 \text{ mm Hg}) - (PaCO_2/0.8) - PaO_2$$

$AaO_2 > 15$ is abnormal suggesting impaired gas exchange due to atelectasis, pneumonia or other causes of ventilation/perfusion mismatch. $AaO_2 \leq 15$ is normal and hypoxemia is due to displacement of alveolar O_2 by CO_2. Therefore, in a child with NMD, hypoxemia in the presence of a normal AaO_2 implies alveolar hypoventilation due to respiratory muscle fatigue.

Assessment of gas exchange is particularly important in patients with advanced disease. Diurnal hypercapnia ($PaCO_2 > 45$ mm Hg) repeatedly measured in a period of time free of chest infections indicates advanced respiratory muscle failure and is associated with a critical prognosis. It should prompt the decision for initiation of noninvasive ventilation [18, 30, 60, 78, 89].

Sleep-Disordered Breathing

SDB is a frequent complication seen in up to 70% of patients with progressive NMD [15, 31, 43, 77, 90–92]. The principle cause of SDB is a disease-related loss of respiratory capacity. This becomes apparent in the setting of physiological sleep-induced reduction of respiratory drive, muscle tone and alveolar ventilation. Respiration is particularly prone to disturbances during rapid eye movement (REM) sleep, the time of maximal muscle hypotonia. This is why inspiratory muscle weakness, especially of the diaphragm, becomes apparent as SDB primarily during REM sleep (fig. 3). Therefore, studying respiration during sleep is an indirect though valuable respiratory function test.

The definition of SDB summarizes disturbances of the respiratory pattern and gas exchange during sleep and includes apnea, hypopnea and hypoventilation with desaturation and CO_2 retention [91, 93–95]. Apneas and hypopneas are defined as cessation or decrease of airflow during sleep lasting longer than two breathing cycles and are accompanied by oxyhemoglobin desaturation >3% [94, 96]. A strict definition of alveolar hypoventilation during sleep does not exist. In children, however, continued carbon dioxide tensions >55 mm Hg are clearly pathological [91, 95]. SDB interferes with normal sleep and is associated with autonomic nervous system dysfunction and neurobehavioral daytime symptoms. Furthermore, nocturnal hypoxemia may cause pulmonary hypertension and cor pulmonale.

The severity of SDB depends on residual lung and inspiratory muscle function. It ranges from transient hypopneas during REM sleep at mild degrees of respiratory muscle weakness to lasting hypoventilation in advanced disease. SDB always precedes manifest diurnal respiratory failure, in most subjects by years, and should be interpreted as an early sign of respiratory muscle failure [31, 77, 90, 92, 97, 98].

VC below 40% is a sensitive and specific threshold for the occurrence of nocturnal hypoventilation and is a clear indication to perform a sleep study. Overnight pulse oximetry or capnography might be sufficient to detect marked SDB. However, these techniques often fail to discover transient hypopneas and apneas that may still cause relevant sleep disturbance and daytime symptoms. Since symptoms might be unspecific and often fail to predict SDB complete polysomnography is indicated if there is a history of unrestful or disturbed sleep or complaints as listed in table 1. This is especially true in children with normal arterial blood gases in whom lung and respiratory muscle test cannot be obtained. In this case sleep studies remain the only technique to assess

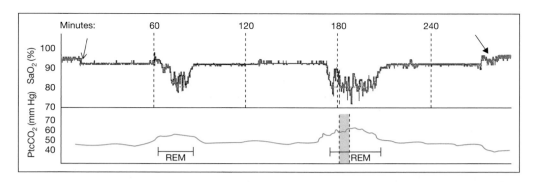

Fig. 3. Nocturnal hypoventilation and severe aggravation during REM sleep. Overnight oximetry and capnometry as details from complete polysomnography. Thin arrow: patient fell asleep; thick arrow: start of noninvasive ventilation. $PtcCO_2$ = Transcutaneous carbon dioxide tension.

respiratory function. In such patients normal polysomnography suggests that VC is still above 40–60% and diaphragm function is still preserved. Such patients are less likely to develop respiratory complications. In contrast, transient hypopneas during REM sleep suggest mild to moderate impaired respiratory function; hypoventilation during REM sleep suggests moderately to severely reduced respiratory function, and hypoventilation in all sleep stages suggests severely reduced respiratory function. Such patients are prone to respiratory complications and should be followed closely.

Timely recognition of SDB is also important as part of the therapy since noninvasive ventilation is available and effective in improving sleep, daytime complaints, quality of life and may also improve survival [17, 30, 99, 100].

Planning Anesthesia and Surgery

NMD patients with impaired respiratory function are prone to experience respiratory failure and severe complications during anesthesia and surgery. The risk is especially high in patients with VC below 50%, diaphragm weakness, preexisting nocturnal hypoventilation and a PCF below

200 liters/min [60, 98, 101, 102]. Therefore, careful preoperative evaluation is mandatory and should include the measurement of VC in the erect and supine positions, PCF, arterial blood gases and overnight pulse oximetry. Frequent complications in NMD patients include difficulties in weaning from mechanical ventilation, severe and prolonged hypoventilation following anesthesia, retention of airway secretions, atelectasis and pneumonia [60, 88, 101–103].

Noninvasive positive pressure ventilation (NIV) for a limited time is especially helpful in the prevention and management of these complications. NIV takes some load off weak inspiratory muscles and augments alveolar ventilation; it thereby counteracts the inevitable side effects of anesthesia and surgery which patients with advanced NMD are unable to compensate. Moreover, NIV is an effective method to overcome acute respiratory deterioration, e.g. due to pneumonia, and may help to prevent reintubation [30, 104–106].

Wherever possible children with an impaired cough should be made familiar with assisted coughing techniques prior to surgery. This therapy should be applied several times a day postoperatively.

References

1 Dubowitz V: Muscle Disorders in Childhood, ed 2. London, Saunders, 1995.

2 Rideau Y, Jankowski LW, Grellet J: Respiratory function in the muscular dystrophies. Muscle Nerve 1981;4/2:155–164.

3 Tangsrud S, Petersen IL, Lodrup-Carlsen KC, Carlsen KH: Lung function in children with Duchenne's muscular dystrophy. Respir Med 2001;9:898–903.

4 McDonald C, Abresch A, Carter G, Fowler W, Johnson E, Kilmer D, et al: Profiles of neuromuscular diseases. Duchenne muscular dystrophy. Am J Phys Med Rehabil 1995;71:S70–S92.

5 Phillips M, Quinlivan R, Edwards RH, Calverley PM: Changes in spirometry over time as a prognostic marker in patients with Duchenne muscular dystrophy. Am J Respir Crit Care Med 2001;164:2191–2194.

6 Hahn A, Bach JR, Delaubier A, Renardel-Irani A, Guillou C, Rideau Y: Clinical implications of maximal respiratory pressure determinations for individuals with Duchenne muscular dystrophy. Arch Phys Med Rehabil 1997;78/ 1:1–6.

7 De Bruin P, Ueki J, Khan Y, Watson A, Pride N: Diaphragm thickness and inspiratory strength in patients with Duchenne muscular dystrophy. Thorax 1997;52:472–475.

8 Koessler W, Wanke T, Winkler G, Nader A, Toifl K, Kurz H, et al: 2 years' experience with inspiratory muscle training in patients with neuromuscular disorders. Chest 2001; 120: 765–769.

9 Hapke E, Meek J, Jacobs J: Pulmonary function in progressive muscular dystrophy. Chest 1972;61/1:41–47.

10 Inkley SR, Oldenburg FC, Vignos PJ Jr: Pulmonary function in Duchenne muscular dystrophy related to stage of disease. Am J Med 1974;56/3:297–306.

11 Kennedy JD, Staples AJ, Brook PD, Parsons DW, Sutherland AD, Martin AJ, et al: Effect of spinal surgery on lung function in Duchenne muscular dystrophy. Thorax 1995;50: 1173–1178.

12 Miller F, Moseley CF, Koreska J: Spinal fusion in Duchenne muscular dystrophy. Dev Med Child Neurol 1992;34:775–786.

13 Baydur A, Gilgoff I, Prentice W, Carlson M, Fischer D: Decline in respiratory function and experience with long-term assisted ventilation in advanced Duchenne's muscular dystrophy. Chest 1990;97;884–889.

14 Canny G, Szeinberg A, Koreska J, Levison H: Hypercapnia in relation to pulmonary function in Duchenne muscular dystrophy. Pediatr Pulmonol 1989;6:169–171.

15 Ragette R, Mellies U, Schwake C, Voit T, Teschler H: Patterns and predictors of sleep disordered breathing in primary myopathies. Thorax 2002;57:724–728.

16 Annane D, Chevrolet JC, Raphael JC: Nocturnal mechanical ventilation for chronic hypoventilation in patients with neuromuscular and chest wall disorders (Cochrane Review). Cochrane Database Syst Rev 2000; 2:CD001941.

17 Eagle M, Baudouin SV, Chandler C, Giddings DR, Bullock R, Bushby K: Survival in Duchenne muscular dystrophy: Improvements in life expectancy since 1967 and the impact of home nocturnal ventilation. Neuromuscul Disord 2002;12:926–929.

18 Simonds AK, Muntoni F, Heather S, Fielding S: Impact of nasal ventilation on survival in hypercapnic Duchenne muscular dystrophy. Thorax 1998;53:949–952.

19 Corrado G, Lissoni A, Beretta S, Terenghi L, Tadeo G, Folia-Manzillo G, et al: Prognostic value of electrocardiograms, ventricular late potentials, ventricular arrhythmias, and left ventricular systolic dysfunction in patients with Duchenne muscular dystrophy. Am J Cardiol 2002;89:838–841.

20 Bushby K, Muntoni F, Bourke JP: 107th ENMC international workshop: The management of cardiac involvement in muscular dystrophy and myotonic dystrophy. 7th–9th June 2002, Naarden, the Netherlands. Neuromuscul Disord 2003;13/2:166–172.

21 Zerres K, Rudnik-Schoneborn S: Natural history in proximal spinal muscular atrophy. Clinical analysis of 445 patients and suggestions for a modification of existing classifications. Arch Neurol 1995;52:518–523.

22 Bach JR, Niranjan V, Weaver B: Spinal muscular atrophy type 1: A noninvasive respiratory management approach. Chest 2000; 117:1100–1105.

23 Souchon F, Simard L, Lebrun S, Rochette C, Lambert J, Vanasse M: Clinical and genetic study of chronic (types II and III) childhood onset spinal muscular atrophy. Neuromuscul Disord 1996;6:419–424.

24 Rodillo E, Marini M, Heckmatt JZ, Dubowitz V: Scoliosis in spinal muscular atrophy: Review of 63 cases. J Child Neurol 1989;4: 118–123.

25 Robinson D, Galasko CS, Delaney C, Williamson J, Barrie J: Scoliosis and lung function in spinal muscular atrophy. Eur Spine J 1995;4:268–273.

26 Chng S, Wong Y, Hui J, Wong H, Ong H, Goh D: Pulmonary function and scoliosis in children with spinal muscular atrophy types II and III. J Paediatr Child Health 2003;39: 673–676.

27 Granata C, Cervellati S, Ballestrazzi A, Corbascio M, Merlini L: Spine surgery in spinal muscular atrophy: Long-term results. Neuromuscul Disord 1993;3/3:207–215.

28 Perez A, Mulot R, Vardon G, Barois A, Gallego J: Thoracoabdominal pattern of breathing in neuromuscular disorders. Chest 1996;110:454–461.

29 Lissoni A, Aliverti A, Tzeng A, Bach JR: Kinematic analysis of patients with spinal muscular atrophy during spontaneous breathing and mechanical ventilation. Am J Phys Med Rehabil 1998;77:188–192.

30 Mellies U, Ragette R, Dohna SC, Boehm H, Voit T, Teschler H: Long-term noninvasive ventilation in children and adolescents with neuromuscular disorders. Eur Respir J 2003;22:631–636.

31 Mellies U, Ragette R, Schwake C, Boehm H, Voit T, Teschler H: Daytime predictors of sleep disordered breathing in children and adolescents with neuromuscular disorders. Neuromuscul Disord 2003;13/2:123–128.

32 Carter G, Abresch A, Fowler W, Johnson E, Kilmer D, McDonald C: Profiles of neuromuscular disease. Spinal muscular atrophy. Am J Phys Med Rehabil 1995;74:S151–S159.

33 Grohmann K, Varon R, Stolz P, Schuelke M, Janetzki C, Bertini E, et al: Infantile spinal muscular atrophy with respiratory distress type 1 (SMARD 1). Ann Neurol 2003;54: 719–724.

34 Brunner H, Nillesen W, van Oost B, Jansen G, Wieringa B, Ropers H-H, et al: Presymptomatic diagnosis of myotonic dystrophy. J Med Genet 1992;29:780–784.

35 Jaspert A, Fahsold R, Grehl H, Claus D: Myotonic dystrophy: Correlation of clinical symptoms with the size of the CTG trinucleotide repeat. J Neurol 1995;242:99–104.

36 White R, Bass S: Myotonic dystrophy and paediatric anaesthesia. Paediatr Anaesth 2003; 13:94–102.

37 Campbell C, Sherlock R, Jacob P, Blayney M: Congenital myotonic dystrophy: Assisted ventilation duration and outcome. Pediatrics 2004; 113:811–816.

38 Rutherford M, Heckmatt J, Dubowitz V: Congenital myotonic dystrophy: Respiratory function at birth determines survival. Arch Dis Child 1989;64/2:191–195.

39 Keller C, Reynolds A, Lee B, Garcia-Prats J: Congenital myotonic dystrophy requiring prolonged endotracheal and non-invasive assisted ventilation: Not a uniformly fatal condition. Pediatrics 1998;101:704–706.

40 Lee S, Chan K, Chow S: Survival of a 30-week baby with congenital myotonic dystrophy initially ventilated 55 days. J Paediatr Child Health 1999;35:313–314.

41 Boogard J, van der Meche F, Hendriks I, Ververs C: Pulmonary function and resting breathing pattern in myotonic dystrophy. Lung 1992;170/3:143–153.

42 Jammes Y, Pouget J, Grimaud C, Serratrice G: Pulmonary function and electromyographic study of respiratory muscles in myotonic dystrophy. Muscle Nerve 1985;8:586–594.

43 Guilleminault C, Shergill RP: Sleep-disordered breathing in neuromuscular disease. Curr Treat Options Neurol 2002;4/2:107–112.

44 Matsumoto H, Osanai S, Onodera S, Akiba Y, Nakano H, Oomatsu H, et al: Respiratory pathphysiology during sleep in patients with myotonic dystrophy. Nihon Kyobu Shikkan Gakkai Zasshi 1990;28:961–970.

45 Nugent A, Smith I, Shneerson J: Domiciliary-assisted ventilation in patients with myotonic dystrophy. Chest 2002;121:459–464.

46 Dohna-Schwake C, Ragette R, Mellies U, Straub V, Teschler H, Voit T: Respiratory function in congenital muscular dystrophy and limb girdle muscular dystrophy 2I. Neurology 2004;62:513–514.

47 Maayan C, Springer C, Armon Y, Bar-Yishay ESY, Godfrey A: Nemaline myopathy as a cause of sleep hypoventilation. Pediatrics 1986;77:390–395.

48 Schweitzer C, Danet V, Polu E, Marchal F, Monin P: Nemaline myopathy and early respiratory failure. Eur J Pediatr 2003;162:216–217.

49 McEntargart M, Parsons G, Buj-Bello A, Biancalana V, Fenton I, Little M, et al: Genotype-phenotype correlations in X-linked myotubular myopathy. Neuromuscul Disord 2002;12:939–946.

50 Zanoteli E, Oliveira A, Schmidt B, Gabbai A: Centronuclear myopathy: Clinical aspects of ten Brazilian patients with childhood onset. J Neurol Sci 1998;158:76–82.

51 Mellies U, Ragette R, Schwake C, Baethmann M, Voit T, Teschler H: Sleep-disordered breathing and respiratory failure in acid maltase deficiency. Neurology 2001;57:1290–1295.

52 Keenan S, Alöexander D, Road J, Ryan C, Oger J, Wilcox P: Ventilatory muscle strength and endurance in myasthenia gravis. Eur Respir J 1995;8:1130–1135.

53 Morita M, Gabbai A, Oliveira A, Penn A: Myasthenia gravis in children. Analysis of 18 patients. Arq Neuropsiquiatr 2001;59/3B:681–685.

54 Keenan S, Alexander D, Road J, Ryan C, Oger J, Wilcox P: Ventilatory muscle strength and endurance in myasthenia gravis. Eur Respir J 1995;8:1130–1135.

55 Spinelli A, Marconi G, Gorini M, Pizzi A, Scano G: Control of breathing in patients with myasthenia gravis. Am Rev Respir Dis 1992;145:1359–1366.

56 Raksadawan N, Kankirawatana P, Balankura K, Prateepratana P, Sangruchi T, Atchaneeyasakul L: Childhood onset myasthenia gravis. J Med Assoc Thai 2002;85(suppl 2):S769–S777.

57 Rabinstein A, Wijdicks E: BiPAP in acute respiratory failure due to myasthenic crisis may prevent intubation. Neurology 2002;59:1647–1649.

58 Iannaccone S, Mills J, Harris K, Herman J, Schochet P, Luckett P: Congenital myasthenic syndrome with sleep hypoventilation. Muscle Nerve 2000;23:1129–1132.

59 McConkey P, Mullens A: Congenital myasthenic syndrome: A rare, potentially treatable cause of respiratory failure in a 'floppy' infant. Anaesth Intensive Care 2000;28:82–86.

60 Wallgren-Pettersson C, Bushby K, Mellies U, Simonds A: 117th ENMC workshop: Ventilatory support in congenital neuromuscular disorders – congenital myopathies, congenital muscular dystrophies, congenital myotonic dystrophy and SMA (II) 4–6 April 2003, Naarden, The Netherlands. Neuromuscul Disord 2004;14/1:56–69.

61 Braun NM, Arora NS, Rochester DF: Respiratory muscle and pulmonary function in polymyositis and other proximal myopathies. Thorax 1983;38:616–623.

62 Samaha FJ, Buncher CR, Russman BS, White ML, Iannaccone ST, Barker L, et al: Pulmonary function in spinal muscular atrophy. J Child Neurol 1994;9:326–329.

63 Nachemson A: A long term follow-up study of non-treated scoliosis. Acta Orthop Scand 1968;39:466–476.

64 Pehrsson K, Danielsson A, Nachemson A: Pulmonary function in adolescent idiopathic scoliosis: A 25 year follow up after surgery or start of brace treatment. Thorax 2001;56:388–393.

65 Kurz LT, Mubarak SJ, Schultz P, Park SM, Leach J: Correlation of scoliosis and pulmonary function in Duchenne muscular dystrophy. J Pediatr Orthop 1983;3:347–353.

66 Miller F, Moseley CF, Koreska J, Levison H: Pulmonary function and scoliosis in Duchenne dystrophy. J Pediatr Orthop 1988;8/2:133–137.

67 Estenne M, Heilporn A, Delhez L, Yernault JC, De Troyer A: Chest wall stiffness in patients with chronic respiratory muscle weakness. Am Rev Respir Dis 1983;128:1002–1007.

68 Gibson GJ, Pride NB, Davis JN, Loh LC: Pulmonary mechanics in patients with respiratory muscle weakness. Am Rev Respir Dis 1977;115:389–395.

69 McCool FD, Mayewski RF, Shayne DS, Gibson CJ, Griggs RC, Hyde RW: Intermittent positive pressure breathing in patients with respiratory muscle weakness. Alterations in total respiratory system compliance. Chest 1986;90:546–552.

70 Fallat RJ, Jewitt B, Bass M, Kamm B, Norris FH Jr: Spirometry in amyotrophic lateral sclerosis. Arch Neurol 1979;36/2:74–80.

71 Vincken WG, Elleker MG, Cosio MG: Flow-volume loop changes reflecting respiratory muscle weakness in chronic neuromuscular disorders. Am J Med 1987;83:673–680.

72 Vincken W, Elleker G, Cosio MG: Detection of upper airway muscle involvement in neuromuscular disorders using the flow-volume loop. Chest 1986;90/1:52–57.

73 Mier-Jedrzejowicz A, Brophy C, Moxham J, Green M: Assessment of diaphragm weakness. Am Rev Respir Dis 1988;137:877–883.

74 Fromageot C, Lofaso F, Annane D, Falaize L, Lejaille M, Clair B, et al: Supine fall in lung volumes in the assessment of diaphragmatic weakness in neuromuscular disorders. Arch Phys Med Rehabil 2001;82/1:123–128.

75 Lechtzin N, Wiener CM, Shade DM, Clawson L, Diette GB: Spirometry in the supine position improves the detection of diaphragmatic weakness in patients with amyotrophic lateral sclerosis. Chest 2002;121:436–442.

76 Miller F, Koreska J: Height measurement of patients with neuromuscular disease and contractures. Dev Med Child Neurol 1992;34/1:55–60.

77 Hukins CA, Hillman DR: Daytime predictors of sleep hypoventilation in Duchenne muscular dystrophy. Am J Respir Crit Care Med 2000;161/1:166–170.

78 Phillips MF, Smith PE, Carroll N, Edwards RH, Calverley PM: Nocturnal oxygenation and prognosis in Duchenne muscular dystrophy. Am J Respir Crit Care Med 1999;160/1:198–202.

79 Fauroux B, Lofaso F: Measurements of respiratory muscle function in children; Hammer J, Eber E (eds): Paediatric Pulmonary Function Testing. Prog Respir Res. Basel, Karger, 2005, vol 33, pp 138–147.

80 American Thoracic Society/European Respiratory Society: ATS/ERS Statement on respiratory muscle testing. Am J Respir Crit Care Med 2002;166:518–624.

81 Gaultier C, Zinman R: Maximal static pressures in healthy children. Respir Physiol 1983;51/1:45–61.

82 Wilson SH, Cooke NT, Edwards RH, Spiro SG: Predicted normal values for maximal respiratory pressures in Caucasian adults and children. Thorax 1984;39:535–538.

83 Mellies U, Schultze S, Schwake C, Ragette R, Teschler H: Respiratory muscle function in 300 healthy children (abstract). Eur Respir J 2001;18(suppl 33):P827.

84 Szeinberg A, Tabachnik E, Rashed N, McLaughlin FJ, England S, Bryan CA, et al: Cough capacity in patients with muscular dystrophy. Chest 1988;94:1232–1235.

85 Stefanutti D, Fitting JW: Sniff nasal inspiratory pressure. Reference values in Caucasian children. Am J Respir Crit Care Med 1999;159/1:107–111.

86 Stefanutti D, Benoist MR, Scheinmann P, Chaussain M, Fitting JW: Usefulness of sniff nasal pressure in patients with neuromuscular or skeletal disorders. Am J Respir Crit Care Med 2000;162:1507–1511.

87 Bach JR: Amyotrophic lateral sclerosis: Predictors for prolongation of life by noninvasive respiratory aids. Arch Phys Med Rehabil 1995;76:828–832.

88 Schmidt-Nowara WW, Altman AR: Atelectasis and neuromuscular respiratory failure. Chest 1984;85:792–795.

89 Simonds AK, Elliott MW: Outcome of domiciliary nasal intermittent positive pressure ventilation in restrictive and obstructive disorders. Thorax 1995;50:604–609.

90 Labanowski M, Schmidt-Nowara W, Guilleminault C: Sleep and neuromuscular disease: Frequency of sleep-disordered breathing in a neuromuscular disease clinic population. Neurology 1996;47:1173–1180.

91 Marcus CL: Sleep-disordered breathing in children. Am J Respir Crit Care Med 2002;164:16–30.

92 Van Lunteren E, Kaminski H: Disorders of sleep and breathing during sleep in neuromuscular disease. Sleep Breath 1999;3/1:23–30.

93 Standards and indications for cardiopulmonary sleep studies in children. American Thoracic Society. Am J Respir Crit Care Med 1996;153:866–878.

94 Cardiorespiratory sleep studies in children. Establishment of normative data and polysomnographic predictors of morbidity. American Thoracic Society. Am J Respir Crit Care Med 1999;160:1381–1387.

95 Marcus CL, Omlin KJ, Basinki DJ, Bailey SL, Rachal AB, von Pechmann WS, et al: Normal polysomnographic values for children and adolescents. Am Rev Respir Dis 1992;146:1235–1239.

96 Schechter MS: Technical report: Diagnosis and management of childhood obstructive sleep apnea syndrome. Pediatrics 2002;109/4:e69.

Neuromuscular Disorders

97 Khan Y, Heckmatt JZ: Obstructive apnoeas in Duchenne muscular dystrophy. Thorax 1994; 49/2:157–161.

98 Sivak ED, Shefner JM, Sexton J: Neuromuscular disease and hypoventilation. Curr Opin Pulm Med 1999;5:355–362.

99 Mellies U, Dohna-Schwake C, Ragette R, Teschler H, Voit T: Nocturnal noninvasive ventilation in pediatric neuromuscular disorders: Impact on sleep and symptoms. Wien Klin Wochenschr 2003;115:855–859.

100 Simonds AK, Ward S, Heather S, Bush A, Muntoni F: Outcome of paediatric domiciliary mask ventilation in neuromuscular and skeletal disease. Eur Respir J 2000;16: 476–481.

101 Bach JR, Zhitnikov S: The management of neuromuscular ventilatory failure. Semin Pediatr Neurol 1998;5:92–105.

102 Schramm CM: Current concepts of respiratory complications of neuromuscular disease in children. Curr Opin Pediatr 2000;12/3: 203–207.

103 Perrin C, Unterborn JN, Ambrosio CD, Hill NS: Pulmonary complications of chronic neuromuscular diseases and their management. Muscle Nerve 2004;29/1:5–27.

104 Antonelli M, Conti G: Noninvasive positive pressure ventilation as treatment for acute respiratory failure in critically ill patients. Crit Care 2000;4/1:15–22.

105 Fortenberry JD, Del Toro J, Jefferson LS, Evey L, Haase D: Management of pediatric acute hypoxemic respiratory insufficiency with bilevel positive pressure (BiPAP) nasal mask ventilation. Chest 1995;108:1059–1064.

106 Padman R, McNamara R: Postoperative pulmonary complications in children with neuromuscular scoliosis who underwent posterior spinal fusion. Del Med J 1990;62: 999–1003.

Dr. Uwe Mellies
Department of Pediatrics and Neuropediatrics
University of Essen, Children's Hospital
Hufelandstrasse 55
DE–45122 Essen (Germany)
Tel. +49 201 723 2118
Fax +49 201 723 2113
E-Mail uwe.mellies@uni-essen.de

Hammer J, Eber E (eds): Paediatric Pulmonary Function Testing.
Prog Respir Res. Basel, Karger, 2005, vol 33, pp 247–254

Paediatric Oncology and Bone Marrow Transplantation

Isa Cerveri[a]   Angelo Corsico[a]   Maria Cristina Zoia[a]   Giovanna Giorgiani[b]

[a]Division of Respiratory Diseases and [b]Department of Paediatrics, University of Pavia,
Istituto di Ricovero e Cura a Carattere Scientifico, 'Policlinico San Matteo', Pavia, Italy

Abstract

The transplantation of haematopoietic stem cells is an established therapy for many chemosensitive or radiosensitive malignancies in both adults and children. Approximately one fifth of the transplants undertaken every year worldwide are performed in paediatric patients and it is estimated that annually a minimum of 1,500–2,000 of these patients will become long-term survivors. Thanks to these transplants, it is now possible that children have a long life expectancy although they are more exposed to the toxicity of treatments than adults. Pulmonary complications account for 10–40% of transplant-related deaths, for significant morbidity and may affect long-term survival and the quality of life of cured patients. Respiratory function tests are particularly useful in children, not least because they are non-invasive, carry no risks, and are reproducible and repeatable over long periods of time for an extended follow-up, constituting an important part of the early identification of lung damage and a method for following up changes over time in order to control the development of any sequelae. Transient reductions in lung volumes and transfer factor approximately 3–6 months after transplantation have been found in many paediatric studies. Both long-term obstructive disease and restrictive disease have been recorded during follow-up periods of 1–13 years. Lung function abnormalities can frequently be present even in the absence of respiratory symptoms; furthermore, respiratory symptoms can be more difficult to detect in children than in adults. The diagnosis of bronchiolitis obliterans, which is currently the most important of the late pulmonary complications, in children is mainly based on lung function tests and imaging without histology; if pulmonary function monitoring is carried out regularly over time, the diagnosis can be made earlier. Particular attention should be given to progressive obstructive airway disease, although less common in children than in adults, because of its poor prognosis. Further long-term studies are needed to ascertain whether lung function abnormalities, in the absence of chronic respiratory symptoms, will become more clinically relevant with increasing age, exposure to smoking and other pollutants and allergens.

Introduction

The transplantation of haematopoietic stem cells is an established therapy for many chemosensitive or radiosensitive malignancies. Haematopoietic stem cells from bone marrow, peripheral blood, or cord blood are used for autologous or allogeneic transplantation. Donors for allogeneic transplants include HLA-identical siblings, other family members, or unrelated volunteers from the vast worldwide donor pools [1].

Over the past 50 years, intensive studies into the use of haematopoietic stem cell transplantation (HSCT) have changed this treatment modality from one that was thought to be doomed by insurmountable complications to one that is now standard therapy for some diseases. Major changes have occurred in HSCT over the last decade. The expansion of unrelated donor pools to a current situation of more than

7.5 million registered donors worldwide, the establishment of cord blood banks in North America and Europe, and the successful introduction of haploidentical HSCT have made allogeneic HSCT available to patients without an HLA-identical sibling donor. New technologies, such as reduced intensity conditioning and improved supportive care, limit early toxicity and make allogeneic HSCT feasible for patients with concomitant organ toxicity. In a recent review, Leiper [2] reports current estimates indicating that more than 30,000 allogeneic and autologous HSCT are undertaken worldwide every year, and that this figure is rising rapidly. Approximately one fifth of these transplants are performed in paediatric patients and it is estimated that a minimum of 1,500–2,000 of these patients annually will become long-term survivors. Improvements in supportive care have made HSCT possible because an ever-increasing number of children survive the effects of the preparative therapy and the subsequent graft-versus-host disease (GVHD) and immaturity of the immune system. Although children with leukaemia constitute an ever-decreasing proportion of those eligible for transplantation because of the success of the initial therapeutic non-transplant treatment they receive, there are still a number of children benefiting from transplantation who have been treated very heavily with alternative therapies [3, 4]. With increasing numbers of long-term survivors, delayed complications, often presenting years after HSCT, are becoming a concern. Late sequelae may arise as a result of the disease for which transplantation was performed or of toxicity associated with the wide variety of conditioning regimens. Most of the latter will include high-dose chemotherapy, alone or accompanied by radiotherapy, in the form of total body irradiation (TBI) or total lymphoid irradiation and/or agents which lead to T cell depletion. The total dose of TBI usually varies from 7.5 Gy, given as a single fraction, up to 15 Gy, given in multiple fractions over a period of 3–4 days. Additional damage may be caused by the toxic effects of some antibiotics and antifungal drugs, or by immunosuppressive agents used to prevent or treat GVHD or by the pathological process of chronic GVHD itself. Other potential variables influencing the impact of late sequelae are the total dose, dose rate and method of fractionation of the radiotherapy, the age and sex of the child, and genetic influences [2].

Pulmonary Complications following Transplantation of Haematopoietic Stem Cells

Cardiac, pulmonary, renal, neurological, and endocrine complications as well as second malignant neoplasms associated with HSCT are of particular clinical concern as they may account for overall morbidity and mortality and may affect the long-term survival and the quality of life of cured patients. Pulmonary complications cause 10–40% of transplant-related deaths [5]. The risks of pulmonary complications depend on the underlying malignancy, the conditioning regimen employed, the type of HSCT and the development of GVHD. Pulmonary complications directly related to HSCT are divided into infectious and non-infectious ones. HSCT patients are distinct from other immunosuppressed patients in that the immunosuppression in the stem cell recipients follows a predictable course over time. This is important as the predictable time course can help to narrow down the differential diagnoses to certain pulmonary complications which characteristically occur at a particular time following HSCT (table 1). An early diagnosis enabling the treatment of the pulmonary complications helps minimize the significant mortality and morbidity. Immunosuppression starts with the conditioning regimen, such as chemotherapy and TBI, usually becoming evident about 1 week before a standard HSCT and profound neutropenia occurs in all patients during the leucopenic phase following HSCT. Neutrophil counts are the first to recover, usually within 2–4 weeks following HSCT, but the lymphocyte count may take months to

Table 1. Pulmonary complications according to the period of time following HSCT

Complications	Early	Late
Non-infectious causes		
Acute pulmonary oedema	++	
Drug reactions	++	
Diffuse alveolar haemorrhage	+	
Pulmonary veno-occlusive disease	+	
Idiopathic pneumonia syndrome	++	+
Bronchiolitis obliterans	+	++
Cryptogenic organizing pneumonia	+	++
Infectious causes		
Bacterial	++	++
Fungal	++	+
CMV	++	+
Herpes virus 6	+	
P. carinii	+	+
Respiratory syncytial virus	+	
Adenovirus	+	

Cerveri/Corsico/Zoia/Giorgiani

GVHD and 45% CMV reactivation; no association was found in this cohort with other previously proposed risk factors, such as a prolonged use of methotrexate, decreased immunoglobulins, increasing recipient age, male gender and lack of human leucocyte antigen matching, and recurrent pulmonary infection [5, 33, 42, 43, 45]. Since the evolution of the disease, despite treatment, is particularly negative with a progressive worsening of respiratory function and a high mortality, early diagnosis is of paramount importance; this can be achieved by systematic regular monitoring of the respiratory function starting from the onset of acute GVHD.

Conclusions

Further long-term studies are needed to ascertain whether lung function abnormalities in the absence of chronic respiratory symptoms will become clinically more relevant with increasing age, exposure to smoking and other pollutants and allergens. In the shorter term, it is permissible to be slightly more optimistic about the effect of HSCT on pulmonary function in the paediatric population than in adults; however, progressive obstructive airway disease, although less common in children than in adults, deserves further attention because of its poor prognosis.

References

1 Gratwohl A, Baldomero H, Horisberger B, Schmid C, Passweg J, Urbano-Ispizua A; Accreditation Committee of the European Group for Blood and Marrow Transplantation (EBMT): Current trends in hematopoietic stem cell transplantation in Europe. Blood 2002;100:2374–2386.
2 Leiper AD: Non-endocrine late complications of bone marrow transplantation in childhood. Part I. Br J Haematol 2002;118:3–22.
3 Trigg ME: Milestones in the development of pediatric hematopoietic stem cell transplantation – 50 years of progress. Pediatr Transplant 2002;6:465–474.
4 Storb R: Allogeneic hematopoietic stem cell transplantation – Yesterday, today, and tomorrow. Exp Hematol 2003;31:1–10.
5 Palmas A, Tefferi A, Myers JL, Scott JP, Swensen SJ, Chen MG, Gastineau DA, Gertz MA, Inwards DJ, Lacy MQ, Litzow MR: Late-onset noninfectious pulmonary complications after allogeneic bone marrow transplantation. Br J Haematol 1998;100:680–687.
6 Wah TM, Moss HA, Robertson RJ, Barnard DL: Pulmonary complications following bone marrow transplantation. Br J Radiol 2003; 76:373–379.
7 Cerveri I, Zoia MC, Fulgoni P, Corsico A, Casali L, Tinelli C, Zecca M, Giorgiani G, Locatelli F: Late pulmonary sequelae after childhood bone marrow transplantation. Thorax 1999;54:131–135.
8 Fanfulla F, Locatelli F, Zoia MC, Giorgiani G, Bonetti F, Spagnolatti L, Cerveri I: Pulmonary complications and respiratory function changes after bone marrow transplantation in children. Eur Respir J 1997;10: 2301–2306.
9 Tanner JM: Growth at Adolescence, ed 2. Oxford, Blackwell, 1962.
10 Rosenthal M, Bain SH, Cramer D, Helms P, Denison D, Bush A, Warner JO: Lung function in white children aged 4 to 19 years. I. Spirometry. Thorax 1993;48:794–802.

11 Rosenthal M, Cramer D, Bain SH, Denison D, Bush A, Warner JO: Lung function in white children aged 4 to 19 years. II. Single breath analysis and plethysmography. Thorax 1993; 48:803–808.
12 Quigley PM, Yeager AM, Loughlin GM: The effects of bone marrow transplantation on pulmonary function in children. Pediatr Pulmonol 1994;18:361–367.
13 Leneveu H, Bremont F, Rubie H, Peyroulet MC, Broue A, Suc A, Robert A, Dutau G: Respiratory function in children undergoing bone marrow transplantation. Pediatr Pulmonol 1999; 28:31–38.
14 Neve V, Foot AB, Michon J, Fourquet A, Zucker JM, Boule M: Longitudinal clinical and functional pulmonary follow-up after megatherapy, fractionated total body irradiation, and autologous bone marrow transplantation for metastatic neuroblastoma. Med Pediatr Oncol 1999;32:170–176.
15 Shaw NJ, Tweeddale PM, Eden OB: Pulmonary function in childhood leukaemia survivors. Med Pediatr Oncol 1989;17:149–154.
16 Jenney ME, Faragher EB, Jones PH, Woodcock A: Lung function and exercise capacity in survivors of childhood leukaemia. Med Pediatr Oncol 1995;24:222–230.
17 Nysom K, Holm K, Olsen JH, Hertz H, Hesse B: Pulmonary function after treatment for acute lymphoblastic leukaemia in childhood. Br J Cancer 1998;78:21–27.
18 Nysom K, Holm K, Hertz H, Hesse B: Risk factors for reduced pulmonary function after malignant lymphoma in childhood. Med Pediatr Oncol 1998;30:240–248.
19 Fulgoni P, Zoia MC, Corsico A, Beccaria M, Georgiani G, Bossi G, Cerveri I: Lung function in survivors of childhood acute lymphoblastic leukaemia. Chest 1999;116:1163–1167.
20 Serota FT, August CS, Koch PA, Fox W, D'Angio GJ: Pulmonary function in patients undergoing bone marrow transplantation. Med Pediatr Oncol 1984;12:137–143.

21 Uderzo C, Rovelli A, Meloni G, Balduzzi A, Pezzini C, Colombini A, Adamoli L, Fraschini D, Locasciulli A, Masera G: Evaluation of late side-effects after bone marrow transplantation in children with leukemia. Bone Marrow Transplant 1991;8: 44–46.
22 Arvidson J, Bratteby LE, Carlson K, Hagberg H, Kreuger A, Simonsson B, Smedmyr B, Taube A, Oberg G, Lonnerholm G: Pulmonary function after autologous bone marrow transplantation in children. Bone Marrow Transplant 1994;14:117–123.
23 Kaplan EB, Wodell RA, Wilmott RW, Leifer B, Lesser ML, August CS: Late effects of bone marrow transplantation on pulmonary function in children. Bone Marrow Transplant 1994;14: 613–621.
24 Nysom K, Holm K, Hesse B, Ulrik CS, Jacobsen N, Bisgaard H, Hertz H: Lung function after allogeneic bone marrow transplantation for leukaemia or lymphoma. Br J Cancer 1996;74:432–436.
25 Johnson FL, Stokes DC, Ruggiero M, Dalla PL, Callihan TR: Chronic obstructive airways disease after bone marrow transplantation. J Pediatr 1984;105:370–376.
26 Kaplan EB, Wodell RA, Wilmott RW, Leifer B, Lesser ML, August CS: Chronic graft-versus-host disease and pulmonary function. Pediatr Pulmonol 1992;14: 141–148.
27 Schultz KR, Green GJ, Wensley D, Sargent MA, Magee JF, Spinelli JJ, Pritchard S, Davis JH, Rogers PC, Chan KW, Phillips GL: Obstructive lung disease in children after allogeneic bone marrow transplantation. Blood 1994;84:3212–3220.
28 Nenadov Beck M, Meresse V, Hartmann O, Gaultier C: Long-term pulmonary sequelae after autologous bone marrow transplantation in children without total body irradiation. Bone Marrow Transplant 1995;16: 771–775.

29 Rovelli A, Pezzini C, Silvestri D, Tana F, Galli MA, Uderzo C: Cardiac and respiratory function after bone marrow transplantation in children with leukaemia. Bone Marrow Transplant 1995;16:571–576.

30 Cerveri I, Fulgoni P, Giorgiani G, Zoia MC, Beccaria M, Tinelli C, Locatelli F: Lung function abnormalities after bone marrow transplantation in children: Has the trend recently changed? Chest 2001;120:1900–1906.

31 Tait RC, Burnett AK, Robertson AG, McNee S, Riyami BM, Carter R, Stevenson RD: Subclinical pulmonary function defects following autologous and allogeneic bone marrow transplantation: Relationship to total body irradiation and graft-versus-host disease. Int J Radiat Oncol Biol Phys 1991;20:1219–1227.

32 Beinert T, Dull T, Wolf K, Holler E, Vogelmeier C, Behr J, Kolb H: Late pulmonary impairment following allogeneic bone marrow transplantation. Eur J Med Res 1996;1:343–348.

33 Soubani AO, Miller KB, Hassoun PM: Pulmonary complications of bone marrow transplantation. Chest 1996;109:1066–1077.

34 Keane TJ, Van Dyk J, Rider WD: Idiopathic interstitial pneumonia following bone marrow transplantation: The relationship with total body irradiation. Int J Radiat Oncol Biol Phys 1981;7:1365–1370.

35 Barrett A, Depledge MH, Powles RL: Interstitial pneumonitis following bone marrow transplantation after low dose rate total body irradiation. Int J Radiat Oncol Biol Phys 1983;9:1029–1033.

36 Twohig KJ, Matthay RA: Pulmonary effects of cytotoxic agents other than bleomycin. Clin Chest Med 1990;11:31–35.

37 Lund MB, Kongerud J, Brinch L, Evensen SA, Boe J: Decreased lung function in one year survivors of allogeneic bone marrow transplantation conditioned with high-dose busulphan and cyclophosphamide. Eur Respir J 1995;8:1269–1274.

38 Tyc VL, Hudson MM, Hinds P, Elliott V, Kibby MY: Tobacco use among pediatric cancer patients: Recommendations for developing clinical smoking interventions. J Clin Oncol 1997;15:2194–2204.

39 Marks DI, Cullis JO, Ward KN, Lacey S, Syzdlo R, Hughes TP, Schwarer AP, Lutz E, Barrett AJ, Hows JM, Batchelor JR, Goldman JM: Allogeneic bone marrow transplantation for chronic myeloid leukemia using sibling and volunteer unrelated donors. A comparison of complications in the first 2 years. Ann Intern Med 1993;119:207–214.

40 Cutler C, Giri S, Jeyapalan S, Paniagua D, Viswanathan A, Antin JH: Acute and chronic graft-versus-host disease after allogeneic peripheral-blood stem-cell and bone marrow transplantation: A meta-analysis. J Clin Oncol 2001;19:3685–3691.

41 Przepiorka D, Anderlini P, Saliba R, Cleary K, Mehra R, Khouri I, Huh YO, Giralt S, Braunschweig I, van Besien K, Champlin R: Chronic graft-versus-host disease after allogeneic blood stem cell transplantation. Blood 2001;98:1695–1700.

42 Clark JG, Schwartz DA, Flournoy N, Sullivan KM, Crawford SW, Thomas ED: Risk factors for airflow obstruction in recipients of bone marrow transplants. Ann Intern Med 1987;107:648–656.

43 Holland HK, Wingard JR, Beschorner WE, Saral R, Santos GW: Bronchiolitis obliterans in bone marrow transplantation and its relationship to chronic graft-v-host disease and low serum IgG. Blood 1988;72:621–627.

44 Prince DS, Wingard JR, Saral R, Santos GW, Wise RA: Longitudinal changes in pulmonary function following bone marrow transplantation. Chest 1989;96:301–306.

45 Schwarer AP, Hughes JM, Trotman DB, Krausz T, Goldman JM: A chronic pulmonary syndrome associated with graft-versus-host disease after allogeneic marrow transplantation. Transplantation 1992;54:1002–1008.

46 Curtis DJ, Smale A, Thien F, Schwarer AP, Szer J: Chronic airflow obstruction in long-term survivors of allogeneic bone marrow transplantation. Bone Marrow Transplant 1995;16:169–173.

47 Sritippayawan S, Keens TG, Horn MV, Starnes VA, Woo MS: What are the best pulmonary function test parameters for early detection of post-lung transplant bronchiolitis obliterans syndrome in children? Pediatr Transplant 2003;7:200–203.

48 Silkoff PE, Caramori M, Tremblay L, McClean P, Chaparro C, Kesten S, Hutcheon M, Slutsky AS, Zamel N, Keshavjee S: Exhaled nitric oxide in human lung transplantation. A noninvasive marker of acute rejection. Am J Respir Crit Care Med 1998;157:1822–1828.

49 De Soyza A, Fisher AJ, Small T, Corris PA: Inhaled corticosteroids and the treatment of lymphocytic bronchiolitis following lung transplantation. Am J Respir Crit Care Med 2001;164:1209–1212.

50 Gabbay E, Walters EH, Orsida B, Whitford H, Ward C, Kotsimbos TC, Snell GI, Williams TJ: Post-lung transplant bronchiolitis obliterans syndrome (BOS) is characterized by increased exhaled nitric oxide levels and epithelial inducible nitric oxide synthase. Am J Respir Crit Care Med 2000;162:2182–2187.

51 Kanamori H, Fujisawa S, Tsuburai T, Yamaji S, Tomita N, Fujimaki K, Miyashita A, Suzuki S, Ishigatsubo Y: Increased exhaled nitric oxide in bronchiolitis obliterans organizing pneumonia after allogeneic bone marrow transplantation. Transplantation 2002;74:1356–1358.

Dr. Isa Cerveri
Division of Respiratory Diseases
IRCCS Policlinico San Matteo
P.le Golgi, 2, IT–27100 Pavia (Italy)
Tel. +39 (0) 382 502611
Fax +39 (0) 382 501359
E-Mail icerveri@smatteo.pv.it

Hammer J, Eber E (eds): Paediatric Pulmonary Function Testing.
Prog Respir Res. Basel, Karger, 2005, vol 33, pp 255–265

....

Long-Term Sequelae of Neonatal Lung Disease

Daniel Trachsel[a]   Allan L. Coates[b]

[a]Division of Intensive Care and Pulmonology, University Children's Hospital,
Basel, Switzerland, [b]Division of Respiratory Medicine, The Hospital for Sick Children,
Toronto, Ontario, Canada

Abstract

In neonatal lung disease, chemical and physical noxious stimuli, microbial aggression, host defence, and an ill-timed exposure to the extrauterine environment all act together in compromising the integrity of the maturing lungs. Pulmonary sequelae, therefore, are determined by the severity of congenital lung disease, but also reflect the multitude of secondary injuries to the newborn child. Various studies have shown that pulmonary function abnormalities in survivors of neonatal lung disease remain highly prevalent despite often favourable clinical outcomes. Mildly impaired compliance, a tendency towards hyperinflation, airway obstruction, and a high prevalence of airway hyperresponsiveness may describe a general pattern of functional remnants in these children. In addition, the possibility of persistently elevated pulmonary artery pressures even in asymptomatic individuals must be kept in mind. Physicians concerned with the follow-up of these patients must be aware of the many extra-pulmonary health issues that need to be regarded. Informed guidance of patients and parents is of importance both in order to prevent stigmatization of these children as overly vulnerable as well as for an early recognition of treatable respiratory problems which might otherwise not be fully apprehended due to a long-standing history of pulmonary disease. With the exception of chronic lung disease of prematurity, long-term follow-up of pulmonary sequelae of neonatal lung diseases so far has referred to children born before the introduction of lung protective ventilation strategies. It thus remains to be seen whether with improved neonatal management and survival of severely sick neonates the profile of long-term pulmonary sequelae will drift towards greater morbidity.

The uniqueness of neonatal lung disease is its temporary coincidence with a vulnerable period of lung maturation. As a consequence, outcome is not only determined by the circulatory and gas exchange capacity of the lungs at birth, but also by the extent of secondary adaptations of the pulmonary architecture to the mostly precocious exposure to extrauterine environment and medical intervention. Before the recognition of oxygen toxicity and barotrauma as important mediators of secondary lung injury [1, 2], long-term outcome of neonatal lung disease was substantially influenced by the aggressiveness of mechanical ventilation and hence the severity of neonatal respiratory distress [3]. The resulting pulmonary sequelae were represented by the histopathological features of classic bronchopulmonary dysplasia (BPD). With the introduction of surfactant therapy and the implementation of lung-protective ventilation strategies, long-term respiratory outcome has become increasingly determined by the size and maturity of the newborn child and by the multitude of comorbidities with pulmonary involvement encountered during infancy and childhood [4–6]. With better survival of more vulnerable very low birth weight (VLBW) infants the prevalence of pulmonary sequelae has not declined as could have been expected from improved management of the more mature neonates [7, 8]. Chorioamnionitis, postnatal infection, and patent ductus arteriosus further augment the risk of secondary lung damage in the prematurely born children [9–12]. If the consequent structural changes are severe enough to cause ongoing compromise of pulmonary function, chronic lung disease (CLD) of infancy results, as defined by prolonged need for oxygen supplementation with or without ventilatory support [13].

Histopathological and Functional Characteristics of Neonatal Lung Disease

The generation of new airways being concluded towards mid-gestation, normal lung development during the last trimester of pregnancy is restricted to airway growth and alveolar multiplication and maturation [14, 15]. Post-mortem studies of young, prematurely born children dying with CLD have shown a markedly reduced number of alveoli with no evidence of compensatory postnatal proliferation, but an arrest of the acinar development in the alveolar saccular and alveolar stage [16–18]. Observations of decreased alveolization in animal models of BPD further corroborated these findings [19, 20]. In addition, alveolar fibrosis was found to be a consistent and prominent feature of children dying with CLD [21]. While earlier studies of infants diagnosed with classic BPD reported a more patchy distribution of heavily fibrosed alveoli side by side with minimally injured but hyperexpanded alveoli [1, 18], newer studies of children dying after the introduction of surfactant instillation showed less but more evenly distributed alveolar fibrosis [18]. Peribronchiolar smooth muscle hypertrophy, fibrosis of the airways, necrotizing bronchiolitis, mucus gland hypertrophy, and acinar arterial thickening are among the other histological features associated with BPD [17, 22, 23]. Although these autopsy findings may describe changes at the worst end of the spectrum, it is felt that similar, though maybe less pronounced changes will be found in survivors of CLD [24].

The consequences of these structural changes are measurable functional abnormalities in many survivors of neonatal lung disease. Recent pulmonary function testing in neonates and young infants with CLD revealed increased levels of functional residual capacity (FRC) by plethysmography and decreased FRC values by nitrogen washout, suggesting the presence of trapped air [25]. Several studies revealed increased airway resistance with a reduction of maximum flows at FRC by more than 50% of predicted, and tidal breathing approaching expiratory flow limitation [26–28]. Specific dynamic compliance may be reduced by more than 50% [29], and work of breathing was reported to be significantly increased [30]. In addition, airway hyperresponsiveness, as reflected by a significant response to bronchodilating

substances, may be present early in CLD [31, 32]. Encouragingly, data retrieved in more recent years point towards less disordered lung function in extremely low birth weight infants surviving modern neonatal intensive care [33].

In the following, long-term outcome of specific neonatal lung diseases will be reviewed focused on pulmonary morbidity. Many survivors, however, have additional health problems involving a variety of other organ systems which cannot be reviewed in this chapter.

Bronchopulmonary Dysplasia and Chronic Lung Disease of Infancy

Evolution of Lung Function from Infancy to Adolescence
Infancy. Longitudinal follow-up studies of children with CLD have generally shown an improvement of airway physiology and elastic properties during infancy and early childhood. Pulmonary compliance was found to improve from 6 to 12 months of age in CLD [5]. Maximum flow rates at FRC were reported to increase significantly within the first two years along with a reduction of airway resistance [34]. Nevertheless, absolute and size-corrected flow rates of infants with BPD remained below those of age- and size-matched controls [26, 27, 35], and infants with CLD reveal slower gas mixing than prematurely born children without CLD at 1 year of age [5]. A minority of children with severe BPD might even fail to improve airway mechanics: a longitudinal study over a 3-year-period found no increment of maximum expiratory flows at 25% of forced vital capacity (FVC) in 6 children with severe BPD requiring more than 9 months of mechanical ventilatory support [36].

Improvement of airway physiology within the first 4 postnatal weeks reflected by a reduction of airway resistance and work of breathing was also reported in non-ventilated low birth weight infants [37]. Recent single institution studies suggested that increased airway resistance in low birth weight infants at the age of 6 months may indeed be independent from mechanical ventilation in the neonatal period [28], although differences in ventilatory support strategies clearly contribute to a high inter-hospital variation of CLD prevalence [38].

Childhood and Adolescence. Lung size increases during the first years of life when the child is growing, and except for the severest cases, respiratory reserve augments. Regardless of still prevailing lung function abnormalities, this is associated with decreasing pulmonary morbidity. While wheezing episodes, chronic coughing and re-admissions to hospital are common in infants and young toddlers with

CLD, tolerance to intermittent respiratory tract infections subsequently improves [39–44]. However, at least one fifth of BPD children may continue to have increased respiratory morbidity beyond 2 years of age [45, 46].

Body plethysmography studies in older children and adolescents generally reveal normal total lung capacities (TLC) [39, 41, 44, 47–49] with some degree of hyperinflation reflected by an increased residual volume (RV) [48, 50] and RV/TLC ratio, respectively [39, 41, 44, 48, 51]. Vital capacity (VC) was found in the lower range of normal [52], and FRC and thoracic gas volumes (TGV) are normal or mildly increased [41, 48, 50, 52–54]. Again, differences between FRC determined by helium dilution and TGV measured with body plethysmography may indicate the presence of trapped air [50]. Consistently, children diagnosed with BPD are more prone to hyperinflation than prematurely born children without BPD [39, 41, 48, 55]. Dynamic pulmonary function measurements frequently show some degree of airway obstruction and reduced dynamic compliance. The latter was reported to be 57% of the control group in BPD at the age of 7.8 years, and 74% in prematurely born children without CLD [54]. FVC may be slightly reduced both in BPD and in VLBW children without BPD [42, 44, 56]. In most cases, forced expiratory volume in 1 s (FEV_1) values lie within the lower normal range or slightly beneath, but a minority have moderate to severe airway obstruction. Cross-sectional studies reported mean FEV_1 values from 64 to 95% and forced mid-expiratory flow ($FEF_{25–75}$) values from 40 to 67% predicted in cohorts of BPD [3, 39, 41, 44, 47, 48, 50, 52, 57–59], and FEV_1 from 83 to 98% and $FEF_{25–75}$ from 75 to 92% in prematurely born subjects without BPD [3, 39, 41, 44, 48, 51, 52, 56, 58, 59].

Risk Profile for Pulmonary Morbidity and Lung Function Abnormalities

Children with BPD were consistently found to be at a higher risk both for chronic respiratory morbidity and for lung function abnormalities compared to preterm-born children without BPD [39, 41, 45, 54]. Birth weight of prematurely born children was found to be one of the strongest predictors of persisting lung function abnormalities [42, 44, 60–62], albeit not for chronic respiratory morbidity [44, 62]. Prematurity, in contrast, has been identified as risk factor for chronic respiratory morbidity [40, 62, 63], with every extra week of pregnancy being reported to reduce the risk of chronic wheezing by 10% [62], but it is controversial as an independent predictor of long-term pulmonary function outcome [44, 60, 63, 64]. Whether a low birth weight of <2,500 g in the absence of prematurity, however, is indeed associated with poor lung function in adolescence is unclear

[65, 66]. Existing data suggest that parental smoking may not increase the risk for chronic respiratory morbidity [41, 54, 56], but the issue is controversial as is the role of mechanical ventilation and oxygen exposure in the neonatal period for predicting lung function abnormalities [41, 42, 44, 48, 51, 56, 64, 67–69].

Airway Hyperresponsiveness

Bronchial hyperresponsiveness (BHR) persisting into late childhood and adolescence has been observed both in children with BPD and prematurely born children without a history of CLD. The prevalence of responsiveness to bronchodilators or hyperresponsiveness to histamine or methacholine challenges was reported in a wide range from 23 to 72% [48, 50–53, 70, 71]. There is considerable controversy regarding the aetiology of BHR in these children. Airway damage during neonatal respiratory therapy has been inculpated by some [59], but others found no association with neonatal history [49, 51, 70]. Airway inflammation does not seem to play a decisive role in BHR outside the atopic setting [72]. Not surprisingly, a positive family history for atopy has been found to interact with the prevalence of BHR in prematurely born children as well. In addition, maternal asthma has been suggested as causative factor of prematurity [70, 73, 74], but a large study found no association between maternal asthma and preterm birth or BHR [75]. However, there seems to be a gender-dependent interrelation between maternal asthma and premature birth. Von Mutius et al. [63], in a study encompassing more than 5,000 children, found prematurity to be associated with asthma in preadolescent girls only. Adding up to this observation is a recent study suggesting that a female fetus has an adverse effect on maternal asthma, which when not treated with inhaled glucocorticosteroids results in reduced fetal growth [76].

Diffusion Capacity of the Lung for Carbon Monoxide, Dependency on Supplemental Oxygen, Pulmonary Hypertension and Exercise Performance

Prolonged oxygen dependency is a criterion of BPD and CLD [13], and likely originates from a multitude of factors including airway obstruction with impaired gas mixing, reduced gas transfer, ventilation perfusion mismatch, and impeded pulmonary circulation. In the long-term perspective, impaired oxygenation is usually not a significant contributor of morbidity. The majority of children are weaned from supplemental oxygen within the first year of life [77]. Exceptions to this include children with very severe BPD, pulmonary hypertension (PHT), and large systemic to pulmonary collateral vessels [78]. The presence of PHT in particular is associated with ongoing respiratory morbidity and high mortality in infants with BPD [79, 80].

Nevertheless, data on the evolution of PHT in BPD are scarce. Within the first year of life, pulmonary artery pressures (PAP) were shown to improve by Doppler echocardiography [81]. One study reported 4 children with BPD followed for PHT by cardiac catheterization to have persistently elevated albeit ameliorating PAP at a mean age of 4.4 years, with a further decrease to supplemental oxygen. These children, however, resided at moderately elevated altitude (1,600 m above sea level) [82]. More recently, 76 survivors of mild to moderate CLD assessed by echocardiogram were reported to have average PAP in the upper normal range at 4 years of age [83]. However, 19% of the children who had abnormal chest radiographs and 39% of those with normal chest radiographs were diagnosed with PHT in this study [83]. Results from exercise studies indicate that PHT is rare later in childhood but might occasionally be present even in asymptomatic individuals [41, 49, 72].

Significant limitations to gas exchange are exceptional in older children with BPD. Although D_{CO} may be lower than in controls, reported mean values invariably lie within the normal range [3, 47, 50, 51, 84–86]. In addition, significant oxygen desaturation during exertion is uncommon in prematurely born children and most likely seen in BPD [52, 58, 60, 84, 85, 87], reflecting an inability of BPD children to increase gas exchange capacity with exercise, as measured by acetylene transfer [85]. Encouragingly, a majority of exercise studies performed in children with BPD and prematurely born children without CLD revealed average exercise capacities in the normal to low-normal range [39, 52, 58, 60, 84], although BPD children may show increased exercise hyperpnea using more of their respiratory reserve [54, 84, 86]. Others, in contrast, found lower ventilatory responses in BPD [88], and some studies reported decreased maximum oxygen consumption in prematurely born children with or without CLD [58, 87, 88]. Exercise-induced asthma was found in 10% of VLBW children [42], and a close correlation between FEV_1 and exercise capacity was observed in BPD [84].

Is CLD/BPD a Disease of Adulthood?

The primary concern for the long-term survival of any child with a paediatric disease is whether or not life expectancy and ability to live independently is adversely affected. Although the study by Northway et al. [3] in young adults who survived BPD as infants revealed relatively mild impairment with a mean FEV_1 of 74.8 ± 2.9% predicted, the individual data showed that 20% had either severe airway obstruction or hyperinflation, and 12% were considered to have severe asthma. Of note, the mean gestational age of 33.2 ± 3.8 weeks and birth weight of 1,894 ± 703 g would, by today's standards, be considered mild degrees of prematurity. The question therefore arises whether these young adults are representative of the more recent BPD survivors. Jacob et al. [48] in their study specifically looked at those with severe disease as defined by a need for supplemental oxygen at 44 weeks post-conceptional age and at the time of hospital discharge. These children had a mean gestational age of 28.7 ± 2.1 weeks and birth weight of 1,110 ± 328 g, reflecting the changing pattern of survival of prematurely born infants between the sixties and eighties. All were born in a period when barotrauma and oxygen exposure was minimized, but before postnatal steroid and surfactant were introduced into neonatal care. The mean requirement for home oxygen was almost 2 years, with 3 infants requiring supplemental oxygen for more than 900 days. At a mean age at follow-up of 10.6 ± 1.7 years, the mean FEV_1 was 63 ± 21% predicted, and in 20% it was ≤40%. Pressure-volume curves were measured in 9 of 15, showing a mixed pattern of curves which were shifted up and flattened, in keeping with a loss of elastic recoil as seen in asthma in some individuals [89], and elevated and steeper than normal in keeping with the radiological picture of hyperinflation and fibrosis in others. The authors speculated that the abnormalities demonstrated in these severely affected children at 11 years of age would be carried into adulthood. Only a few longitudinal studies have been published investigating the potential for improvement of lung function from mid childhood onwards. In a study of children with BPD, an increasing FEV_1 from 63 ± 11 to 72 ± 16% was found from age 7–10 years, while RV and RV/TLC remained elevated [50]. Another study in prematurely born children with a history of CLD but normal FEV_1 and only mildly reduced FEF_{25-75} showed normalization of hyperinflation in the period from 8–15 years of life [71].

Starting out as an adult with severe airway obstruction would suggest that the loss of elastic recoil that accompanies the aging process could result in severe respiratory impairment at a young age. The effects of smoking could accelerate these changes resulting in the appearance of chronic obstructive pulmonary disease (COPD) at a much earlier age than would be expected in the term-born population. With a rate of premature birth in the order of 7%, if only 1% of prematurely born children had 'severe' BPD, this would still yield a disease prevalence of the same order of magnitude as cystic fibrosis. In other words, severe CLD/BPD is becoming an 'adults' disease and questions regarding birth should be part of any respiratory history in an adult.

In summary for a vast majority of CLD/BPD survivors, growth is associated with increasing respiratory reserve and significant clinical improvement. The characteristic functional sequelae comprise mild airway obstruction with reduced flow rates and some degree of air trapping. In addition, dynamic compliance measurements suggest that the lungs remain slightly stiffer. As is commonly found in survivors of neonatal lung disease, the prevalence of BHR is high, which should be accounted for when evaluating follow-up data. Pulmonary circulation similarly improves with growth, but PAP should be expected to remain elevated even in asymptomatic individuals. Although some might use more of their respiratory reserve during exercise, physical capacity is normal in most survivors of CLD. It is noteworthy, however, that all cohorts of CLD survivors contain some individuals with severe residual compromise of ventilatory and circulatory function, especially among those diagnosed with BPD.

Congenital Diaphragmatic Hernia

Intrauterine displacement of abdominal organs into the thoracic cavity in children with congenital diaphragmatic hernia (CDH) is associated with bilateral pulmonary hypoplasia, which is characterized by a numerical reduction of airways, alveoli, and vascular generations [90–93]. As in BPD, histological follow-up is only available from children who eventually died, thus presumably representing the severest end of the spectrum. These studies revealed compensatory emphysematous changes on both sides, and some catch-up growth by increased alveolization was described on the contralateral side in CDH [91, 94, 95].

Due to their reduced pulmonary reserve, infants with CDH are more prone to pulmonary exacerbation from viral respiratory tract infections than normal babies [96, 97]. A high prevalence of gastro-esophageal reflux additionally contributes to chronic pulmonary morbidity early in the lives of these children [98–100]. With increasing age, however, infection-related pulmonary morbidity tends to decrease [96], and most children will have little restriction in their daily activities in the long-term, though some remain more susceptible to respiratory disease [101–104].

Pulmonary function tests in later childhood and adolescence mostly showed normal TLC [101, 105–107], but in general revealed some degree of airway obstruction with a tendency of hyperinflation, reflected by increased RV/TLC [105, 106]. Decreased chest wall compliance may contribute to higher RV, as scoliosis and chest deformities such

as pectus excavatum are frequent in CDH [103, 108]. Cross-sectional follow-up studies typically show FEV_1 values distributed over a wide range, with the means of FEV_1 situated in the lower normal range [101, 107, 109], or slightly beneath [97, 102, 105, 106]. In addition, there is a high prevalence of airway hyperresponsiveness in these children [102, 105]. As most studies did not report spirometry data after bronchodilation, fixed airway obstruction might be less frequent than suggested. In agreement with the relatively mild abnormalities of airway mechanics, air entry to both lungs assessed by nuclear ventilation scans frequently normalizes even in children with severe respiratory distress in the neonatal period, although some side differences of the ventilation rate may remain detectable [97, 101, 110, 111].

While respiratory variables improve in childhood, pulmonary circulation shows much less potential for catch-up growth. Histologically, medial and adventitial thickening of acinar arteries and veins and the absence of normal postnatal arterial remodelling are consistent features early after CDH repair [112–114]. On a functional level, PHT causes ongoing pulmonary morbidity in some CDH patients even after resolution of ventilatory insufficiency [96, 115], and PHT has been reported in as many as 38% of patients with repaired CDH at 3.2 ± 1.4 years of age [116]. Persistence of scintigraphic perfusion asymmetries and ventilation perfusion mismatch in adolescent CDH survivors who had severe neonatal respiratory distress suggest limited developmental reserve of the ipsilateral pulmonary vascular bed [97, 103, 111]. It is unclear, however, how many adolescent CDH survivors have abnormal pulmonary pressures. Echocardiographic studies in adolescent patients born between 1960 and 1976 did not reveal evidence of persisting PHT [101]. Exercise studies may show reduced physical capacity in a number of CDH patients, but life style and stigmatization probably contribute to lower exercise performance in these patients [104, 106].

In conclusion, similarly to survivors of CLD, children with CHD usually are asymptomatic by adolescence, but on average show mild residual hyperinflation and some airway obstruction on pulmonary function testing. There is, however, a wide range from completely normal measurements in many to severely compromised lung function in a few individuals. Residual chest wall deformities might impede respiratory forces and the capability to fully exhale. Again, there is a high prevalence of BHR persisting into adolescence. Perfusion to the ipsilateral lung remains reduced in most patients, and exercise capacity may be slightly impaired. However, the prevalence of PHT later in childhood in CDH patients is unknown.

Congenital Malformations of the Lung

Pulmonary sequestration, congenital cystic adenomatoid malformation, bronchogenic and other foregut cysts, and congenital lobar emphysema (CLE) are among the more frequently encountered congenital malformations of the lung. These lesions may present early in life with respiratory distress due to space-occupational effects, or they may be found later by chance on chest imaging films done for other reasons or because of secondary complications, such as chronic cough, wheezing, blue spells, infection, pneumothorax, haemorrhage, or malignant transformation [117–119]. Successful conservative management is being advocated in CLE with mild or no symptoms [120], but for other clinically silent malformations the expectant approach remains controversial [121–125]. If symptoms occur, interventional therapy by surgical resection or, more recently, embolization for pulmonary sequestration, is generally accepted as the treatment of choice [126–128].

Long-term follow-up studies are largely focused on the capacity of the remaining lung to compensate for the loss of tissue after pulmonary resection. This implies that the surrounding lung is generally considered to be normal [129], although not much systematic information is available on this issue. Studies in rats and foxhounds suggested that augmented alveolar multiplication indeed occurs after pneumonectomy in very young animals, while in older individuals the loss of lung tissue is compensated by distension of the existing air space only [130, 131]. Work done in beagles, however, at a 5-year follow-up after pneumonectomy failed to document a difference in alveolar count between early and late resection [132]. This would imply that the age of resection had relatively little relevance to the long-term pulmonary outcome [133].

In humans, follow-up studies predominantly relate to clinical, radiographic, and pulmonary function evaluation. The majority of patients without associated extrapulmonary pathology do not suffer from increased morbidity once the malformation is successfully removed [126, 127, 134–136]. Resection of up to three segments seems to have little impact on lung volumes and dynamic measures [137]. It has been speculated that some compensatory lung growth occurs in young infants after resection based on the observation that residual lung volumes were higher than what would have been expected from the proportion of lung tissue removed [138]. However, the observed 10% reduction of lung volumes corresponds to the amount of volume loss found after lobectomy in adults [139]. In addition, a study comparing conservatively and surgically treated infants with CLE found no significant differences in lung function at 10 years of age [120]. Mild to moderate elevation of RV and FRC commonly found after lobectomy favours the concept that overexpansion of the residual lung contributes to compensation of volume loss [120, 140]. This is further corroborated by the scintigraphic finding of reduced perfusion to the lung field of the resected lobe [140]. Limited information on exercise performance indicates, however, that lobectomy does not, in the long-term, significantly affect physical capacity in children and adults [138, 141, 142]. It is well understood, that pulmonary function and exercise performance are more compromised in the rare cases were removal of an entire lung is required.

In summary, long-term follow-up findings in patients with localized congenital lung malformations depend on the capacity of the remaining lung to compensate for the volume loss after resection of the malformation. Lobectomy is usually well tolerated by young children with an expected functional volume loss in the range of 10%, which does not significantly affect respiratory health and exercise capacity. In the rare cases where larger parts must be removed, the function of gas exchange as well as pulmonary circulation will be compromised. Early resection might induce some compensatory alveolization, but existing data are not solid enough to justify the risk of a surgical intervention in the neonatal period in infants who are stable enough to allow some growth and adaptation to extrauterine life before surgery.

Meconium Aspiration Syndrome

Meconium aspiration syndrome (MAS) is diagnosed when respiratory distress develops in a neonate who was delivered through meconium-stained amniotic fluid. Inflammation, bronchial obstruction, surfactant dysfunction, and pulmonary vascular dysregulation contribute to the complex pathogenesis and account for the patchy radiological appearances of this syndrome [143]. MAS is very uncommon in prematurely born children and, hence, an arrest of pulmonary development as seen in association with prematurity is unexpected [144]. Instead, histopathological changes from MAS rather resemble the pattern of lung injury seen in patients with acute respiratory distress syndrome, with areas of atelectasis being in direct vicinity to overinflated districts, resulting in uneven exposure to oxygen and barotrauma.

There is limited information on long-term pulmonary sequelae of MAS. Clinically, these children may have an increased risk for recurrent cough and wheezing, but most are completely asymptomatic following recovery from MAS [145–147]. Mild cases who are manageable without

Table 1. Considerations regarding the pulmonary follow-up of survivors of various neonatal lung diseases

	CLD/BPD	CDH	Cong. malformation	MAS
General considerations	Standardized follow-up programmes recommended for high prevalence of comorbidities	Standardized follow-up programmes recommended for high prevalence of comorbidities	Follow-up mandatory for conservatively managed cases	Regular follow-up warranted in rare cases only
RSV prophylaxis	Recommended according to (inter-)national guidelines	Not recommended for lack of scientific data	Not recommended for lack of scientific data	Not recommended for lack of scientific data
Sleep monitoring	Recommended for infants with oxygen dependency, suspected apnoeas, or persisting PHT	Recommended for infants with oxygen dependency, suspected apnoeas, or persisting PHT	Recommended for infants with oxygen dependency, suspected apnoeas, or persisting PHT	Recommended for infants with oxygen dependency, suspected apnoeas, or persisting PHT
Pneumococcal vaccine	No specific recommendation besides (inter-)national guidelines	No specific recommendation outside (inter-)national guidelines	No specific recommendation outside (inter-)national guidelines	No specific recommendation outside (inter-)national guidelines
Radiographic follow-up	Recommended until stable appearance and in case of ongoing respiratory morbidity: Aspiration? Bronchial wall thickening? Pulmonary circulation?	Recommended until stable appearance and in case of ongoing respiratory morbidity: Aspiration? Bronchial wall thickening? Pulmonary circulation? Missed associated lung malformation? Relapse of DH? Scoliosis?	Recommended until stable appearance. High index of suspicion for complications in conservatively managed cases	Recommended until stable appearance
Lung function testing	5–7 years: pre- and post-bronchodilator spirometry suggested even in asymptomatic individuals. 10–12 years: follow-up recommended, may consider bronchial challenge	5–7 years: pre- and post-bronchodilator spirometry suggested even in asymptomatic individuals. 10–12 years: follow-up recommended, may consider bronchial challenge	5–7 years: recommended for children with significant neonatal respiratory distress, in-cluding pre- and post-bronchodilator spirometry	5–7 years: pre- and post-bronchodilator spirometry suggested for children with significant neonatal respiratory distress
Echocardiography	Follow-up until normalized. Consider scheduled follow-up into adolescence for lack of published data on evolution of PAP, at least in individuals with abnormal lung function	Follow-up until normalized. Consider scheduled follow-up into adolescence for lack of published data on evolution of PAP in all individuals	Follow-up until normalized. Consider scheduled follow-up for pneumonectomy	Follow-up until normalized
Exercise testing	Not recommended routinely	Not recommended routinely	Not recommended routinely	Not recommended routinely
Gastro-esophageal reflux	High index of suspicion	High index of suspicion	No published data. High index of suspicion in individuals fulfilling criteria of CLD/BPD	No published data. High index of suspicion in individuals fulfilling criteria of CLD/BPD

CLD = chronic lung disease; BPD = bronchopulmonary dysplasia; CDH = congenital diaphragmatic hernia; Cong. = congenital; MAS = meconium aspiration syndrome; PHT = pulmonary hypertension; DH = diaphragmatic hernia; PAP = pulmonary artery pressure.

invasive ventilation are not likely to suffer from significant pulmonary lung function abnormalities later in childhood [148]. Those requiring mechanical ventilation may subsequently have a higher prevalence of airway hyperresponsiveness as described for survivors of other neonatal lung diseases, but not all studies concur [145–147]. In addition, some found MAS survivors to be at risk of hyperinflation (mean RV/TLC of 30%, range 18–54), and decreased closing volumes were described in these subjects [147]. Recent follow-up of a cohort of 17 adolescents surviving severe MAS requiring extracorporeal membrane oxygenation has revealed exercise-induced bronchoconstriction in 41% of subjects, with mild air trapping evident after exercise [149]. Encouragingly, no significant differences in aerobic capacity were found compared to controls.

Although children with MAS may have severe lung disease as neonates, existing data suggests that little residual compromise of pulmonary function persists in the long-term. Reported abnormalities include a higher prevalence of hyperinflation and BHR.

Suggestions for Follow-Up of Survivors of Neonatal Lung Disease

Authors' considerations regarding long-term management of survivors of the neonatal lung pathologies discussed above are summarised in table 1. For more detailed recommendations regarding survivors of CLD and BPD, please refer to published statements [4].

References

1 Northway WH Jr, Rosan RC, Porter DY: Pulmonary disease following respirator therapy of hyaline-membrane disease. N Engl J Med 1967;276:357–368.

2 O'Brodovich HM, Mellins RB: Bronchopulmonary dysplasia: Unresolved neonatal acute lung injury. Am Rev Respir Dis 1985;132:694–709.

3 Northway WH Jr, Moss RB, Carlisle KB, Parker BR, Popp RL, Pitlick PT, Eichler I, Lamm RL, Brown BW: Late pulmonary sequelae of bronchopulmonary dysplasia. N Engl J Med 1990;323:1793–1799.

4 American Thoracic Society: Statement on the care of the child with chronic lung disease of infancy and childhood. Am J Respir Crit Care Med 2003;168:356–396.

5 Merth IT, de Winter JP, Zonderland HM, Borsboom GJJM, Quanier PH: Pulmonary function in infants with neonatal chronic lung disease with or without hyaline membrane disease at birth. Eur Respir J 1997;10:1606–1613.

6 Sinkin RA, Cox C, Phelps DL: Predicting risk for bronchopulmonary dysplasia: Selection criteria for clinical trials. Pediatrics 1990;86:728–736.

7 Manktelow BN, Draper ES, Annamalai S, Field S: Factors affecting the incidence of chronic lung disease of prematurity in 1987, 1992, and 1997. Arch Dis Child Fetal Neonatal Ed 2001;85:F33–F35.

8 Parker RA, Lindstrom DP, Cotton RB: Improved survival accounts for most, but not all, of the increase in bronchopulmonary dysplasia. Pediatrics 1992;90:663–668.

9 Gonzales A, Sosenko IR, Chandar J, Hummler H, Claure N, Bancalari E: Influence of infection on patent ductus arteriosus and chronic lung disease in premature infants weighing 1000 grams or less. J Pediatr 1996;128:470–478.

10 Rojas MA, Gonzalez A, Bancalari E, Claure N, Poole C, Silva-Neto G: Changing trends in the epidemiology and pathogenesis of neonatal chronic lung disease. J Pediatr 1995;126:605–610.

11 Van Marter LJ, Dammann O, Allred EN, Leviton A, Pagano M, Moore M, Martin C: Chorioamnionitis, mechanical ventilation, and postnatal sepsis as modulators of chronic lung disease in preterm infants. J Pediatr 2002;140:171–176.

12 Watterberg KL, Demers LM, Scott SM, Murphy S: Chorioamnionitis and early lung inflammation in infants on whom bronchopulmonary dysplasia develops. Pediatrics 1996;97:210–215.

13 Jobe AH, Bancalari E: Bronchopulmonary dysplasia. Am J Respir Crit Care Med 2001;163:1723–1729.

14 Zeltner TB, Caduff JH, Gehr P, Pfenninger J, Burri PH: The postnatal development and growth of the human lung. I. Morphometry. Respir Physiol 1986;67:247–267.

15 Hislop A, Reid L: Development of the acinus in the human lung. Thorax 1974;29:90–94.

16 Hislop AA, Wigglesworth JS, Desai R, Aber V: The effects of preterm delivery and mechanical ventilation on human lung growth. Early Hum Dev 1987;15:147–164.

17 Margraf LR, Tomashefski JF Jr, Bruce MC, Dahms BB: Morphometric analysis of the lung in bronchopulmonary dysplasia. Am Rev Respir Dis 1991;143:391–400.

18 Husain AN, Siddiqui NH, Stocker JT: Pathology of arrested acinar development in postsurfactant bronchopulmonary dysplasia. Hum Pathol 1998;29:710–717.

19 Albertine KH, Jones GP, Starcher BC, Bohnsack JF, Davis PL, Cho SC, Carlton DP, Bland RD: Chronic lung injury in preterm lambs: Disordered respiratory tract development. Am J Respir Crit Care Med 1999;159:945–958.

20 Coalson JJ, Winter V, deLemos RA: Decreased alveolarization in baboon survivors with bronchopulmonary dysplasia. Am J Respir Crit Care Med 1995;152:640–646.

21 Stocker JT: Pathologic features of long-standing 'healed' bronchopulmonary dysplasia. Hum Pathol 1986;17:943–961.

22 Thibeault DW, Truog WE, Ekekezie II: Acinar arterial changes with chronic lung disease of prematurity in the surfactant era. Pediatr Pulmonol 2003;36:482–489.

23 Bonikos DS, Bensch KG, Northway WH Jr, Edwards DK: Bronchopulmonary dysplasia: The pulmonary pathologic sequel of necrotizing bronchiolitis and pulmonary fibrosis. Hum Pathol 1976;7:643–666.

24 Hislop AA: Bronchopulmonary Dysplasia: Pre- and postnatal influences and outcome. Pediatr Pulmonol 1997;23:71–75.

25 Wauer RR, Maurer T, Nowotny T, Schmalisch G: Assessment of functional residual capacity using nitrogen washout and plethysmographic techniques in infants with and without bronchopulmonary dysplasia. Intensive Care Med 1998;24:469–475.

26 Iles R, Edmunds AT: Assessment of pulmonary function in resolving chronic lung disease of prematurity. Arch Dis Child Fetal Neonatal Ed 1997;76:F113–F117.

27 Tepper RS, Morgan WJ, Cota K, Taussig LM: Expiratory flow limitation in infants with bronchopulmonary dysplasia. J Pediatr 1986;109:1040–1046.

28 Yuksel B, Greenough A, Green S: Lung function abnormalities at 6 months of age after neonatal intensive care. Arch Dis Child 1991;66:472–476.

29 Gerhardt T, Hehre D, Feller R, Reifenberg L, Bancalari E: Serial determination of pulmonary function in infants with chronic lung disease. J Pediatr 1987;110:448–456.

30 Wolfson MR, Bhutani VK, Shaffer TH, Bowen FW Jr: Mechanics and energetics of breathing helium in infants with bronchopulmonary dysplasia. J Pediatr 1984;104:752–757.

31 Motoyama EK, Fort MD, Klesh KW, Mutich RL, Guthrie RD: Early onset of airway reactivity in premature infants with bronchopulmonary dysplasia. Am Rev Respir Dis 1987; 136:50–57.

32 Gomez-Del Rio M, Gerhardt T, Hehre D, Feller R, Bancalari E. Effect of a beta-agonist nebulization on lung function in neonates with increased pulmonary resistance. Pediatr Pulmonol 1986;2:287–291.

33 Fitzgerald DA, Mesiano G, Brosseau L, Davis GM: Pulmonary outcome in extremely low birth weight infants. Pediatrics 2000;105: 1209–1215.

34 Farstad T, Brockmeier F, Bratlid D: Cardiopulmonary function in premature infants with bronchopulmonary dysplasia – A 2-year follow up. Eur J Pediatr 1995;154:853–858.

35 De Boeck K, Smith J, Van Lierde S, Devlieger H: Response to bronchodilators in clinically stable 1-year-old patients with bronchopulmonary dysplasia. Eur J Pediatr 1998;157:75–79.

36 Mallory GB, Chaney H, Mutich RL, Motoyama EK: Longitudinal changes in lung function during the first three years of premature infants with moderate to severe bronchopulmonary dysplasia. Pediatr Pulmonol 1991;11:8–14.

37 Abbasi S, Bhutani VK: Pulmonary mechanics and energetics of normal, non-ventilated low birth weight infants. Pediatr Pulmonol 1990;8:89–95.

38 Van Marter LJ, Allred EN, Pagano M, Sanocka U, Parad R, Moore M, Susser M, Paneth N, Leviton A: Do clinical markers of barotrauma and oxygen toxicity explain interhospital variation in rates of chronic lung disease? Pediatrics 2000;105:1194–1201.

39 Gross SJ, Iannuzzi DM, Kveselis DA, Anbar RD: Effect of preterm birth on pulmonary function at school age: A prospective controlled study. J Pediatr 1998;133:188–192.

40 Korhonen P, Koivisto AM, Ikonen S, Laippala P, Tammela O: Very low birthweight, bronchopulmonary dysplasia and health in early childhood. Acta Paediatr 1999;88:1385–1391.

41 Hakulinen AL, Heinonen K, Länsimies E, Kiekara O: Pulmonary function and respiratory morbidity in school-aged children born prematurely and ventilated for neonatal respiratory distress. Pediatr Pulmonol 1990;8: 226–232.

42 McLeod A, Ross P, Mitchell S, Tay D, Hunter L, Hall A, Paton J, Mutch L: Respiratory health in a total very low birth weight cohort and their classroom controls. Arch Dis Child 1996;74:188–194.

43 Wong YC, Beardsmore CS, Silverman M. Pulmonary sequelae of neonatal respiratory distress in very low birth weight infants: A clinical and physiological study. Arch Dis Child 1982;57:418–424.

44 Kitchen WH, Olinski A, Doyle LW, Ford GW, Murton LJ, Slonim L, Callanan C: Respiratory health and lung function in 8-year-old children of very low birth weight: A cohort study. Pediatrics 1992;89: 1151–1158.

45 Palta M, Sadek M, Barnet JH, Evans M, Weinstein MR, McGuiness G, Peters ME, Gabbert D, Fryback D, Farrell P: Evaluation of criteria for chronic lung disease in surviving very low birth weight infants. J Pediatr 1998;132:57–63.

46 Kitchen WH, Ford GW, Doyle LW, Richards AL, Kelly EA: Health and hospital readmission of very-low-birth-weight and normal-birth-weight children. Am J Dis Child 1990; 144:2213–2218.

47 de Kleine MJK, Roos CM, Voorn WJ, Jansen HM, Koppe JG: Lung function 8–18 years after intermittent positive pressure ventilation for hyaline membrane disease. Thorax 1990;45:941–946.

48 Jacob SV, Coates AL, Lands LC, MacNeish CF, Riley SP, Hornby L, Outerbridge EW, Davis GM, Williams RL: Long-term pulmonary sequelae of severe bronchopulmonary dysplasia. J Pediatr 1998;133:193–200.

49 MacLusky IB, Stringer D, Zarfen J, Smallhorn J, Levison H: Cardiorespiratory status in long-term survivors of prematurity, with and without hyaline membrane disease. Pediatr Pulmonol 1986;2:94–102.

50 Blayney M, Kerem E, Whyte H, O'Brodovich H: Bronchopulmonary dysplasia: Improvement in lung function between 7 and 10 years of age. J Pediatr 1991;118:201–206.

51 Galdès-Sebaldt M, Sheller JR, Grogaard J, Stahlman M: Prematurity is associated with abnormal airway function in childhood. Pediatr Pulmonol 1989;7:259–264.

52 Andreasson B, Lindroth M, Mortensson W, Svenningsen NW, Jonson B: Lung function eight years after neonatal ventilation. Arch Dis Child 1989;64:108–113.

53 Ahrens P, Zielen S, Stover B, von Loewenich V, Hofmann D: Pulmonary sequelae of long-term ventilation of very low birth weight premature infants. Results of a follow-up study of 6-to-9-year-old children. Klin Pädiatr 1991;203:366–371.

54 Parat S, Moriette G, Delaperche M-F, Escourrou P, Denjean A, Gaultier C: Long-term pulmonary functional outcome of bronchopulmonary dysplasia and premature birth. Pediatr Pulmonol 1995;20: 289–296.

55 Wheeler WB, Castile RG, Brown ER, Wohl MEB: Pulmonary function in survivors of prematurity. Am Rev Respir Dis 1984;129:A218.

56 Mieskonen S, Eronen M, Malmberg LP, Turpeinen M, Kari MA, Hallman M: Controlled trial of dexamethasone in neonatal chronic lung disease: An 8-year follow-up of cardiopulmonary function and growth. Acta Paediatr 2003;92:896–904.

57 Giacoia GP, Venkataraman PS, West-Wilson KI, Faulkner MJ: Follow-up of school-age children with bronchopulmonary dysplasia. J Pediatr 1997;130:400–408.

58 Kilbride HW, Gelatt MC, Sabath RJ: Pulmonary function and exercise capacity for ELBW survivors in preadolescence: Effect of neonatal chronic lung disease. J Pediatr 2003;143:488–493.

59 Pelkonen AS, Hakulinen AL, Turpeinen M: Bronchial lability and responsiveness in school children born very preterm. Am J Respir Crit Care Med 1997;156:1178–1184.

60 Bader D, Ramos AD, Lew CD, Platzker AC, Stabile MW, Keens TG: Childhood sequelae of infant lung disease: Exercise and pulmonary function abnormalities after bronchopulmonary dysplasia. J Pediatr 1987;110: 693–699.

61 Barker DJP, Godfrey KM, Fall C, Osmond C, Winter PD, Shaheen SO: Relation of birth weight and childhood respiratory infection to adult lung function and death from chronic obstructive disease. BMJ 1991;303: 671–675.

62 Rona RJ, Gulliford MC, Chinn S: Effects of prematurity and intrauterine growth on respiratory health and lung function in childhood. BMJ 1993;306:817–820.

63 von Mutius E, Nicolai T, Martinez FD: Prematurity as a risk factor for asthma in preadolescent children. J Pediatr 1993;123:223–229.

64 Chan KN, Noble-Jamieson CM, Elliman A, Bryan EM, Silverman M: Lung function in children of low birth weight. Arch Dis Child 1989;64:1284–1293.

65 Matthes JWA, Lewis PA, Davies DP, Bethel JA: Birth weight at term and lung function in adolescence: No evidence for programmed effect. Arch Dis Child 1995;73:231–234.

66 Seidman DS, Laor A, Gale R, Stevenson DK, Danon YL: Is low birth weight a risk factor for asthma during adolescence? Arch Dis Child 1991;66:584–587.

67 Chan KN, Wong YC, Silverman M: Relationship between infant lung mechanics and childhood lung function in children of very low birth weight. Pediatr Pulmonol 1990;8: 74–81.

68 Coates AL, Desmond K, Willis D, Nogrady MB: Oxygen therapy and long-term pulmonary outcome of respiratory distress syndrome in newborns. Am J Dis Child 1982; 136:892–895.

69 Tammela OK, Linna OV, Koivisto ME: Long-term pulmonary sequelae in low birth weight infants with and without respiratory distress syndrome. Acta Paediatr Scand 1991;80: 542–544.

70 Chan KN, Elliman A, Bryan E, Silverman M: Clinical significance of airway responsiveness in children of low birthweight. Pediatr Pulmonol 1989;7:251–258.

71 Koumbourlis AC, Motoyama EK, Mutich RL, Mallory GB, Walczak SA, Fertal K: Longitudinal follow-up of lung function from childhood to adolescence in prematurely born patients with neonatal chronic lung disease. Pediatr Pulmonol 1996;21:28–34.

72 Mieskonen ST, Malmberg LP, Kari MA, Pelkonen AS, Turpeinen MT, Hallman NMK, Sovijärvi ARA: Exhaled nitric oxide at school age in prematurely born infants with neonatal chronic lung disease. Pediatr Pulmonol 2002;33:347–355.

73 Giffin F, Greenough A, Yuksel B: Prediction of respiratory morbidity in the third year of life in children born prematurely. Acta Paediatr 1994;83:157–158.

74 Bertrand JM, Riley SP, Popkin J, Coates AL: The long-term pulmonary sequelae of prematurity: The role of familial airway hyperactivity and the respiratory distress syndrome. N Engl J Med 1985;312:742–745.

75 Chan KN, Noble-Jamieson CM, Elliman A, Bryan EM, Aber VR, Silverman M: Airway responsiveness in low birth weight children and their mothers. Arch Dis Child 1988;63:905–910.

76 Murphy VE, Gibson PG, Giles WB, Zakar T, Smith R, Bisits AM, Kessell CG, Clifton VL: Maternal asthma is associated with reduced female fetal growth. Am J Respir Crit Care Med 2003;168:1317–1323.

77 Hudak BB, Allen MC, Hudak ML, Loughlin GM: Home oxygen therapy for chronic lung disease in extremely low-birth-weight infants. Am J Dis Child 1989;143:357–360.

78 Abman SH: Monitoring cardiovascular function in infants with chronic lung disease of prematurity. Arch Dis Child Fetal Neonatal Ed 2002;87:F15–F18.

79 Fouron JC, Le Guennec JC, Villemant D, Perreault G, Davignon A: Value of echocardiography in assessing the outcome of bronchopulmonary dysplasia of the newborn. Pediatrics 1980;65:529–535.

80 Goodman G, Perkin RM, Anas NG, Sperling DR, Hicks DA, Rowen M: Pulmonary hypertension in infants with bronchopulmonary dysplasia. J Pediatr 1988;112:67–72.

81 Subhedar NV, Shaw NJ: Changes in pulmonary arterial pressure in preterm infants with chronic lung disease. Arch Dis Child Fetal Neonatal Ed 2000;82:F243–F247.

82 Berman WJr, Katz R, Yabek SM, Dillon T, Fripp RR, Papile LA: Long-term follow-up of bronchopulmonary dysplasia. J Pediatr 1986;109:45–50.

83 Fitzgerald D, Evans N, Van Asperen P, Henderson-Smart D: Subclinical persisting pulmonary hypertension in chronic lung disease. Arch Dis Child Fetal Neonatal Ed 1994;70:F118–F122.

84 Jacob SV, Lands LC, Coates AL, Davis GM, MacNeish CF, Hornby L, Riley SP, Outerbridge EW: Exercise ability in survivors of severe bronchopulmonary dysplasia. Am J Respir Crit Care Med 1997;155:1925–1929.

85 Mitchell SH, Teague WG, Robinson A: Reduced gas transfer at rest and during exercise in school-age survivors of bronchopulmonary dysplasia. Am J Respir Crit Care Med 1998;157:1406–1412.

86 Pianosi PT, Fisk M: Cardiopulmonary exercise performance in prematurely born children. Respir Res 2000;47:653–658.

87 Pianosi P, Pelech A: Stroke volume during exercise in cystic fibrosis. Am J Respir Crit Care Med 1996;153:1105–1109.

88 Santuz P, Baraldi E, Zaramella P, Filippone M, Zacchello F: Factors limiting exercise performance in long-term survivors of bronchopulmonary dysplasia. Am J Respir Crit Care Med 1995;152:1284–1289.

89 Zapletal A, Desmond KJ, Demizio D, Coates AL: Lung recoil and the determination of airflow limitation in cystic fibrosis and asthma. Pediatr Pulmonol 1993;15:13–18.

90 Areechon W, Reid L: Hypoplasia of the lung with congenital diaphragmatic hernia. Br Med J 1963;1:230–233.

91 Beals DA, Schloo BL, Vacanti JP, Reid LM, Wilson JM: Pulmonary growth and remodeling in infants with high-risk congenital diaphragmatic hernia. J Pediatr Surg 1992;27:997–1002.

92 Geggel RL, Murphy JD, Langleben D, Crone RK, Vacanti JP, Reid LM: Congenital diaphragmatic hernia: arterial structural changes and persistent pulmonary hypertension after surgical repair. J Pediatr 1985;107:457–464.

93 Kitagawa M, Hislop A, Boyden EA, Reid L: Lung hypoplasia in congenital diaphragmatic hernia. A quantitative study of airway, artery, and alveolar development. Br J Surg 1971;58:342–346.

94 Hislop A, Reid L: Persistent hypoplasia of the lung after repair of congenital diaphragmatic hernia. Thorax 1963;31:452–455.

95 Thurlbeck WM, Kida K, Langston C, Cowan MJ, Kitterman JA, Tooley W, Bryan H: Postnatal lung growth after repair of diaphragmatic hernia. Thorax 1979;34:338–343.

96 Jaillard SM, Pierrat V, Dubois A, Truffert P, Lequien P, Wurtz AJ, Storme L: Outcome at 2 years of infants with congenital diaphragmatic hernia: A population-based study. Ann Thorac Surg 2003;75:250–256.

97 Muratore CS, Kharasch V, Lund DP, Sheils C, Friedman S, Brown C, Utter S, Jaksic T, Wilson JM: Pulmonary morbidity in 100 survivors of congenital diaphragmatic hernia monitored in a multidisciplinary clinic. J Pediatr Surg 2001;36:133–140.

98 Kieffer J, Sapin E, Berg A, Beaudoin S, Bargy F, Helardot PG: Gastroesophageal reflux after repair of congenital diaphragmatic hernia. J Pediatr Surg 1995;30:1330–1333.

99 Koot VC, Bergmeijer JH, Bos AP, Molenaar JC: Incidence and management of gastroesophageal reflux after repair of congenital diaphragmatic hernia. J Pediatr Surg 1993;28:48–52.

100 Van Meurs KP, Robbins ST, Reed VL, Karr SS, Wagner AE, Glass P, Anderson KD, Short BL: Congenital diaphragmatic hernia: Long-term outcome in neonates treated with extracorporeal membrane oxygenation. J Pediatr 1993;122:893–899.

101 Freyschuss U, Lannergren K, Frenckner B: Lung function after repair of congenital diaphragmatic hernia. Acta Paediatr Scand 1984;73:589–593.

102 Vanamo K, Rintala R, Sovijarvi A, Jaaskelainen J, Turpeinen M, Lindahl H, Louhimo I: Long-term pulmonary sequelae in survivors of congenital diaphragmatic defects. J Pediatr Surg 1996;31:1096–1100.

103 Falconer AR, Brown RA, Helms P, Gordon I, Baron JA: Pulmonary sequelae in survivors of congenital diaphragmatic hernia. Thorax 1990;45:126–129.

104 Zaccara A, Turchetta A, Calzolari A, Iacobelli B, Nahom A, Lucchetti MC, Bagolan P, Rivosecchi M, Coran AG. Maximal oxygen consumption and stress performance in children operated on for congenital diaphragmatic hernia. J Pediatr Surg 1996;31:1092–1095.

105 Ijsselstijn H, Tibboel D, Hop WJ, Molenaar JC, de Jongste JC: Long-term pulmonary sequelae in children with congenital diaphragmatic hernia. Am J Respir Crit Care Med 1997;155:174–180.

106 Marven SS, Smith CM, Claxton D, Chapman J, Davies HA, Primhak RA, Powell CVE: Pulmonary function, exercise performance, and growth in survivors of congenital diaphragmatic hernia. Arch Dis Child 1997;78:137–142.

107 Wohl MEB, Griscom NT, Striedler DJ, Schuster SR, Treves S, Zwerdling RG: The lung following repair of congenital diaphragmatic hernia. J Pediatr 1977;90:405–414.

108 Vanamo K, Peltonen J, Rintala R, Lindahl H, Jaaskelainen J, Louhimo I: Chest wall and spinal deformities in adults with congenital diaphragmatic defects. J Pediatr Surg 1996;31:851–854.

109 Wischermann A, Holschneider AM, Hubner U: Long-term follow-up of children with diaphragmatic hernia. Eur J Pediatr Surg 1995;5:13–18.

110 Jeandot R, Lambert B, Brendel AJ, Guyot M, Demarquez JL: Lung ventilation and perfusion scintigraphy in the follow up of repaired congenital diaphragmatic hernia. Eur J Nucl Med 1989;15:591–596.

111 Nagaya M, Akatsuka H, Kato J, Niimi N, Ishiguro Y: Development in lung function of the affected side after repair of congenital diaphragmatic hernia. J Pediatr Surg 1996;31:349–356.

112 Shehata SM, Tibboel D, Sharma HS, Mooi WJ: Impaired structural remodelling of pulmonary arteries in newborns with congenital diaphragmatic hernia: A histological study of 29 cases. J Pathol 1999;189:112–118.

113 Thibeault DW, Haney B: Lung volume, pulmonary vasculature, and factors affecting survival in congenital diaphragmatic hernia. Pediatrics 1998;101:289–295.

114 Yamataka T, Puri P: Pulmonary artery structural changes in pulmonary hypertension complicating congenital diaphragmatic hernia. J Pediatr Surg 1997;32:387–390.

115 Kinsella JP, Parker TA, Ivy DD, Abman SH: Noninvasive delivery of inhaled nitric oxide therapy for late pulmonary hypertension in newborn infants with congenital diaphragmatic hernia. J Pediatr 2003;142:397–401.

116 Schwartz IP, Bernbaum JC, Rychik J, Grunstein M, D'Agostino J, Polin RA: Pulmonary hypertension in children following extracorporeal membrane oxygenation therapy and repair of congenital diaphragmatic hernia. J Perinatol 1999;19:220–226.

117 Evrard V, Ceulemans J, Coosemans W, De Baere T, De Leyn P, Deneffe G, Devlieger H, De Boeck C, Van Raemdonck D, Lerut T: Congenital parenchymatous malformations of the lung. World J Surg 1999;23:1123–1132.

118 Granata C, Gambini C, Balducci T, Toma P, Michelazzi A, Conte M, Jasonni V: Bronchioloalveolar carcinoma arising in congenital cystic adenomatoid malformation in a child: A case report and review on malignancies originating in congenital cystic adenomatoid malformation. Pediatr Pulmonol 1998;25:62–66.

119 MacSweeney F, Papagiannopoulos K, Goldstraw P, Sheppard MN, Corrin B, Nicholson AG: An assessment of the expanded classification of congenital cystic adenomatoid malformations and their relationship to malignant transformation. Am J Surg Pathol 2003;27:1139–1146.

120 Eigen H, Lemen RJ, Waring WW: Congenital lobar emphysema: Long-term evaluation of surgically and conservatively treated children. Am Rev Respir Dis 1976;113:823–831.

121 Adzick NS, Harrison MR, Crombleholme TM, Flake AW, Howell LJ: Fetal lung lesions: Management and outcome. Am J Obstet Gynecol 1998;179:884–889.

122 Laberge JM, Flageole H, Pugash D, Khalife S, Blair G, Filiatrault D, Russo P, Lees G, Wilson RD: Outcome of the prenatally diagnosed congenital cystic adenomatoid lung malformation: A Canadian experience. Fetal Diagn Ther 2001;16:178–186.

123 Marshall KW, Blane CE, Teitelbaum DH, van Leeuwen K: Congenital cystic adenomatoid malformation: Impact of prenatal diagnosis and changing strategies in the treatment of the asymptomatic patient. Am J Roentgenol 2000;175:1551–1554.

124 Thorpe-Beeston JG, Nicolaides KH: Cystic adenomatoid malformation of the lung: Prenatal diagnosis and outcome. Prenat Diagn 1994;14:677–688.

125 Van Raemdonck D, De Boeck K, Devlieger H, Demedts M, Moerman P, Coosesmans W, Deneffe G, Lerut T: Pulmonary sequestration: A comparison between pediatric and adult patients. Eur J Cardio-Thorac Surg 2001;19:388–395.

126 Bogers AJJC, Hazebroek FWJ, Molenaar J, Bos E: Surgical treatment of congenital bronchopulmonary disease in children. Eur J Cardiothorac Surg 1993;7:117–20.

127 Ribet ME, Copin M-C, Gosselin BH: Bronchogenic cysts of the lung. Ann Thorac Surg 1996;61:1636–1640.

128 Wesley JR, Heidelberger KP, DiPietro MA, Cho KJ, Coran AG: Diagnosis and management of congenital cystic disease of the lung in children. J Pediatr Surg 1986;21:202–207.

129 Mentzer SJ, Filler RM, Phillips J. Limited pulmonary resections for congenital cystic adenomatoid malformation of the lung. J Pediatr Surg 1992;27:1410–1413.

130 Holmes C, Thurlbeck WM: Normal lung growth and response after pneumonectomy in rats at various ages. Am Rev Respir Dis 1979;120:1125–1136.

131 Takeda S, Hsia CC, Wagner E, Ramanathan M, Estrera AS, Weibel ER: Compensatory alveolar growth normalizes gas-exchange function in immature dogs after pneumonectomy. J Appl Physiol 1999;86:1301–1310.

132 Davies P, McBride J, Murray GF, Wilcox BR, Shallal JA, Reid L: Structural changes in the canine lung and pulmonary arteries after pneumonectomy. J Appl Physiol 1982;53:859–864.

133 Zach MS, Eber E: Adult outcome of congenital lower respiratory tract malformations. Thorax 2001;56:65–72.

134 Bratu I, Flageole H, Chen M-F, Di Lorenzo M, Yazbeck S, Laberge JM: The multiple facets of pulmonary sequestration. J Pediatr Surg 2001;36:784–790.

135 Cass DL, Crombleholme TM, Howell LJ, Stafford PW, Ruchelli ED, Adzick NS: Cystic lung lesions with systemic arterial blood supply: A hybrid of congenital cystic adenomatoid malformation and bronchopulmonary sequestration. J Pediatr Surg 1997;32:986–990.

136 Pinter A, Kalman A, Krsza L, Verebely T, Szemledy F: Long-term outcome of congenital cystic adenomatoid malformation. Pediatr Surg Int 1999;15:332–335.

137 Holschneider AM, Schlachtenrath R, Knoop U: Follow-up examination results and changes in pulmonary function following lung resection in childhood. Z Kinderchir 1990;45:349–350.

138 Frenckner B, Freyschuss U: Pulmonary function after lobectomy for congenital lobar emphysema and congenital cystic adenomatoid malformation. A follow-up study. Scand J Thorac Cardiovasc Surg 1982;16:293–298.

139 Bolliger CT, Jordan P, Soler M, Stulz P, Tamm M, Wyser C, Gonon M, Perruchoud AP: Pulmonary function and exercise capacity after lung resection. Eur Respir J 1996;9:415–421.

140 Werner HA, Pirie GE, Nadel HR, Fleisher AG, LeBlanc JG: Lung volumes, mechanics, and perfusion after pulmonary resection in infancy. J Thorac Cardiovasc Surg 1993;105:737–742.

141 Nugent A-M, Stelle IC, Carragher AM, McManus K, McGuigan JA, Gibbons JRP, Riley MS, Nicholls DP: Effect of thoracotomy and lung resection on exercise capacity in patients with lung cancer. Thorax 1999;54:334–338.

142 Pelletier C, Lapointe L, LeBlanc P: Effects of lung resection on pulmonary function and exercise capacity. Thorax 1990;45:497–502.

143 Cleary GM, Wiswell TE: Meconium-stained amniotic fluid and the meconium aspiration syndrome. An update. Pediatr Clin North Am 1998;45:511–529.

144 Matthews TG, Warshaw JB: Relevance of the gestational age distribution of meconium passage in utero. Pediatrics 1979;64:30–31.

145 MacFarlane PI, Heaf DP: Pulmonary function in children after neonatal meconium aspiration syndrome. Arch Dis Child 1988;63:368–372.

146 Nüsslein TG, Benzing M, Riedel F, Rieger CH: Meconium aspiration in the newborn infant – Lack of long-term pulmonary sequelae. Klin Pädiatr 1994;206:369–371.

147 Swaminathan S, Quinn J, Stabile MW, Bader D, Platzker ACG, Keens TG: Long-term pulmonary sequelae of meconium aspiration syndrome. J Pediatr 1989;114:356–361.

148 Stevens JC, Eigen H, Wysomierski D: Absence of long-term pulmonary sequelae after mild meconium aspiration syndrome. Pediatr Pulmonol 1988;5:74–81.

149 Boykin AR, Quivers ES, Wagenhoffer KL, Sable CA, Chaney HR, Glass P, Bahrami KR, Short BL: Cardiopulmonary outcome of neonatal extracorporeal membrane oxygenation at ages 10–15 years. Crit Care Med 2003;31:2380–2384.

Daniel Trachsel, MD
Division of Intensive Care and Pulmonology
University Children's Hospital
Postal Box CH-4005 Basel (Switzerland)
Tel. +41 61 685 6565
Fax +41 61 685 5004
E-Mail daniel.trachsel@ukbb.ch

Hammer J, Eber E (eds): Paediatric Pulmonary Function Testing.
Prog Respir Res. Basel, Karger, 2005, vol 33, pp 266–281

....

Pulmonary Function Testing in the Neonatal and Paediatric Intensive Care Unit

J. Hammer[a]   C.J.L. Newth[b]

[a]Division of Intensive Care and Pulmonology, University Children's Hospital Basel, Basel, Switzerland;
[b]Department of Anesthesiology and Critical Care Medicine, Children's Hospital Los Angeles, University of Southern California, Los Angeles, Calif., USA

Abstract

The philosophy of mechanical ventilation has changed substantially over the past few decades, which also changed the expectations of what information should be available to help with the ventilator management of critically ill infants and children. Many techniques have been developed to investigate the various aspects of respiratory function in intubated children such as the elastic properties and volumes of the lung, and the degree of airway obstruction or hyperinflation, and the response to ventilatory strategies or therapeutic interventions. The potential value of integrating pulmonary function tests into routine intensive care unit (ICU) care is manifold, although there exists no evidence that the availability of such data makes a real difference to outcome. Pulmonary function testing offers a great educational tool for any critical care physician to acquire the physiological background necessary for rational ventilation of sick children. Awareness of the pitfalls of these measurements and knowledge of their limitations are crucial for correct interpretation of such data. This chapter reviews the most common techniques currently applied in paediatric intensive care, discusses their shortcomings and usefulness in assessing intubated children, and provides a guide for data interpretation.

Introduction

The marked improvement in microprocessor technology and the development of new lung function tests allow those involved in the care of critically ill infants and children to obtain novel measurements and gain new perspectives in both the assessment and management of respiratory failure. The lack of cooperation, the size of the subjects to be studied in this age group, and their cardiorespiratory instability from critical illness demand miniaturization and special adjustments of both methods and apparatus. Pulmonary function testing offers the potential advantage of integrating measurements of lung function into routine intensive care unit (ICU) management. At present, the only evidence available that pulmonary function tests can influence outcome is limited to the relatively simple measure of tidal volume. Significant differences in mortality from ARDS have been demonstrated based on the measurement and control of tidal volume [1]. It is important to define the physiological basis underlying new techniques to clarify exactly what parameters these tests can and cannot measure. The ATS/ERS Working Group on Infant Lung Function Testing has recently emphasized the importance of setting standards for performance and measurement conditions to achieve international consensus, to enable multicentre collaborative studies, and to establish normal reference data [2, 3].

Measurement conditions in the ICU environment differ substantially from those encountered in the outpatient laboratories. The large variety of ventilation modes and the different strategies used result in many more variables that must be considered. Study conditions, however, can be extremely well controlled in intubated infants by the use of sedation and neuromuscular blockade so that lung function can be measured without the influence of respiratory muscle activity. Coefficients of variation of repeated measurements are commonly lower when compared to analogous measurements in spontaneously breathing infants. Hence, pulmonary function tests are much more sensitive in detecting a statistically significant alteration in pulmonary function in response to any therapeutic intervention in intubated patients. Pulmonary function testing in intubated patients requires ideally that there be no leak around the endotracheal tube (ETT) in order to obtain reliable and representative measurements. Main et al. [4] showed that accurate 'on-line' resistance and compliance measurements could be obtained with a leak of up to 18% difference between inspired and exhaled tidal volumes. In most patients a leak can be eliminated by applying gentle cricoid pressure or by the use of a cuffed ETT. It has been recently demonstrated that the new generation of cuffed ETT can be safely used in children without increasing the risk of subglottic injury, provided they are correctly sized and cuff pressure is closely monitored [5].

It is not the intent of this chapter to justify as 'useful' or 'essential' any of the techniques which will be discussed. Justification for the routine use of a diagnostic or monitoring tool is commonly very difficult, if there is no scientific evidence that its application is associated with a reduction in morbidity, mortality or costs. On the other hand, any bedside pulmonary function test that improves our understanding of the disease process can be justified, if there is neither risk for nor deleterious effect on the patient.

Purpose of Pulmonary Function Testing in the ICU

With the increasing sophistication and complexity of neonatal and paediatric respiratory care, the philosophy of mechanical ventilation has changed substantially over the past few decades. Simultaneously, this also changed the expectations of what information should be available to guide mechanical ventilation. When the first infant ventilators were designed, the time-cycled, pressure-limited mode was the only realistic manner for mechanical ventilation of neonates and infants. Technically, these infant ventilators were very simple and comparable to 'reversed vacuum cleaners' that delivered unknown tidal volumes, because measurements of such low volumes were not feasible. Personal experience was a major determinant of success in those days. Today, the approach to infant mechanical ventilation is guided increasingly by understanding of the underlying respiratory pathophysiology and has moved away from the cookbook-type strategies based on local and historical tradition. The goal of mechanical ventilation is to provide adequate oxygenation and ventilation with the least risk for ventilator-induced injury and with the smallest amount of patient discomfort. Although good ventilator management is still based on clinical experience and knowledge of the conditions producing respiratory failure, much can be learned from objective measures of pulmonary function.

Rational monitoring of mechanical ventilation requires knowledge of the mechanical characteristics of both the patient and the machine. It has been suggested that the minimum physiological information needed for successful use of a mechanical ventilator requires the measurement of at least four parameters: (1) $P_{ET}CO_2$ (or $PaCO_2$), (2) SaO_2 (or PaO_2), (3) mechanical time constant of the respiratory system, and (4) functional residual capacity (FRC) [6].

Today, additional information such as the lower and upper inflection points (LIP and UIP) of the pressure-volume (PV) curve or the measurement of intrinsic positive end-expiratory pressure (PEEP) is desired to facilitate ventilator management. Current ventilator strategies attempt to target mechanical ventilation to the area between the LIP and UIP of the PV curve. The area above the UIP can be regarded as a zone of overdistension. The avoidance of overinflation has led to the strategy of permissive hypercapnia that limits airway pressure and tidal volume while permitting respiratory acidosis. The area below the LIP can be described as the zone where derecruitment and atelectasis occur. The so-called 'open lung concept' suggests that all recruitable lung tissue should be opened up and kept open during the entire ventilatory cycle. High-pressure recruitment manoeuvres have been advocated to open up the lung. Most involve the transient use of sustained inflations with high inflation pressures. PEEP is then applied to maintain ventilation above the critical closing pressure of the lung. Hence, the determination of the lower and UIP of the PV curve may help to decrease the risk of ventilator-induced lung injury.

The problem with 'intrinsic PEEP', which usually occurs in obstructive airway disease, is that gas trapped in the airways exerts a positive pressure, and the patient must generate a much higher negative inspiratory pressure in order for air to flow and trigger the ventilator. This hugely increases the work of breathing. The increased work of breathing associated with intrinsic PEEP can be offloaded by applying PEEP at a level close to the intrinsic PEEP to the airway. The measurement of intrinsic PEEP may help to improve patient-ventilator interaction and to decrease the work of breathing needed for triggering the ventilator. Unfortunately, a minimally invasive and accurate pulmonary function tool that offers an easy guide to the most gentle but effective ventilation is still missing.

The clinical benefit expected from pulmonary function tests in ventilated patients is not only to help with ventilator management, but also to understand the features and the severity of the disturbance in respiratory function, to assist in the assessment of therapeutic interventions and in the monitoring of the progression or the resolution of pulmonary disease (table 1). Nevertheless, the major benefit of pulmonary function testing today is related to objective assessments of scientific investigations in this field and not to clinical management.

Methods Used to Measure Pulmonary Function in the ICU

There is a whole battery of tests available to assess all the different aspects of pulmonary function in ventilated children such as pulmonary mechanics, maximum expiratory flow-volume (MEFV) curves, lung volumes, ventilation inhomogeneity, and work of breathing (table 2). This chapter will concentrate on current methods to assess respiratory mechanics, forced expiration, lung volumes and ventilation inhomogeneity. Measurements of work of breathing and thoraco-abdominal asynchrony are discussed in the chapter by Newth and Hammer [7]. It must be emphasized that almost all of these tests are used as research tools and have not found their way into routine clinical practice.

Measurements of Respiratory Mechanics

Measurements of respiratory mechanics examine the physics of moving air into and out of the lungs and describe the movements of the respiratory pump and the forces applied to it in a mathematical fashion. Most techniques for measuring respiratory mechanics assume that the respiratory system can be modelled by a single balloon on a pipe. This assumption can be described by the general equation of motion for a linear single compartment model as $P = V/C + RV' + IV''$, where P = driving pressure, V = volume change, C = compliance, R = resistance, V' = airflow, I = inertance and V'' = volume acceleration. For most practical applications the contribution of inertance is negligible at normal ventilation frequencies [8]. Hence, the calculation of compliance and resistance which reflect the mechanical properties of the respiratory system requires the measurement of flow, volume and pressure.

Many different techniques have been used to measure dynamic or static respiratory mechanics in ventilated

Table 1. Potential clinical value of pulmonary function testing in neonatal and paediatric intensive care

Purpose	Goal
Assessment of pulmonary pathophysiology	Detection of disease states
	Assessment of disease severity
	Guidance for ventilator management
	Time constant and FRC (end-expiratory volume)
	Avoid breath stacking by inadequately short expiratory times
	Choice of mode of ventilation
	Avoid HFOV in the presence of obstructive airway disease
	Inflection points of the PV curve
	Set PIP and PEEP
Assessment of therapeutic interventions	Bronchodilator therapy, surfactant, positioning (prone vs. supine), lung recruitment manoeuvres
Longitudinal monitoring	Documention of disease progression or resolution
	Acute respiratory failure (e.g. RDS → CLD)
	Chronic respiratory failure (e.g. children on home ventilation)
	Weaning from ventilation
	Prediction of outcome (?)
	Prediction of length of ventilation (e.g. RSV-associated pneumonia vs. bronchiolitis)

CLD = Chronic lung disease; HFOV = high-frequency oscillatory ventilation; PIP = positive inspiratory pressure; RDS = respiratory distress syndrome; RSV = respiratory syncytial virus.

children – so many that dealing with them in detail would go far beyond the scope of this chapter. The measurements can be classified as dynamic when obtained during rhythmic breathing, or as static (passive) when respiratory muscles are inactive during the test procedure. Passive refers to a relaxed state of respiratory muscles so that flow and pressure are solely determined by lung and airway mechanics, and not by muscle force. What follows is a brief discussion of the most common techniques currently used in ventilated children. For methodological details, the reader is referred to the chapter by Davis et al. [9] or original papers.

Pulmonary Graphics and Dynamic Measurements

Most modern ventilators today provide measurements of tidal volume, flow and pressure with on-line visualization of

Table 2. Pulmonary function tests used in neonatal and paediatric intensive care

Respiratory function characteristic	Technique

Respiratory mechanics	Dynamic measurements
	  Mead-Whittenberger
	   technique
	  MLR
	  FOT
	Passive measurements
	  Single breath occlusion
	  (Quasi)static PV curves
	  Interrupter technique

Forced expiration	FD technique
Lung volumes (FRC, TLC)	N_2 washout, helium dilution SF_6 washin-washout Respiratory inductance plethysmography
Ventilation inhomogeneity	Multiple breath washout Lung clearance index EIT
Measurement of work of breathing	Oesophageal pressure (pressure-rate product) Oxygen consumption
Measurement of thoraco-abdominal asynchrony	Respiratory inductance plethysmography

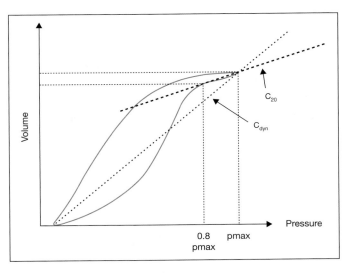

Fig. 1. Flattening of the dynamic inspiratory PV curve at end inspiration is a sign of lung overdistension. This can be quantified by calculation of the ratio of the calculated compliance for the terminal 20% of inspiration divided by the compliance value for the entire breath (C_{20}/C_{dyn} ratio). A ratio <0.8 suggests overdistension of the lung.

pulmonary graphics such as tidal breathing PV and FV loops. Although these measurements provide continuous real time data of ventilatory function, they are accurate in ventilated children only when measured at the airway opening without incorporating the mechanical characteristics of the ventilator circuit [4]. Pulmonary graphics are not helpful in calculating physiological lung function indices, but provide a real time display of patient-ventilator interaction at the bedside. Correct interpretation of pulmonary graphics requires pattern recognition, similar to other types of monitoring in the ICU (e.g., electrocardiography) rather than a profound understanding of pulmonary physiology. During volume-controlled ventilation, an inconsistent shape of the pressure-time waveform may alert the clinician that the patient demand exceeds the set flow (ventilator output). The inspection of the dynamic PV curve allows identification of volume changes outside the linear portion of the PV curve. Flattening of the dynamic inspiratory PV curve at end inspiration is a sign of lung overdistension. This can be quantified by calculation of the ratio of the calculated compliance for the terminal 20% of inspiration divided by the compliance value for the entire breath (C_{20}/C_{dyn} ratio, see fig. 1) [10].

The flow-time curve may help to detect the presence of inadvertent PEEP, when expiratory flow fails to return to zero before delivery of the next breath. Visual observation of the shape of the FV loop may be helpful to detect expiratory airflow obstruction (concave expiratory limb) or a partially obstructed ETT (linear inspiratory limb).

Dynamic compliance (C_{dyn}) and resistance (R_{dyn}) are commonly derived from such ventilator measurements using the Mead-Whittenberger technique which calculates these indices from two points of zero flow at end expiration and end inspiration. This technique does not provide accurate measurements of respiratory mechanics in most ventilated infants, because it assumes that C_{dyn} and R_{dyn} are constant throughout the respiratory cycle. Furthermore, zero flow conditions are only very briefly achieved during mechanical ventilation at end expiration and end inspiration, so that such pressure measurements also incorporate flow-resistive forces.

The classic technique to measure lung compliance under dynamic conditions ($C_{L,dyn}$) is based on the measurements of flow, volume and oesophageal pressure (P_{oes}) [11]. If P_{oes} is measured between the points of zero flow at end inspiration and end expiration, then the resistive element is cancelled out and $C_{L,dyn}$ can be easily calculated. However, this technique requires the placement of an oesophageal catheter, and the accuracy of such measurements in sick intubated children is controversial [12, 13]. During spontaneous breathing, the changes in pleural pressure generated by the respiratory muscles occur in the negative direction during inspiration, while airway opening pressure remains at zero throughout the breathing cycle. In contrast, during positive pressure ventilation with no spontaneous breathing, most of the applied pressure at the airway opening is used to stretch the lungs and to overcome the resistance to airflow. Changes in pleural pressure are usually very small, occur in the positive direction and reflect chest wall compliance. However, chest wall compliance is usually very high in neonates and infants, and its contribution can often be neglected [14, 32]. Regardless of the mode of breathing, $C_{L, dyn}$ can be calculated by relating transpulmonary pressure to corresponding changes in volume.

With recent advances in computer technology, the data collected during the entire breathing cycle can be used to calculate mechanics by multiple linear regression (MLR) analysis [15]. A computer calculates C_{dyn} and R_{dyn} to provide the best fit of the single compartment model with the measured data. In contrast to the traditional technique where the calculation of mechanics is based on only two measurement points, this approach produces a weighted average of C_{dyn}, R_{dyn}, and end-expiratory alveolar pressure [16].

Measurements derived from dynamic PV curves are probably the most widely used measures of respiratory mechanics in the ICU, but have quite marked limitations even when measured at the airway opening. C_{dyn} is very dependent on the ventilator settings (PEEP, respiratory rate) and preceding recruitment and derecruitment manoeuvres which shift the location on the full PV curve of the respiratory system [17, 18]. Similarly, R_{dyn} may be markedly influenced by the size of the ETT used, and the head position of the infant. In a recent paediatric study, respiratory mechanics were determined by MLR based on either airway pressure (thus including the resistance of the ETT) or tracheal pressure. Resistance was found to be slightly higher in the pressure-controlled than in the volume-controlled mode. The ventilatory modes had no effect on the determination of compliance. Elimination of the flow-dependent resistance of the ETT preserved the differences between the modes. The authors concluded that using MLR analysis compliance is not affected by the actual ventilator mode, whereas resistance is [19].

Static Measurements
Methods to measure static compliance (C_{rs}) and resistance (R_{rs}) are based on relaxation of both inspiratory and expiratory muscles during brief airway occlusions during exhalation. Muscle relaxation is achieved either by invoking the Hering-Breuer inflation reflex or by use of neuromuscular blockade.

The most widely used method is the passive deflation technique [20–22]. This technique involves measuring pressure during occlusion of the airway at end inspiration and fitting a straight line to the FV curve obtained during the subsequent passive exhalation [23, 24]. If there is no muscle activity during exhalation, the expiratory time constant (T_{rs}) or emptying time of the respiratory system will be entirely dependent on the mechanical properties of the lung and is the product of C_{rs} and R_{rs}. Thus, both C_{rs} and R_{rs} can be obtained from a single breath. The determination of T_{rs} gives some idea of how rapidly the lung empties following a mechanical breath. A single time constant is defined as the time required to exhale 63% of the tidal volume. Three time constants are needed to exhale 95% of the delivered tidal volume. This permits the determination of expiratory times allowing complete exhalation or the detection of rate settings which lead to inadvertent PEEP. This technique has clear limitations because it models the lungs as a single compartment. If the lung does not behave like a single compartment (as confirmed in children with severe ARDS), such curvilinear slopes cannot be accurately described by one single slope [25].

The interrupter technique which uses a single occlusion during expiration allows partitioning of respiratory resistance into airway resistance and the visco-elastic properties of the lung. The former is calculated from the initial rapid rise in pressure after occlusion and the flow measured prior to occlusion. The latter is derived from the secondary rise in pressure to a plateau which represents stress recovery within the tissues and the chest wall, and 'pendelluft' [26]. Further techniques to assess passive respiratory mechanics in the ICU use multiple occlusions which can either be performed by interrupting multiple breaths at different volumes or by multiple interruptions of a single expiration [27]. C_{rs} is calculated from the slope of the volume-pressure data. None of these methods have found widespread application in the paediatric ICU.

Endotracheal Tube
Another important issue in ventilated patients is the effect of the ETT [28, 29]. The ETT bypasses the upper airway and acts as a high non-linear resistance. Hence, measurements of respiratory mechanics will automatically include ETT resistance (R_{ett}). These effects are further aggravated by secretions, kinking, changes in the shape of the tube in vivo, and leaks around uncuffed tubes. Endotracheal suctioning shortly before measuring will prevent the effect of secretions [30]. In vitro experiments have used empirical equations to characterize the pressure-flow

relationships of ETTs, mostly based on Rohrer's law: $R_{ett} = K_1 + K_2 V'$, where K_1 and K_2 are constants, and V' is flow. These constants have been determined for paediatric tubes from in vitro experiments. Thus, the airway opening pressure can be corrected for the pressure drop across the tubes [31]. Alternatively, direct measurement of tracheal pressure at the distal end of the tracheal tube allows assessing respiratory mechanics without the ETT [32]. Nevertheless, for most clinical situations it will be acceptable to use results including the tube, since the ETT is part of the respiratory system of the ventilated patient.

Normal Data

There is still a great lack of normal values for C_{rs} and R_{rs} in intubated infants and children. According to our studies, such normal data lie in the range of 0.8–1.2 ml/cm H_2O/kg for C_{rs} and 0.04–0.08 ml/cm H_2O/s (up to 1.0 with ETT <3.5 mm ID) for R_{rs} [33].

Assessment of the Static PV Curve

The static PV curve of the respiratory system is characterized by an initial concave segment ending at the LIP which is thought to reflect the critical opening pressure for the majority of alveoli. Above this point, the PV curve turns into a straight segment of maximal compliance until the curve flattens at the UIP. Above this point static compliance decreases in response to alveolar overdistension (fig. 2).

Many authors have advocated the construction of static PV curves with a large air-filled 'super-syringe' in order to determine LIP and UIP to adjust ventilator pressures. In this technique, the lungs are inflated stepwise from residual volume (RV) to total lung capacity (TLC). Each volume step is maintained for 2–3 s until a stable plateau airway pressure is recorded, thereby excluding the dynamic resistive forces of the respiratory system. The method has many disadvantages if applied to critically ill patients. It is time consuming, cumbersome, difficult to standardize, the patient must be paralyzed (i.e. no spontaneous breaths) and is at risk for oxygen desaturation.

A much easier alternative to assess PV relationships is the recording of quasi-static PV curves using the low-flow inflation technique. A low-flow insufflation is performed in the volume-controlled mode set with a prolonged low-flow inspiration of 6 s (T_I/T_{tot} of 0.5) and with a tidal volume to result in an expected peak insufflation pressure of approximately 40 cm H_2O. The relatively low flow rate reduces the resistive pressure component during insufflation. This technique allows detecting overdistension by inspection of the curve. Overdistension can also be detected by fitting a second-order polynomial equation to the recorded data

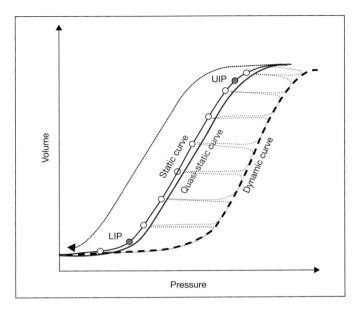

Fig. 2. PV curves of the lung. The static inspiratory PV curve is constructed by stepwise inflation with a super-syringe while the quasi-static inspiratory curve is obtained by low-flow inflation. The dynamic curve is recorded during uninterrupted inspiration during mechanical ventilation and includes the resistive forces of the respiratory system. The dotted line with an arrow on the left represents the passive deflation limb on exhalation and is the same for all manoeuvres.

points ($\Delta V = a + bP + cP^2$, where coefficients a, b, and c are constants). A negative non-linear coefficient c indicates a decreasing slope with increasing volume, i.e. overdistension [34]. Current data suggest that this technique is superior to the calculation of the C_{20}/C_{dyn} ratio of dynamic PV loops to detect ventilator-induced overdistension.

Conceptually, the LIP and UIP on a static PV curve might be a rational guide to determining best PEEP and PIP during mechanical ventilation. It is, however, important to understand that the PV curve is the sum of numerous lung regions with potentially widely varying differences in their mechanical properties. Recruitment of alveoli also occurs throughout much of the steep part of the PV curve in injured lungs. Hence, it may be overly simplistic to assume that the measured LIP and UIP represent the ideal points to set ventilator pressures.

Forced Expiration

The measurement of MEFV relationships is one of the most valuable clinical tests in the assessment of pulmonary function. Its history goes back to John Hutchinson [35] who defined vital capacity (VC) and established its linear

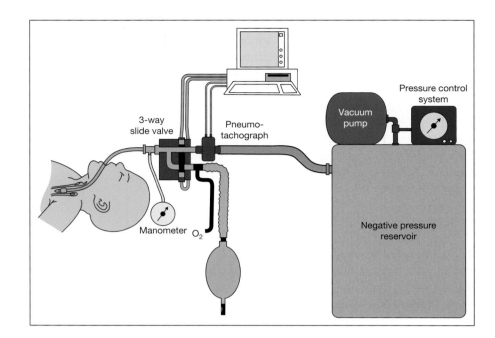

Fig. 3. FD apparatus.

relationship to height. In 1947, Tiffeneau and Pinelli [36] recognized that volume-time measurements during forced vital capacity (FVC) manoeuvres are very sensitive in detecting obstructive airway disease. The FVC manoeuvre is standardized by having subjects perform a maximum inspiration to TLC followed by a maximum effort expiration to RV allowing the recording of MEFV curves. Forced expirations can also be initiated from a partial inspiration to a volume below TLC allowing the recording of partial expiratory flow-volume curves.

Intubated infants and children can be forced to exhale rapidly only by use of an external pressure source. This is best achieved by exposing the airways to negative pressure resulting in rapid lung deflation. Negative pressure application to the airways was first used in animals and excised lung preparations to examine the physiological mechanisms of forced expirations [37–39]. The technique and apparatus necessary to generate MEFV curves in intubated infants by forced deflation (FD), in other words airway evacuation by suction, was first described in 1977 [40]. This technique is now regarded as the gold standard to examine maximal flow characteristics in intubated and critically ill infants [41] since it was validated that (1) FD reliably achieves flow limitation in intubated infants with normal lungs below 25% FVC with -40 cm H_2O or greater airway opening pressures [42] and (2) maximum expiratory flows are not influenced by an appropriately sized ETT at lung volumes below 25% FVC [43].

The technique has been used to describe pathophysiological alterations of different lung diseases and to assess therapeutic interventions such as bronchodilator therapy in critically ill children [25, 44–49].

Measurement Procedure (fig. 3)

Before and between the deflations the patient is manually ventilated via the side port of a three-way directional sliding valve placed at the proximal end of the ETT by squeezing a 0.5-litre Jackson-Rees anaesthesia bag filled from a continuous wall oxygen supply. Manual ventilation is controlled by a wall manometer at approximately the same inspiratory pressures as on mechanical ventilation.

For the test procedure, the lungs are inflated by squeezing the breathing bag to $+40$ cm H_2O inflation pressure, defined as TLC. Present knowledge of PV relationships under the condition of neuromuscular blockade in infants and children supports the recommended definition of TLC at $+40$ cm H_2O inspiratory pressure [42, 50, 51]. To eliminate breath-hold time as a variable and to establish a consistent volume history, it is important to use the same inflation procedure for all manoeuvres [52, 53]. Therefore, inflation pressures are held static for at least 3 s, after which a three-way directional sliding valve placed at the proximal end of the ETT is electronically activated to open the airways to a 100-litre-capacity, constant negative pressure source of -40 cm H_2O deflation pressure. The lungs are deflated until expiratory flow ceases at RV or for no longer than 3 s. Prolonged exposure to the negative pressure source is prevented by an electronic control system. The resulting MEFV curve is measured by a pneumotachograph which is attached to the ETT or tracheostomy tube. Usually, a minimum of four manoeuvres is recorded, and the manoeuvre achieving the highest FVC is analyzed. As for all pulmonary function tests in subjects with artificial airways it is important that no leak occurs during the testing procedure. This is best achieved by using a cuffed ETT. Throughout the procedure the individual is usually under neuromuscular blockade and sedation, and monitored by pulse oximetry, electrocardiography and capnography.

Physiological and Technical Considerations

The advantage of this technique is that full MEFV curves can be generated and that the study conditions are well controlled. In contrast to measurements of respiratory mechanics, FD does not rely upon any modelling assumption. Presetting the same volume history by maintaining constant inflation (to TLC) and deflation pressures results in MEFV curves that are almost perfectly reproducible. Flow limitation consistently occurs for flows at and below 25% FVC by applying a negative airway opening pressure of -40 cm H_2O in intubated infants with normal lungs. However, it is important to realize that the application of excessive negative pressure to the airway opening may influence airway calibre resulting in lower maximum expiratory flows, a phenomenon referred to as negative effort dependence. We observed such behaviour beyond airway opening pressures of -40 cm-H_2O [54, 55]. This phenomenon is explained by the effect of longitudinal tension on airway compliance [56]. This implies that it is necessary to titrate the deflation pressure, especially if there is a disease process likely to increase the tendency for airway collapse in small infants (e.g., bronchomalacia, bronchiolitis). In such situations, comparison of the MEFV curve obtained using the standardized deflation pressure of -40 cm H_2O with a passive expiration curve from TLC (or MEFV curves obtained with lower driving pressures) is strongly recommended in order to detect negative effort dependence.

Pressurization of flow meters is an inevitable problem when generating forced expirations with this technique. Preliminary studies suggest that measurements obtained by screen-type pneumotachographs are slightly affected by pressures in the range used for FD manoeuvres. Hot wire anemometers or ultrasonic flow sensors may be the preferred measuring devices [57, 58].

Another concern is that the deflation manoeuvre may cause bronchoconstriction, an increase in lung tissue resistance, and atelectasis analogous to the effect of endotracheal suctioning. Such effects, however, are easily reversed by performing a recruitment manoeuvre after suctioning, as previously demonstrated by others [59, 60]. We have demonstrated that inflating the lungs to TLC before the FD manoeuvres not only prevents or offsets possible adverse effects on respiratory mechanics caused by applying negative pressure to the airways, but also recruits previously collapsed lung units in anaesthetized and intubated children with lung disease [18]. Hence, the FD manoeuvre may increase subsequent measurements of respiratory system compliance. This implies that testing sequences should be the same each time when different pulmonary function tests are used to assure that changes in lung function are not related to short-term alterations in volume history, but reflect changes related to therapeutic interventions or alterations in the disease process.

Interpretation, Normal Data

Analysis of the MEFV curve allows measurements of pulmonary function which are independent of the mode of mechanical ventilation such as the measurements of FVC and maximum expiratory flows at 25 and 10% FVC (MEF_{25} and MEF_{10}). MEF_{50} is affected by the diameter of the ETT and meaningless as an index of airway function [41]. The coefficient of variation for repeated measurements is in the range of 7–16% for MEF_{25} and MEF_{10}, and 3–8% for FVC [18, 45]. Normal values of MEFV curves generated by FD are available on only a small number of healthy infants and those published are all reported in relation to body weight (table 3) [33, 61]. Normal data still needs to be defined in a larger study population and should probably be reported in relation to length analogous to adult standards. Height may also be more robust in the presence of growth disorders or different nutritional status.

Visual pattern recognition adds valuable information to the interpretation of results obtained by measuring MEFV curves. While obstructive lung disease results in a typical curvilinear, concave pattern of the expiratory FV loop, normal lungs and those with restrictive disease are characterized by convex loop patterns. Bronchodilator responsiveness can be readily assessed in intubated infants with obstructive airway disease (fig. 4).

Measurement of Lung Volumes (FRC)

The FRC is the only lung volume that can be accurately and repeatedly measured in ventilated patients of all ages. Other lung volumes such as TLC, VC, and RV can also be measured, but these techniques are rarely employed.

Table 3. Published normal values for FD

	Full-term neonates [61]	Infants and children [33]
Number	16	26
Age	1–13 days	1–36 months
FVC, ml/kg	46.1 (27–61)	55.3 (42–76)
MEF_{25}, ml/kg/s	44.4 (19–73)	35 (16–60)
MEF_{10}, ml/kg/s	14.9 (8–25)	8.7 (5–20)

Data are means with the range in parentheses. MEF_{25} = Maximal expiratory flow at 25% of FVC; MEF_{10} = maximal expiratory flow at 10% of FVC.

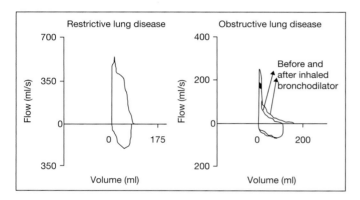

Fig. 4. Characteristic patterns of FD MEFV curves obtained in restrictive lung disease (e.g., ARDS, pneumonia) and obstructive airway disease (e.g., bronchiolitis, asthma). The benefits of inhaled bronchodilators on pulmonary function can be objectively assessed by analysis of FD curves [adapted from 44].

Plethysmographic methods are cumbersome, impractical and even potentially unsafe for ventilated, sick children and are rarely used in the ICU environment [62]. There are several gas dilution techniques described to measure FRC in ventilated children: the closed-circuit helium (He) dilution technique, the open-circuit nitrogen (N_2) washout or the open-circuit sulphur hexafluoride (SF_6) washin/washout. The basics of FRC measurements by gas dilution are covered in the chapter by Gustaffson and Ljungberg [63]. This chapter will focus on the particular aspects of measuring FRC in children on mechanical ventilation.

Helium Dilution

The setup for a closed-circuit He dilution method to measure FRC on ventilated patients has been described by Heldt and Peters [64]. The patient is connected via the

ETT and a sliding valve to both a bag (which is situated inside a transparent plexiglass box) and to the ventilator. In the pretest position the patient is ventilated directly by the ventilator through the valve. The bag, which contains a known amount of gas with known He concentration (and thus a known amount of helium), is sealed and is not connected to the patient. At end exhalation the valve is switched so that the patient is directly connected only to the He-containing bag while the ventilator ventilates the box surrounding the bag and compresses the bag accordingly. The patient is thus ventilated by the bag which is externally compressed by the ventilator cycle. Once equilibration of He concentration between the lungs and the bag is achieved, FRC can be calculated in the same way as in non-ventilated subjects. This technique is applicable to patients on very high inspired oxygen concentrations ($FiO_2 = 0.97$). Unfortunately, most thermal conductivity based He analyzers are inaccurate when O_2 concentrations are very high and must be carefully calibrated. Leak-free connections are crucial for accurate lung volume measurements by He dilution in intubated children. Fox et al. [65] described a method to correct for leaks during He dilution.

Nitrogen Washout

This technique is based on washing out the N_2 from the lungs by giving the subject 100% O_2 to breathe. If the amount of N_2 washed out is measured and the initial alveolar N_2 concentration is known, then the lung volume from which point the washout started can be derived. N_2 washout techniques can be divided into breath-by-breath and bias flow washout systems. The breath-by-breath N_2 washout technique measures the instantaneous N_2 concentration and air flow during each breath at the airway opening and has not been applied to ventilated patients. The bias flow N_2 washout method uses a mixing chamber and represents the gold standard of measuring FRC by N_2 washout in ventilated children. In this open-circuit method, the patient is connected to two ventilators separated by a slider valve at the proximal end of the ETT (fig. 5). At FRC, the patient is switched from his regular ventilator to the second washout ventilator delivering 100% O_2 with the same settings. The washout ventilator is also used for calibration. The gas leaving that ventilator via the exhalation port is routed through a mixing chamber, and the falling N_2 concentration is then analyzed continuously by a mass spectrometer or an N_2 analyzer. The volume of N_2 exhaled (VN_{2test}) is determined by integration with respect to time of the instantaneous N_2 concentration flowing in the exhalation circuit multiplied by the instantaneous flow

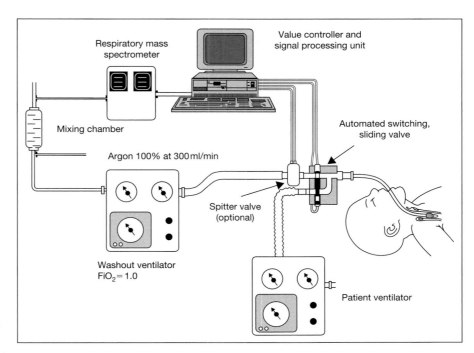

Fig. 5. Bias flow N_2 washout system to measure FRC in ventilated children.

(fig. 6). The test is complete when the N_2 concentration is stable at zero, similar to the start of the test.

This method is crucially dependent on the measurement of gas flow during calibration and during the test. In order to overcome this difficulty, Sivan et al. [66] used the respiratory mass spectrometer, already 'in-line' for measuring the instantaneous N_2 concentration, to record the minute ventilation (V'e) by the argon dilution technique [67]. FRC is then calculated according to the following equation:

$$VN_{2_{test}} = \frac{V'e_{test}}{V'e_{cal}} \times \frac{VN_{2_{cal}}}{\int [N_2]_{cal} \times dt} \times \int [N_2]_{test} \times dt$$

The ratio $V'e_{test}/V'e_{cal}$ is obtained from V'e measured by the argon dilution technique (utilizing a respiratory mass spectrometer) during the calibration and the test. The ratio $VN_2cal /[N_2]_{cal} \times dt$ is defined during the calibration procedure. The system is calibrated by means of a precision syringe filled with known amounts of room air attached to the washout ventilator in place of the patient's ETT. Two-point calibration is used, at volumes below and above the estimated FRC. The plunger of the syringe is pushed back by the washout ventilator and advanced by the technician. The gas leaving the washout ventilator is analyzed as described. Corrections for additional dead space during calibration have to be made.

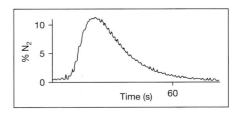

Fig. 6. Typical N_2 washout curve. FRC is calculated from the area under the curve.

As an alternative, it is much easier to use an intermittent flow ventilator (e.g., Siemens Servo 900C) with settings matched to the patient's ventilator of the same type. The washout ventilator is calibrated at the same minute ventilation delivered to the patient (volume-controlled ventilation), and since the 'calibration' and 'test' (patient) V'e are the same, there is no need to measure V'e and to apply the ratio mathematics since the ratio is equal to 1. In this situation, the mass spectrometer can be replaced by a simple N_2 analyzer.

This technique has been shown to be accurate and reproducible with a coefficient of variation for repeated measurements of less than 6.5% [66]. The technique, however, has some limitations and disadvantages:

1. The method is time-consuming and requires bulky equipment such as an expensive respiratory mass

spectrometer (except in the special circumstance noted above) and a second ventilator. Repeated measurements are necessary and both the argon dilution and N_2 washout systems must be independently calibrated.

2. It is limited to patients at $FiO_2 < 0.75$.
3. Breathing 100% O_2 repeatedly for such tests may have toxic effects on preterm infants. This can be modified by using heliox (helium-oxygen) gas mixtures [68, 69].
4. When the patient is washed out with a constant flow ventilator, the washed-out N_2 is diluted in a very large volume of gas resulting in very low concentrations of N_2 which may decrease the accuracy. A splitter isolation valve (see fig. 5) placed at the end of the ETT which directs only the gas exhaled from the patient to the mixing chamber solves this problem.
5. All gas dilution techniques for FRC measurements are particularly susceptible to inaccuracies from leaks in the system (e.g., use of uncuffed ETT)

In practice, the system has been shown to be applicable also to ventilated preterm infants with $FiO_2 \leq 0.75$ and with FRC as low as 20 ml [69]. It has also been demonstrated that lung volumes above FRC such as TLC can be reliably measured by this technique and that FRC measurements reasonably reflect true FRC [70, 71]. For infants and children, in our laboratory, we normally perform three tests (at least two) and accept the mean of the data if the spread is within 2 ml/kg body weight.

SF$_6$ Washout

Recently, techniques using SF_6 as a tracer have become more popular. This method was first described in 1985 in adults [72]. It is an open-circuit tracer gas washout employing a device for dispensing SF_6 into the inspiratory limb of the ventilator circuit, a fast SF_6 infrared analyzer, a pneumotachograph and a computer. The dispensing device delivers SF_6 into the airway in proportion to inspiratory flow so that the inspired SF_6 is held constant, usually at about 0.5%. At the end of washin, the alveolar SF_6 concentration is obtained as the mean concentration during expiration of the second half of the tidal volume. Washout is started simply by stopping SF_6 infusion between two inspirations, and is considered complete when the mean expired SF_6 concentration in the last five breaths is less than 0.001%. The concentration of SF_6 is measured breath-by-breath and the expired SF_6 volume is calculated by integrating SF_6 flow (area under the curve). FRC is determined by dividing the expired SF_6 volume by the end-tidal SF_6 concentration before washout. The value obtained is converted to BTPS conditions and the apparatus dead space is subtracted. Rebreathing of SF_6 from the pneumotachograph or ventilatory circuit also needs to be taken into consideration for FRC calculation.

If SF_6 is delivered from a dispensing unit at a constant rate to the inspiratory limb of the ventilator circuit, the technique is crucially dependent on a constant flow of the inspired air. This is most easily achieved with constant flow ventilators which allow the regulation of bias flow. Several technical modifications of the initial system have been described. SF_6 can be delivered at a constant level irrespective of the inspiratory flow pattern with a piezoelectric valve delivering SF_6 in short pulses and a microprocessor modulating the pulse frequency of the valve in proportion to flow [73, 74]. Another system modified for small volume lungs delivers pure SF_6 via a side port into the constant flow of humidified gas entering the pneumatic unit of the ventilator [75]. The newest development of the SF_6 washout technique involves the use of a mainstream ultrasonic flow meter which can measure flow and tracer gas concentration of the inspiratory and expiratory gas simultaneously with the same ultrasonic signal [76]. The concentration of SF_6 or any tracer gas can be estimated from the molar mass (grams per mole) signal of the ultrasonic flow meter during an inert gas washin or washout. Molar mass can be computed from transit times and temperature along the sound transmission path. The transit time can be measured with high accuracy, and its value is directly proportional to the density of the gas. It has been demonstrated in an animal model that FRC can be accurately measured by this technique and that results can be compared to standard methods such as the bias flow N_2 washout technique [77]. This system, which is the only one currently commercially available, depends also on a constant circuit flow which excludes its use with intermittent-flow ventilators. Breath-by-breath systems have the additional advantage of providing information on ventilation distribution. The different indices to describe ventilation inhomogeneity, such as the lung clearance index or moment ratio analysis, are described in further detail in the chapter of Gustaffson and Ljungberg [63]. Schibler and Henning [78] have described that simple indices of ventilation inhomogeneity can demonstrate improved ventilation distribution by the application of PEEP (fig. 7). The coefficient of variation for repeated measurements in mechanically ventilated children is around 2–9% and less than 6.6% in adults [79]. The technique has been applied to mechanically ventilated neonates and children in several further studies [62, 80, 81].

Normal Data

FRC reference values for mechanically ventilated infants without underlying lung disease are available for only a

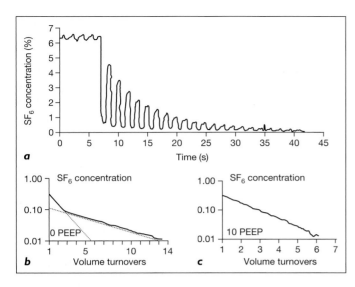

Fig. 7. *a* Typical SF_6 washout in a child on ventilatory support. *b* A washout curve with PEEP at 0 cm H_2O. *c* A washout curve with PEEP at 10 cm H_2O. The washout curve at zero PEEP has an initial fast-declining component followed by a second slower one. With increased PEEP of 10 cm H_2O, only one component of the washout curve can be detected [adapted from 78].

limited number of infants and children. FRC values from spontaneously breathing healthy infants are inaccurate as reference data for several reasons. The nasopharynx, which contributes to total dead space in spontaneously breathing infants, is bypassed by the ETT. Sedation and paralysis may reduce FRC, which is further dependent on the mode of ventilation (e.g., PEEP). Normal FRC reported for 26 sedated and paralyzed children measured at PEEP of 2–4 cm H_2O by N_2 washout was 23.7 ± 1.5 ml/kg (mean ± SE) [44]. Thorsteinsson et al. [80] reported normal lung volume data for 48 anaesthetized and paralyzed infants and children by SF_6 washout. Mean ± SD FRC was 20 ± 5 ml/kg in infants and 26 ± 6 ml/kg in older children. They also measured inspiratory capacity at +30 cm H_2O by spirometry to determine TLC. Mean ± SD TLC (defined at +30 cm H_2O inspiratory pressure) was 52 ± 13 ml/kg in infants and 87 ± 11 ml/kg in older children. The calculated regression equations for FRC and TLC were:

FRC = −113 + 32.5 × weight (kg), r = 0.95

FRC = 0.0025 × length (mm), r = 0.97

TLC = −278 + 99.8 × weight (kg), r = 0.98.

TLC measured by N_2 washout in 14 ventilated children (mean ± SE age = 20 ± 5 months) without lung disease at

+40 cm H_2O inspiratory pressure was 66.4 ± 3.8 ml/kg (mean ± SE) [71]. TLC in this study was higher than the data reported by Thorsteinsson et al. [80] for infants of similar age and weight. This can be explained by the observation that the flat portion of the PV curve is not reached with +30 cm H_2O inspiratory pressure under conditions of neuromuscular blockade [50]. Hence, TLC should be defined at +40 cm H_2O inspiratory pressure in intubated infants and children.

Developing Techniques

Forced Oscillation Technique

A novel promising method to assess dynamic respiratory mechanics in intubated children is the forced oscillation technique (FOT) superimposing sinusoidal pressure oscillations on tidal breathing [82, 83]. This technique can be applied during normal ventilation provided the measured frequencies are well above the respiratory rate. For routine clinical applications of FOT, oscillation frequency is chosen in a medium frequency range of about 4–30 Hz. This technique assesses respiratory impedance, which simplistically can be conceived as a generalization of resistance. Respiratory impedance is described by two components: respiratory resistance (R_{rs}) and reactance (X_{rs}). The measure of R_{rs} is independent of the oscillation frequency. By contrast, X_{rs} depends highly on the oscillation frequency, and is a measure of the elastic properties (of the airways, lung tissue and thoracic wall) and the inertial properties (of the whole respiratory system and the gas in the airways). Hence, modification of oscillation frequencies facilitates the study of different pathophysiological aspects of respiratory mechanics. For instance, the low-frequency FOT using oscillatory signals <2 Hz allows the study of respiratory tissue properties in addition to respiratory resistance. At present, there are very few studies that assessed this technique in ventilated infants. Its great potential lies in the assessment of changes in lung mechanics resulting from recruitment manoeuvres and pressure changes during high-frequency oscillation [84]. Respiratory impedance measurements by the low-frequency FOT have to be performed during short intervals of suspended mechanical ventilation in intubated and paralyzed children [85]. In contrast, high-frequency oscillation measurements above ~100 Hz are much less affected by tissue properties and may provide a better measure of airway characteristics, including airway wall compliance. These measurements can be performed during assisted ventilation. Nevertheless, no commercial systems are yet available to assess respiratory mechanics by FOT in ventilated children [for the application of the FOT in spontaneously breathing children see 86].

Respiratory Inductance Plethysmography and Lung Volume Assessment

The use of respiratory inductance plethysmography to assess tidal breathing and thoraco-abdominal asynchrony is described in the chapters of Carlsen and Carlsen [87] and Newth and Hammer [7] in further detail. Recently, respiratory inductance plethysmography measurements have been used to assess lung volume changes during high-frequency oscillation in animal models [88, 89]. The technique can also be used to construct full PV curves during high-frequency oscillation [90]. The clinical relevance of monitoring lung volume changes during HFOV in infants and children has yet to be determined.

Electrical Impedance Tomography

Another exciting technology is electrical impedance tomography (EIT), used to assess changes in regional lung function. The method is based on the premise that the movement of air, blood, and extravascular fluid modifies the electrical properties of lung tissue [91]. In this technique, surface electrodes are placed circumferentially around the chest wall, and each electrode sequentially transmits and receives an electrical micro-current. Within a particular cross-sectional plane, harmless electrical currents are driven across the thorax in a rotating pattern, generating a potential gradient at the surface, which is then transformed into a two-dimensional image of the electric impedance distribution within the thorax. The dynamic behaviour and the qualitative information extracted from these images can be compared to dynamic CT studies or ventilation scintigraphy [92, 93].

The technique has the potential to monitor imbalances of regional ventilation and to assess regional lung function. It has been used to assess regional PV relationships, and to study the effect of traditional recruitment manoeuvres and high-frequency oscillatory ventilation on regional ventilation in animal models of acute lung injury [94–97]. Initial clinical experience with EIT in critically ill children demonstrated that the technology can identify changes in regional lung ventilation in response to modified ventilator settings and/or asymmetrical surfactant instillation [98]. At present, the EIT technology has limitations with respect to motion artefacts and low spatial resolution. It fails to provide such precise morphologic information as can be obtained by CT or magnetic resonance imaging. Nevertheless, EIT is a promising non-invasive technique that could be useful to assess pulmonary function of critically ill patients at the bedside [99].

Conclusion

There is no question that measurements of pulmonary function have increased our understanding of the effects of diseases and therapy on the respiratory system of ventilated infants and children. Unfortunately, there exist hardly any data about the cost-effectiveness or the impact on outcome of measuring pulmonary function in critically ill infants and children. It has been demonstrated that mechanical ventilation with a lower tidal volume than traditionally used results in decreased mortality and increases the number of days without ventilator use in adult patients with ARDS [1]. Studies using pulmonary function tests in critically ill children have mainly focused on answering physiological questions or evaluating the immediate efficacy of treatment modalities. Studies looking at the benefit of pulmonary function testing for clinical management are few. In one example, it has been shown that measurements of lung function in infants with respiratory syncytial virus-induced respiratory failure allow the construction of a lung injury score which is very helpful in predicting the duration of mechanical ventilation [44].

The authors have no doubt that pulmonary function testing is an essential educational tool for any critical care physician who wants to acquire the physiological background necessary for rational ventilation of sick children. The choice of a particular ventilator strategy depends on the underlying pathophysiology. High-frequency oscillatory ventilation, for example, performs very poorly in children with severe obstructive airway disease. There is, however, not a single pulmonary function parameter that satisfactorily describes the complete respiratory physiology of ventilated patients. The selection of the appropriate tests depends highly on the clinical question to be answered. More work is required to standardize and evaluate techniques in the clinical setting before pulmonary function equipment will be commercially available and introduced into standard ventilator management. The application of old and new pulmonary function tests may eventually improve our interpretation of disease processes and the responses to therapy. Furthermore, incorporation of sophisticated pulmonary function tests, which go beyond simple measures of respiratory mechanics, into the ventilator apparatus (for example, the continuous assessment of FRC) may eventually improve ventilator management. At present, the best monitors are still physicians and nurses, who integrate all of the physiological parameters with the known pathophysiology, and the role of the bedside intensivist remains as the heart of good ventilator management [100].

References

1 Ventilation with lower tidal volumes as compared with traditional tidal volumes for acute lung injury and the acute respiratory distress syndrome. The Acute Respiratory Distress Syndrome Network. N Engl J Med 2000;342: 1301–1308.

2 American Thoracic Society/European Respiratory Society: Respiratory mechanics in infants: Physiologic evaluation in health and disease. Am Rev Respir Dis 993;147:474–496.

3 Taussig LM: From the mouths of babes... Am Rev Respir Dis 1993;147:254–255.

4 Main E, Castle R, Stocks J, James I, Hatch D: The influence of endotracheal tube leak on the assessment of respiratory function in ventilated children. Intensive Care Med 2001;27: 1788–1797.

5 Newth CJL, Rachman B, Patel N, Hammer J: The use of cuffed versus uncuffed endotracheal tubes in pediatric intensive care. J Pediatr 2004;144:333–337.

6 Shannon DC: Rational monitoring of respiratory function during mechanical ventilation of infants and children. Intensive Care Med 1989;15(suppl 1):S13–16.

7 Newth CJL, Hammer J: Measurements of thoraco-abdominal asynchrony and work of breathing in children; Hammer J, Eber E (eds): Paediatric Pulmonary Function Testing. Prog Respir Res. Basel, Karger, 2005, vol 33, pp 148–156.

8 Turner MJ, MacLeod IM, Rothberg AD: Effect of airway inertia on linear regression estimates of resistance and compliance in mechanically ventilated infants: A computer model study. Pediatr Pulmonol 1991;11:147–152.

9 Davis SD, Gappa M, Rosenfeld M: Respiratory mechanics; Hammer J, Eber E (eds): Paediatric Pulmonary Function Testing. Prog Respir Res. Basel, Karger, 2005, vol 33, pp 20–33.

10 Fisher JB, Mammet MC, Coleman M, Bing DR, Boros SJ: Identifying lung overdistension during mechanical ventilation by using volume-pressure loops. Pediatr Pulmonol 1988; 5:10–14.

11 Mead J, Whittenberger JL: Physical properties of human lungs measured during spontaneous respiration. J Appl Physiol 1952;5: 779–796.

12 LeSouëf PN, Lopes JM, England SJ, Bryan MH, Bryan AC: Influence of chest wall distortion on esophageal pressure. J Appl Physiol 1983;55:353–358.

13 Heaf DP, Turner H, Stocks J, Helms P: The accuracy of esophageal pressure measurements in convalescent and sick intubated infants. Pediatr Pulmonol 1986;2:5–8.

14 Davis GM, Coates AL, Papageorgiou A, Bureau MA: Direct measurement of static chest wall compliance in animal and human neonates. J Appl Physiol 1988;65:1093–1098.

15 Bhutani VK, Sivieri EM, Abbasi S, Shaffer TH: Evaluation of neonatal pulmonary mechanics and energetics: A two factor least mean square analysis. Pediatr Pulmonol 1988;4:150–158.

16 Lanteri CJ, Kano S, Nicolai T, Sly PD: Measurement of dynamic respiratory mechanics in neonatal and pediatric intensive care: The multiple linear regression technique. Pediatr Pulmonol 1995;19:29–45.

17 Rimensberger PC, Cox PN, Frndova H, Bryan AC: The open lung during small tidal volume ventilation: Concepts of recruitment and 'optimal' positive end-expiratory pressure. Crit Care Med 1999;27:1946–1952.

18 Hammer J, Patel N, Newth CJ: Effect of forced deflation maneuvers upon measurements of respiratory mechanics in ventilated infants. Intensive Care Med 2003;29:2004–2008.

19 Kessler V, Guttmann J, Newth CJ: Dynamic respiratory system mechanics in infants during pressure and volume controlled ventilation. Eur Respir J 2001;17:115–121.

20 Zin WA, Pengelly LD, Milic-Emili J: Single-breath method for measurement of respiratory mechanics in anesthetized animals. J Appl Physiol 1982;52:1266–1271.

21 Olinsky A, Bryan MH, Bryan AC: A simple method of measuring total respiratory system compliance in newborn infants. S Afr Med J 1976;50:128–130.

22 Guslits BG, Wilkie RA, England SJ, Bryan AC: Comparison of methods of measurement of compliance of the respiratory system in children. Am Rev Respir Dis 1987;136: 727–729.

23 Mortola JP, Fisher JT, Smith B, Fox G, Weeks S: Dynamics of breathing in infants. J Appl Physiol 1982;52:1209–1215.

24 LeSouëf PN, England SJ, Bryan AC: Passive respiratory mechanics in newborns and children. Am Rev Respir Dis 1984;129:727–729.

25 Newth CJL, Stretton M, Deakers TW, Hammer J: Assessment of pulmonary function in the early phase of ARDS in pediatric patients. Pediatr Pulmonol 1997;23:169–175.

26 Sly PD, Bates JHT: Computer analysis of physical factors affecting the use of the interrupter technique in infants. Pediatr Pulmonol 1988;4:219–224.

27 Fletcher ME, Dezateux CA, Stocks J: Respiratory compliance in infants – A preliminary evaluation of the multiple interrupter technique. Pediatr Pulmonol 1992;14:118–125.

28 Sullivan M, Paliotta J, Saklad M: Endotracheal tube as a factor in measurement of respiratory mechanics. J Appl Physiol 1976; 41:590–592.

29 Wright PE, Marini JJ, Bernard GR: In vitro versus in vivo comparison of endotracheal tube airflow resistances. Am Rev Respir Dis 1989;140:10–16.

30 Prendiville A, Thomson A, Silverman M: Effects of tracheobronchial suction on respiratory resistance in intubated preterm infants. Arch Dis Child 1986;61:1178–1183.

31 Guttmann J, Eberhard L, Fabry B, Bertschmann W, Wolff G: Continuous calculation of intratracheal pressure in tracheally intubated patients. Anesthesiology 1993;79: 503–513.

32 Sondergaard S, Karason S, Hanson A, Nilsson K, Hojer S, Lundin S, Stenqvist O: Direct measurement of intratracheal pressure in pediatric respiratory monitoring. Pediatr Res 2002; 51:339–345.

33 Hammer J, Numa A, Patel N, Newth CJL: Normal values for pulmonary function in intubated infants (abstract). Am J Respir Crit Care Med 1995;151:A439.

34 Neve V, de la Roque ED, Leclerc F, Leteurtre S, Dorkenoo A, Sadik A, Cremer R, Logier R: Ventilator-induced overdistension in children: Dynamic versus low-flow inflation volume-pressure curves. Am J Respir Crit Care Med 2000;162:139–147.

35 Hutchinson J: On the capacity of lungs and on the respiratory function with view of establishing a precise and easy method of detecting diseases by spirometer. Trans Med Soc Lond 1846;29:137–252.

36 Tiffeneau R, Pinelli A: Air circulant et air captif dans l'exploration de la fonction ventilatoire pulmonaire. Paris Med 1947;133: 624–628.

37 Jones JG, Fraser RB, Nadel JA: Prediction of maximum expiratory flow rate from area-transmural pressure curve of compressed airway. J Appl Physiol 1975;38:1002–1011.

38 Jones JG, Fraser RB, Nadel JA: Effect of changing airway mechanics on maximum expiratory flow. J Appl Physiol 1975;38: 1012–1021.

39 Elliott EA, Dawson SV: Test of wave-speed theory of flow limitation in elastic tubes. J Appl Physiol 1977;43:516–522.

40 Motoyama EK: Pulmonary mechanics during early postnatal years. Pediatr Res 1977; 11:220–223.

41 Hammer J, Newth CJL: Influence of endotracheal tube diameter on forced deflation flow-volume curves in rhesus monkeys. Eur Respir J 1997;10:1870–1873.

42 Hammer J, Newth CJL: Effort and volume dependence of forced deflation flow-volume relationships in intubated infants. J Appl Physiol 1996;80:345–350.

43 Hammer J: Forced expiratory flow analysis in infants and preschool children. Eur Respir Mon 1997;5:1–26.

44 Hammer J, Numa A, Newth CJL: Acute respiratory distress syndrome induced by respiratory syncytial virus. Pediatr Pulmonol 1997; 23:176–183.

45 Hammer J, Numa A, Newth CJL: Albuterol responsiveness in infants with respiratory failure due to RSV infection. J Pediatr 1995; 127:485–490.

46 Mallory GB, Motoyama AK, Koumbourlis AC, Mutich RL, Nakayama DK: Bronchial reactivity in infants in acute respiratory failure with viral bronchiolitis. Pediatr Pulmonol 1989;6:253–259.

47 Motoyama EK, Fort MD, Klesh KW, Mutich RL, Guthrie RD: Early onset of airway reactivity in premature infants with bronchopulmonary dysplasia. Am Rev Respir Dis 1987; 136:50–57.

48 Koumbourlis AC, Mutich RL, Motoyama EK: Contribution of airway hyperresponsiveness to lower airway obstruction after extracorporeal membrane oxygenation for meconium aspiration syndrome. Crit Care Med 1995;23:749–754.

49 Mallory GB, Chaney H, Mutich RL, Motoyama EK: Longitudinal changes in lung function during the first three years of premature infants with moderate to severe bronchopulmonary dysplasia. Pediatr Pulmonol 1991;11:8–14.

50 Hammer J, Newth CJL: Effect of lung volume on forced expiratory flows during rapid thoracoabdominal compression in infants. J Appl Physiol 1995;78:1993–1997.

51 Thorsteinsson A, Larsson A, Jonmarker C, Werner O: Pressure-volume relations of the respiratory system in healthy children. Am J Respir Crit Care Med 1994;150:421–430.

52 D'Angelo E, Prandi E, Milic-Emili J: Dependence of maximal flow-volume curves on time course of preceding inspiration. J Appl Physiol 1993;75:1155–1159.

53 Sette L, Del Col G, Comis A, Milic-Emili J, Rossi A, Boner AL: Effect of pattern of preceding inspiration on FEV1 in asthmatic children. Eur Respir J 1996;9:1902–1906.

54 Newth CJ, Amsler B, Anderson GP, Morley J: The effects of varying inflation and deflation pressures on the maximal expiratory deflation flow-volume relationship in anesthetized rhesus monkeys. Am Rev Respir Dis 1991; 144:807–813.

55 Hammer J, Sivan Y, Deakers TW, Newth CJ: Flow limitation in anesthetized rhesus monkeys: A comparison of rapid thoracoabdominal compression and forced deflation techniques. Pediatr Res 1996;39:539–546.

56 Wilson TA: Modeling the effect of axial bronchial tension on expiratory flow. J Appl Physiol 1978;45:659–665.

57 Hammer J, Stenzler A, Newth CJL: Forced deflation in intubated infants: Effect of pressurization on measurements by pneumotachygraph and mass flow sensor. Am J Respir Crit Care Med 1995;151:A439.

58 Hammer J, Schibler A, Newth CJ: Measurements of forced expiratory flows and volumes in intubated monkeys: Pneumotachograph versus ultrasonic flow meter. Am J Respir Crit Care Med 2003;167:A 507.

59 Lu Q, Capderou A, Cluzel P, Mourgeon E, Abdennour L, Law-Koune JD, Straus C, Grenier P, Zelter M, Rouby JJ: A computed tomographic scan assessment of endotracheal suctioning-induced bronchoconstriction in ventilated sheep. Am J Respir Crit Care Med 2000;162:1898–1904.

60 Sigurdsson S, Svantesson C, Larsson A, Jonson B: Elastic pressure-volume curves indicate derecruitment after a single deep expiration in anaesthetised and muscle-relaxed healthy man. Acta Anaesthesiol Scand 2000; 44:980–984.

61 LeSouëf PN, Castile R, Turner DJ, Motoyama E, Morgan WJ: Forced expiratory maneuvers; in Stocks J, Sly PD, Tepper RS, Morgan WJ (eds): Infant Respiratory Function Testing. New York, Wiley-Liss, 1996, pp 379–409.

62 Edberg KE, Sandberg K, Silberberg A, Ekstrom-Jodal B, Hjalmarson O: Lung volume, gas mixing, and mechanics of breathing in mechanically ventilated very low birth weight infants with idiopathic respiratory distress syndrome. Pediatr Res 1991;30: 496–500.

63 Gustafsson PM, Ljungberg H: Measurement of functional residual capacity and ventilation inhomogeneity by gas dilution techniques; Hammer J, Eber E (eds): Paediatric Pulmonary Function Testing. Prog Respir Res. Basel, Karger, 2005, vol 33, pp 54–65.

64 Heldt GP, Peters RM: A simplified method to determine functional residual capacity during mechanical ventilation. Chest 1978;74: 492–496.

65 Fox WW, Schwartz JG, Shaffer TH: Effects of endotracheal tube leaks on functional residual capacity determination in intubated neonates. Pediatr Res 1979;13:60–64.

66 Sivan Y, Deakers TW, Newth CJL: An automated bedside method for measuring functional residual capacity by N_2 washout in mechanically ventilated children. Pediatr Res 1990;28:446–450.

67 Davies NJH, Denison DM: The measurement of metabolic gas exchange and minute volume by mass spectrometry alone. Respir Physiol 1979;36:261–267.

68 Poets CF, Rau GA, Gappa M, Seidenberg J: Comparison of heliox and oxygen as washing gases for the nitrogen washout technique in preterm infants. Pediatr Res 1996;39: 1099–1102.

69 Hentschel R, Suska A, Volbracht A, Brune T, Jorch G: Modification of the open circuit N_2 washout technique for measurement of functional residual capacity in premature infants. Pediatr Pulmonol 1997;23:434–441.

70 Sivan Y, Hammer J, Newth CJL: Measurement of high lung volumes by nitrogen washout method. J Appl Physiol 1994;77: 1562–1564.

71 Hammer J, Numa A, Newth CJL: Total lung capacity by N_2 washout from high and low lung volumes in ventilated infants and children. Am J Respir Crit Care Med 1998;158:526–531.

72 Jonmarker C, Jansson L, Jonson B, Larsson A, Werner O: Measurement of functional residual capacity by sulfur hexafluoride washout. Anesthesiology 1985;63:89–95.

73 Larsson A, Linnarsson D, Jonmarker C, Jonson B, Larsson H, Werner O: Measurement of lung volume by sulfur hexafluoride washout during spontaneous and controlled ventilation: Further development of a method. Anesthesiology 1987;67: 543–550.

74 Vilstrup CT, Bjorklund LJ, Larsson A, Lachmann B, Werner O: Functional residual capacity and ventilation homogeneity in mechanically ventilated small neonates. J Appl Physiol 1992;73:276–283.

75 Schulze A, Schaller P, Töpfer A, Kirpalani H: Measurement of functional residual capacity by sulfur hexafluoride in small-volume lungs during spontaneous breathing and mechanical ventilation. Pediatr Res 1994;35:494–499.

76 Schibler A, Henning R: Measurement of functional residual capacity in rabbits and children using an ultrasonic flow meter. Pediatr Res 2001;49:581–588.

77 Schibler A, Hammer J, Isler R, Buess C, Newth CJ: Measurement of lung volume in mechanically ventilated monkeys with an ultrasonic flow meter and the nitrogen washout method. Intensive Care Med 2004;30:127–132.

78 Schibler A, Henning R: Positive end-expiratory pressure and ventilation inhomogeneity in mechanically ventilated children. Pediatr Crit Care Med 2002;3:124–128.

79 Thorsteinsson A, Jonmarker C, Larsson A, Vilstrup C, Werner O: Functional residual capacity in anesthetized children: Normal values and values in children with cardiac anomalies. Anesthesiology 1990;73:876–881.

80 Thorsteinsson A, Larsson A, Jonmarker C, Werner O, Thorsteinsson A, Larsson A, Jonmarker C, Werner O: Pressure-volume relations of the respiratory system in healthy children. Am J Respir Crit Care Med 1994;150:421–430.

81 Edberg KE, Ekström-Jodal B, Hallman M, Hjalmarson O, Sandberg K, Silberberg A: Immediate effects on lung function of instilled human surfactant in mechanically ventilated newborn infants with IRDS. Acta Paediatr Scand 1990;79:750–755.

82 Navajas D, Farre R: Forced oscillation assessment of respiratory mechanics in ventilated patients. Crit Care 2001;5:3–9.

83 Oostveen E, MacLeod D, Lorino H, Farre R, Hantos Z, Desager K, Marchal F; ERS Task Force on Respiratory Impedance Measurements: The forced oscillation technique in clinical practice: Methodology, recommendations and future developments. Eur Respir J 2003;22:1026–1041.

84 Pillow J, Sly P, Hantos Z: Monitoring of lung volume recruitment and derecruitment using oscillatory mechanics during high frequency oscillatory ventilation in the preterm lamb. Pediatr Crit Care Med 2004; 5:172–180.

85 Peták F, Babik B, Asztalos T, Hall GL, Deák ZI, Sly PD, Hantos Z: Airway and tissue mechanics in anesthetized paralyzed children. Pediatr Pulmonol 2003;35:169–176.

86 Hall GL, Brookes IM: Techniques for measurement of lung function in toddlers and preschool children; Hammer J, Eber E (eds): Paediatric Pulmonary Function Testing. Prog Respir Res. Basel, Karger, 2005, vol 33, pp 66–77.

87 Lødrup C, Carlsen KC, Carlsen KH: Tidal breathing measurements; Hammer J, Eber E (eds): Paediatric Pulmonary Function Testing. Prog Respir Res. Basel, Karger, 2005, vol 33, pp 10–19.

88 Weber K, Courtney SE, Pyon KH, Chang GY, Pandit PB, Habib RH: Detecting lung overdistention in newborns treated with high-frequency oscillatory ventilation. J Appl Physiol 2000;89:364–372.

89 Habib RH, Pyon KH, Courtney SE: Optimal high-frequency oscillatory ventilation settings by nonlinear lung mechanics analysis. Am J Respir Crit Care Med 2002;166:950–953.

90 Brazelton TB, Watson KF, Murphy M, Al-Khadra E, Thompson JE, Arnold JH: Identification of optimal lung volume during high-frequency oscillatory ventilation using respiratory inductive plethysmography. Crit Care Med 2001;29:2349–2359.

91 Nopp P, Rapp E, Pfutzner H, Nakesch H, Ruhsam C: Dielectric properties of lung tissue as a function of air content. Phys Med Biol 1993;38:699–716.

92 Victorino JA, Borges JB, Okamoto VN, Matos GF, Tucci MR, Caramez MP, Tanaka H, Sipmann FS, Santos DC, Barbas CS, Carvalho CR, Amato MB: Imbalances in regional lung ventilation: A validation study on electrical impedance tomography. Am J Respir Crit Care Med 2004;169:791–800.

93 Hinz J, Neumann P, Dudykevych T, Andersson LG, Wrigge H, Burchardi H, Hedenstierna G: Regional ventilation by electrical impedance tomography: A comparison with ventilation scintigraphy in pigs. Chest 2003;124:314–322.

94 Kunst PW, Bohm SH, Vazquez de Anda G, Amato MB, Lachmann B, Postmus PE, de Vries PM: Regional pressure volume curves by electrical impedance tomography in a model of acute lung injury. Crit Care Med 2000;28/1:178–183.

95 Kunst PW, Vazquez de Anda G, Bohm SH, Faes TJ, Lachmann B, Postmus PE, de Vries PM: Monitoring of recruitment and derecruitment by electrical impedance tomography in a model of acute lung injury. Crit Care Med 2000;28:3891–3895.

96 van Genderingen HR, van Vught AJ, Jansen JR: Estimation of regional lung volume changes by electrical impedance pressures tomography during a pressure-volume maneuver. Intensive Care Med 2003;29:233–240.

97 van Genderingen HR, van Vught AJ, Jansen JRC: Regional lung volume during high-frequency oscillatory ventilation by electrical impedance tomography. Crit Care Med 2004;32:787–794.

98 Frerichs I, Schiffmann H, Hahn G, Hellige G: Non-invasive radiation-free monitoring of regional lung ventilation in critically ill infants. Intensive Care Med 2001;27:1385–1394.

99 Hedenstierna G: Using electric impedance tomography to assess regional ventilation at the bedside. Am J Respir Crit Care Med 2004;169:777–778.

100 DeNicola LK, Kissoon N, Abram HS Jr, Sullivan KJ, Delgado-Corcoran C, Taylor C: Noninvasive monitoring in the pediatric intensive care unit. Pediatr Clin North Am 2001;48:573–588.

Prof. Dr. med. Jürg Hammer
Division of Intensive Care and Pulmonology
University Children's Hospital Basel
Römergasse 8
CH–4005 Basel (Switzerland)
Tel. +41 61 685 65 65
Fax +41 61 685 50 59
E-Mail juerg.hammer@unibas.ch

Author Index

Subject Index

Chronic lung disease of infancy (CLD)
    follow-up of survivors 261
    lung function evolution from infancy to
        adolescence 256, 257
    pathophysiology 256
    pulmonary sequelae
        adult survivor trends 258, 259
        bronchial hyperresponsiveness 257
        gas exchange 257, 258
        risk profile 257
Cold air hyperventilation challenge, bronchial
    hyperresponsiveness assessment 130, 131
Congenital diaphragmatic hernia (CDH)
    clinical features 259
    follow-up of survivors 261
    pulmonary sequelae 259
Congenital lobar emphysema (CLE)
    follow-up of survivors 261
    pulmonary sequelae 260
Cystic fibrosis (CF)
    bronchial hyperresponsiveness 219, 220
    exhaled breath condensate analysis
        195, 196
    gene mutations 218
    infant pulmonary function testing
        86, 87, 217
    lung transplantation and monitoring
        220
    lung volume measurements 113, 217
    monitoring with pulmonary function tests
        217–219
    pathophysiology and lung function
        effects 215–217
Cytokines, exhaled breath condensate
    analysis 193

Electrical impedance tomography (EIT),
    intensive care unit 278
Electromyography (EMG)
    expiratory muscle strength assessment
        144, 145
    inspiratory muscle strength assessment
        143
Equation of lung motion 21
Esophageal manometry, dynamic respiratory
    mechanics measurement in infants
    balloon or catheter placement 28, 29
    data analysis 29
    equipment 27, 28
    infant preparation 27
    prospects 84
    technique 29
Exercise testing
    bronchial hyperresponsiveness
        assessment
        equipment 129
        principles 129

protocols 130
lung transplant recipients 230
tidal flow volume 17
Exhaled breath condensate (EBC)
    clinical prospects 198, 199
    collection 191, 192
    contents 190
    findings
        asthma 194, 195
        cystic fibrosis 195, 196
        primary ciliary dyskinesia 196, 197
    markers and assays
        cytokines 193
        hydrogen peroxide 192
        8-isoprostane 192
        leukotrienes 193
        reactive nitrogen species 192, 193
    pH measurement 193, 194
Exhaled nitric oxide, *see* Nitric oxide
Expiratory muscle strength, *see* Respiratory
    muscle function
Expiratory volume clamping, passive
    respiratory mechanics measurement in
    infants 27

FEV_1
    asthma 204, 205, 208
    cystic fibrosis 217–220
    pediatric spirometry interpretation and
        reporting 99, 100
Forced oscillation technique (FOT)
    asthma evaluation in preschoolers 211
    child preparation 72
    clinical applications
        airway reactivity 73, 74
        baseline airway obstruction 73
    data analysis and reporting 72, 73
    equipment 71, 72
    impedance data collection 72
    intensive care unit 277
    low-frequency technique 83
    overview 70, 71
    quality control 72
    reference data 73
    technical aspects 71
Forced vital capacity (FVC)
    intensive care unit measurement 272, 273
    pediatric spirometry interpretation and
        reporting 99
Functional residual capacity (FRC)
    definition 104
    intensive care unit measurements
        helium dilution 274
        nitrogen washout 274–276
        overview 273, 274
        reference values 276, 277
        sulfur hexafluoride washout 276

measurement in infants, *see* Gas dilution
    techniques; Whole-body
    plethysmography
physiology in infants 54, 55
variability of measurements 112

Gas dilution techniques
    clinical applications in infants 63, 64
    gas trapping 62, 111, 112
    helium dilution
        closed-circuit helium dilution 55
        multiple-breath helium dilution 109,
            110
        single-breath helium dilution 110
    indications
        asthma 112, 113
        congenital disorders 114
        cystic fibrosis 113
        restrictive lung disease 114
    indices of ventilation inhomogeneity
        58–62, 111, 112
    inert marker gases 55
    intensive care unit measurements
        helium dilution 274
        nitrogen washout 274–276
        overview 273, 274
        reference values 276, 277
        sulfur hexafluoride washout 276
    lung volume measurements 64
    mass conservation principle 109
    normative data for functional residual
        capacity and ventilation
        inhomogeneity 63
    prospects 84
    washout methods
        bias flow nitrogen washout 56
        breath-by-breath washout 56–58
        multiple-breath nitrogen washout
            110, 111
        single-breath nitrogen washout 111
        sulfur hexafluoride washout 111
Graft-versus-host disease (GVHD),
    pulmonary complications 251–253

Helium dilution, *see* Gas dilution techniques
Hematopoietic stem cell transplantation
    (HSCT)
    indications 247, 248
    matching 248
    phases following transplantation
        early phase 249
        late phase 249
        neutropenic phase 249
    pulmonary complications 248, 249
    pulmonary function testing in recipients
        obstructive disease 252, 253
        outcomes in children 250, 251

Nasal nitric oxide, *see* Nitric oxide
Neuromuscular disorders (NMD)
   anesthesia and surgery planning 243
   clinical features
      congenital muscular dystrophies 236
      Duchenne muscular dystrophy 234
      myasthenia gravis 236
      myopathies 236
      myotonic dystrophy 235
      spinal muscular atrophy 234, 235
      spinal muscular atrophy with
         respiratory distress 235
   evaluation
      guidelines for periodic testing
         236–238
      history and physical examination 238
      pulmonary function testing
         238–240
      respiratory muscle function testing
         145, 240–242
   lung diffusing capacity measurement
      162, 242
   sleep-disordered breathing 242, 243
NIOX®, exhaled nitric oxide measurement
   170
Nitric oxide (NO)
   exhalation measurement
      advantages 177, 178
      asthma
         Child Asthma Research and
            Education Network 176
         control assessment 173–176
         diagnostic value 172, 173, 176
         latent airway inflammation
            173, 174
         NIOX® monitoring 170
         preschool disease detection 174
         severity 173
         wheezy infants 174
      clinical use prospects 166, 167, 178
      collection
         single breath on-line 167, 168
         tidal breathing 168–170
      diurnal variation 171
      epidemiological studies
         air pollution 176
         tobacco exposure studies 176
      equipment 167
      factors affecting in children 171
      feasibility 171
      limitations 178
      mean levels 170
      multiple exhalation flow technique
         176, 177
      reproducibility 170, 171, 177
      standardization 170
   nasal nitric oxide
      diagnostic utility 186, 187

factors affecting levels 185, 186
   functions 182
   measurement
      analyzer 183
      humming and sinus ventilation
         assessment 185
      standard technique 183–185
      terminology and units 182, 183
   normal values in children 186
   origins 182
   synthesis 181, 182

Obstructive airway disease (OAD)
   hematopoietic stem cell transplant
      recipients 252, 253
   lung diffusing capacity 161
   tidal flow volume measurements
      diagnostic utility 15
      intervention monitoring 15–17
Occlusion techniques, passive respiratory
   mechanics measurement in infants
   equipment 23, 24
   infant preparation 23
   modifications 26, 27
   multiple occlusion technique
      data analysis 26
      methodology 25, 26
   single occlusion technique
      data analysis 25
      methodology 24

Peak cough flow (PCF), neuromuscular
   disorder evaluation 242
pH, exhaled breath condensate analysis
   193, 194
Phase angle, *see* Work of breathing
Phrenic nerve conduction, inspiratory
   muscle strength assessment 141
Plethysmography, *see also* Respiratory
   inductive plethysmography
   calibration 106
   data analysis 107
   equipment
      barometric plethysmograph 105
      volume displacement plethysmograph
         105, 106
   indications
      asthma 112, 113
      congenital disorders 114
      cystic fibrosis 113
      restrictive lung disease 114
   infants, *see* Whole-body plethysmography
   interpretation
      airway resistance 108
      thoracic gas volume 107, 108
   measurement

airway resistance 106, 107
      thoracic gas volume 106, 107
   principles
      airway resistance 104, 105
      thoracic gas volume 104
   prospects 114, 115
   relationship between thoracic gas volume
      and airway resistance 109
   time constant measurements 106
   variability of measurements 112
Pneumotachography, tidal flow volume
   measurement in infants and children
   11, 12
Preschool children lung function testing
   forced oscillation technique 70–74
   interrupter technique 67–70
   overview 66, 67
   prospects 74
Pressure-rate product, *see* Work of
   breathing
Pressure-time product, *see* Work of
   breathing
Primary ciliary dyskinesia (PCD)
   exhaled breath condensate analysis
      196, 197
   nasal nitric oxide measurement 187

Rapid thoracoabdominal compression (RTC)
   techniques
   asthma evaluation 209, 210
   infant preparation 35
   physiological background 34, 35
   raised volume RTC technique
      applications 41
      data analysis and interpretation 40, 41
      limitations 41
      multiple inflation technique
         equipment 39
         procedure 39, 40
      overview 38
      pumping technique
         equipment 38
         procedure 39
   tidal volume RTC technique
      applications 37
      equipment 35, 36
      historical perspective 35
      interpretation 36, 37
      limitations 37
      procedure 36
Reactive nitrogen species, exhaled breath
   condensate analysis 192, 193
Reference equations, ventilatory function
   testing in school-age children
   checklist for selection 123
   importance 118, 119
   independent variables

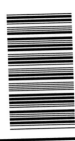

BLACKWELL'S
BOOK SERVICES

Order Type: 104 NTAS

Customer
Name: University Of Calif San Francisco

Customer SSFM
Alpha Code
& Number: 152500006

Del
Add: 02

BBS Order
Number: C294898

Customer
Order Number:

Dept:
Customer
Order Date: 28-Apr-2005

Fund
Number: a
List Price 152.75

ISBN: 3805577532

Title: **PAEDIATRIC PULMONARY FUNCTION TESTING**

Author:

Sub-Title:

Order
Qty: 1

Shipped
Qty: 1

Publisher: Karger.

Series Title:

Spine Title:

Volume Number:

Publication Year: 2005

No. of Volumes: 001

Format: Hardback

Document Text:

npanying Material: .